Manual of
Human
Anatomy
Dissection

Manual of
Human
Anatomy
Dissection

Krishna Garg
MBBS MS PhD FIMSA FIAMS FAMS FASI

Legend of Anatomy   Nation's Who's Who   Member and Fellow, Academy of Medical Sciences
Fellow, Indian Academy of Medical Specialists   Fellow, International Medical Science Academy
Fellow, Anatomical Society of India   Lifetime Achievement Awardee   DMA Distinguished Service Awardee

Ex-Professor and Head, Department of Anatomy
Lady Hardinge Medical College, New Delhi

Medha Joshi
MBBS, FCGP

Ex-Lecturer in Anatomy
Krishna Dental College and HD Dental College
Ghaziabad, Uttar Pradesh
Guest Faculty
Pt Deendayal Upadhyaya National Institute of Persons with Physical Disabilities, New Delhi
and Amar Jyoti Institute of Physiotherapy, Delhi

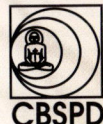

CBSPD

CBS Publishers & Distributors Pvt Ltd

New Delhi • Bengaluru • Chennai • Kochi • Kolkata • Lucknow • Mumbai
Hyderabad • Jharkhand • Nagpur • Patna • Pune • Uttarakhand

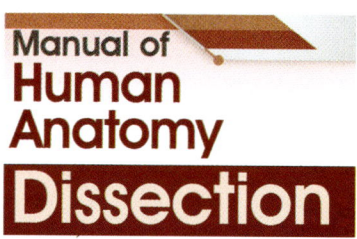

ISBN: 978-93-89688-00-9

First Edition: 2021
 Reprint: 2021, 2022
 Revised Reprint: 2024

Published by Satish Kumar Jain and produced by Varun Jain for

CBS Publishers & Distributors Pvt Ltd

4819/XI Prahlad Street, 24 Ansari Road, Daryaganj, New Delhi 110 002, India
Ph: 011-23289259, 23266861   Website: www.cbspd.com
                                    e-mail: delhi@cbspd.com

Corporate Office: 204 FIE, Industrial Area, Patparganj, Delhi 110 092, India
Ph: 011-4934 4934   Fax: 011-4934 4935   e-mail: publishing@cbspd.com;
                                              publicity@cbspd.com

Branches

• **Bengaluru:** Seema House 2975, 17th Cross, KR Road, Banasankari 2nd Stage, Bengaluru 560 070, Karnataka, India
  Ph: +91-80-26771678/79   Fax: +91-80-26771680   e-mail: bangalore@cbspd.com
• **Chennai:** 7, Subbaraya Street, Shenoy Nagar, Chennai 600 030, Tamil Nadu, India
  Ph: +91-44-26680620, 26681266   Fax: +91-44-42032115   e-mail: chennai@cbspd.com
• **Kochi:** 42/1325, 1326, Power House Road, Opp KSEB, Power House, Ernakulum Kochi 682 018, Kerala, India
  Ph: +91-484-4059061-65,67   Fax: +91-484-4059065   e-mail: kochi@cbspd.com
• **Kolkata:** 147, Hind Ceramics Compound, 1st Floor, Nilgunj Road, Belghoria, Kolkata-700056, West Bengal, India
  Ph: +033-25633055, 033-25633056   e-mail: kolkata@cbspd.com
• **Lucknow:** Basement, Khushnuma Complex, 7 Meerabai Marg (Behind Jawahar Bhawan), Lucknow-226001, UP, India
  Ph: +0522-4000032   e-mail: tiwari.lucknow@cbspd.com
• **Mumbai:** PWD Shed, Gala no 25/26, Ramchandra Bhatt Marg, Next to JJ Hospital Gate no. 2, Opp. Union Bank of India, Noorbaug, Mumbai-400009, Maharashtra, India
  Ph: 022-66661880/89   e-mail: mumbai@cbspd.com

Representatives

| • | Hyderabad | 0-9885175004 | • | Jharkhand | 0-9811541605 | • | Nagpur | 0-8692091830 |
| • | Patna | 0-9334159340 | • | Pune | 0-9664372571 | • | Uttarakhand | 0-9716462459 |

Printed at Magic International Pvt. Ltd., Greater Noida, UP, India

Preface

*I learn anatomy not from books but from dissections,
not from the tenets of philosophers but from the fabric of nature.*
—William Harvey

Dissection is but one of the means of learning anatomy. Dissection of an animal is the learning of zoology while dissection of a human cadaver is the learning of anatomy.

Dissection is a time-tested means of learning anatomy for centuries despite the technological advances. Dissection is a very specialised scientific procedure and is different from an "autopsy" or "postmortem". During the anatomical dissection, the medical student, under the instructions of an experienced teacher, works slowly and steadily, identifying various structures. As of now, it takes almost one year during the preclinical course to dissect the whole body and there is a definite procedure to perform the dissection of any region. For this we have some Indian books which give steps of dissection with the hand-drawn/computer-drawn diagrams taken from textbooks of anatomy and are not the actual dissection photographs/diagrams; defeating the whole exercise of dissection. A few foreign atlases are available with beautiful dissection photographs but these look "too good to be true" for our milieu.

Mr SK Jain, Chairman and Managing Director, CBS Publishers & Distributors, proposed a "Dissector of anatomy". After many deliberations, considering the real requirements of MBBS students, we decided to give the entire dissection in one volume only. The highlight of the volume would be to provide "actual ordinary dissection photographs" as seen in the dissection halls of a medical college.

There have been a multitude of hurdles in obtaining the "actual dissected specimens" from various sources. We could have taken specimens from any good museum, but these would be "too real for actual ordinary dissection specimen" as museum specimens are the artwork of senior teachers and technicians.

The first group of teachers to help us in this difficult and tough endeavour was the Principal, Rama Medical College, Kanpur. Later, assistance came from Bakson Homeopathic Medical College and Hospital, Greater Noida, UP. We have emphasised on the *dissection* photographs, not on illustrations giving only *theoretical* knowledge.

Actual dissection specimens were also available from DDU National Institute for Persons with Physical Disabilities, New Delhi, where we performed the dissection ourselves and took requisite photographs. Some photographs were also taken from Subharti Medical College, Meerut.

Towards the end of three years' ongoing struggle AIIMS-Raipur pitched in, giving us the remaining photographs as the work on the Manual got completed. Despite all these efforts, a few diagrams are still hand- or computer-drawn, which we will like to replace in the future editions.

The aim of this dissector is to reach, locate and identify the structures in a particular region. Their full description is beyond the scope of this book and has to be learnt from a standard textbook of anatomy, e.g. BD Chaurasia's *Human Anatomy*, 9th edn, Vols 1–4. It has been done deliberately to limit the size of the book, avoiding repetition of theoretical text material. Thus this Manual on dissection is a supplement to the textbook of anatomy. It should be able to provide holistic, useful, photographic memory for students during long happy clinical years.

Steps of dissection are given in a simplified way with as many "ordinary dissection photographs" as possible to make the whole exercise easy and interesting. It will make many senior students or doctors nostalgic about their days in the dissection hall.

In the majority of medical colleges there is a shortage of cadavers and scarcity of time. In most of the medical institutions there are 20–30 students for one region being dissected and the time allocated to study of anatomy is hardly one year.

In this dissector the text of dissection is divided into Introduction and six sections, i.e. •Upper Limb, •Thorax, •Lower Limb, •Abdomen and Pelvis, •Head and Neck, and •Brain.

The chapter on introduction relates to getting the cadaver, embalming procedure, maintaining and caring for the cadaver and finally disposing its parts. It also includes various instruments for dissection.

Every section is divided into various chapters. Each chapter starts with "learning objectives" and "overview", providing the bird's eyeview of the particular topic. These are followed by "steps of dissection" and actual photographs of the concerned area. Emphasis has been given on the structures visible only. The chapter ends with a few *viva voce* examination questions to help in relearning the topic. This procedure is followed in all the chapters of a section. At the end of each section 10–15 *spots* are given. These are important from "examination point of view". This is the simple procedure followed in the present book.

Only authentic way to learn anatomy is to draw, draw and draw coloured diagrams and marking structures on your body.

We would be highly obliged if our worthy teachers of anatomy send us the dissected photographs of any region of the body. These can be added later in the future printings of the Manual to improve its quality and would be thankfully acknowledged.

We are reminded of the quotation:

If I hear, I forget
If I see, I remember
and
If I do, I understand

Wishing you happy understanding and learning of anatomy

Krishna Garg
Medha Joshi

Acknowledgements

Idea is the main and most important component of any project. The idea for the present book, i.e. dissection manual, was provided by none other than Mr SK Jain, Chairman and Managing Director, CBS Publishers & Distributors. It was his brain-child given to us about four years back. For the idea to sink in deep, develop methodology and implementing it in right ernest has taken this much time.

The text writing was done in one volume only. The problematic part was to procure "actual ordinary dissection photographs". First help for this was provided by Prof RK Srivastava, the then Principal, Rama Medical College, Kanpur, and two of his colleagues, Prof Shirin Jahan and Mr Kiran Kumar P. Over a period of time some photographs were provided by Dr Rashmi Bhardwaj of Mahaveer Tirthankar Medical College; Prof Satyam Khare and Prof Shilpi Jain of Subharti Medical College; and Prof Sushant Rit and Dr Yash Mehra of Bakson Homeopathic College, Greater Noida. Lastly, to cap it all tremendous assistance poured in from Prof Manisha B Sinha and Prof DK Sharma, Department of Anatomy, under the guidance of Prof Nitin Nagarkar, Director, AIIMS-Raipur. We would like to thank Dr Puneet Kaur for her valuable inputs from time to time. A special thank you to Dr Amritpal Singh, for his beautiful sketch. Thanks to Dr Gayatri Rath, Dr PS Mittal and Dr Mrudula Chandrupatla for their kind help. We are grateful to Rekha Garg for her technical guidance.

We are very grateful to Mr SK Jain, Mr Varun Jain, Mr YN Arjuna, Ms Ritu Chawla, Ms Jyoti Kaur, Mr Sanjay Chauhan, Mr Kshirodh Sahoo and Mr Neeraj Prasad, for their valuable guidance and help.

We are highly obliged to the Almighty and each and everyone who gave us timely helping hand during this difficult and tough endeavour. We hope and pray for continuous guidance and support from all members of anatomy fraternity.

Thanking everyone once again.

Krishna Garg
Medha Joshi

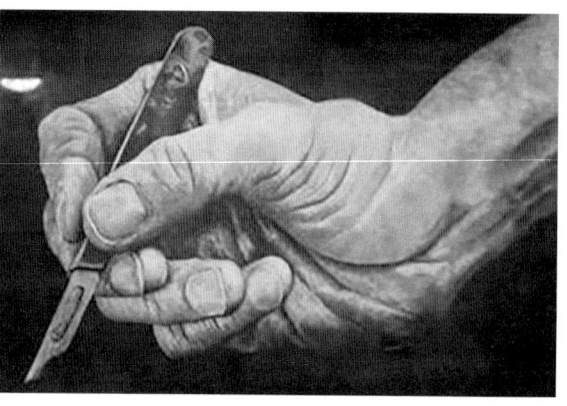

Contents

Section IV: Abdomen and Pelvis

Section V: Head and Neck

Section VI: Brain

The Speaking Cadaver

I am nameless

I am casteless

I have no religion

You do not know who are my friends

Nor do you know my foes

But of one thing be rest assured

I will be your anatomy teacher

Serve you through thick and thin

Take care of me, learn from me

And I shall be your life-long guide

Uphold My Honour and I Shall Uphold Yours

Poem contributed by Puneet Kaur

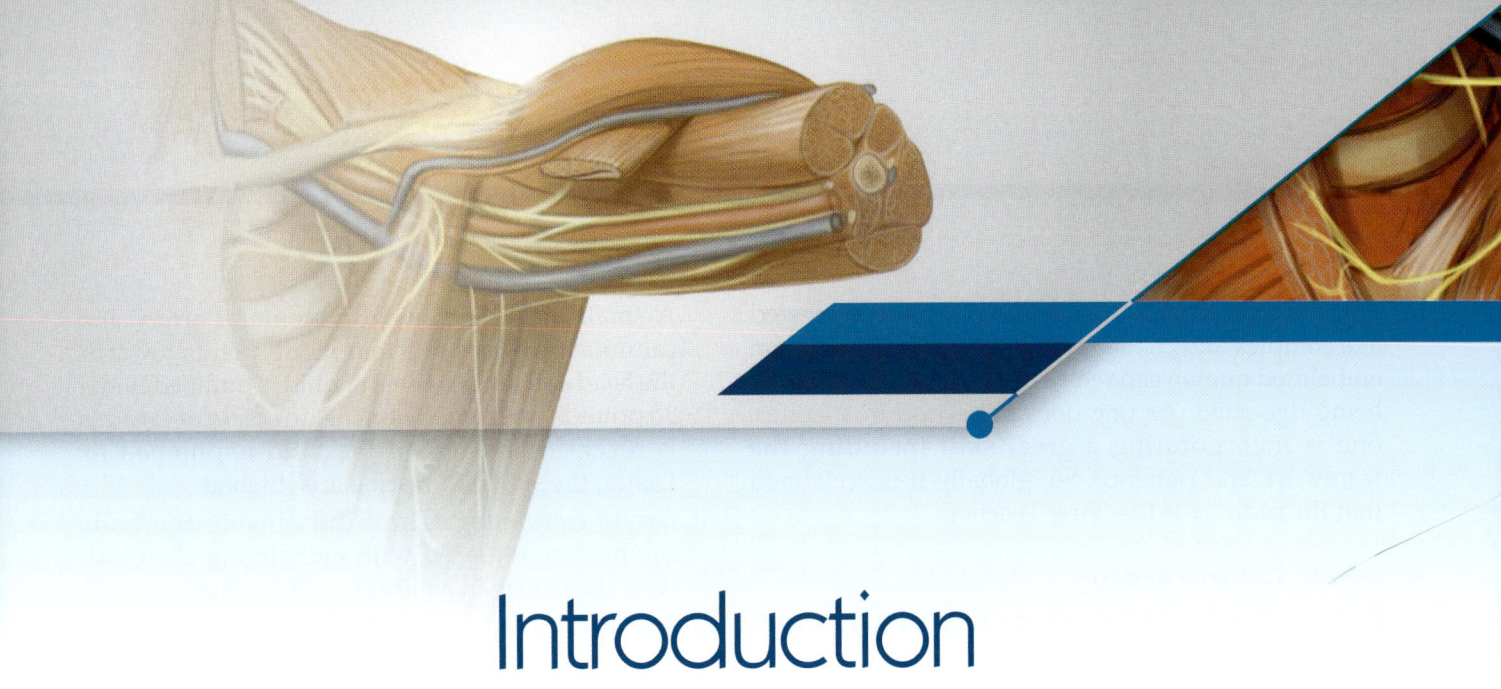

Introduction

INTRODUCTION

Language of Dissection

Dissect means to cut apart. One is very scared of dissection to begin with. Slowly one starts liking it.

Anatomical dissection: It is the procedure/technique to visualise the interior of the human dead body/cadaver.

Zoology is a science to learn the structure of the animal kingdom, while in anatomy one learns the gross, microscopic and ultramicroscopic structure of the human body.

Blunt dissection: A procedure by which various structures are separated by a probe. This method just separates without any injury to any body part. It may also be done by using the scissors, as some connective tissues need to be cut to clean the nerves and blood vessels.

Scalpel/sharp dissection: It is done for cutting a soft structure. Beginners must not use sharp dissection on their own. They should do it under the guidance of their teacher.

Clean the fat: Under the skin lies the superficial fascia which mainly contains fat intermingled with cutaneous nerves, arteries, veins and lymph nodes. Fat lobules must be picked by forceps and put in a tray. One should be careful of not cutting an artery/nerve/vein.

Clean the muscle: The fascia over the muscle must be removed gently with forceps and scalpel. Slowly and steadily the borders and surfaces of the muscle are cleaned. Now the surfaces of the muscle are cleaned revealing the fibres.

Cleaning the vessel/nerve: With probe and blunt forceps, the connective tissue and fat around these structures are removed enabling them to be seen properly in their entire course including their branches.

Cutting the vein: The blood clots in the veins make them wider. These veins overlie the nerves and arteries. To see the nerves and arteries, the vein is ligated with black thread at two ends. Then the vein is cut close to the ligatures, removed and put in the adjacent tray. Now the deeper structures can be comfortably cleaned and visualised.

Retract: To pull a structure to one side so that deeper structures can be seen.

Reflect the skin: To cut the skin along the lines of incision and separate it from underlying fascia by blunt dissection. Then fold it from the cut edge to one side so that fascia is visualised.

Cut/transect: To actually cut a muscle/tendon/vessel/bone in two parts so that deep structures can be viewed properly.

Cadaver as a First Teacher

Once a senior secondary school student with biology gets admission in a medical college, she/he is renamed as a medical student who is mentally prepared to study for about 10 years before becoming a specialized doctor. During the first professional year a medical student needs to study anatomy, physiology and biochemistry.

1

From time immemorial, anatomy has been viewed as a complex and challenging subject to be learnt from embalmed human cadaver who is slowly and steadily being dissected. As one does dissection in a group, one is incorporating a great skill including the teamwork and patience. So, globally it is acclaimed that the cadaver is the 'First Teacher'.

How to Obtain a Cadaver

Cadaver is a dead human body used in scientific or medical research.

Earlier and even at present, unclaimed dead bodies usually belonging to poor strata are taken by the police. Police personnel inform the medical college (anatomy department) to collect the body. Even if postmortem has been done, the body is taken by the anatomy department for the dissection of the limbs. For the last decade or so many persons make a 'Will' to donate their bodies. To promote this scheme, many anatomy departments give it as a news item in the local newspapers. The department puts the photograph of the voluntary donor outside the Dissection Hall.

Preservation of the Cadavers

The dead body starts putrefying and decaying within few hours after death depending on the weather. To prevent this, bodies are embalmed with formalin mixture. Procedure of embalming takes few hours to complete.

Embalming is also done if a dead body or cadaver is to be transported to a distant place in the country or abroad.

Embalming can be done as: (i) arterial embalming, (ii) cavity embalming, (iii) hypodermic embalming and (iv) surface embalming.

Embalming fluid—the fluid is prepared by thoroughly mixing up 5 litres of formalin (40%), 2 litres of spirit, 1 litre of glycerine, sodium chloride, etc.

The cadaver is put in a supine position on a table. It is shaved and cleaned.

i. *Procedure for arterial embalming:* A 6 cm long vertical incision is given in the upper medial side of thigh. After reflecting skin and fasciae, femoral sheath is incised to visualise the femoral artery. The prepared embalming fluid is put in the embalming machine which is connected to a cannula.

A small nick is given in the femoral artery and cannula introduced so that its tip points towards the head end and 8.5 litres of fluid is pumped under 20 pounds pressure. Then the direction of cannula is reversed and rest of the fluid is pumped in. Lastly, the skin and fasciae are stitched.

ii. *Cavity embalming:* The fluids inside the body cavities are replaced with embalming chemicals with the use of an aspirator and trochar.

iii. *Hypodermic embalming:* Injection of embalming fluid into tissues with the help of syringe and needle. It is done in an area where arterial fluid has not reached.

iv. *Surface embalming:* Preserves areas on skin damaged by accidents or skin donations.

Embalming and Ethics

The decision for embalming is taken by close relatives usually when there is a 'Will' to the same effect. This trend is 'catching up' and some people are 'making a Will' to donate their body for education or research to the department of anatomy. Earlier and even now many bodies are the 'unclaimed ones'.

Care of the cadaver: The cadaver has to be handled with care and respect. Only the part being dissected is kept open and exposed, rest is to be covered by a sheet. After dissection the dissecting part must also be covered. Palms and soles are wrapped till their dissection is reached. Over the weekend or a holiday, the cadaver or the body is put in a formalin tank to be taken out after the weekend. There is always an irritating smell of formalin causing watering of eyes but it gets over within 30–40 minutes. Detached limbs are to be wrapped up by a bandage to prevent drying. If fungus is seen on a part, it must be removed by using dilute carbolic acid. "You care for the cadaver, he or she takes care of your learning anatomy".

So, a cadaver, a dead human body is showing his internal features to help you learn anatomy and cadaver is the first teacher. The students of University of Taiwan are told about the family of the cadaver. They visit the family to pay their respects as their deceased family member is assisting them to become a doctor for treating the patients.

Many institutions start their anatomy dissection classes with a prayer to thank Almighty for giving them a body to learn. At a college in Mumbai, the cadaveric oath is administered to first year medical undergraduates who pledge to honour the dignity and integrity of the human remains that they are about to work on. Anatomical memorial services are held in Mayo Medical College, Rochester, USA, enable students to reflect on the lives of the departed souls who facilitated their education. The cadaver in addition to teaching anatomy also teaches to work in a team. Even after many years of dissection one remembers colleagues of your dissection table and the happy hours spent together. We must all remember that the cadaver was one of us and deserve great respect. Cadaver not only teaches gross anatomy but also surface anatomy and embryology from dissection of the foetuses.

Disposal of the cadaver: The remains of the cadaver are buried in the burial ground attached to the department of anatomy.

The cadaver continues to be a teacher in Forensic Medicine. Here the cause of death has to be established by postmortem so that guilty persons may be punished.

Dress code for the students: All students must wear an apron/overall, a cap, gloves and closed shoes to prevent injuring oneself from a scalpel, knife, etc.

While cutting bones one should wear glasses/goggles to protect the eyes against flying chips of the bones.

These young students look like "young inexperienced surgeons" who are keen to learn new methods.

Dissection Instruments

Large instruments like hammer, saw, chisel, etc. are provided in the department. Every medical student must have the following instruments in his/her dissection box.

Scalpel: The scalpel is used for giving incisions. It should have a detachable blade of 3–4 cm. Scalpel blade should be sharp and scalpel handle need to be metallic. Care must be taken not injure oneself (Figs 1a to c).

Forceps: Forceps are used to hold the part being dissected (Fig. 2a to c). One pair should be serrated tip forceps for lifting the skin, nerve, artery or vein, etc. Another pair should be blunt forceps for holding the structure firmly while dissection is being done. Size of the forceps may be 7.5 to 15 cm.

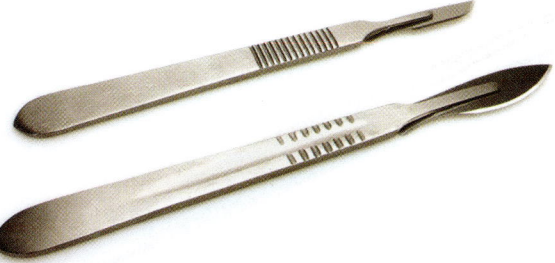

Fig. 1a: Scalpel with blade

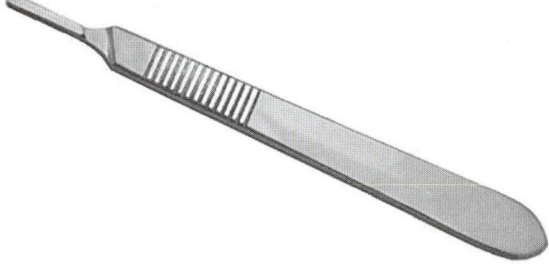

Fig. 1b: Scalpel handle

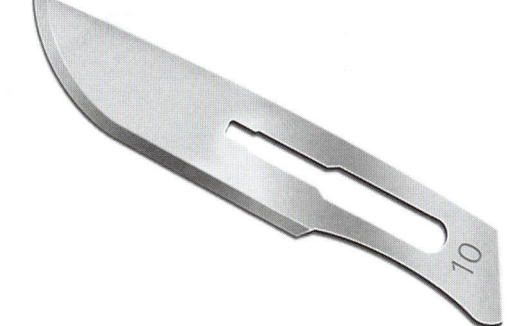

Fig. 1c: Scalpel blade

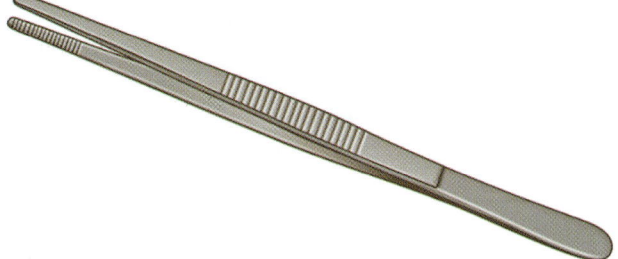

Fig. 2a: Toothed forceps

Probe: It is useful for doing blunt dissection and for cleaning the dissecting region (Fig. 4).

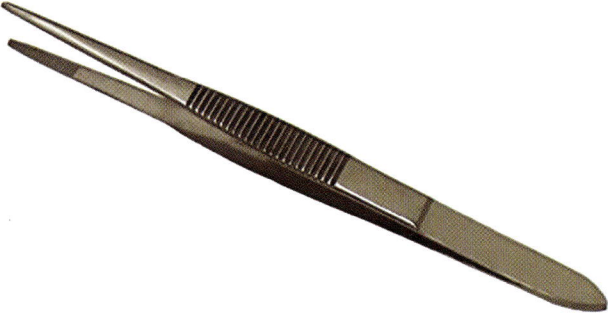

Fig. 2b: Blunt forceps

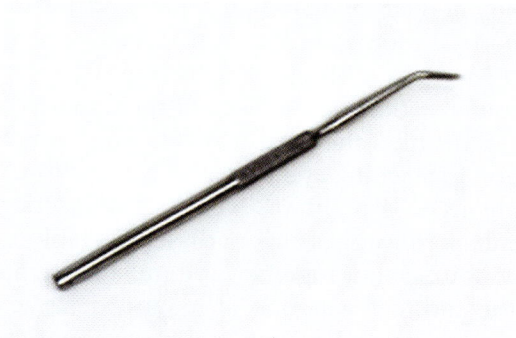

Fig. 4: Probe

Hand lens: The hand lens is required to magnify the smaller structures for better and correct identification (Fig. 5).

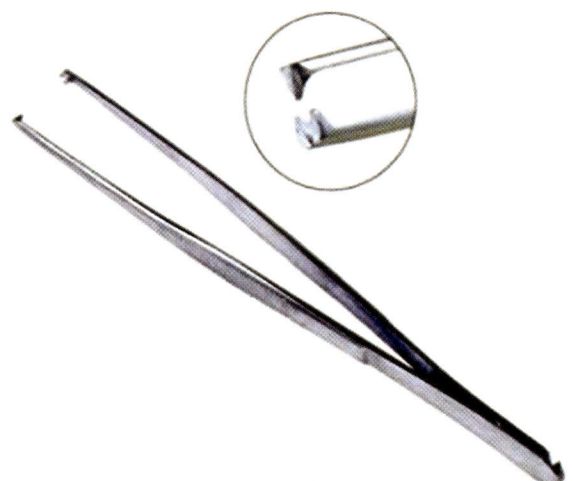

Fig. 2c: Pointed forceps

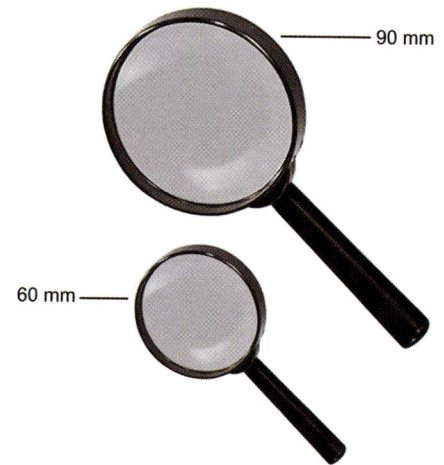

90 mm

60 mm

Scissors: A pair of small scissors is necessary for cutting a small structure (Fig. 3). Another pair of big scissors (15 cm) is also required at times.

Fig. 5: Hand lens

Skin marking pencil: This is used for marking the skin incisions (Fig. 6).

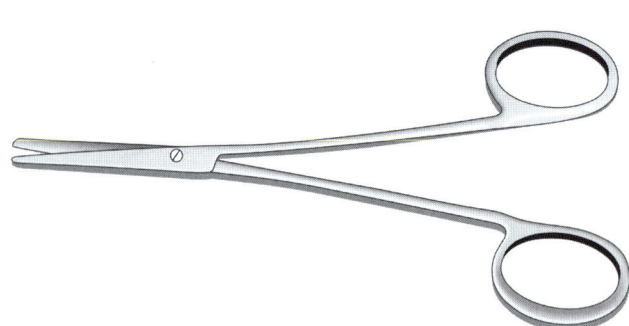

Fig. 3: Scissors

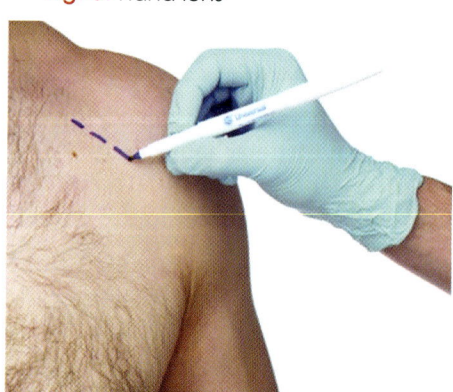

Fig. 6: Skin marking pencil/pen

REVIEW

It is this dead body that will teach the young bright medical/dental students. So the saying "Dead Teach The Living" is absolutely right. Even the skeletons/loose bones prepared from the dead bodies are teaching the medical personnel. As of now synthetic bones are available. In later years, autopsy of the dead patient, with consent, teaches the clinicians and senior medical students. The findings guide them all for improved treatment.

The cadaver "keeps quiet" as its main aim is not to complain but to let one learn at ones own pace and learn well, to enable one to treat future patients better and in a humane manner.

The cadaver may actually be enjoying the company of young talkative students, as it probably never had such an opportunity during its life time.

For the last few years, people have voluntarily started donation their bodies after death. Earlier these used to be of poor people who could not afford to get the last rites done.

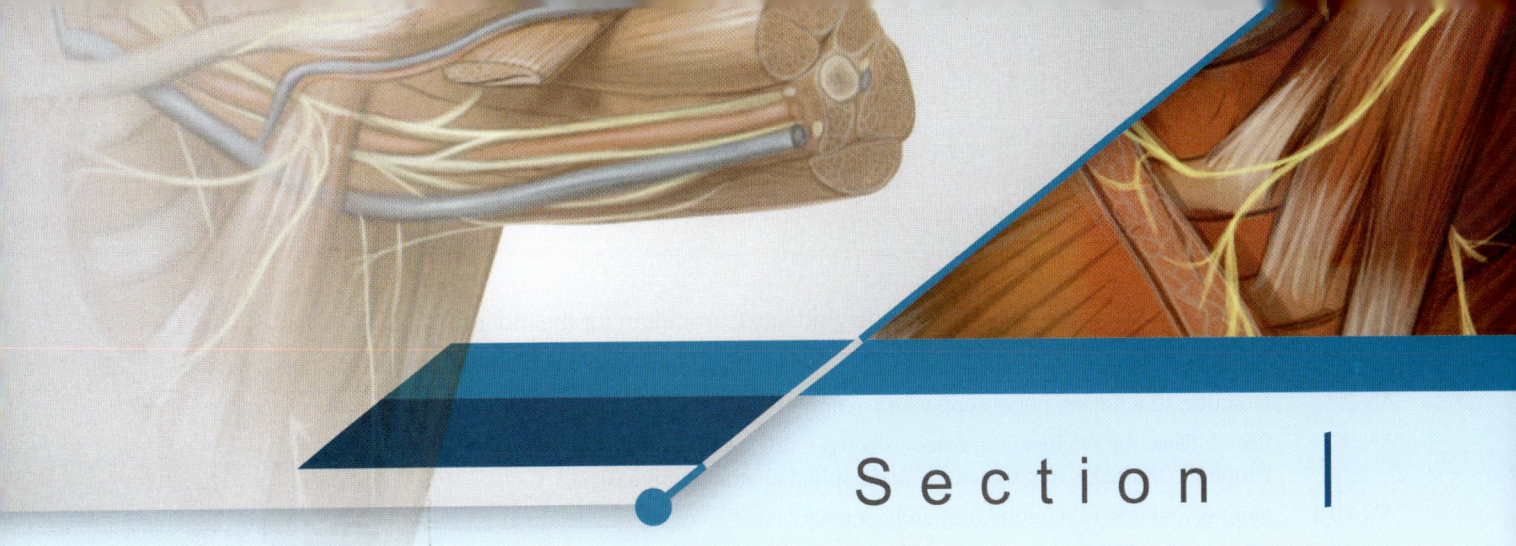

Section |

Upper Limb

Index of Competencies (Competency based Undergraduate Curriculum for the Indian Medical Graduate 2018;1:44–80)

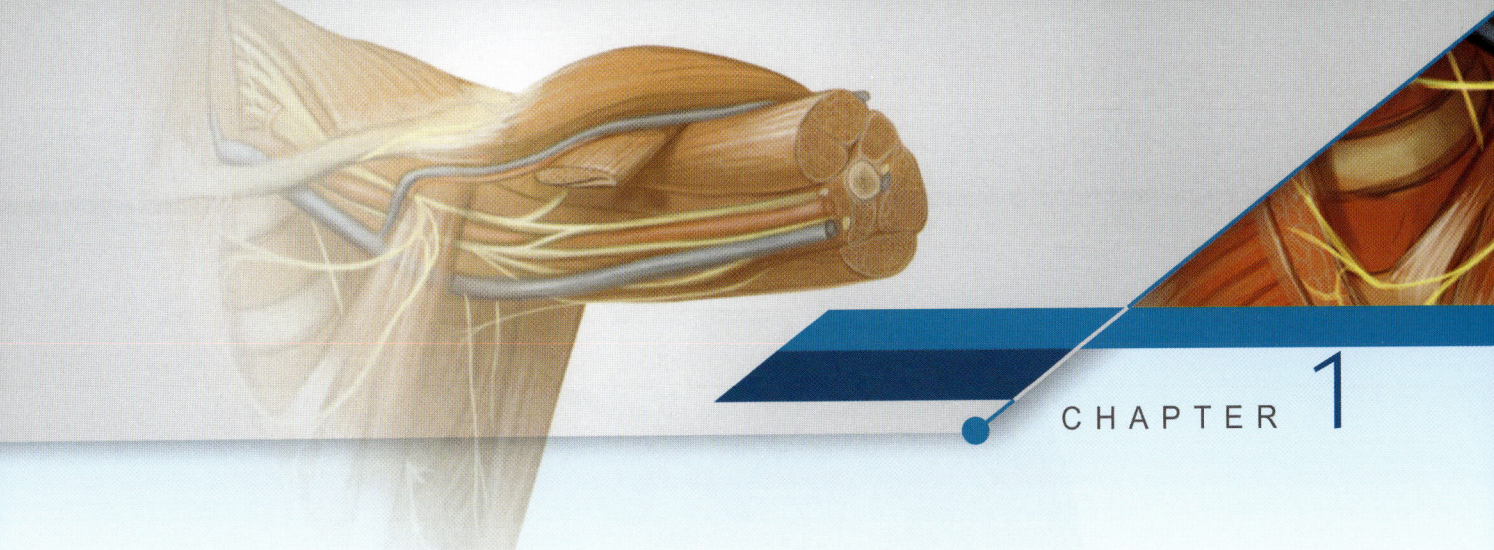

Pectoral Region

Learning Objectives

One should be able to

1. Mark proximal and distal attachments of pectoralis major, pectoralis minor and serratus anterior muscles.
2. Show the actions of clavicular and sternocostal parts of pectoralis major separately including actions of the muscle as a whole.
3. Show the position of scapula in case of injury to the nerve to serratus anterior.
4. Palpate all four quadrants of mammary gland.
5. Show how to feel various groups of lymph nodes in the axilla.

OVERVIEW

The pectoral region (part of the upper limb) lies on the front of thoracic wall, i.e. in relation to sternum, clavicle and the upper ribs. This region contains a very important gland—mammary gland in addition to the pectoral muscles. Skin of the pectoral region is innervated by C3, C4 nerves and T2–T6 nerves as the ventral rami of C5–C8 and T1 have been pulled up in the developing upper limb.

Mammary gland is important from clinical point of view as its cancer is a very common disease which has the potential to spread to a wide area via the lymphatics. Early diagnosis is the key to best line of treatment. Self examination of the glands on a monthly basis is the only way for its diagnosis.

Pectoralis major is the main muscle forming the bed for the mammary gland. This muscle has extensive origin from clavicle, sternum and costal cartilages and gets inserted by bilaminar tendon into lateral lip of intertubercular sulcus of humerus. It is innervated by both medial and lateral pectoral nerves and has an important role in the movements of shoulder joint.

Deep to pectoralis major lies triangular pectoralis minor muscle.

STEPS OF DISSECTION

- Mark the following points (Fig. 1.1).
    i. Centre of the suprasternal notch
    ii. Xiphoid process
    iii. 7 o'clock position at the margin of areola (left side), and 5 o'clock position at the margin of areola (right side)
    iv. Lateral end of clavicle.
- Give an incision vertically down from the first point to the second which joins the centre of the suprasternal notch to the xiphoid process in the midsagittal plane. From the lower end of this line, extend the incision upward and laterally till you reach to the third point on the areolar margin.
- Encircle the areola and carry the incision upwards and laterally till the anterior axillary fold is reached.
- Continue the line of incision downwards along the medial border of the upper arm till its junction of

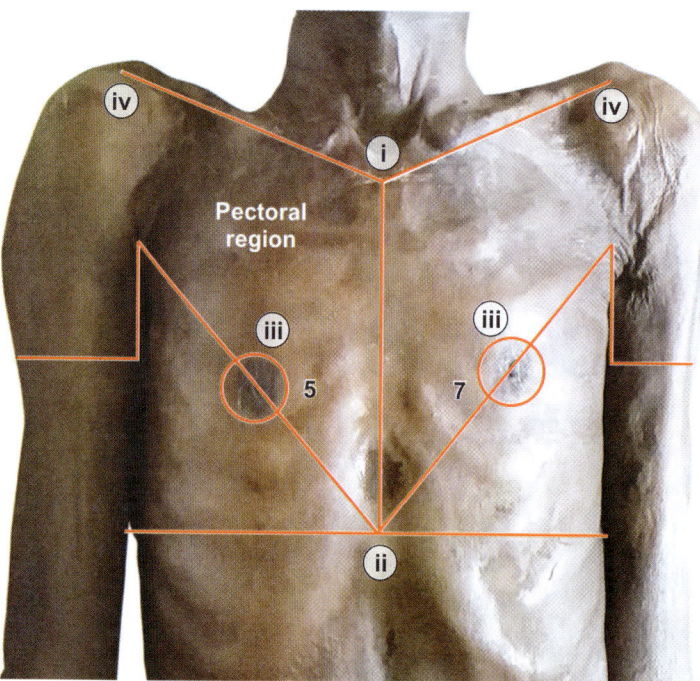

Fig. 1.1: Lines of incision

upper one-third and lower two-thirds. Extend this incision transversely across the arm.

- Make another incision horizontally from the xiphoid process across the chest wall till the posterior axillary line (Fig. 1.2).
- Lastly, give horizontal incision from the centre of suprasternal notch to the lateral (acromial) end of the clavicle.
- Reflect the two flaps of skin towards the upper limb.

CUTANEOUS NERVES

- Supraclavicular nerves—medial, intermediate and lateral descend over the clavicle to supply the skin of 1st intercostal space and skin over upper half of deltoid. These are branches of cervical plexus (C3, C4).
- Anterior cutaneous branches of intercostal nerves with perforating branches of internal thoracic artery.
- Lateral cutaneous branches of intercostal nerves emerge along midaxillary line to divide into anterior and posterior branches. Lateral cutaneous branch of 2nd intercostal nerve is large and is called intercostobrachial nerve. It supplies skin of floor of axilla and medial side of arm.

Competency achievement: The student should be able to:

AN 9.2 Breast: Describe the location, extent, deep relations, structure, age changes, blood supply, lymphatic drainage, microanatomy and applied anatomy of breast.

MAMMARY GLANDS/BREAST

- Study the mammary gland (breast) lying on the pectoralis major muscle (Figs 1.2 and 1.3).

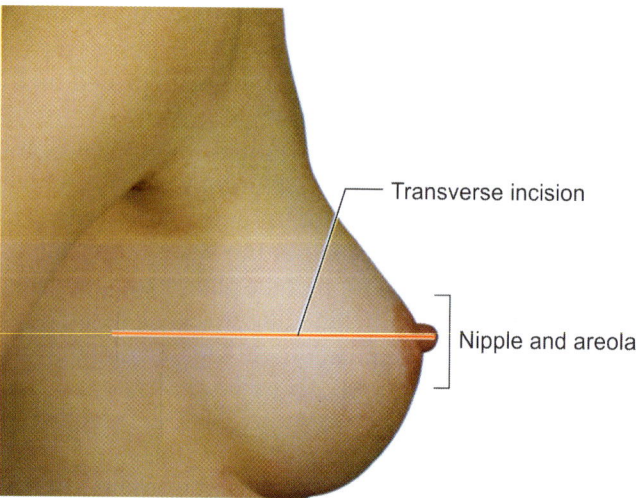

Transverse incision

Nipple and areola

Fig. 1.2: Transverse incision through nipple and breast till posterior axillary line

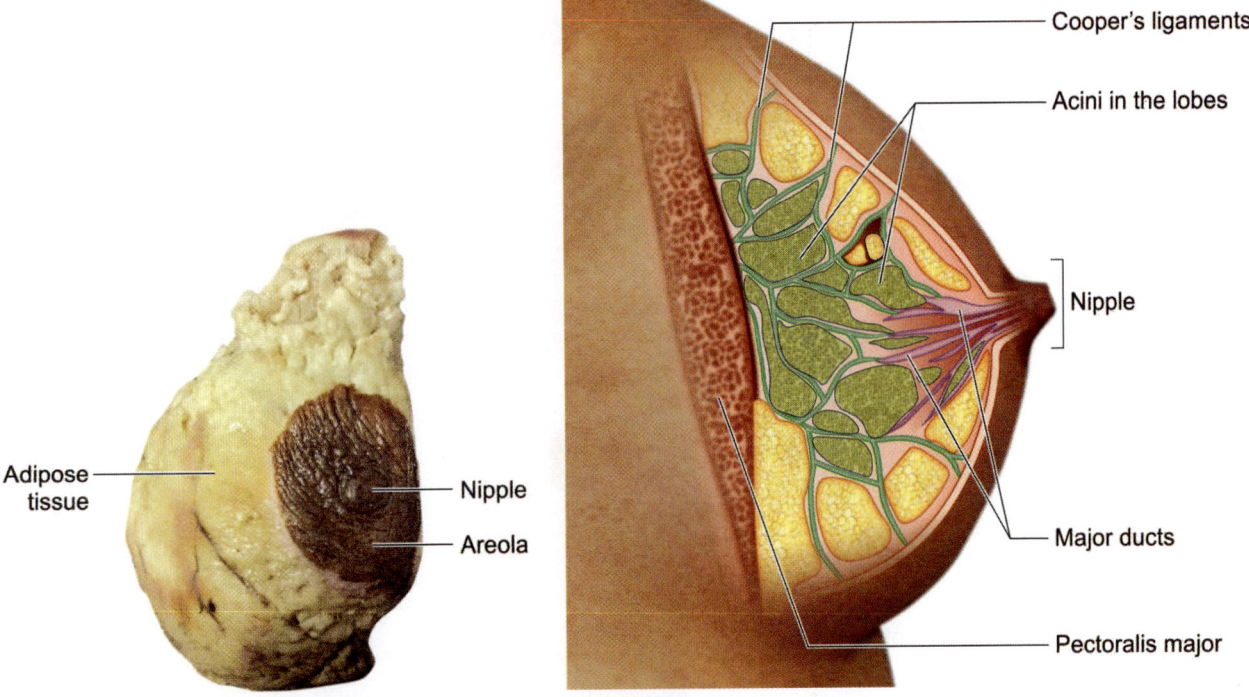

Fig. 1.3: Gross and macroscopic features of mammary gland

- Examine the vertical and transverse extent of gland lying in the superficial fascia. A small part may be seen extending into the axilla.
- Identify the nipple and areola. Make a transverse cut through the nipple and gland till the posterior axillary line.
- Look for lobes and ducts of the gland. The Cooper's/suspensory ligaments are fibrous bands which extend from the nipple and skin of breast to the deep fascia of pectoralis major (Fig. 1.3).
- See that the gland is lying mainly on the pectoralis major and to a little extent on external oblique muscle of abdomen and serratus anterior muscle. These three muscles—pectoralis major, external oblique and serratus anterior—form the bed for the mammary gland.
- Lymphatic drainage of mammary gland needs good understanding as diagnosis and prognosis of breast cancer depends upon its lymphatic spread.

Competency achievement: The student should be able to:

AN 9.1 Describe attachment, nerve supply and actions of pectoralis major and pectoralis minor muscles.

PECTORAL MUSCLES

- Identify deep fascia over pectoralis major. It is continuous with periosteum of sternum and clavicle. Laterally, it gets continuous with fascia covering the deltoid muscle by passing over the infraclavicular fossa and deltopectoral groove. Further it curves at inferolateral border of pectoralis major to get continuous with the axillary fascia. Axillary fascia extends between pectoralis major and latissimus dorsi muscles. When the arm is abducted by the deltoid, axillary fascia gets lifted into the axilla to form the armpit.
- Demarcate the deltopectoral groove by removing the deep fascia. Identify the cephalic vein (which drains into axillary vein), a small artery (branch of thoracoacromial artery), and a few lymph nodes (Fig. 1.4a).
- The pectoralis major arises from clavicle, anterior aspect of sternum, 1–6 costal cartilages and aponeurosis of external oblique muscle of abdomen. It is inserted by a bilaminar tendon into lateral lip of intertubercular sulcus of humerus.
- Divide the clavicular head of the muscle and reflect it laterally. Clavicular part is innervated by lateral

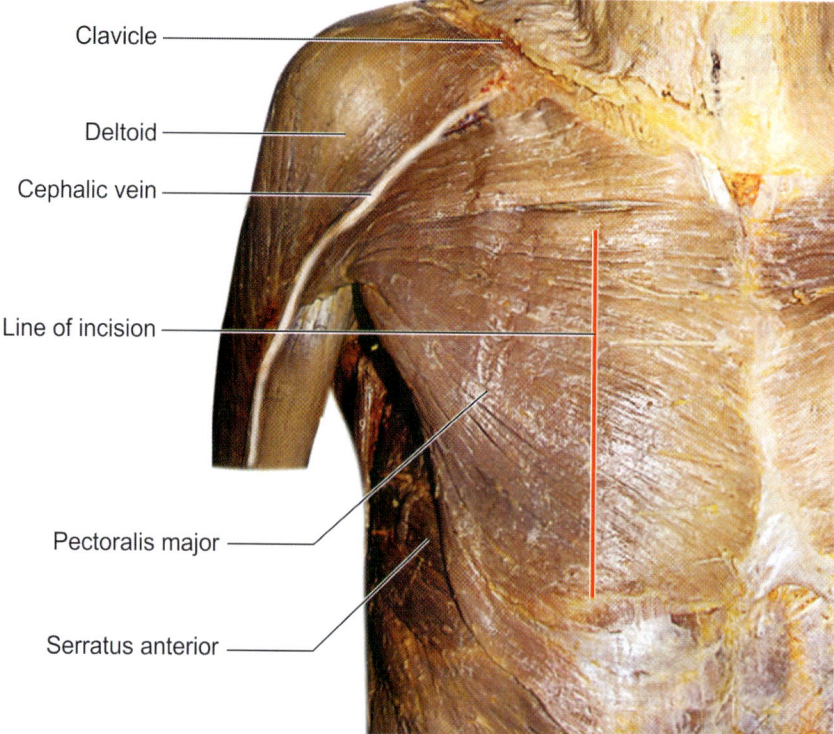

Clavicle

Deltoid

Cephalic vein

Line of incision

Pectoralis major

Serratus anterior

Fig. 1.4a: Deltopectoral groove with cephalic vein

pectoral nerve and sternocostal part by medial pectoral nerve.

- Make a vertical incision 5–6 cm from lateral border of sternum and reflect its sternocostal head laterally.
- Identify the triangular pectoralis minor muscle under central part of pectoralis major muscle. It arises from 3rd, 4th and 5th costochondral junctions and gets inserted on the medial border of coracoid process of scapula (Fig. 1.4b). It is innervated by both medial and lateral pectoral nerves. Lateral thoracic artery runs along the inferolateral border of this muscle to supply this muscle and the mammary gland.
- Note the clavipectoral fascia extending between upper border of pectoralis minor and clavicle (Fig. 1.5). This fascia splits to enclose the small sub-clavius muscle situated below the clavicle. Sub-clavius extends between 1st costochondral junction and inferior surface of clavicle. It is supplied by nerve to subclavius and acts as a cushion for axillary artery and brachial plexus.

- Identify the structures piercing clavipectoral fascia (Fig. 1.5). These are:
  a. Cephalic vein
  b. Thoracoacromial artery
  c. Lateral pectoral nerve
  d. Some lymph vessels

Competency achievement: The student should be able to:
AN 10.11 Describe and demonstrate attachment of serratus anterior with its action.

- Also identify serratus anterior muscle on the side of chest wall getting inserted into costal surface of medial border of scapula deep to the subscapularis. This muscle arises as slips from middle of the outer surfaces of 1st–8th ribs. Its lower slips interdigitate with the external oblique muscle. It is inserted into medial border and inferior angle of costal surface of scapula (Fig. 1.6). It is supplied by long thoracic nerve. The muscle keeps the scapula in contact with chest wall and supports the scapula. It is protractor of shoulder girdle.

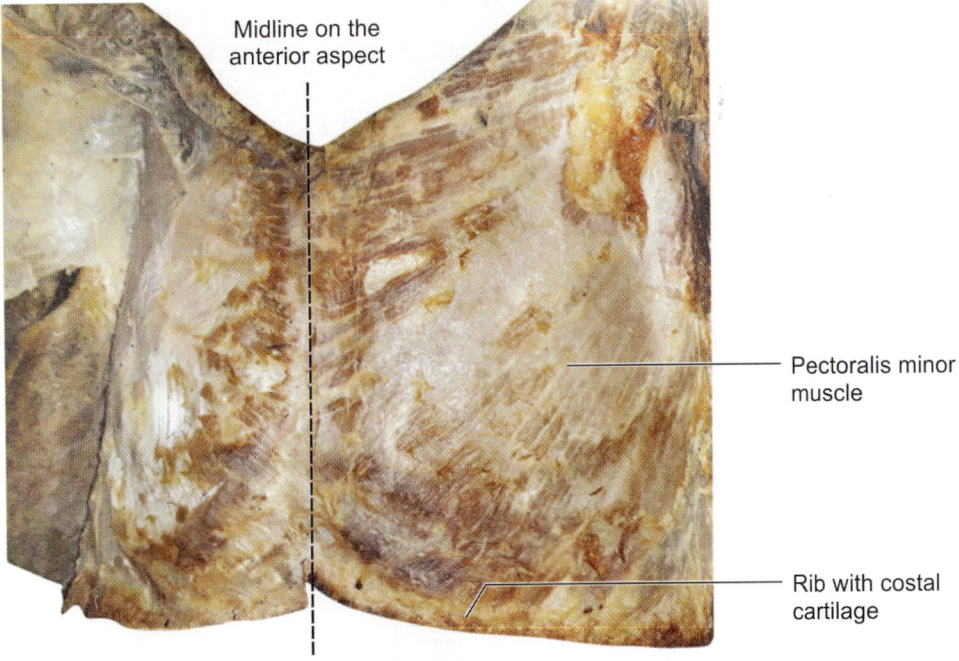

Fig. 1.4b: Pectoralis minor muscle

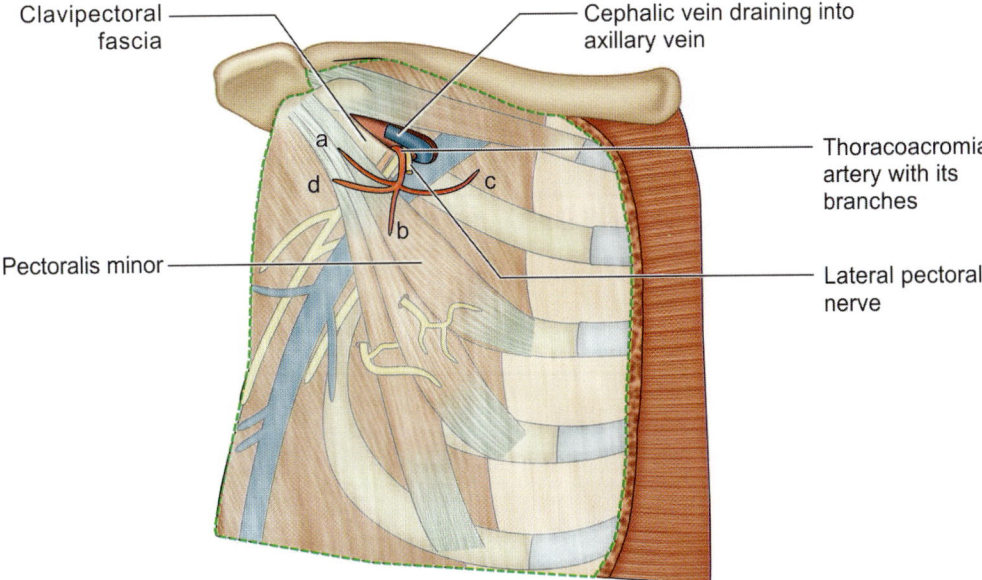

Fig. 1.5: Structures percing clavipectoral fascia. Branches of thoracoacromial artery: a: Acromial, b: pectoral, c: clavicular, d: deltoid

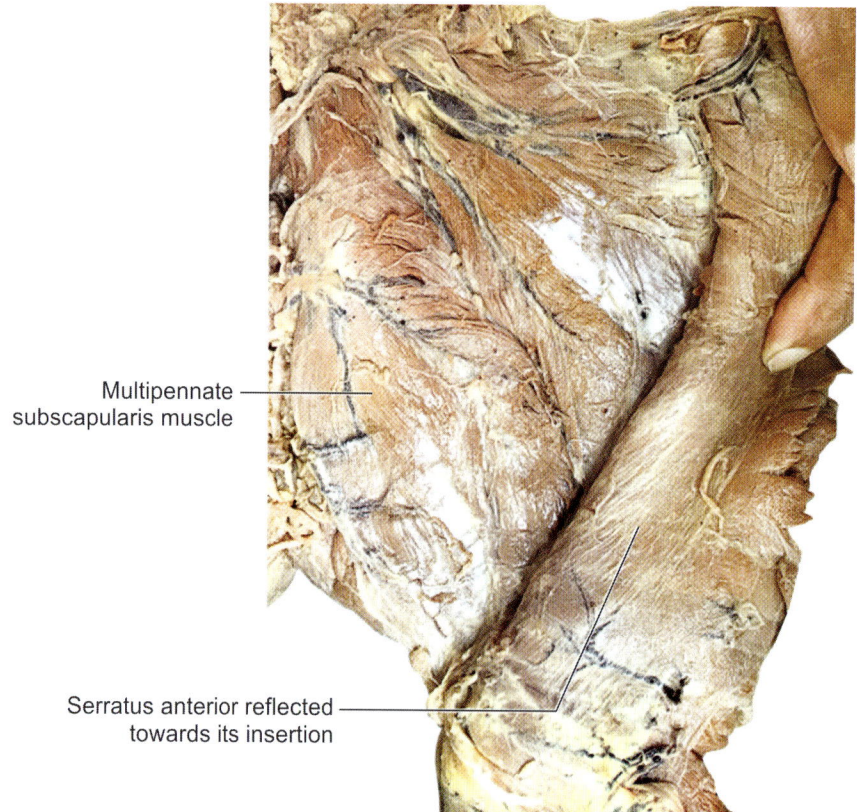

Multipennate
subscapularis muscle

Serratus anterior reflected
towards its insertion

Fig. 1.6: Right serratus anterior muscle

- What muscles form the deep relations of the mammary gland?
- What structures pierce the clavipectoral fascia?
- How does one examine the clavicular and sternocostal heads of pectoralis major muscle?
- Which muscle divides the axillary artery in three parts?

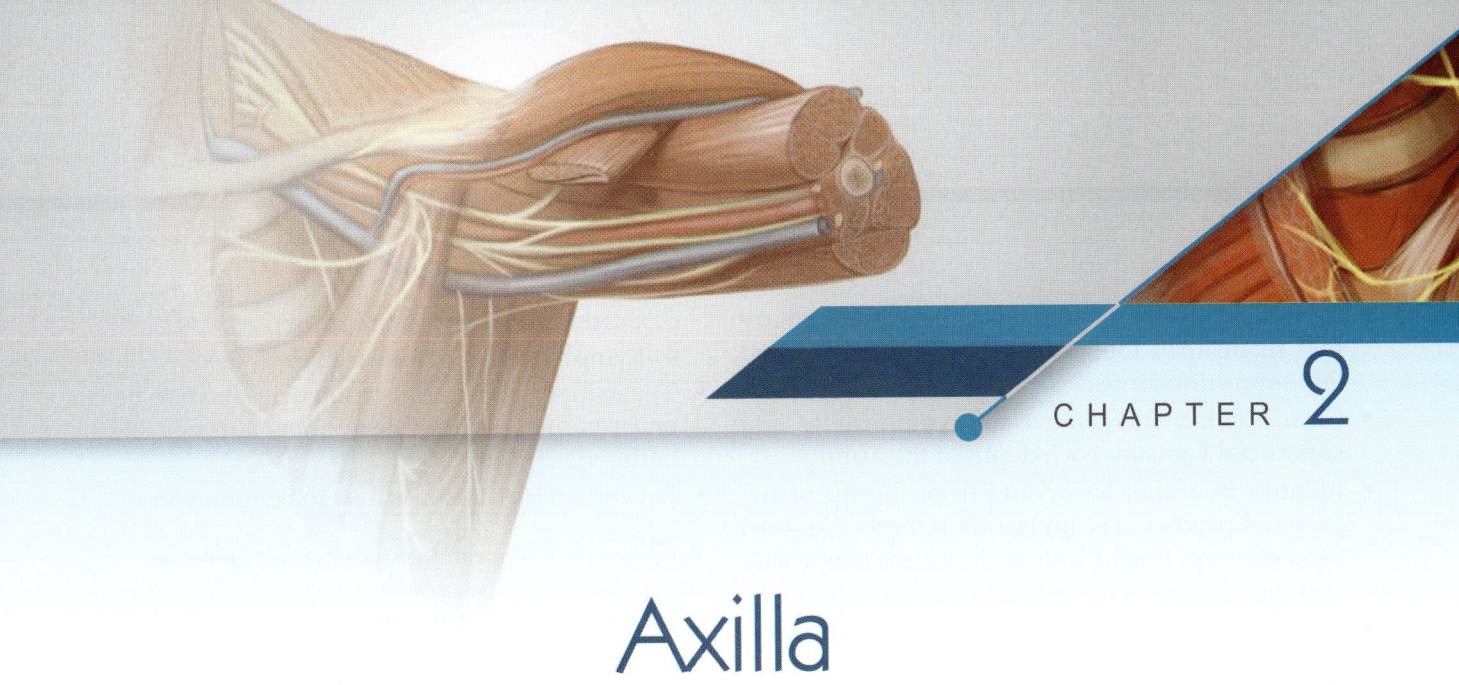

Axilla

Learning Objectives

One should be able to

1. Identify the three trunks of brachial plexus.
2. Identify the formation of three cords of brachial plexus.
3. Identify the three branches of lateral cord, five branches of medial cord and five branches of posterior cord of brachial plexus.
4. Name the branches of axillary artery

OVERVIEW

The axilla is a pyramidal shaped space between the lateral side of upper thoracic wall and medial aspect of upper limb. It comprises a truncated apex formed by clavicle, upper border of scapula and outer border of 1st rib.

Its base or floor is formed by skin and axillary fascia extending between pectoralis major and latissimus dorsi muscles.

Anterior wall is formed by pectoralis major, pectoralis minor and clavipectoral fascia.

Posterior wall is constituted by big latissimus dorsi twisting around teres major muscle and subscapularis present on the costal surface of scapula.

Narrow lateral wall is formed by shaft of humerus in the region of bicipital groove and two muscles, i.e. coracobrachialis medially and short head of biceps brachii laterally. Both muscles arise from the tip of coracoid process of scapula.

Medial wall is formed by upper four ribs with their intercostal muscles and upper 3–4 digitations of serratus anterior muscle.

Competency achievement: The student should be able to:

AN 10.1 Identify and describe boundaries and contents of axilla.

STEPS OF DISSECTION

- Place a rectangular wooden block under the neck and shoulder region of cadaver. Ensure that the block supports the body firmly.
- Abduct the limb at right angles to the trunk; and strap the wrist firmly on block projecting towards your side (Fig. 2.1).

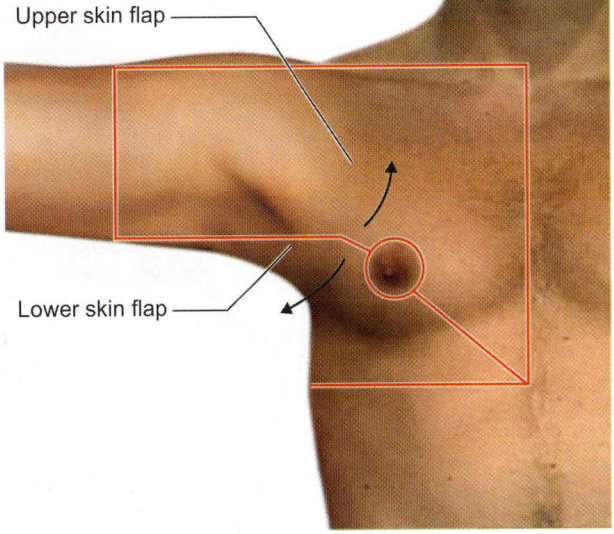

Upper skin flap

Lower skin flap

Fig. 2.1: Lines of incision of axilla

- Reflect the lower skin flap till the posterior axillary fold, made up by the subscapularis, teres major, and latissimus dorsi muscles.
- Clean the fat, and remove the lymph nodes and superficial veins to reach depth of the armpit.
- Identify two muscles arising from the tip of the coracoid process of scapula; out of these, the short head of biceps brachii muscle lies on the lateral side and the coracobrachialis on the medial side.
- The pectoral muscles with the clavipectoral fascia form anterior boundary of the region. Look for upper three intercostal muscles and serratus anterior muscle which make the medial wall of axilla.
- Clean and identify the axillary vessels. Trace the course of the branches of the axillary artery.
- Reflect the upper skin flap on the arm till the incision already given at its junction of upper one-third and lower two-thirds.
- Pectoralis major is reflected laterally and pectoralis minor is reflected superiorly.
- *Identify contents of axilla:*
  1. Axillary sheath around axillary vessels and brachial plexus. It is thin over the vein.
  2. Axillary artery and its branches with medially placed axillary vein with its tributaries (Fig. 2.2a).
  3. Cords and branches of brachial plexus.
  4. Lymph nodes, fat and areolar tissue.
- The axillary vein and its tributaries have to be cut and removed so that nerves and arteries can be better visualised.
- Fat and areolar tissue is also to be removed

Competency achievement: The student should be able to:

AN 10.4 Describe the anatomical groups of axillary lymph nodes and specify their areas of drainage.

- Note the position of the lymph nodes before these are sacrificed. These are:
  1. Anterior or pectoral along lateral thoracic vessels (Fig. 2.2a).
  2. Posterior or subscapular along subscapular vessels.
  3. Lateral group lies along and medial to axillary vein.
  4. Central group in relation the fat of the axilla.
  5. Apical group lies deep to clavipectoral fascia along axillary vessels.
- To remove axillary vein, cut at the point of union of cephalic with axillary vein in infraclavicular fossa. Next cut the axillary vein at outer border of 1st rib. Lastly cut the vein at lower border of teres major. Now the whole axillary vein can be removed including tributaries of the vein. This makes the

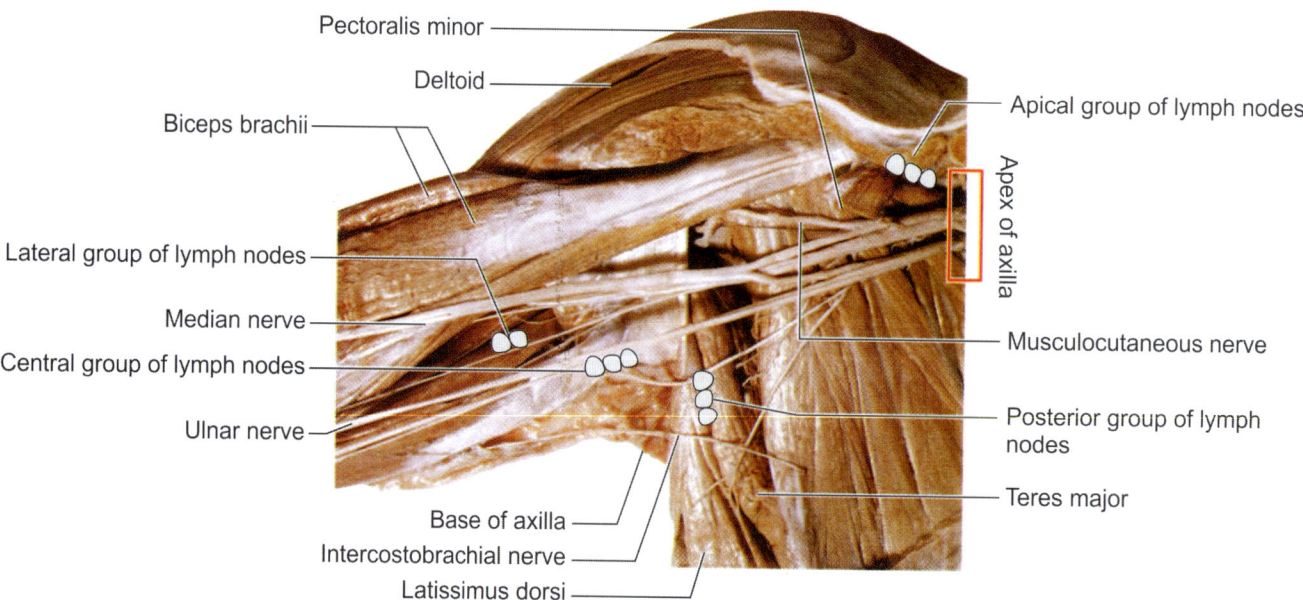

Fig. 2.2a: Apex and base of axilla with axillary lymph nodes

Pectoralis minor
muscle with
pectoral branch of
thoracoacromial
artery

Pectoral fascia
reflected

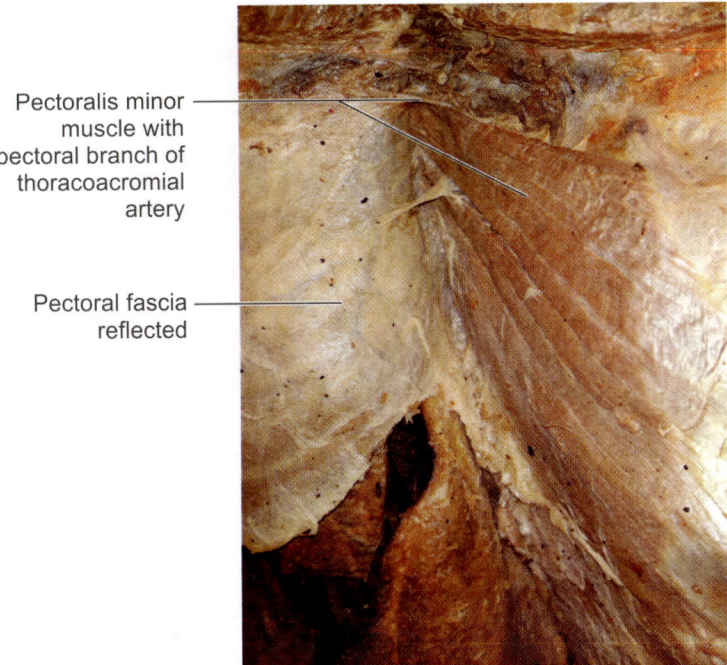

Fig. 2.2b: Pectoralis minor muscle

axilla less crowdy and clear for the branches of axillary artery and of brachial plexus to be traced to their destinations.

- See the axillary artery extending from the outer border of 1st rib to lower border of teres major muscle. Observe that it is crossed by pectoralis minor muscle dividing the artery into three parts:
  - 1st part, medial to muscle
  - 2nd part, posterior to muscle
  - 3rd part, lateral to muscle.
- Identify branches of:
  - 1st part: Superior thoracic is given off near the apex of axilla. It supplies upper two intercostal spaces and mammary gland.
  - 2nd part
    1. Thoracoacromial/acromiothoracic is given off behind pectoralis minor and comes at the medial or upper border of the muscle. The artery pierces clavipectoral fascia and divides into four branches:

    i. Acromial runs towards acromion process.
    ii. Pectoral supplies the pectoral muscles and breast (Fig. 2.2b).
    iii. Clavicular goes towards clavicle to supply bone and muscle (*see* Fig. 1.5).
    iv. Deltoid runs in deltopectoral groove to supply the muscle.
    2. Lateral thoracic runs along inferolateral border of pectoralis minor to supply it as well as the mammary gland (Fig. 2.3).
  - 3rd part
    1. Subscapular artery: It is the largest branch of axillary artery. It supplies muscles of posterior axillary wall (Fig. 2.3).
    2. Posterior circumflex humeral artery: It passes posterior to surgical neck of humerus with the axillary nerve. Both these are contents of quadrangular space.
    3. Anterior circumflex humeral artery: It is smaller than the posterior artery. It passes deep to tendon of long head of biceps brachii along the anterior aspect of humerus. Both these arteries anastomose laterally.

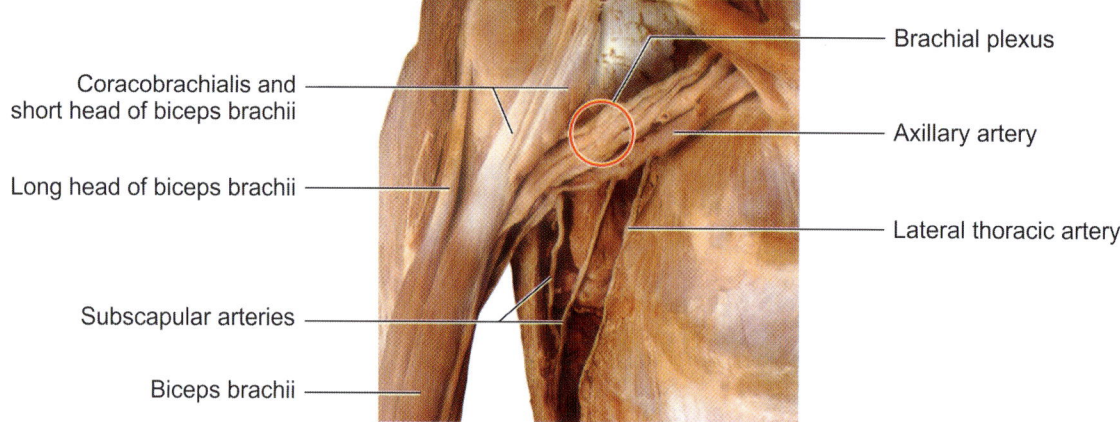

Coracobrachialis and
short head of biceps brachii

Long head of biceps brachii

Subscapular arteries

Biceps brachii

Brachial plexus

Axillary artery

Lateral thoracic artery

Fig. 2.3: Some branches of axillary artery

Competency achievement: The student should be able to:

AN 10.3 Describe, identify and demonstrate formation, branches, relations, area of supply of branches, course and relations of terminal branches of brachial plexus.

BRACHIAL PLEXUS

Brachial plexus is formed by ventral primary rami of C5–C8 and T1 nerves. These are also called roots. Five roots join to form 3 trunks, upper, middle and lower. Each trunk divides into an anterior and a posterior division. These divisions from 3 cords, which give 13 branches. Four branches are given by roots and upper trunk. So there are 17 branches from brachial plexus.

For details *see* BD Chaurasia's *Human Anatomy*. Look for the cords and branches of brachial plexus which are encountered in the axilla. The cords are related to 1st and 2nd parts of axillary artery while the branches are related to its 3rd part (Figs 2.4 to 2.8).

1. Identify the lateral cord. It lies lateral to 2nd part of axillary artery. Its branches are:
   i. Musculocutaneous nerve as the lateral branch of the plexus. It arises from the lateral cord. Trace the musculocutaneous nerve up till the lateral cord.
   ii. Other branch of lateral cord is the lateral root of median nerve. Trace it to the median nerve.

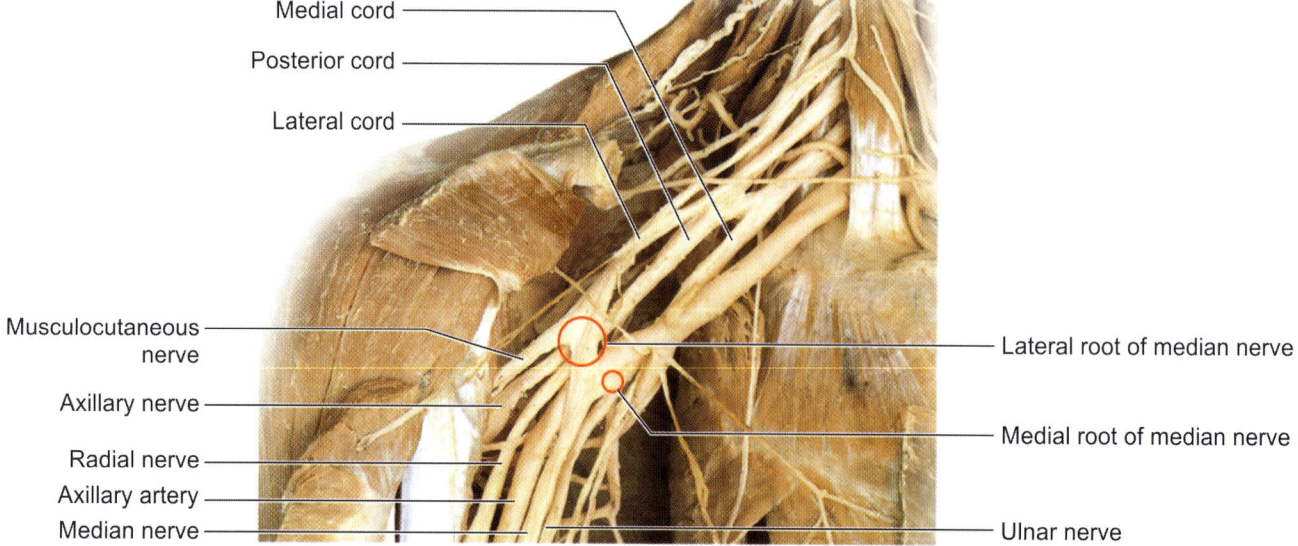

Medial cord

Posterior cord

Lateral cord

Musculocutaneous
nerve

Axillary nerve

Radial nerve

Axillary artery

Median nerve

Lateral root of median nerve

Medial root of median nerve

Ulnar nerve

Fig. 2.4: Main branches of brachial plexus

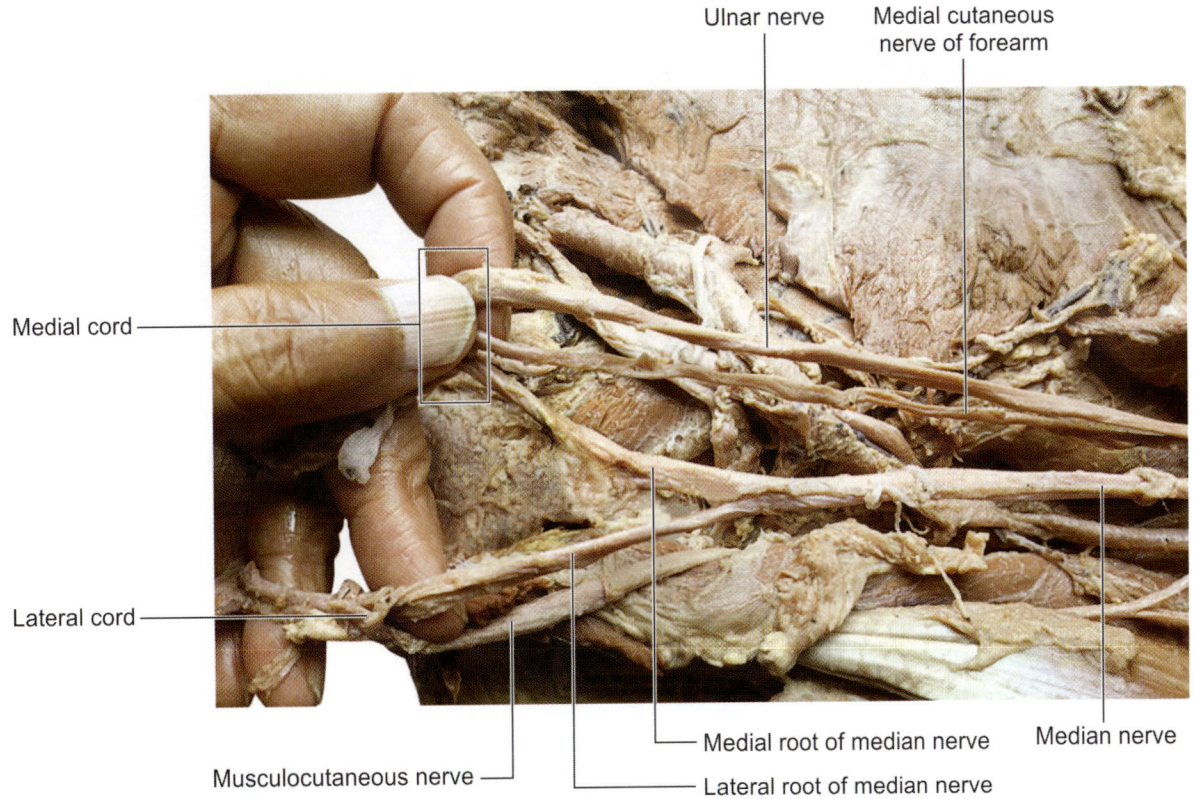

Ulnar nerve

Medial cutaneous nerve of forearm

Medial cord

Lateral cord

Musculocutaneous nerve

Medial root of median nerve

Lateral root of median nerve

Median nerve

Fig. 2.5: Some cords of brachial plexus, musculocutaneous nerve and roots of median nerve

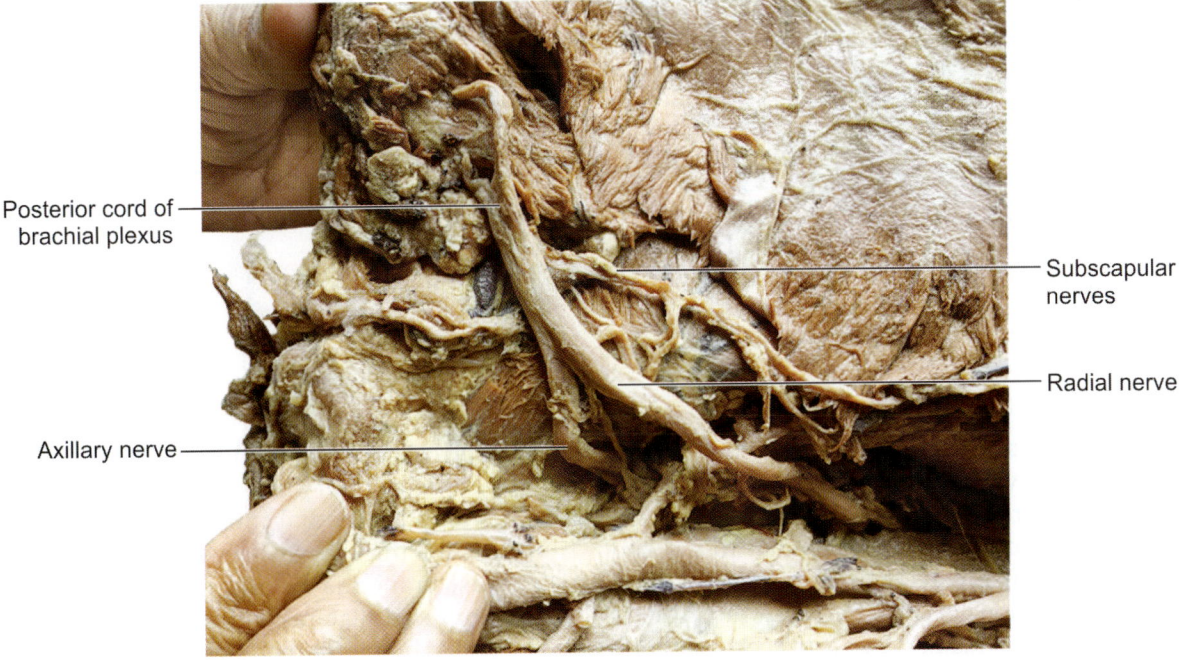

Posterior cord of brachial plexus

Subscapular nerves

Radial nerve

Axillary nerve

Fig. 2.6: Branches of posterior cord of brachial plexus

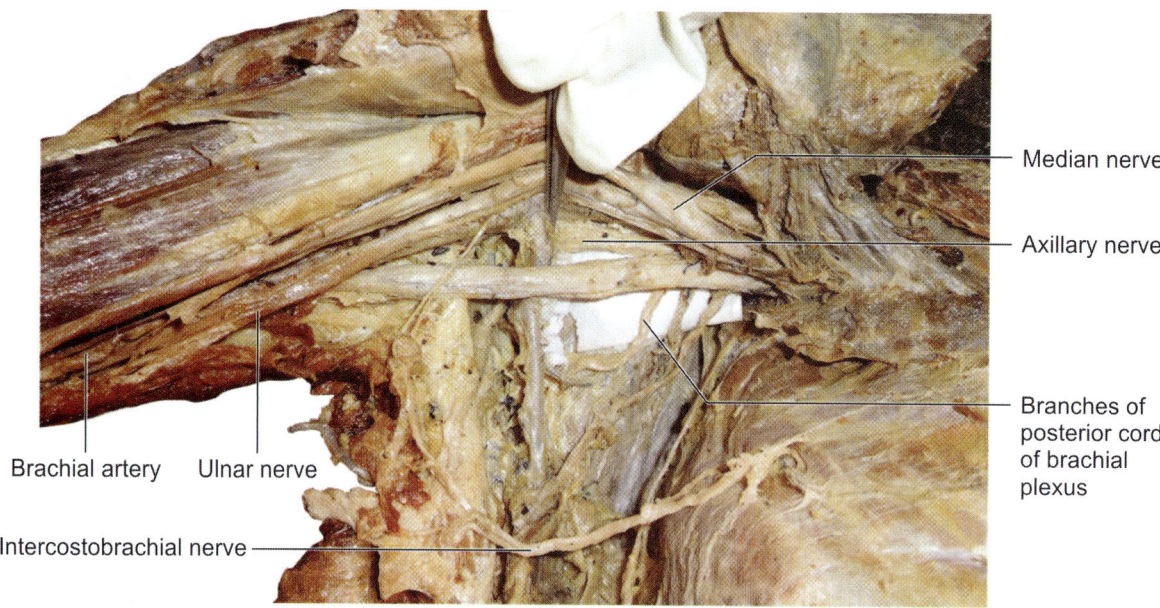

Fig. 2.7: Branches of posterior cord of brachial plexus, with median and ulnar nerves

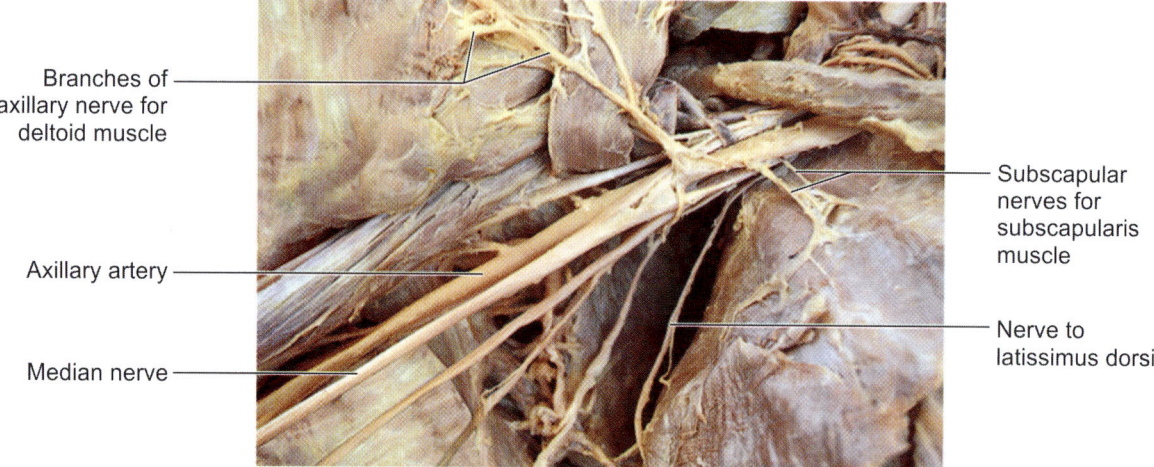

Fig. 2.8: Branches of posterior cord of brachial plexus

iii. A smaller branch of the lateral cord is lateral pectoral nerve for the two pectoral muscles. It is the first branch of lateral cord.
2. Identify the medial cord lying medial to the 2nd part of axillary artery. Its branches are:
  i. Medial pectoral nerve for two pectoral muscles.
  ii. Medial cutaneous nerve of arm seen medial to axillary vein.

iii. Medial cutaneous nerve of forearm lying between axillary artery and axillary vein.
iv. Behind the medial cutaneous nerve of forearm lies the thick ulnar nerve.
  v. Last branch is medial root of median nerve. Appreciate lateral and medial cords and their united branch as modified letter "M". The upper two ends represent the lateral and medial cords.

The lower three ends represent the musculo-cutaneous, median and ulnar nerves (Fig. 2.5).

3. Identify the thickest cord, the posterior cord of brachial plexus behind axillary artery. Retract the axillary artery, lateral and medial cords to visualise the posterior cord and its following branches:
   i. Upper subscapular for innervating subscapularis muscle (Figs 2.6 to 2.8).
   ii. Thoracodorsal nerve for supplying the latissimus dorsi muscle.
   iii. Lower subscapular for supplying the subscapularis and teres major muscles.
   iv. Axillary nerve coursing through the quadrangular space to supply the deltoid and teres minor muscles.
   v. Radial nerve is the continuation of the posterior cord. It passes through the lower triangular space to reach posterior to humerus; lying anterior to teres major and latissimus dorsi muscles.

- Observe that the posterior wall of axilla is formed by subscapularis, teres major and latissimus dorsi muscles.
- Subscapularis fills up the subscapular fossa of scapula and is inserted into lesser tubercle of humerus.
- Observe the attachments of the following muscles of this region: Subscapularis, teres major, latissimus dorsi and serratus anterior.

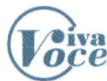

Viva Voce

- Name the muscles forming posterior wall of axilla. Which nerves supply these muscles.
- Name the branches of axillary artery.
- Which is the largest branch of axillary artery?
- Name the branches of lateral cord of brachial plexus.
- Name the branches of medial cord of brachial plexus.
- Name the branches of posterior cord of brachial plexus.
- Which is the thickest branch of brachial plexus?

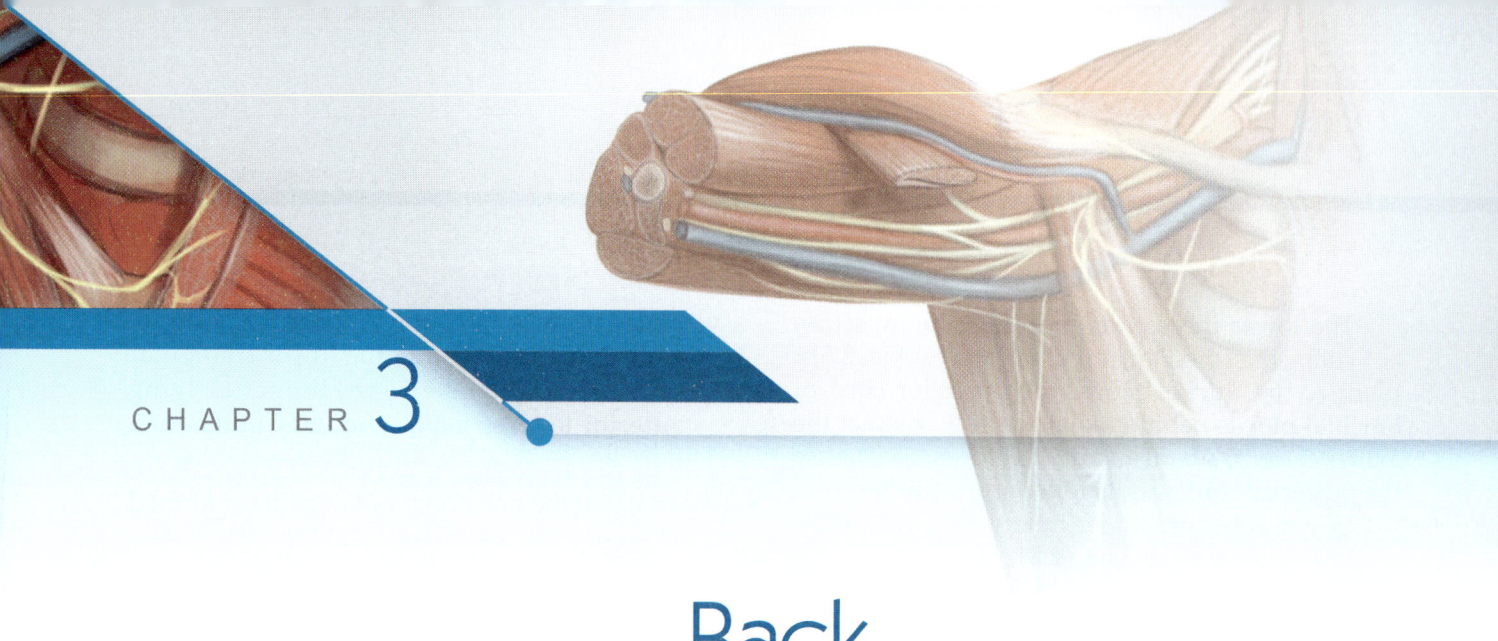

CHAPTER 3

Back

Learning Objectives

One should be able to

1. Show actions of upper, middle and lower fibres of the important trapezius muscle.
2. Show the action of trapezius in conjunction with serratus anterior during overhead abduction of shoulder joint.
3. Identify the triple relation of latissimus dorsi with teres major.
4. Show the actions of latissimus dorsi muscle.

OVERVIEW

The skin of back is thicker than that of the front. Nerves innervating the skin of back are posterior primary rami of lower cervical nerves.

Main muscles are trapezius—the shrugging muscle and the latissimus dorsi—the coughing muscle. Many muscles, nerves, vessels, etc. lie deep to trapezius, which is innervated by spinal root of accessory nerve. The proprioceptive fibres are from C3 and C4 nerves.

Competency achievement: The student should be able to:

AN 10.8 Describe, identify and demonstrate the position, attachment, nerve supply and actions of trapezius and latissimus dorsi.

STEPS OF DISSECTION

- Identify the external occipital protuberance (i) of the skull (Fig. 3.1).
- Draw a line in the midline from (ii) the protuberance to the spine of the last thoracic (T12) vertebra.
- Make incision along this line.
- Extend the incision from its lower end to the deltoid tuberosity (iii) on the humerus which is present on lateral surface about the middle of the arm. Note that the arm is placed by the side of the trunk.
- Make another incision along a horizontal line from seventh cervical spine—vertebra prominens (iv) to the acromion process of scapula (v).
- Reflect the skin flap laterally. The skin of back is thicker than the skin on front of the body. It is supplied by posterior primary rami of spinal nerves.
- See that the fasciae are deep to the skin. Deep to the fascia are two superficial muscles.
- Identify the attachments of trapezius muscle in the upper part of back and that of latissimus dorsi in the lower part (Fig. 3.2a and b).
- Clean areolar tissue from surface of trapezius muscle. Define the inferolateral border of the muscle. Trapezius is attached to external occipital protuberance, superior nuchal line, ligamentum nuchae, spines of 7th cervical and spines of T1–T12 vertebrae. It comprises three distinct parts. These are:
  - Upper part is attached to posterior surface of lateral 1/3rd of clavicle. It elevates the scapula,

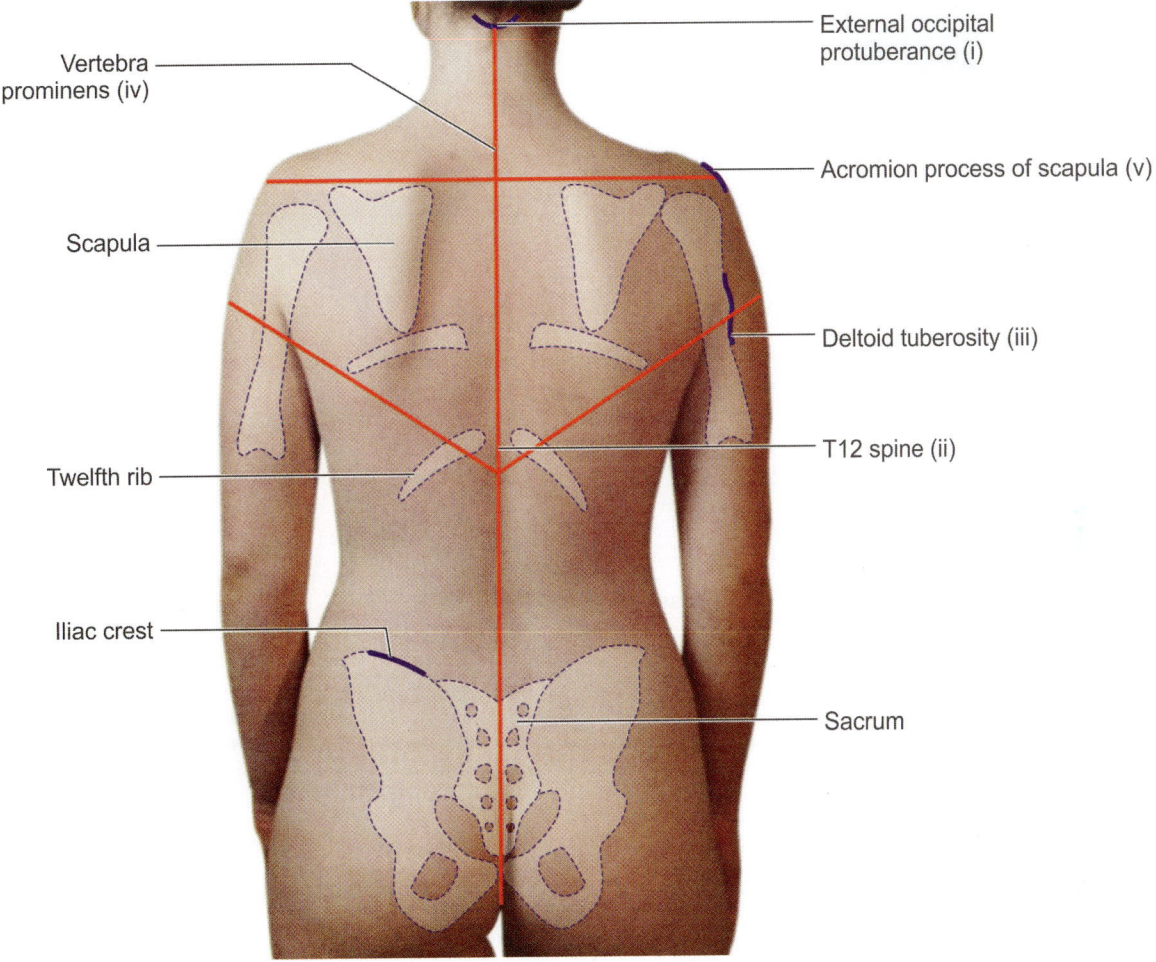

Vertebra prominens (iv)

External occipital protuberance (i)

Acromion process of scapula (v)

Scapula

Deltoid tuberosity (iii)

T12 spine (ii)

Twelfth rib

Iliac crest

Sacrum

Fig. 3.1: Lines of incision of back

i.e. causes shrugging of the shoulder. Trapezius is also known as "shrugging muscle".

- Middle part is attached to medial border of acromion process and upper border of crest of spine of scapula. It retracts the scapula.
- The lower part is attached to the apex of triangular area at the medial end of the spine of scapula. The upper and lower fibres act with serratus anterior to rotate the scapula round the chest wall and cause abduction of arm beyond 90°.
- Separate the trapezius muscle from deeper muscles by putting a forceps deep to its inferolateral border.
- Clean and identify the flat latissimus dorsi muscle in the lower part of the trunk (Fig. 3.2b). The attachments of this muscle are to the spines of T7– T12 vertebrae, thoracolumbar fascia, posterior 1/3rd of outer lip of ventral segment of iliac crest, lower four ribs and inferior angle of scapula. The muscle is inserted into the floor of inter-tubercular sulcus of humerus. As it passes upwards it is intimately related to teres major muscle.

- The muscle is innervated by thoracodorsal nerve, a branch of posterior cord of brachial plexus. The arterial supply reaches via a branch of subscapular artery of 3rd part of axillary artery. The muscle causes extension, adduction and medial rotation of shoulder joint.
- Insert a forceps deep to the superior border of the muscle to remove the loose tissue deep to it.
- Cut the muscle 5 cm lateral to its medial attachment and reflect the muscle laterally. The part of the muscle arising from the lower ribs and inferior angle of scapula may not be disturbed.

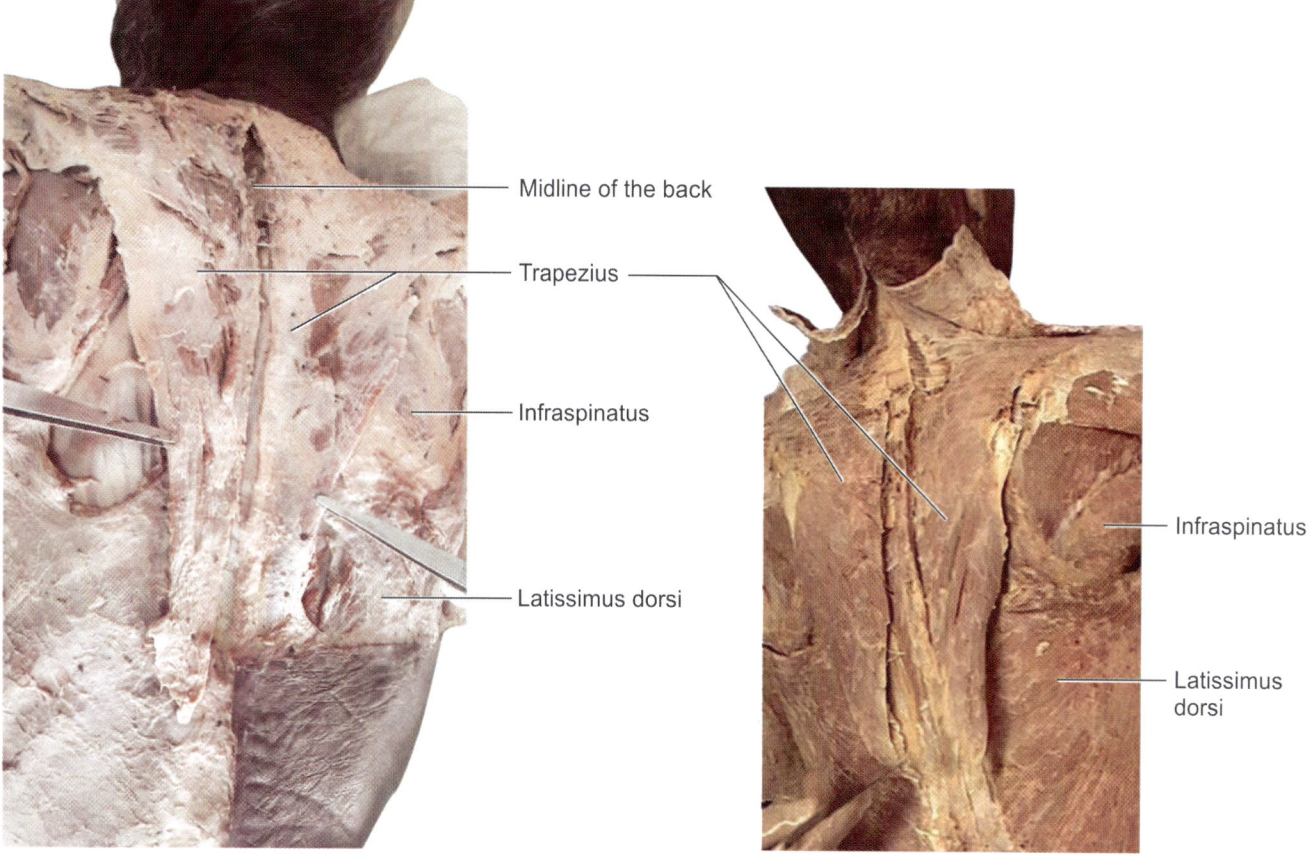

Fig. 3.2a: Superficial muscles of the back   **Fig. 3.2b:** Trapezius and latissimus dorsi muscles

This muscle is first behind, then below and finally is inserted in front of teres major muscle. So it has triple relation to teres major. Both the muscles form part of posterior wall of axilla.

- Cut vertically through trapezius 5 cm lateral to vertebral spines. Divide lateral part of muscle horizontally between the clavicle and spine of scapula. Reflect it laterally to identify accessory nerve and superficial branch of transverse cervical artery and vein.
- Look for suprascapular nerve and vessels deep to trapezius muscle, towards the scapular notch.

MUSCLES DEEP TO TRAPEZIUS

Levator scapulae: This muscle elevates the scapula with upper fibres of trapezius. Its proximal attachment is from the transverse processes of C1–C4 vertebrae. The distal attachment is to dorsal aspect of medial border of scapula from its superior angle to the root of spine. It is innervated by dorsal scapular nerve (C5). This nerve is accompanied by deep branch of transverse cervical artery. Both these lie on the deep surface of the muscle (Fig. 3.3).

Rhomboid minor lies just inferior to levator scapulae at its scapular attachment. The muscle arises from ligamentum nuchae and spines of C7 and T1 vertebrae. It is attached to the dorsal aspect of root of spine of scapula.

Rhomboid major lies below rhomboid minor. It is attached to spines of T2–T5 vertebrae and inserted on dorsal aspect of medial border of scapula from its root to its inferior angle. Both rhomboids are rhombus (◊) shaped muscles and are innervated by dorsal scapular nerve (C5). The arterial supply is from deep branch of transverse cervical artery. Both these muscles are retractors of scapula.

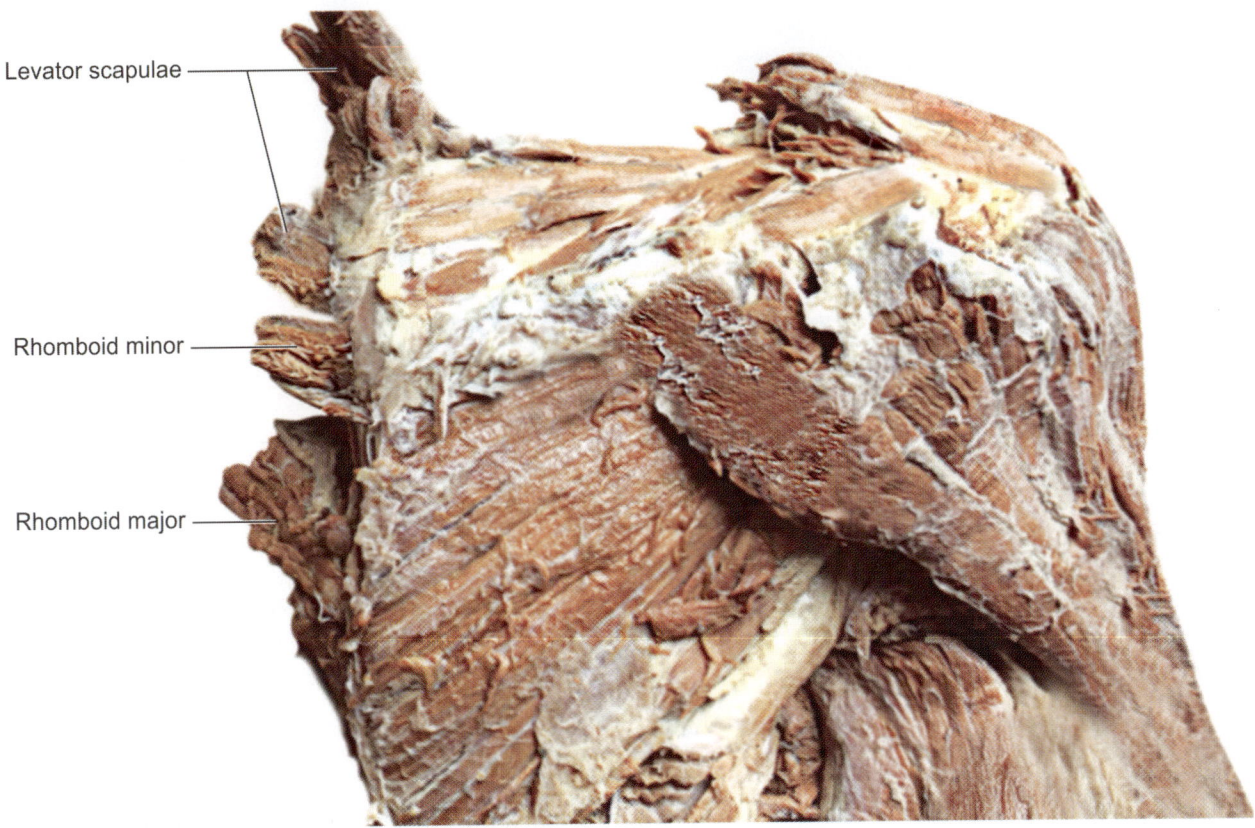

Levator scapulae

Rhomboid minor

Rhomboid major

Fig. 3.3: Deeper muscles of the back

- Cut through levator scapulae muscle midway between its two attachments and identify dorsal scapular nerve with its accompanying blood vessels. Identify rhomboid minor from rhomboid major muscle.
- Revise attachments of latissimus dorsi muscle.

DETACHMENT OF LIMB

- For detachment of the limb, muscles which need to be incised are trapezius, levator scapulae, rhomboid minor and major, serratus anterior, latissimus dorsi and sternocleidomastoid.
- The sternoclavicular joint is opened to free clavicle from the sternum. Upper limb with clavicle and scapula is removed en bloc.

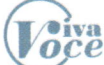
iva Voce

- Mark the insertion of trapezius on the scapula.
- Give the attachments of latissimus dorsi muscle.
- What nerves supply the trapezius and latissimus dorsi muscles?

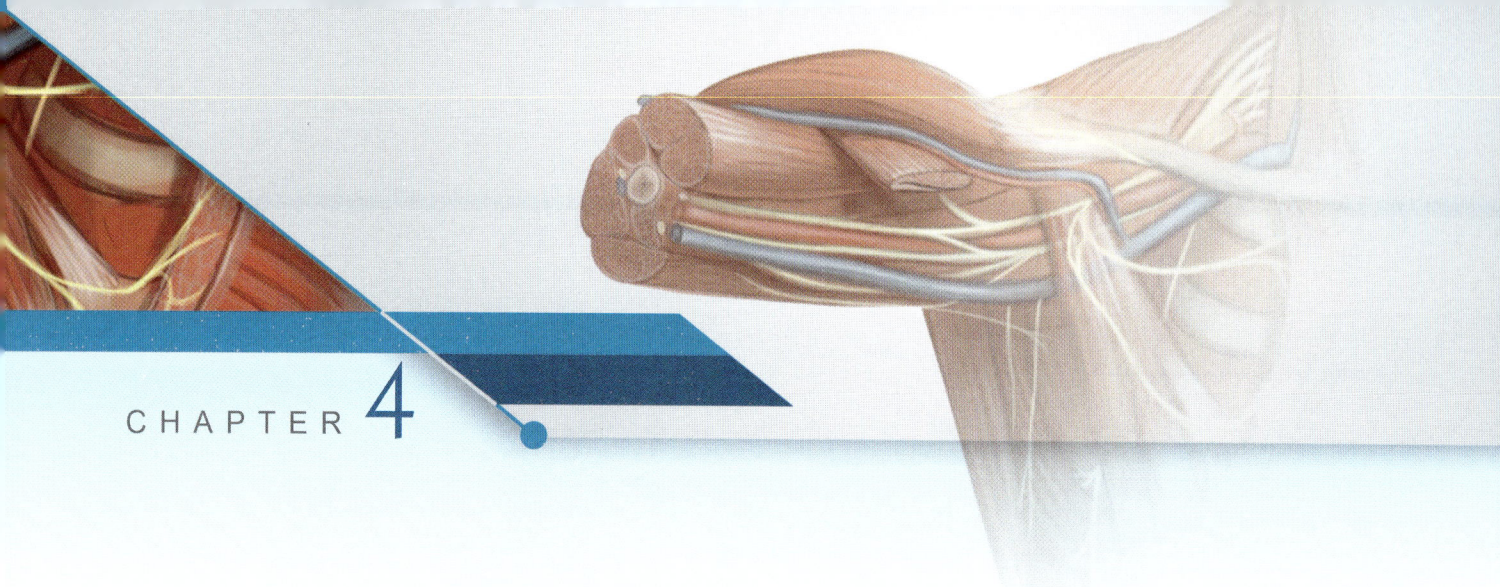

CHAPTER 4

Scapular Region

One should be able to

1. Identify the four boundaries of the quadrangular space and look for its contents.
2. Locate the upper triangular space with its contents.
3. Identify the boundaries and contents of lower triangular space.
4. Lastly identify the three arteries running along each of the three borders of scapula.

OVERVIEW

The scapular region is characterised by the deltoid muscle and some muscles under cover of deltoid. These are supraspinatus, infraspinatus, teres minor and teres major on dorsal aspect of scapula and subscapularis on costal aspect of scapula.

Competency achievement: The student should be able to:

AN 10.10 Describe and identify the deltoid and rotator cuff muscles.

STEPS OF DISSECTION

- Define the borders of the big triangular deltoid muscle covering the shoulder joint region (*see* Fig. 3.3). See it arising from anterior surface of lateral 1/3rd of clavicle, lateral surface of acromion and lower border of the crest of spine of scapula. The acromial fibres are multipennate. Observe that four septa are attached to the acromion process and three septa are attached to the deltoid tuberosity of the humerus. In between these septa are a huge volume of fibres of deltoid muscle. These cause powerful actions of the muscle.

- Detach the muscle close to the bones from its origin and reflect it downwards and laterally towards its insertion.
- The axillary/circumflex nerve accompanied by posterior circumflex humeral vessels lie on the deep surface of the muscle. The axillary nerve supplies the deltoid muscle—the most important abductor of the shoulder joint. It also supplies the small teres minor muscle.
- Long head of triceps brachii is seen running vertically between the scapula and humerus. Teres major lies anterior to the long head while teres minor lies posterior to it. Long head form boundaries of the three intermuscular spaces as described later (Fig. 4.1).
- See the supraspinatus lying above the spine of scapula. Clean it and cut it medial to suprascapular notch. Separate the two parts, identify supra-scapular nerve and vessels entering supraspinous fossa of scapula. The suprascapular nerve innervates the supraspinatus and infraspinatus.
- Identify infraspinatus in the infraspinous fossa. The muscle is attached to the middle impression of greater tubercle of humerus (Fig. 4.2).

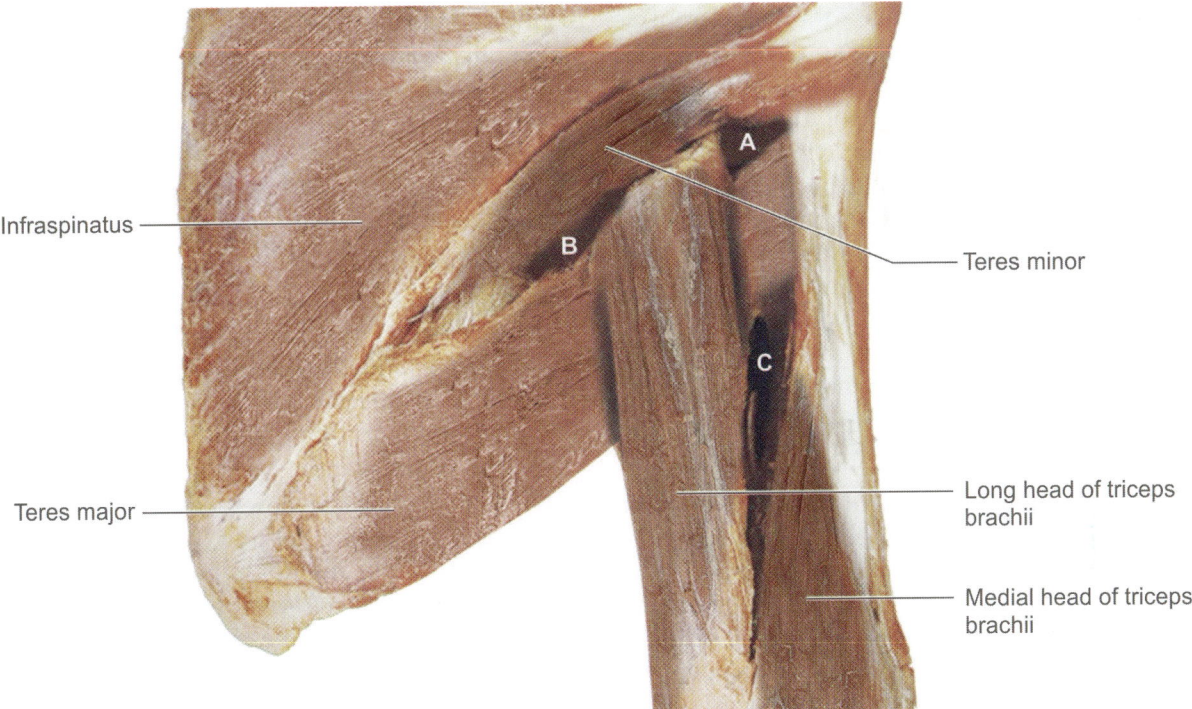

Infraspinatus

Teres major

A

B

C

Teres minor

Long head of triceps brachii

Medial head of triceps brachii

Fig. 4.1: Intermuscular spaces: A—quadrangular space; B—upper triangular space; C—lower triangular space

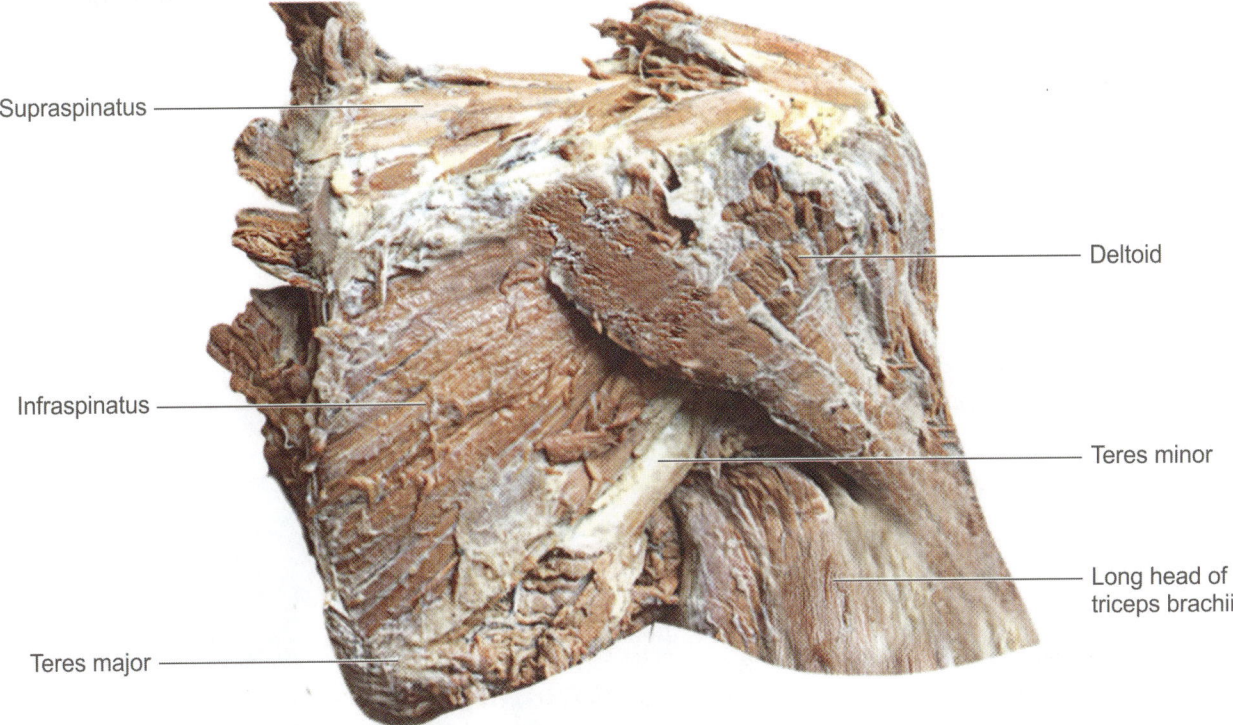

Supraspinatus

Infraspinatus

Teres major

Deltoid

Teres minor

Long head of triceps brachii

Fig. 4.2: Muscles attached to the scapula

- See the teres minor which is a thin small muscle attached to lateral border of scapula by two slips. Its lateral attachment (insertion) is on the lower impression of greater tubercle of humerus.
- Identify teres major muscle as it is bigger than teres minor. Its medial attachment is from the oval facet on the inferior angle of dorsal surface of scapula. Its lateral attachment is on to the medial lip of intertubercular sulcus of humerus. This muscle forms the lowest limit of the axilla. It also forms part of posterior boundary of axilla. Teres major adducts and medially rotates the shoulder joint.

INTERMUSCULAR SPACES

- The quadrangular intermuscular space is a space in between the scapular muscles. The quadrangular space is bounded by teres minor above and teres major below; by the long head of triceps muscle medially and the surgical neck of humerus laterally. The axillary nerve accompanied with posterior circumflex humeral vessels lie in this space. Identify the nerve to the teres minor muscle.
- Another intermuscular space, the upper triangular space should be dissected. It is bounded by the teres minor muscle medially, long head of triceps laterally, and teres major muscle below.
- Define the attachments of infraspinatus and cut muscle at the neck of scapula and reflect it on both sides.
- Look for structures under cover of deltoid muscle. These are bones, joints, vessels, nerves, bursae, etc. Learn them well.
- Identify a lower triangular space which is bounded above by the lower border of teres major muscle, medially by the long head of triceps brachii and laterally by the medial border of humerus. The radial nerve and profunda brachii vessels pass through the space.
- Dissect and identify the arteries taking part in the anastomoses around scapula. These are suprascapular along upper border, deep branch of transverse cervical (dorsal scapular) along medial border and circumflex scapular along lateral border of scapula.
- Observe that the intermuscular spaces are related to long head of triceps brachii muscle (Fig. 4.3). The three intermuscular spaces are:

a. Quadrangular space (Fig. 4.1)

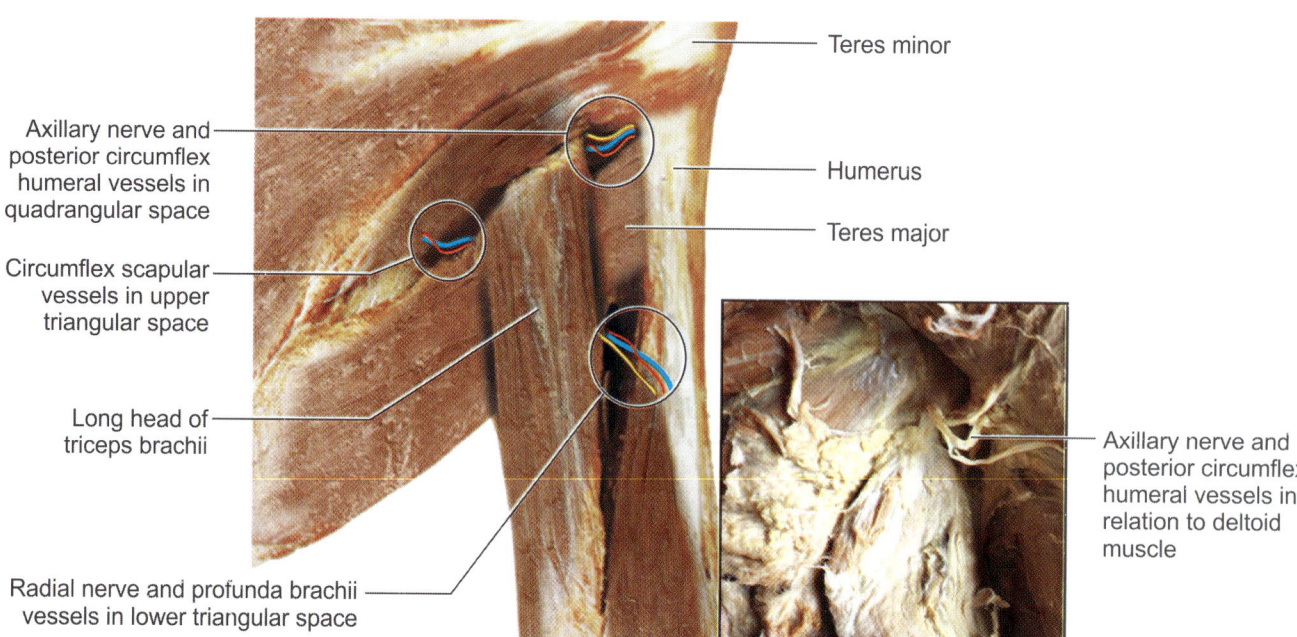

Axillary nerve and posterior circumflex humeral vessels in quadrangular space

Circumflex scapular vessels in upper triangular space

Long head of triceps brachii

Radial nerve and profunda brachii vessels in lower triangular space

Teres minor

Humerus

Teres major

Axillary nerve and posterior circumflex humeral vessels in relation to deltoid muscle

Fig. 4.3: Contents of three intermuscular spaces

b. Upper triangular space

c. Lower triangular space

Boundaries of quadrangular space

- Above: Teres minor
- Below: Teres major
- Medial: Long head of triceps brachii
- Lateral: Surgical neck of humerus

Contents of quadrangular space are: Axillary or circumflex nerve accompanied by posterior circumflex humeral vessels. The nerve innervates most important deltoid muscle and teres minor muscle. The nerve to teres minor has a pseudo-ganglion (Fig. 4.3).

Boundaries of upper triangular space

- Medial: Teres minor
- Lateral: Long head of triceps brachii
- Inferior: Teres major

Contents of upper triangular space: Circumflex scapular vessels only (Fig. 4.3).

Boundaries of lower triangular space

- Above: Lower border of teres major
- Medial: Long head of triceps brachii
- Lateral: Medial border of humerus

Contents of lower triangular space are:

1. Radial nerve, the thickest branch of brachial plexus supplying the extensors of elbow, wrist and digits (Fig. 4.3).
2. Profunda (deep) brachii vessels accompany the radial nerve.

- Dissect and identify the arteries taking part in the anastomoses around scapula. These are supra-scapular along upper border, deep branch of transverse cervical (dorsal scapular) along medial border and circumflex scapular along lateral border of scapula.

Rotator Cuff

It is formed by tendons of insertion of subscapularis, supraspinatus, infraspinatus and teres minor muscles (Fig. 4.4).

ANASTOMOSES AROUND SCAPULA

Arteries participating are:

1. Suprascapular along the upper border. It is a branch of thyrocervical trunk. The trunk arises from 1st part of subclavian artery.
2. Deep branch of transverse cervical runs along medial border deep to levator scapulae, rhomboid

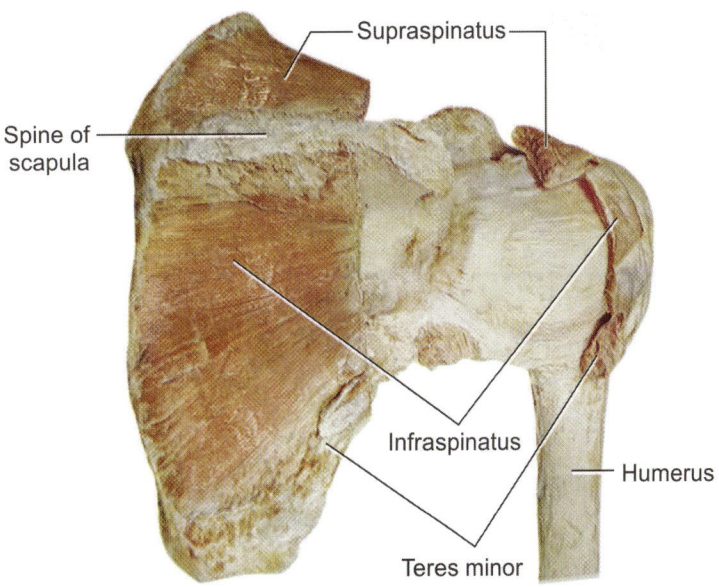

Fig. 4.4: Muscles forming part of rotator cuff

minor and rhomboid major muscles. It is a branch of transverse cervical which is also a branch of thyrocervical trunk.

3. Circumflex scapular passes along lateral border of scapula. It is a branch of subscapular artery of 3rd part of axillary artery.

Understand that this anastomoses is between branches of 1st part of subclavian artery and 3rd part of axillary artery. In case of blockage of 2nd or 3rd part of subclavian artery or 1st and 2nd parts of axillary artery, the arterial supply to the upper limb will be taken care of by this anastomoses.

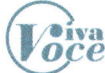

Viva Voce

- What type of fibres is the middle fibres of deltoid muscle?
- Name the muscles forming rotator cuff of shoulder.
- Name the boundaries of quadrangular space and give its contents.
- What does the word 'profunda' mean?

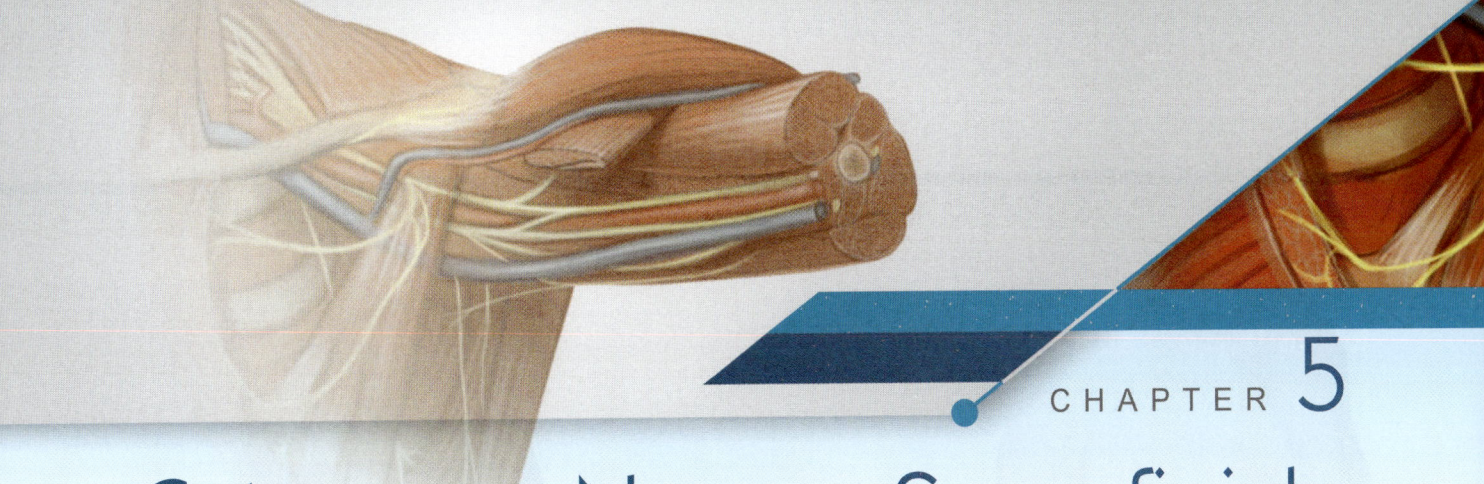

CHAPTER 5

Cutaneous Nerves, Superficial Veins and Lymphatic Drainage

Learning Objectives

One should be able to

1. Study the distribution of cutaneous nerves on the anterior and posterior aspects of the upper limb.
2. Learn the position of various groups of lymph nodes.
3. Identify the superficial veins on the dorsum of hand. Trace these veins to the front of forearm, cubital fossa, upper arm and axilla.

OVERVIEW

Skin of upper limb is mostly supplied by branches of brachial plexus formed by ventral primary rami of C5–C8 and T1 nerves. Only the part of the proximal part is innervated by a branch of supraclavicular nerve (ventral rami of C3, C4 segments of spinal cord) and a branch of T2 segment. This nerve is called intercostobrachial nerve (*see* Fig. 2.7).

Dermatome is area of skin supplied by ventral and dorsal primary rami of both right and left sides of a single spinal segment. This holds true only in the region of trunk. The limbs are not supplied by dorsal primary rami. C5 and C6 segments innervate the lateral side of upper limb; C7 the distal part, i.e. the hand and C8 and T1 supply the medial side.

Since nails develop along the tip of fingers and later lie on the dorsal aspects of digits, these carry their nerves from the region of palm.

Competency achievement: The student should be able to:

AN 11.3 Describe the anatomical basis of venepuncture of cubital veins.

STEPS OF DISSECTION

- Make one horizontal incision in the arm at its junction of upper one-third and lower two-thirds segments and a vertical incision through the centre of arm and forearm till the wrist where another transverse incision is given (*see* Fig. 6.1).
- Reflect the skin on either side on the front as well as on the back of the limb. Use this huge skin flap to cover the limb after the dissection.

CUTANEOUS VEINS

- The skin of palm is not incised to prevent drying of the structures present there.
- From the middle of the back of the wrist make an incision to the centre of the middle finger and reflect the skin on either side. The dorsum of hand will show veins in the superficial fascia.

Dorsal venous plexus is seen superficial to the extensor tendons on the dorsum of hand (Fig. 5.1). It is formed by:

i. Three dorsal metacarpal veins
ii. One dorsal digital vein from medial side of little finger

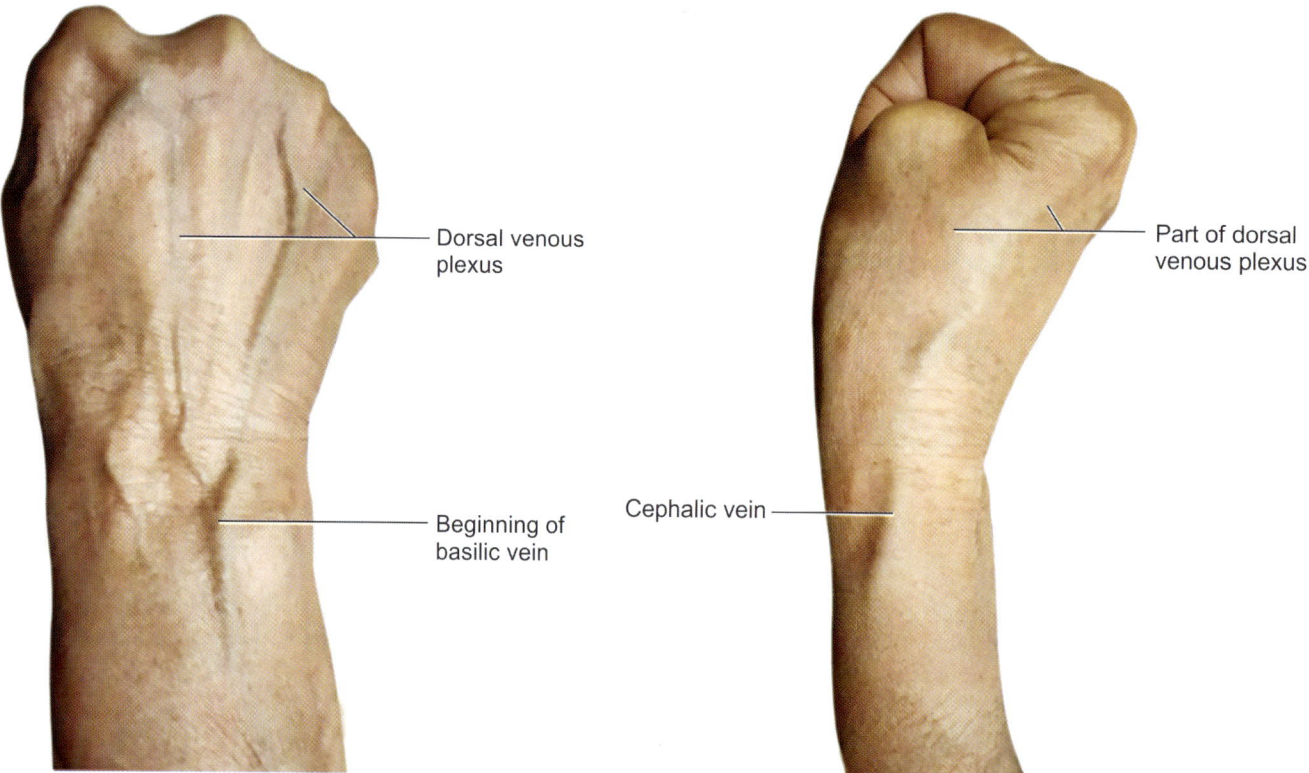

Fig. 5.1: Dorsal venous plexus and beginning of basilic vein

Fig. 5.2: Beginning of cephalic vein in anatomical snuff box

iii. One dorsal digital vein from lateral side of index finger

iv. Two dorsal digital veins from the thumb

Cephalic vein starts from the lateral end of dorsal venous plexus, reaches the *anatomical snuff box*, curves and comes to front of forearm (Fig. 5.2). Then it runs upwards to the elbow and along lateral border of biceps brachii, enters deltopectoral groove by piercing deep fascia at lower border of pectoralis major. Then it runs up till infraclavicular fossa where it pierces clavipectoral fascia to join axillary vein (*see* Fig. 1.4a).

Just below the elbow, median cubital vein is given off which crosses elbow joint to drain into basilic vein above elbow (Fig. 5.3a and b).

Basilic vein starts from the medial end of dorsal venous plexus, runs to the medial border of forearm where it winds around medial border and runs up along medial border of biceps brachii muscle. It pierces the deep fascia at middle of arm to join brachial vein which lies along medial side of brachial artery. It continues as axillary vein at the lower border of teres major (Fig. 5.3a and b).

Median cubital vein: It joins cephalic and basilic veins. It is separated from brachial artery by bicipital aponeurosis. It is connected to deep veins through a perforator vein. It is commonly used for venipuncture

- Lift the superficial veins. Many of these are connected to deep veins via perforating veins which pass through the deep fascia.

Cutaneous Nerve Supply of the Upper Limb

All the cutaneous nerves are not always seen. The nerve supply of regions of upper limb is:

- *Arm and axilla:* The lateral surface of upper 1/3rd of arm is innervated by lateral supraclavicular nerve. The axilla is innervated by intercostobrachial nerve (T2) (*see* Fig. 2.2a and 2.7).

  The lower 2/3rd of arm is innervated by:
  - Medial cutaneous nerve of arm (Fig. 5.3a)
  - Posterior cutaneous nerve of arm
  - Lateral cutaneous nerve of arm (Fig. 5.3a)
- *Forearm*
  - Lateral cutaneous nerve of forearm

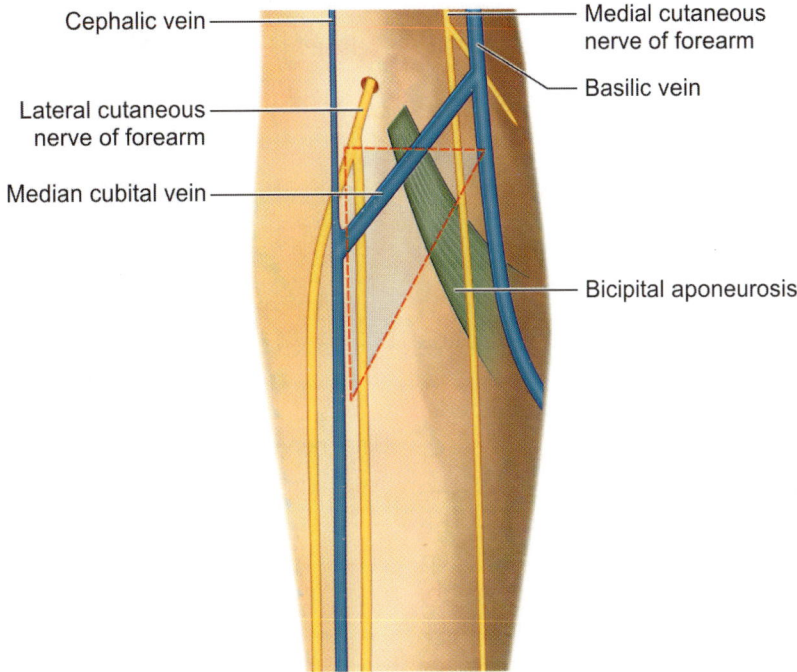

Fig. 5.3a: Superficial veins anterior to the elbow joint (schematic)

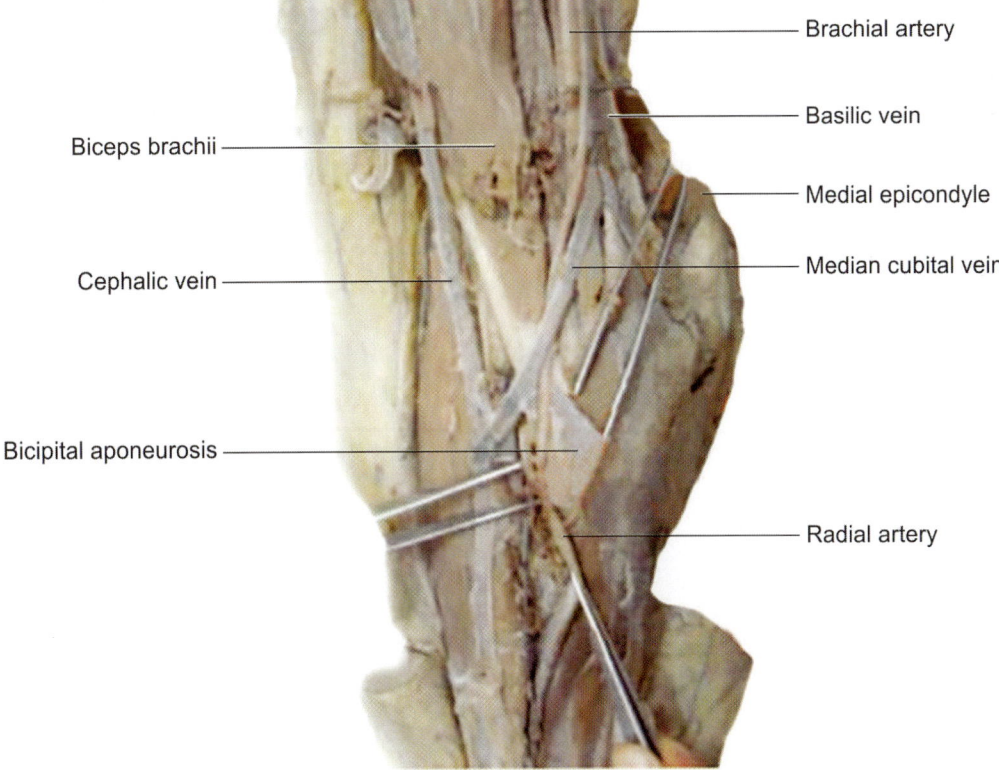

Fig. 5.3b: Superficial veins anterior to the elbow joint

- – Posterior cutaneous nerve of forearm
- – Medial cutaneous nerve of forearm
- *Palm*
  - – Lateral 2/3rd by median nerve
  - – Medial 1/3rd by ulnar nerve
- *Dorsum of hand*
  - – Lateral 1/2 by radial nerve
  - – Medial 1/2 by ulnar nerve
- *Digits*
  - – Lateral 3½ median including their nail beds (Fig. 5.3c).
  - – Medial 1½ ulnar nerve including their nail beds.

LYMPH VESSELS

Lymphatic channels run along two sets—the superficial lymphatics which run with veins and deep ones along the blood vessels. Lymph from upper limb, pectoral region and back till the level of umbilicus drain into the axillary lymph nodes.

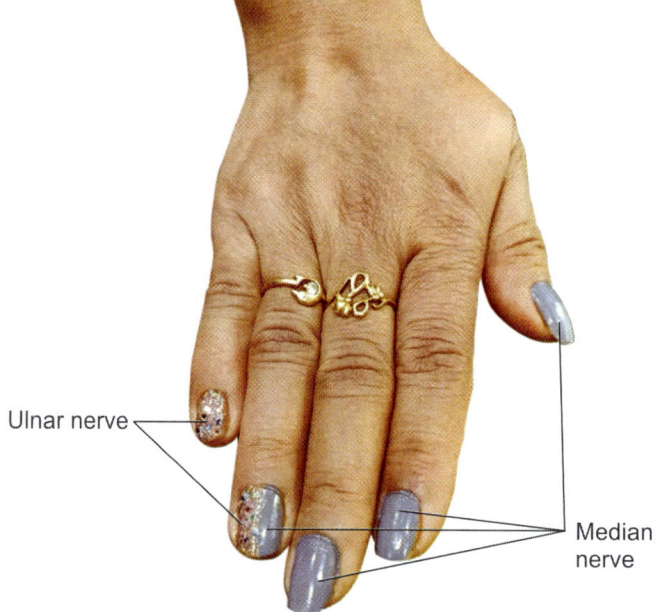

Fig. 5.3c: Nerve supply of nail beds

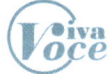

- In which box cephalic vein lies on the lateral side of the wrist?
- What is the importance of median cubital vein?
- What fascia is pierced by cephalic vein before it drains into a big vein?
- Which are the commonly used veins for venipuncture?

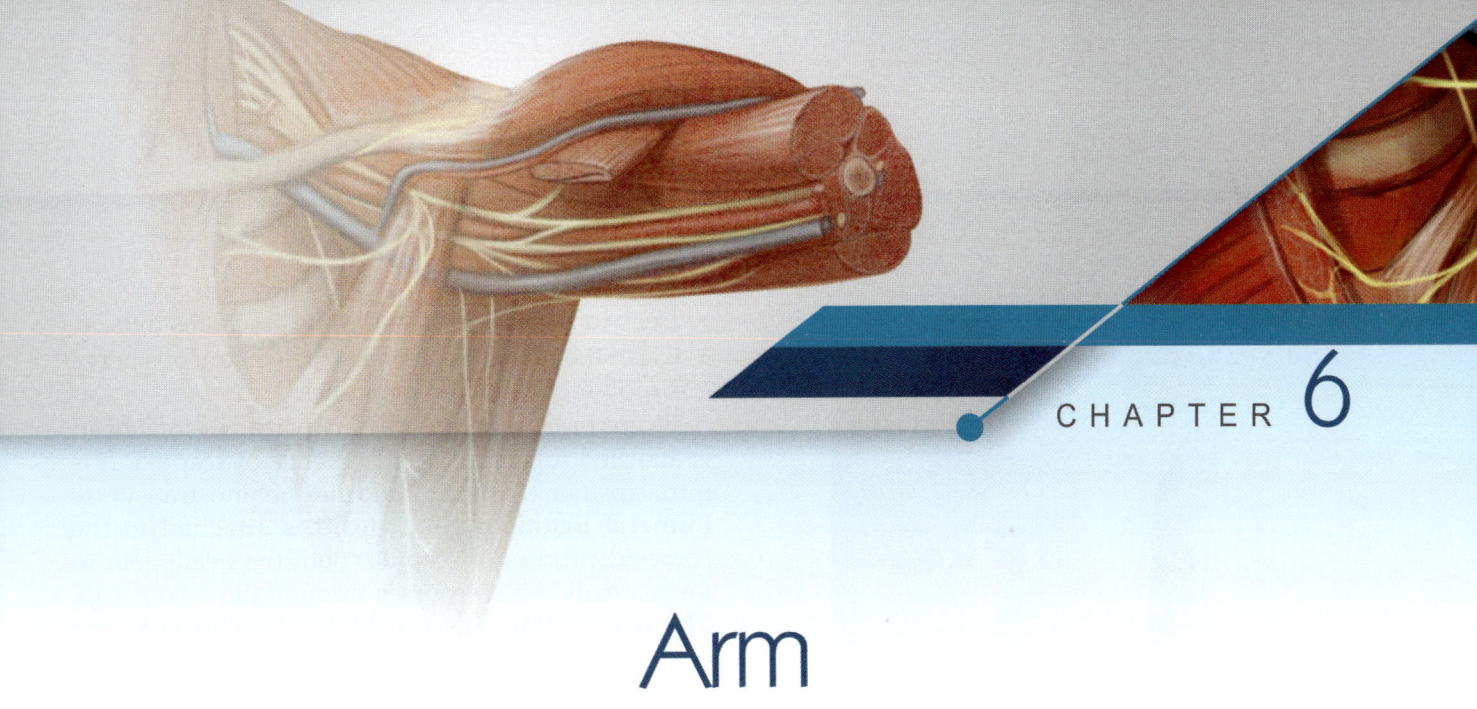

Arm

OVERVIEW

Next to the reflection of skin is the superficial fascia with cutaneous nerves. These are branches of medial cord of brachial plexus (medial cutaneous nerve of arm), intercostobrachial (ventral ramus of T2) and lower lateral cutaneous nerve of arm (radial nerve). Their names indicate the area innervated.

DEEP FASCIA

The deep fascia of arm is continuous with the fascia covering deltoid, latissimus dorsi and axillary fascia. In the lower half of arm, the fascia is thickened forming lateral and medial intermuscular septa, dividing the arm into an anterior and a posterior compartment. The deep fascia is continuous distally with the deep fascia of the forearm.

A. The anterior compartment contains:
   a. Three muscles—coracobrachialis, biceps brachii and brachialis.
   b. Brachial artery and its branches.
   c. Three nerves—musculocutaneous, median and ulnar.

B. Posterior compartment contains:
   a. Three heads of a huge triceps brachii muscle
   b. Radial nerve and its branches
   c. Profunda brachii vessels

Competency achievement: The student should be able to:
AN 11.1 Describe and demonstrate muscle groups of upper arm with emphasis on biceps and triceps brachii.

Steps of Dissection

- Make an incision in the middle of deep fascia of the upper arm right down up to the elbow joint (Fig. 6.1).
- Reflect the flap sideways. On each side in the lower half of arm look and identify the intermuscular septa. These are the lateral and medial septa.
- The most prominent muscle seen is the biceps brachii with two heads—the tendinous laterally placed long head and the muscular medially placed short head (Fig. 6.2a).
- Medial to short head of biceps brachii is coracobrachialis. This is pierced by the musculocutaneous nerve.

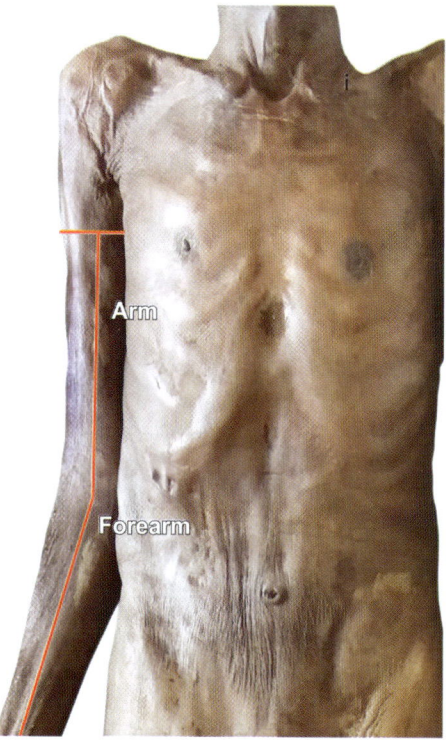

Fig. 6.1: Lines of incision on the arm

- Deep to the biceps brachii is the brachialis muscle.
- Clean the branches of the musculocutaneous nerve supplying all the three muscles.

Biceps brachii comprises of two heads—long head is attached to supraglenoid tubercle of scapula. It is intracapsular (Fig. 6.2b) and lies behind transverse humeral ligament. Short head is attached to the coracoid process of scapula. Both the heads join to form a belly which courses through the whole arm. The distal attachment of biceps brachii is to the posterior surface of radial tuberosity with a bursa intervening. It is not attached to humerus, but covers the whole humerus. It is attached to the bones proximal and distal to humerus.

Coracobrachialis extends between the coracoid process of scapula and the middle of medial border of humerus.

- Cut through the middle of biceps brachii muscle. Identify the brachialis muscle deep to it.

Brachialis spans over the lower half of humerus, crosses the elbow joint to be inserted to the anterior surface of coronoid process of ulna.

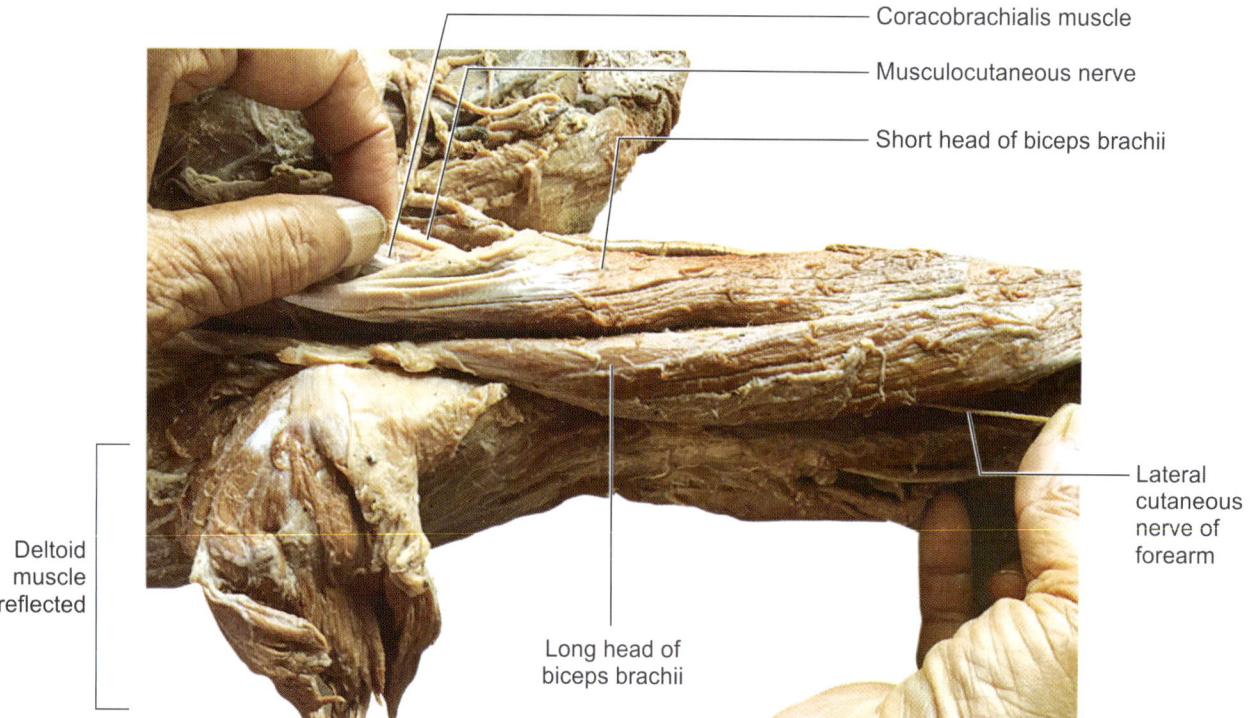

Fig. 6.2a: Muscles and nerves of front of arm

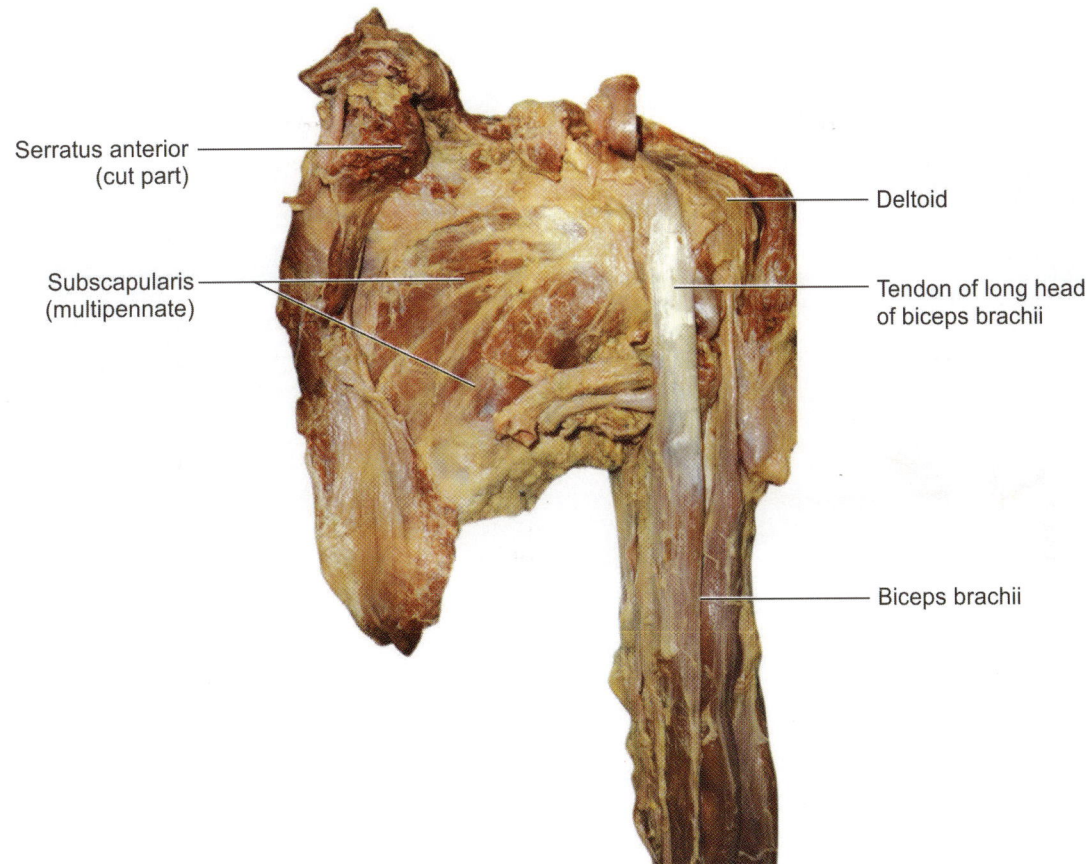

Serratus anterior
(cut part)

Subscapularis
(multipennate)

Deltoid

Tendon of long head
of biceps brachii

Biceps brachii

Fig. 6.2b: Muscles on costal aspect of scapula with muscles on front of arm

Competency achievement: The student should be able to:
AN 11.2 Identify and describe origin, course, relations, branches (or tributaries), termination of important nerves and vessels in arm.

Musculocutaneous nerve (C5–C7) is the nerve of the arm supplying all the three muscles (Fig. 6.2a). It arises from the lateral cord of brachial plexus. It gives a branch to coracobrachialis, pierces it to lie in the fascia between biceps brachii and brachialis. It gives branches to both heads of biceps brachii and brachialis. It exits brachialis 5 cm above the elbow joint to continue as lateral cutaneous nerve of forearm which accompanies cephalic vein.

• Next look for median nerve made by two roots, lateral and medial. Medial root crosses the axillary artery to join the lateral root to form the median nerve (*see* Fig. 2.6).

Median nerve lies on lateral side of proximal part of brachial artery. There it crosses the brachial artery

anteriorly at middle of arm and runs alongside the medial aspect of the artery. Both median nerve and brachial artery cross the elbow joint to enter the cubital fossa.

Branch to pronator teres is given by the median nerve in the arm.

• Look and follow the ulnar nerve from the medial cord of brachial plexus.

It is placed medially in the upper part of the arm. At the level of middle of arm, it pierces the medial intermuscular septum to lie in the posterior compartment and then behind the medial epicondyle of humerus where it is easily palpable (Fig. 6.3). Ulnar nerve is accompanied by superior ulnar collateral artery, a branch of brachial artery.

The ulnar nerve does not give any branches in the arm.

• Identify the medial cutaneous nerve of forearm, a branch of medial cord of brachial plexus. It lies in

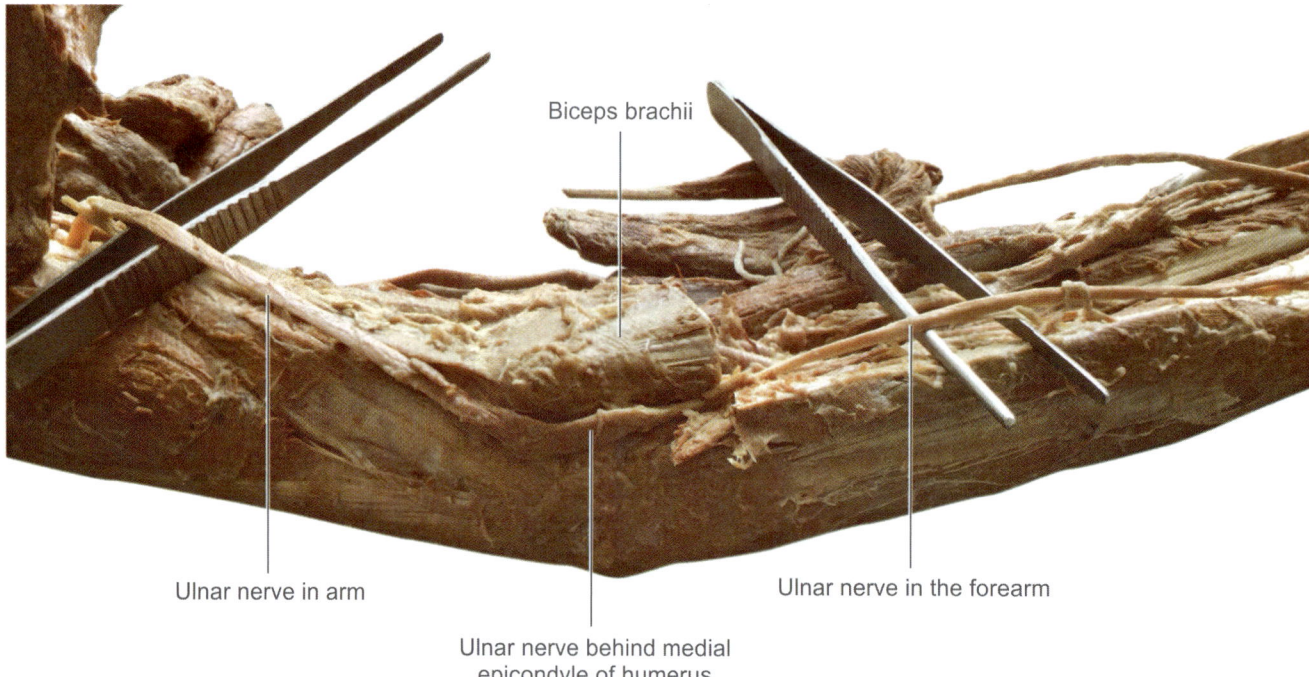

Biceps brachii

Ulnar nerve in arm

Ulnar nerve behind medial
epicondyle of humerus

Ulnar nerve in the forearm

Fig. 6.3: Course of ulnar nerve in arm behind medial epicondyle and in the forearm

the superficial fascia and accompanies the basilic vein.

- Lastly identify and clean the important brachial artery.

Brachial artery starts at the lower border of teres major as a continuation of axillary artery (Fig. 6.4). Here it lies on the medial side of humerus and is crossed by median nerve anteriorly. The nerve and artery enter the cubital fossa. The artery ends by dividing into radial and ulnar arteries at the neck of radius.

- *Identify the branches of brachial artery:*
  1. Profunda brachii—largest branch. It accompanies radial nerve in the lower triangular space, passes through the radial sulcus of humerus in the posterior compartment of arm. Below the middle of humerus identify its two branches which lie on anterior and posterior aspects of the lateral epicondyle of humerus.
  2. Superior ulnar collateral just above the middle of humerus accompanying the ulnar nerve. It lies behind medial epicondyle.

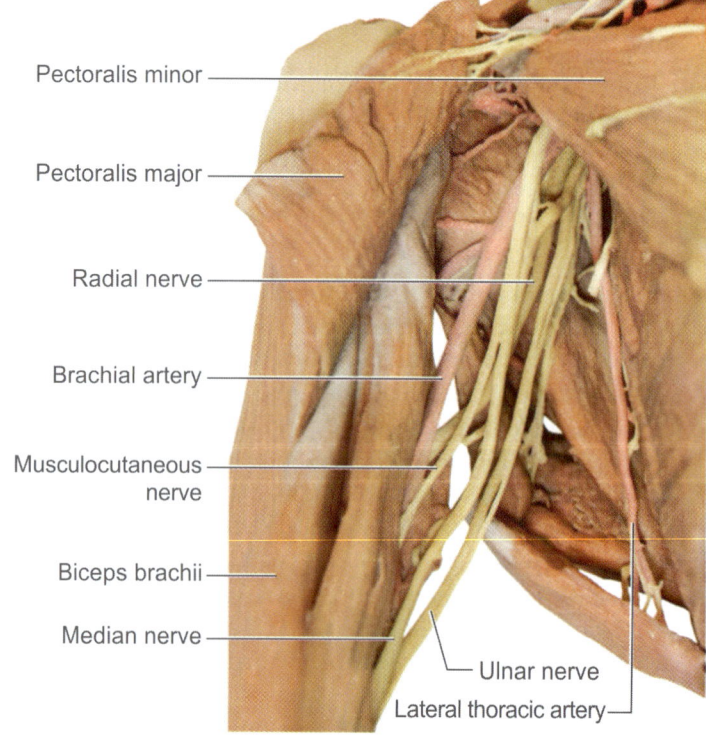

Pectoralis minor

Pectoralis major

Radial nerve

Brachial artery

Musculocutaneous
nerve

Biceps brachii

Median nerve

Ulnar nerve

Lateral thoracic artery

Fig. 6.4: Brachial artery with main branches of brachial plexus

3. Nutrient artery to humerus—given at middle of humerus. It enters the nutrient foramen to supply the inner two-thirds of cortex and bone marrow.

4. Inferior ulnar collateral artery arises a little above the medial epicondyle and lies anterior to it.

5. Numerous muscular and cutaneous branches are also given.

The two branches of profunda brachii and superior and inferior ulnar collateral arteries take part in the anastomoses around the elbow joint.

Brachial artery is universally auscultated to measure blood pressure in the upper limb.

> *Competency achievement:* The student should be able to:
> **AN 11.5** Identify and describe boundaries and contents of cubital fossa.

CUBITAL FOSSA

Cubital fossa is a shallow depression just below and anterior to the elbow joint. It contains veins and brachial artery. Veins are used for venepuncture and artery for measuring blood pressure.

Steps of Dissection

Identify the boundaries of cubital fossa are as follows:

- **Base**—imaginary line joining anterior aspects of lateral and medial epicondyles of humerus.
- **Lateral boundary**—brachioradialis (Fig. 6.5)
- **Medial boundary**—pronator teres (with its two heads). The median nerve leaves the fossa by passing between the two heads. Ulnar artery passes deep to both the heads of pronator teres.
- **Apex**—point where brachioradialis crosses the insertion of pronator teres on the maximum convexity at lateral surface of radius.
- **Floor**—brachialis in upper part (Fig. 6.5) and supinator in lower part.
- **Roof**—deep fascia supplemented on medial side by bicipital aponeurosis which separates the median cubital vein from brachial artery.

Superficial fascia containing parts of cephalic vein laterally, basilic vein medially and whole of median cubital vein. The two big veins are accompanied by cutaneous nerves (*see* Fig. 5.3a).

Identify contents from medial to lateral side. These are:

1. Median nerve with its muscular branches (Fig. 6.6)

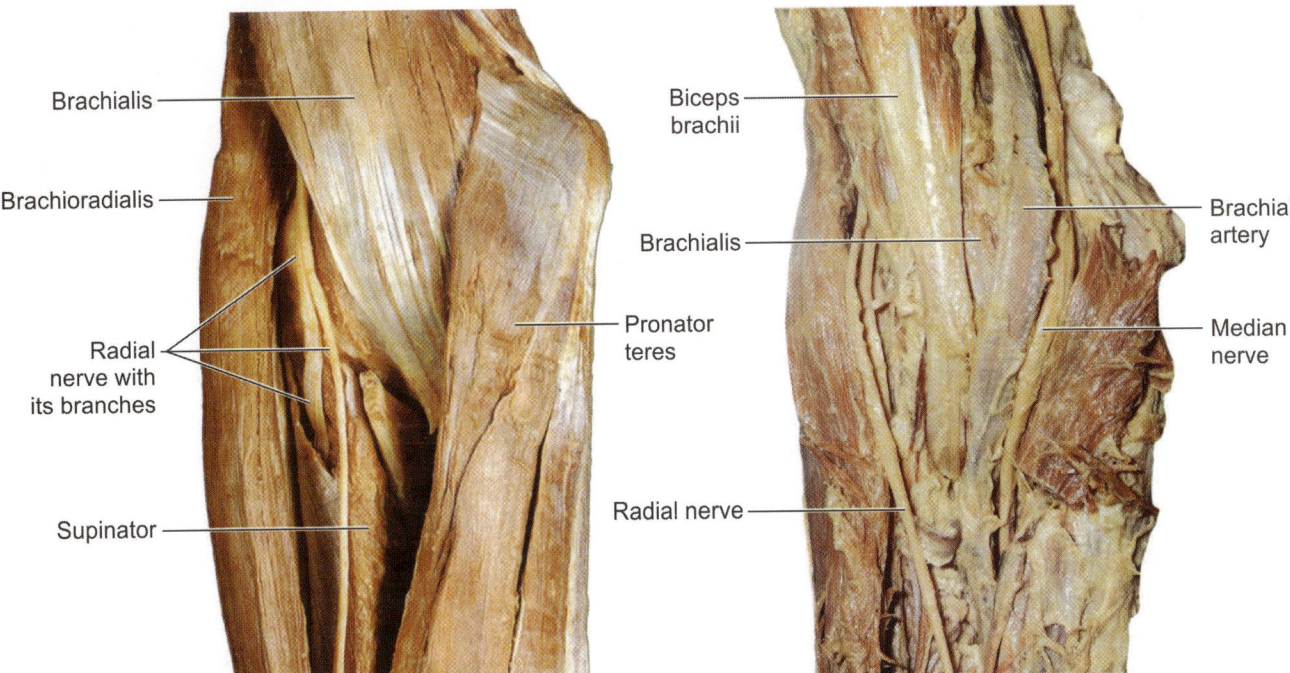

Fig. 6.5: Structures forming boundaries and floor of cubital fossa. Radial nerve with its branches also seen

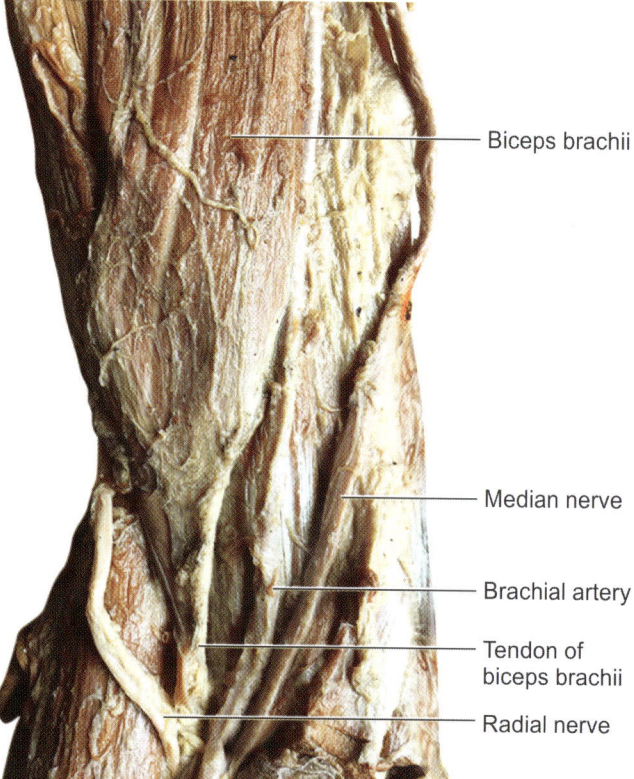

Biceps brachii

Median nerve

Brachial artery

Tendon of
biceps brachii

Radial nerve

Fig. 6.6: Contents of cubital fossa

Triceps Brachii

Long head arises from the infraglenoid tubercle of scapula. It was also noted while dissecting the intermuscular spaces in scapular region (*see* Fig. 4.1).

Lateral head is attached to a ridge on upper posterior surface of humerus superolateral to radial sulcus.

Big medial head is attached to large lower and medial portion of humerus inferomedial to the radial sulcus (Fig. 6.7).

Long and lateral heads form the superficial part of muscle, while medial head forms the deep part.

2. Brachial artery in upper part and its two terminal divisions with their branches in the lower part.
3. Tendon of biceps brachii passing towards its insertion.
4. Radial nerve lies on lateral epicondyle. In the cubital fossa, radial nerve ends by dividing into a thick muscular deep branch and a thin sensory superficial branch.

POSTERIOR COMPARTMENT OF ARM

The posterior compartment contains the huge triceps brachii muscle and radial nerve accompanied by profunda brachii artery.

Steps of Dissection

- The detached limb is placed in prone position.
- Make a longitudinal incision in the middle and reflect and remove the whole fascia making triceps fully visible.

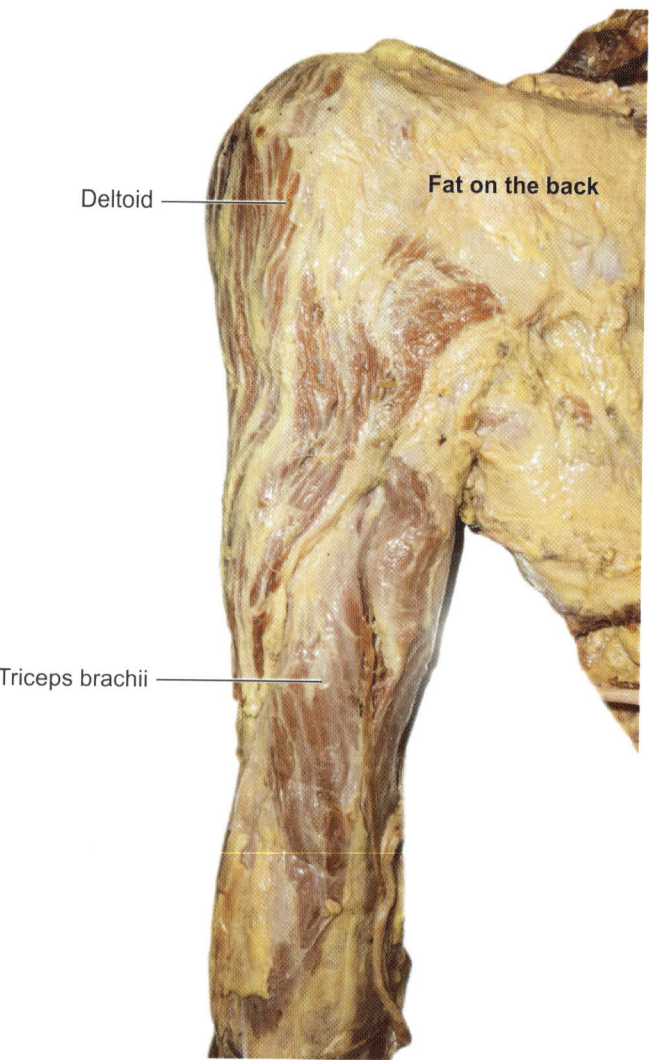

Deltoid

Fat on the back

Triceps brachii

Fig. 6.7: Triceps brachii muscle

The muscle is attached distally to the posterior part of upper surface of olecranon process of ulna.

Triceps brachii is the chief active extensor of elbow joint which can also be extended passively by gravity.

- Identify teres major, presents anterior to long head of triceps brachii.
- Separate with scalpel the long and lateral heads of triceps to see radial nerve in the radial sulcus of humerus. The nerve pierces the lateral inter-muscular septum from posterior to anterior side to enter deep part of lower lateral part of arm (Figs 6.8 and 6.9).

- Identify following branches of radial nerve:
  - *Axilla:* Branches for long and medial heads of triceps brachii and one cutaneous branch
  - *Radial sulcus:* Branches to lateral and medial heads of triceps brachii and anconeus, and two cutaneous branches.
  - *Lower lateral part:* Branches to brachioradialis, extensor carpi radialis longus and proprioceptive fibres to brachialis.
- Identify anconeus as a small muscle between lateral epicondyle of humerus and lateral surface of olecranon process of ulna. It is supplied by radial nerve and helps in extension of elbow joint.

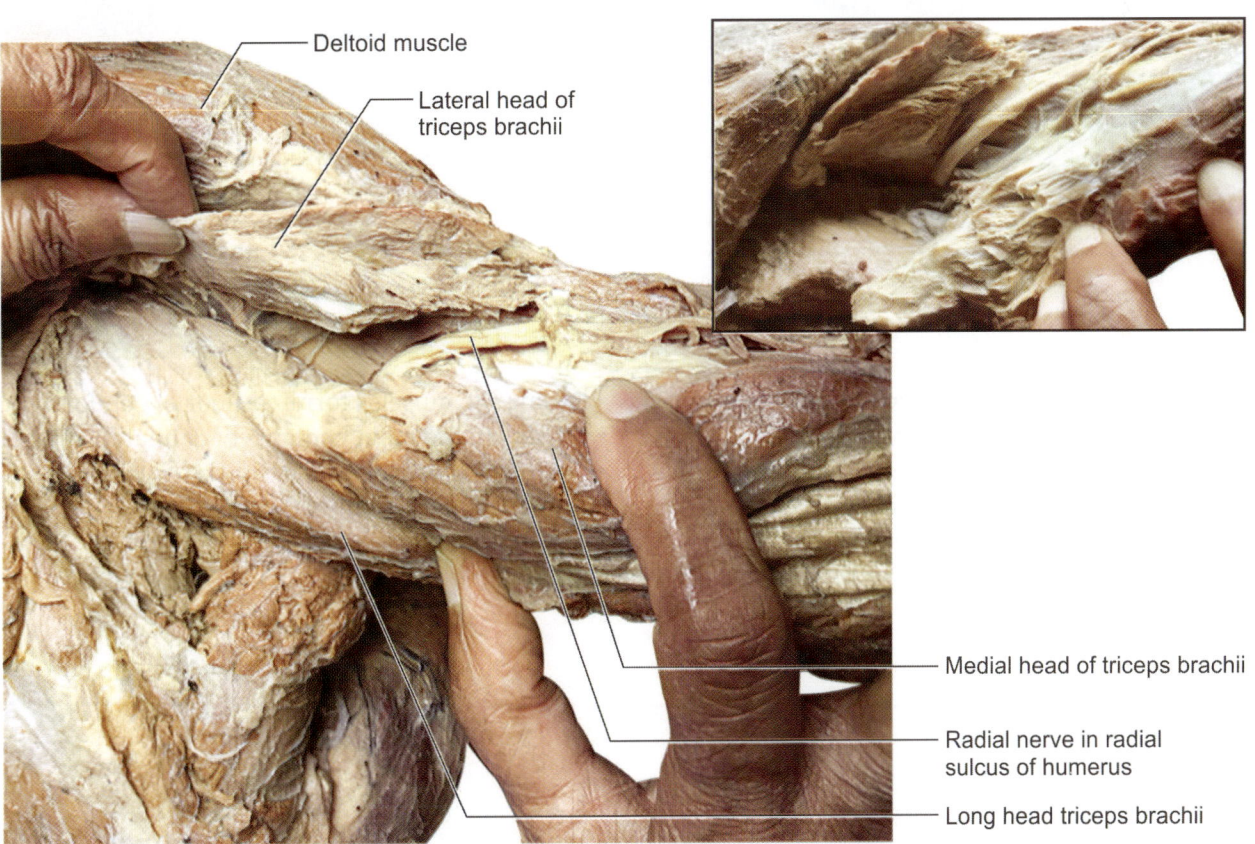

Deltoid muscle

Lateral head of triceps brachii

Medial head of triceps brachii

Radial nerve in radial sulcus of humerus

Long head triceps brachii

Fig. 6.8: Radial nerve in the radial groove of humerus

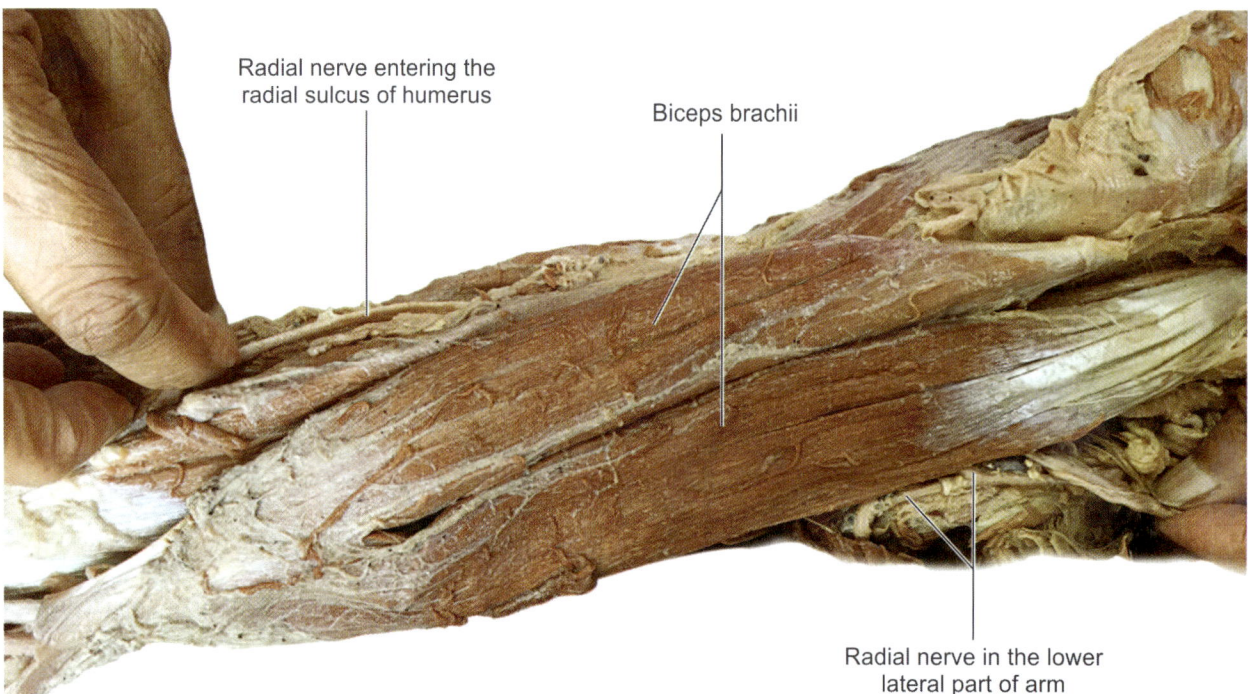

Radial nerve entering the
radial sulcus of humerus

Biceps brachii

Radial nerve in the lower
lateral part of arm

Fig. 6.9: Radial nerve entering and leaving the radial sulcus

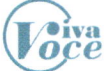 **Viva Voce**

- What is root value of musculocutaneous nerve.
- Name the muscles supplied by musculocutaneous nerve.
- Name the branches of brachial artery. What is the clinical importance of brachial artery?
- Name the muscles forming floor of cubital fossa.
- What are the main contents of cubital fossa?
- Name the heads of triceps brachii muscle and show their origins and insertion.
- What does word "profunda" mean?

Forearm and Hand

OVERVIEW

Forearm extends from elbow joint to the wrist joint. Cubital fossa lies on the upper part of front of forearm. It has been described with the arm. The bones of forearm comprise of the lateral radius and medial ulna, united by the interosseous membrane. There are eight muscles in the front of forearm—5 superficial and 3 deep. The back of forearm contains 12 muscles.

Bones of the palm are 1–5 metacarpal bones. These are numbered from lateral to medial side. 1st metacarpal is shortest, stout and rotated medially. In between the metacarpals are the interosseous spaces.

The metacarpals articulate proximally with the distal row of carpal bones. 1st metacarpal articulates with distal surface of trapezium to form the 1st carpometacarpal joint—a unique synovial joint of saddle variety. 2nd metacarpal articulates with trapezoid, 3rd with capitate, 4th and 5th articulate with hamate.

In the palm, the prominence on the side of the thumb is called thenar eminence and that on medial side is called hypothenar eminence.

In between the two eminences is the tendon of palmaris longus which expands in a triangular manner to form the palmar aponeurosis. The aponeurosis protects the underlying vessels and nerves. It shows four longitudinal bands one each for 2nd–5th digits. These bands continue with fibrous flexor sheaths of the four medial digits.

The fascia of the hypothenar eminence shows a small muscle—the palmaris brevis. This small muscle is to be incised and reflected medially.

Competency achievement: The student should be able to:

AN 12.1 Describe and demonstrate important muscle groups of ventral forearm with attachments, nerve supply and actions.

STEPS OF DISSECTION

- The detached upper limb is placed in the supine position.
- The skin has already been reflected.

  The superficial fascia contains medial cutaneous nerve of forearm from medial cord of brachial plexus, lateral cutaneous nerve of forearm (continuation of musculocutaneous nerve) and posterior cutaneous nerve, a branch of radial nerve. It also contains parts of cephalic and basilic veins. (*see* Fig. 5.1)

- Cut through the superficial and deep fasciae to expose the superficial muscles of the forearm.
- Identify these five muscles. These are from lateral to medial side, pronator teres getting inserted into middle of radius, flexor carpi radialis reaching till the wrist, palmaris longus continuing with palmar aponeurosis, flexor digitorum superficialis passing through the palm and most medially the flexor carpi ulnaris getting inserted into the pisiform bone (Fig. 7.1).

SUPERFICIAL MUSCLES

Pronator teres lies most laterally. It arises from medial epicondyle (superficial head) and medial border of coronoid process of ulna (deep head) to get inserted into lateral surface of radius in its middle.

Flexor carpi radialis lies medial to pronator teres. It arises from medial epicondyle of humerus and spans the whole of forearm. Its distal attachment is to base of 2nd metacarpal bone. Radial pulse is palpated just lateral to the tendon of this muscle.

Palmaris longus runs medial to flexor carpi radialis. It lies between medial epicondyle of humerus towards wrist and continues with palmar aponeurosis in the palm. Median nerve lies lateral to palmaris longus close to the wrist.

Flexor digitorum superficialis arises from medial epicondyle of humerus, medial side of coronoid process (humeroulnar head) and anterior oblique line of radius (radial head). The muscle forms an arch along its upper border. It passes towards wrist and enters palm deep to flexor retinaculum. Rest will be seen in the palm.

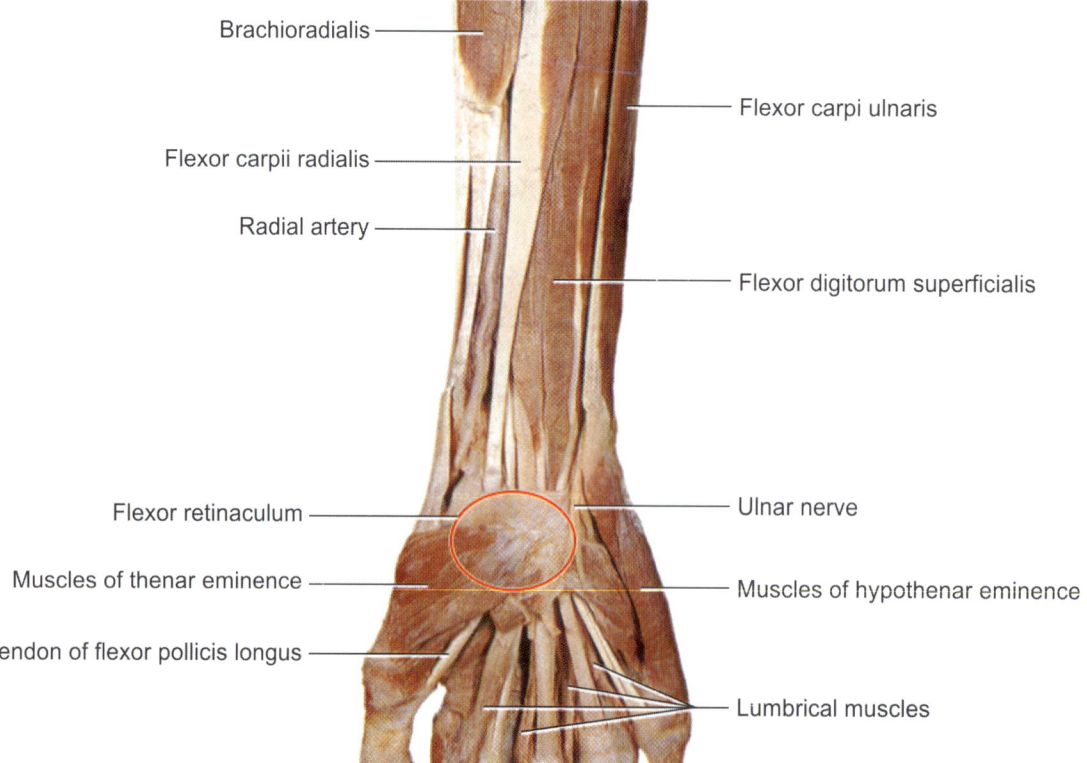

Fig. 7.1: Some muscles of front of forearm and flexor retinaculum

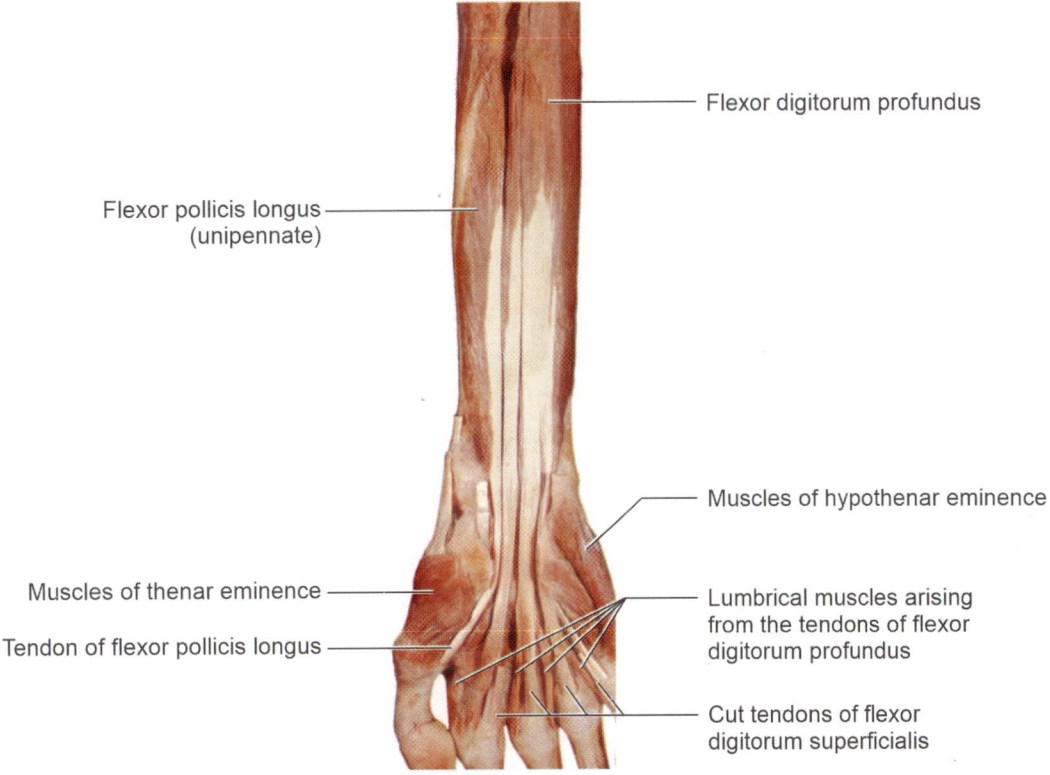

Flexor digitorum profundus

Flexor pollicis longus
(unipennate)

Muscles of hypothenar eminence

Muscles of thenar eminence

Lumbrical muscles arising
from the tendons of flexor
digitorum profundus

Tendon of flexor pollicis longus

Cut tendons of flexor
digitorum superficialis

Fig. 7.2: Two deep muscles of front of forearm

Flexor carpi ulnaris is the most medial muscle. It arises from medial epicondyle of humerus and posterior border of ulna till the wrist to be attached to pisiform bone. Ulnar vessels and nerve lie deep to it.

• Cut through the origin of superficial muscles of forearm at the level of medial epicondyle of humerus and reflect them distally. This will expose the three deep muscles, e.g. flexor pollicis longus, flexor digitorum profundus and pronator quadratus (Figs 7.2 and 7.3).

DEEP LAYER OF MUSCLES

Flexor pollicis longus is a **unipennate** muscle. Its proximal attachment is to anterior surface of radius. Its tendon passes deep to flexor retinaculum to be inserted into base of distal phalanx of the 1st digit/thumb (Fig. 7.2).

Flexor digitorum profundus (hybrid or composite muscle) envelops most of the anterior and medial surfaces of ulna right till its posterior border. It lies on the medial side of forearm. Near the wrist it divides into four tendons which course deep to flexor retinaculum to be inserted in the palm (Fig. 7.3).

Pronator quadratus lies horizontally in the distal part of forearm. It is attached to both the radius and ulna bones (Fig. 7.3). Flexor carpi radialis, palmaris longus, flexor carpi ulnaris and flexor pollicis longus lie anterior to this muscle. These muscles need to be retracted to visualise pronator quadratus.

Competency achievement: The student should be able to:

AN 12.2 Identify and describe origin, course, relations, branches (or tributaries), termination of important nerves and vessels of forearm.

• Having dissected the superficial and deep group of muscles of the forearm, identify the terminal branches of the brachial artery, e.g. ulnar and radial arteries and their branches

• Radial artery follows the direction of brachial artery.

• Ulnar artery passes obliquely deep to heads of pronator teres and then vertically till the wrist.

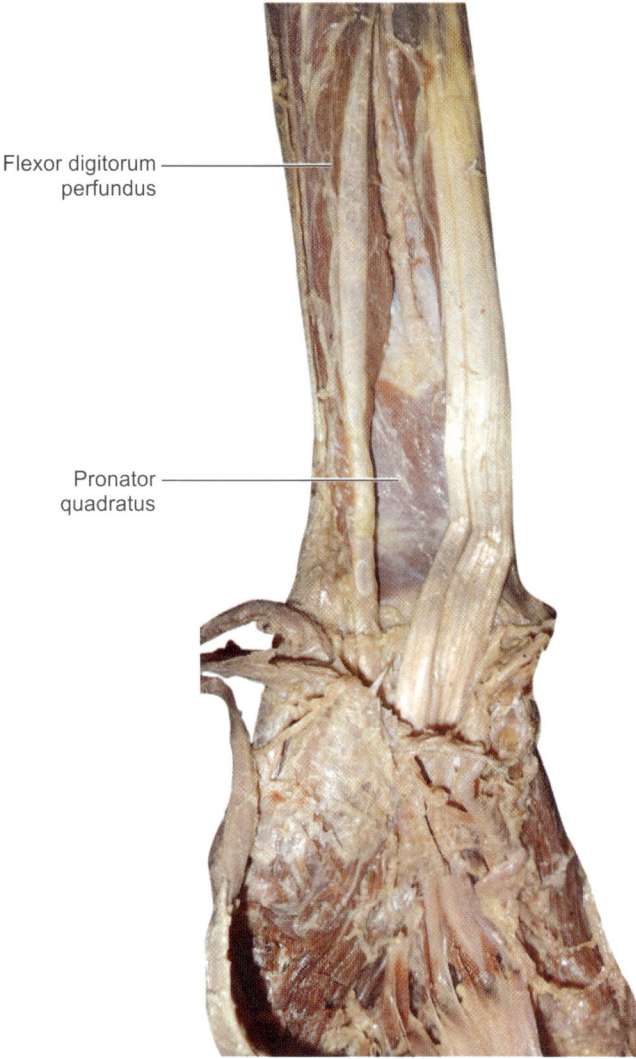

Flexor digitorum perfundus

Pronator quadratus

Fig. 7.3: Pronatur quadratus—a deep muscle of front of forearm

Carefully look for common interosseous branch of ulnar artery and its anterior and posterior branches.

ARTERIES OF FRONT OF FOREARM

- Identify and clean brachial artery in the cubital fossa.
- Look for its two terminal branches, the lateral smaller one is radial artery and the larger medial is the ulnar artery.
- Clean the radial artery and its muscular and cutaneous branches (Fig. 7.4).
- Identify pronator teres, flexor digitorum superficialis, flexor pollicis longus and pronator

quadratus muscles. Pronator quadratus forms the bed for the radial artery.

- Identify the radial artery just above the wrist lying between tendons of flexor carpi radialis and brachioradialis. From here see the artery curving laterally towards anatomical snuff box.
- Look for radial recurrent artery in proximal part of forearm. It ascends up to anastomose with a branch of profunda brachii artery anterior to lateral epicondyle of humerus.
- Look for superficial palmar branch of radial artery in distal part of forearm. It descends into the palm superficial to thenar muscles to take part in the superficial palmar arch.
- Identify the ulnar artery being given off from brachial artery. The artery passes deep to both heads of pronator teres. Trace the artery entering the forearm as it lies deep to the arch formed by flexor digitorum superficialis muscle.
- Clean the artery along its whole course till it lies on the medial aspect of flexor retinaculum covered by its superficial slip (Fig. 7.4). There it divides into a superficial and deep branch.

Branches of ulnar artery are:

1. Anterior and posterior ulnar recurrent arteries for anastomoses at the medial epicondyle.
2. Several muscular branches
3. Common interosseous branch which divides into anterior interosseous and posterior interosseous arteries. The anterior interosseous artery along with anterior interosseous nerve lies on the interosseous membrane, only the artery pierces it in lower part and reaches back of forearm.

NERVES OF FRONT OF FOREARM

- Median nerve is the chief nerve of the forearm. It enters the forearm by passing between two heads of pronator teres muscle (Fig. 7.4).
- Its anterior interosseous branch is given off as it is leaving the cubital fossa.
- Identify median nerve stuck to the fascia on the deep surface of flexor digitorum superficialis muscle. Thus, the nerve lies superficial to the flexor digitorum profundus.
- Dissect the anterior interosseous nerve as it lies on the interosseous membrane between flexor pollicis

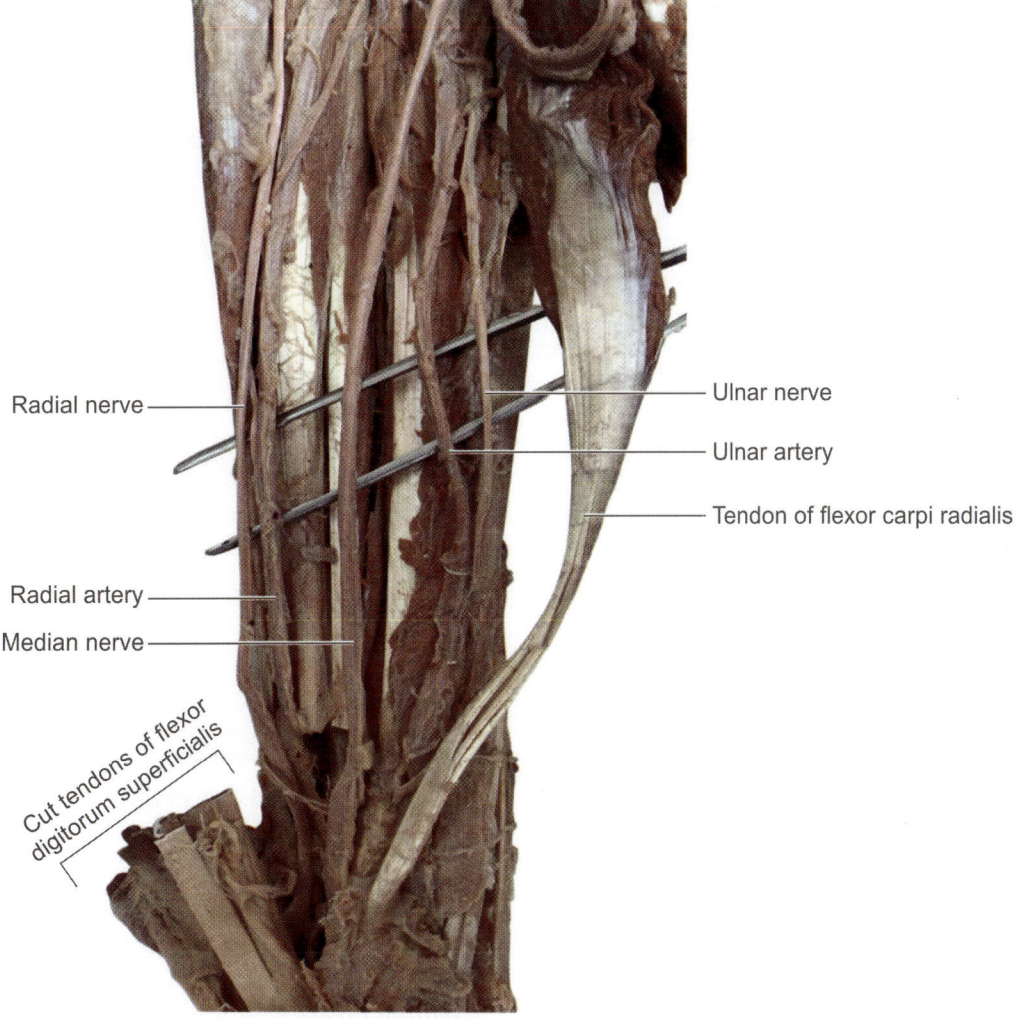

Radial nerve

Ulnar nerve

Ulnar artery

Tendon of flexor carpi radialis

Radial artery

Median nerve

Cut tendons of flexor digitorum superficialis

Fig. 7.4: Nerves and arteries of front of forearm

longus and flexor digitorum profundus muscles.

- Identify the ulnar nerve situated behind medial epicondyle. Trace it vertically down till flexor retinaculum (*see* Fig. 6.3).

- Trace the radial nerve and its two branches in the lateral part of cubital fossa. Its deep branch is muscular and superficial branch is cutaneous (*see* Fig. 6.5).

Median Nerve

It is the chief nerve of forearm

- Identify it in the medial part of cubital fossa, where it supplies three out of five superficial muscles (*see* Fig. 6.6). One muscle is supplied in the arm.

- Trace the nerve as it lies between two heads of pronator teres and then deep to arch of flexor digitorum superficialis. See the nerve lying on the deep surface of flexor digitorum superficialis.

- Clean the fascia around the nerve. Follow the nerve distally near the wrist (Fig. 7.4) where it lies lateral to tendon of palmaris longus. It gives a palmar cutaneous branch.

- Identify anterior interosseous branch of median nerve. It lies on a deeper plane, between flexor pollicis longus and flexor digitorum profundus and then deep to pronator quadratus muscle where it ends. So the nerve supplies 6½ muscles, four superficial; flexor pollicis longus, pronator quadratus and lateral half of flexor digitorum profundus (2½ muscles).

Ulnar Nerve

Ulnar nerve was seen and palpated behind medial epicondyle of humerus (*see* Fig. 6.3). *It is not a content of cubital fossa*. The nerve lies between the two heads of flexor carpi ulnaris and soon joins ulnar artery to lie on its medial side. Both descend vertically deep to flexor carpi ulnaris lying on flexor digitorum profundus till the flexor retinaculum (Fig. 7.4).

In the forearm it gives following branches:
1. Dorsal cutaneous branch
2. Palmar cutaneous branch
3. Muscular branches to flexor carpi ulnaris and medial half of flexor digitorum profundus.
4. Its terminal branches are superficial and deep, to be seen in the palm.

Radial Nerve

Radial nerve was seen to divide into its two terminal branches in the cubital fossa (*see* Fig. 6.5). Follow the deep branch which innervates extensor carpi radialis brevis and supinator, passes through supinator to reach the back of forearm. The superficial branch runs vertically downwards. Identify it and see it running on lateral side of radial artery in middle one-third of forearm only (Fig. 7.4). In the lower one-third, it winds laterally to back of forearm and lies in the anatomical snuff box. It is entirely cutaneous in nature.

> *Competency achievement:* The student should be able to:
> **AN 12.3** Identify and describe flexor retinaculum with its attachments.

PALMAR ASPECT OF WRIST AND HAND

At the wrist the skeleton comprises eight small bones. These are scaphoid, lunate, triquetral and pisiform in the proximal row from lateral to medial side. The distal row comprises trapezium, trapezoid, capitate and hamate (hook). The flexor retinaculum is a thickening of deep fascia to keep the structures in place. With the concavity of carpal bones, it creates a carpal tunnel.

Steps of Dissection

- A horizontal incision at the distal crease of front of the wrist has already been made (Fig. 7.5, position 1).

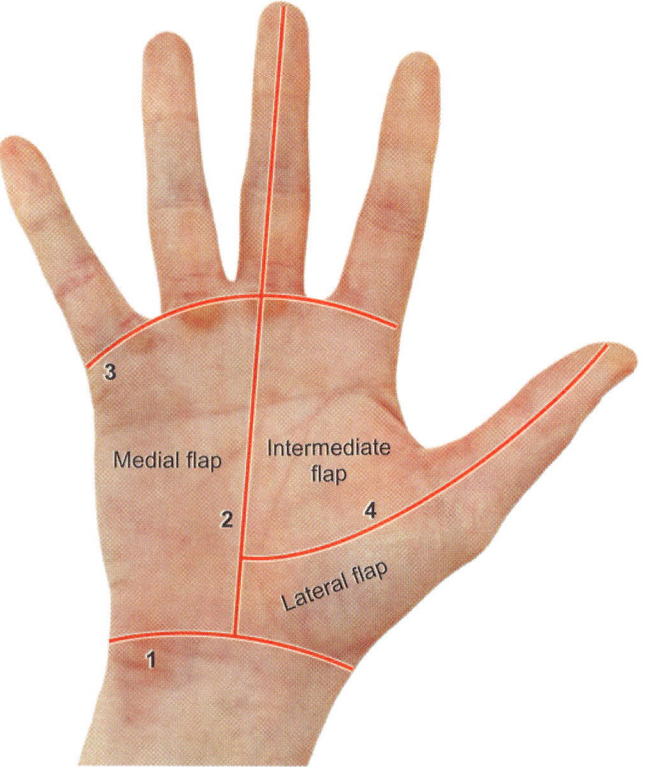

Fig. 7.5: Incisions in the palm

- Make a vertical incision from the centre of the above incision through the palm to the centre of the middle finger (Fig. 7.5, position 2).
- Make one horizontal incision along the distal palmar crease (Fig. 7.5, position 3).
- Make an oblique incision starting 3 cm distal to incision no. 2 and extend it till the tip of the distal phalanx of the thumb (Fig. 7.5, position 4).
- Thus the skin of the palm gets divided into three areas. Reflect the skin of lateral and medial flaps on their respective sides. The skin of the intermediate flap is reflected distally towards the distal palmar crease. Further the skin of middle finger is to be reflected on either side.

Superficial fascia and deep fascia
- Remove the superficial fascia to clean the underlying deep fascia.
- Deep fascia is modified to form the flexor retinaculum at wrist, palmar aponeurosis in the palm, and fibrous flexor sheaths in the digits. Identify the structures on its superficial surface.

Divide the flexor retinaculum between the thenar and hypothenar eminences, carefully preserving the underlying median nerve and long flexor tendons.

- Identify long flexor tendons enveloped in their synovial sheaths including the digital synovial sheaths.

- Clean and identify the attachments of flexor retinaculum (Fig. 7.1). Laterally, it is attached to scaphoid (boat-shaped) and on trapezium to the lips of groove for flexor carpi radialis. Medially, it is attached to pisiform and hook of hamate. Its small superficial slip is also attached to pisiform.

- Identify the structures superficial to flexor retinaculum. From lateral to medial, these are:
    - Palmar cutaneous branch of median nerve
    - Tendon of palmaris longus
    - Palmar cutaneous branch of ulnar nerve

    - Ulnar artery and ulnar nerve. These two are under a thin superficial slip of flexor retinaculum.
- Incise the flexor retinaculum in its middle and reflect the parts on each side.

Identify the four tendons of flexor digitorum superficialis (Fig. 7.6) and four tendons of flexor digitorum profundus on a deeper plane. See that these tendons are enclosed in a synovial sheath called ulnar bursa. Lateral to the ulnar bursa is the most important content of carpal tunnel—the median nerve. Deep to the median nerve is the tendon of flexor pollicis longus enclosed in a synovial sheath—the radial bursa. Most lateral structure within the flexor retinaculum is tendon of flexor carpi radialis (Fig. 7.6).

Pressure on the median nerve due to any reason results in clinical condition called "Carpal tunnel syndrome". There is pain and abnormal sensations in lateral 3½ digits with weakness of the thenar muscles.

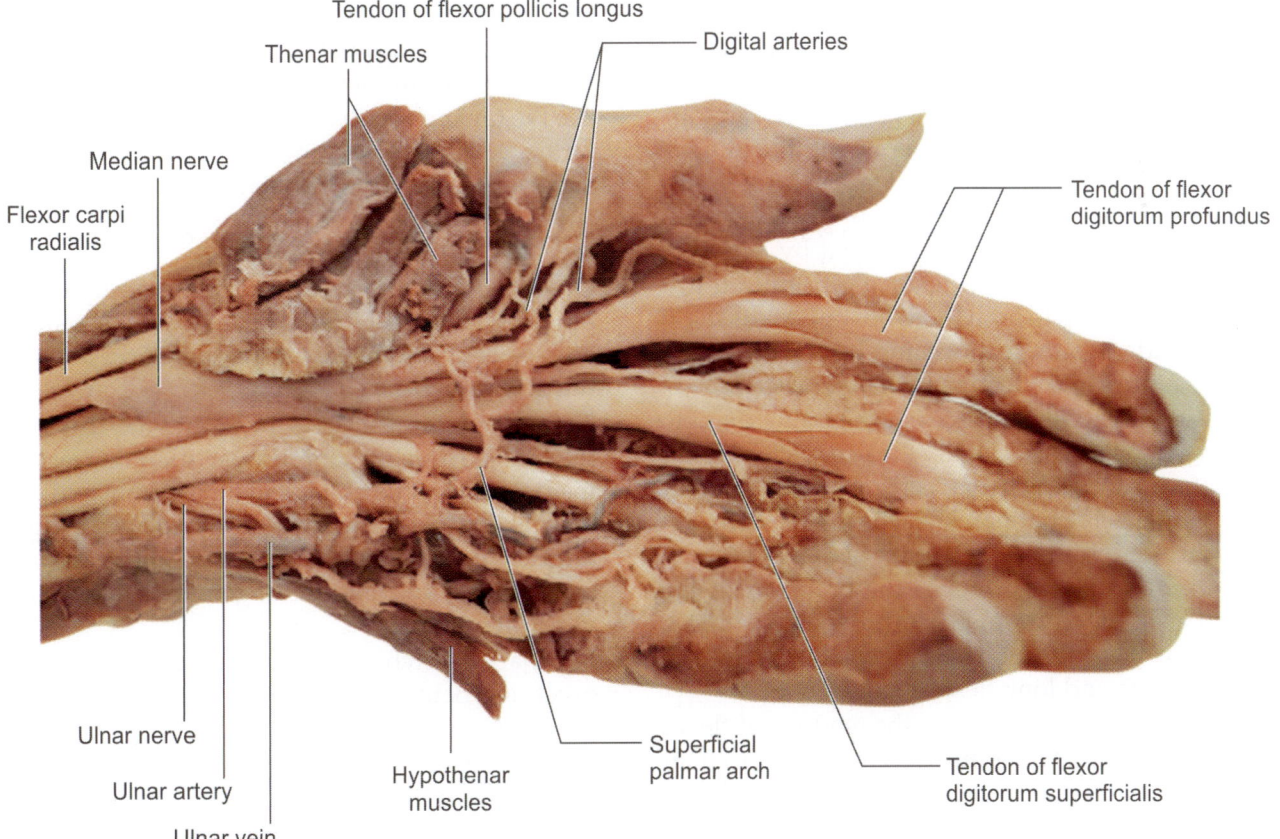

Fig. 7.6: Structures passing through the carpal tunnel. Superficial palmar arch also seen

THE PALM

Competency achievement: The student should be able to:

AN 12.7 Identify and describe course and branches of important blood vessels and nerves in hand.

Steps of Dissection

- Clean the thenar and hypothenar muscles. Carefully preserve the median nerve and superficial and deep branches of ulnar nerve which supply these muscles.
- Abductor pollicis brevis is the lateral muscle; flexor pollicis brevis is the medial one. Both these form the superficial lamina. The deeper lamina is constituted by opponens pollicis.
- Cut through the abductor pollicis brevis and flexor pollicis brevis to expose the opponens pollicis. These three muscles constitute the muscles of thenar eminence, supplied by thick recurrent branch of median nerve.
- Incise flexor pollicis brevis in its centre and reflect its two parts. This will reveal the tendon of flexor pollicis longus and adductor pollicis on a deeper plane.
- On the medial side of hand, identify thin palmaris brevis muscle in the superficial fascia. It receives a twig from the superficial branch of ulnar nerve.
- Hypothenar eminence is comprised by abductor digiti minimi medially, flexor digiti minimi just lateral to it. Deep to both these lies opponens digiti minimi. Identify these three muscles and trace their nerve supply from deep branch of ulnar nerve.
- Between the two eminences of the palm, deep to palmar aponeurosis, identify the superficial palmar arch formed mainly by superficial branch of ulnar and superficial palmar branch of radial artery. Identify its common and proper digital branches.
- Clean, dissect and preserve the branches of the median nerve and superficial division of ulnar nerve in the palm lying between the superficial palmar arch and long flexor tendons.
- Lying on a deeper plane are the tendons of flexor digitorum superficialis muscle. Dissect the peculiar mode of its insertion in relation to that of tendon of flexor digitorum profundus.
- Cut through the tendons of flexor digitorum superficialis 5 cm above the wrist. Divide both ends of

superficial palmar arch. Reflect them distally towards the metacarpophalangeal joints.
- Identify four tendons of flexor digitorum profundus diverging in the palm with four delicate muscles, the lumbricals, arising from them. Dissect the nerve supply to these lumbricals. The first and second are supplied from median and third and fourth from the deep branch of ulnar nerve.
- Divide the flexor digitorum profundus 5 cm above the wrist and reflect it towards the metacarpophalangeal joints. Trace one of its tendons to its insertion into the base of distal phalanx of one finger
- The central palmar aponeurosis continues with thinner fascia on thenar and hypothenar eminences.
- Detach palmar aponeurosis carefully from the subjacent structures, starting proximally and slowly going distally.
- See the superficial palmar arch lying deep to the aponeurosis in the central part (Fig. 7.6). Look for recurrent branch of median nerve passing towards the thenar eminence.
- Identify superficial palmar arch chiefly formed by the superficial branch of the ulnar artery.
- See the ulnar artery lying on the superficial surface of the flexor retinaculum, where it divides into a superficial and a deep branch. Appreciate how the superficial branch forms the superficial palmar arch.
- Look for a small contribution from superficial palmar branch of radial artery which usually crosses over the thenar muscles to form a part of the palmar arch.
- Clean and identify the branches of this arch (Fig. 7.6). These are one proper digital artery for medial side of little finger and three common digital arteries each of which divide into two proper digital arteries to supply adjacent sides of little and ring fingers; ring and middle fingers and middle and index fingers.
- See that this arch supplies seven digital branches exception being to the thumb and lateral side of index finger.
- On the medial side of palm, find the ulnar nerve superficial to the flexor retinaculum. Dissect its superficial and deep branches (Fig. 7.10b). See that superficial branch innervates palmaris brevis muscle and gives digital branches to medial 1½

fingers. These also innervate medial 1½ nail beds and distal phalanges on the dorsum of hand.

- Clean median nerve as it lies deep to flexor retinaculum in the carpal tunnel (Fig. 7.7). As it enters palm, medial to thenar eminence, look for its recurrent branch which supplies three muscles of thenar eminence, i.e. abductor pollicis brevis, flexor pollicis brevis and opponens pollicis. Identify its additional two branches—lateral and medial. Trace the lateral branch giving two digital branches to the thumb and one to lateral side of index finger including first lumbrical muscle.
- Trace the medial branch dividing into two common digital branches. Each of them divides into two proper digital branches in the distal part of palm for adjoining sides of index and middle fingers; and middle and ring fingers. The digital nerve for middle finger innervates 2nd lumbrical muscle.
- Revise that median nerve gives sensory innervation to lateral 3½ digits or 7/10 sides of five digits, including their nail beds.
- See that division of common digital nerves into two proper digital nerves is proximal to the division of common digital artery into two proper digital arteries.

Competency achievement: The student should be able to:
AN 12.5 Identify and describe small muscles of hand. Also describe movements of thumb and muscles involved.

Thenar Muscles

- Identify abductor pollicis brevis laterally placed, flexor pollicis brevis medially placed on the lateral side of hand. Deep to both these muscles, identify opponens pollicis (Fig. 7.6).
- To see the opponens pollicis, incise both the superficial muscles in centre and reflect them on either side. See the opponens pollicis attached to whole length of lateral side of 1st metacarpal bone.

Hypothenar Muscles

- Identify hypothenar muscles along medial side of palm (Fig. 7.7). These are:
  - Abductor digiti minimi, and
  - Flexor digiti minimi, both are superficial
  - Opponens digiti minimi is deep.
- Look for a twig of deep branch of ulnar nerve to innervate all three muscles.

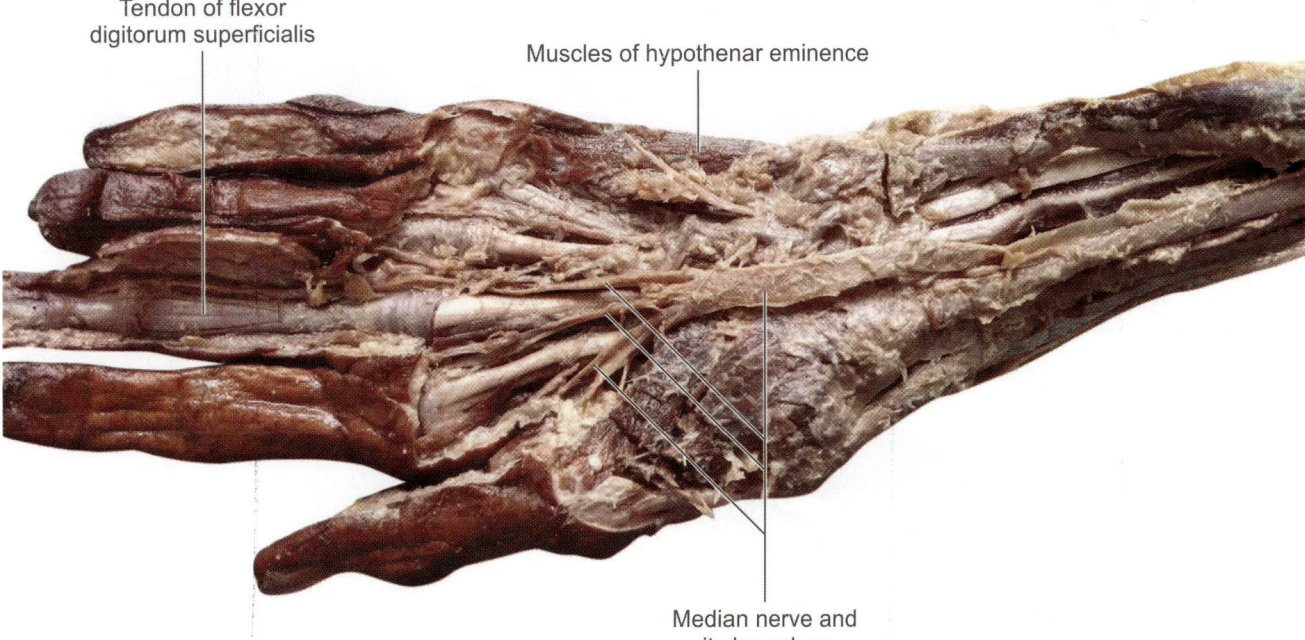

Fig. 7.7: Median nerve and its branches in the palm

Tendons Reaching the Digits

- Identify four tendons of flexor digitorum superficialis and four tendons of flexor digitorum profundus (Figs 7.6 and 7.8b). See that these are enclosed in a single synovial sheath—ulnar bursa.
- Trace the tendon of flexor pollicis longus from the carpal tunnel, medial to thenar eminence to pass distally to the distal phalanx of thumb. It is enclosed in a single synovial sheath—radial bursa.
- Look for insertion of flexor pollicis longus into base of distal phalanx of thumb (Fig. 7.6).
- Trace the four tendons of flexor digitorum superficialis distally in the palm. See that each tendon bifurcates into two slips each. These two slips embrace the tendon of flexor digitorum profundus (Fig. 7.8a). The two slips cross proximal interphalangeal joint to be inserted into sides of shaft of 2nd phalanx of the respective digits (Fig. 7.6).

- Incise these four tendons at the wrist and reflect them distally towards the phalanges.
- Now identify the deeper flexor digitorum profundus tendon also dividing into four tendons. Each passes between two slips of flexor digitorum superficialis and then courses straight to be inserted into bases of distal phalanges of all four digits (Fig. 7.6).
- Look for the four lumbrical muscles arising from the four tendons of flexor digitorum profundus (Fig. 7.8a). 1st and 2nd are unipennate and 3rd and 4th are bipennate.
- Adductor pollicis—define borders of two heads of adductor pollicis muscle. These are the transverse head and oblique head which join to be attached to medial side of base of proximal phalanx of thumb (Fig. 7.9).

Deep Palmar Arch and Deep Branch of Ulnar Nerve

- Identify and clean deep palmar arch formed by radial artery (Fig. 7.10a).

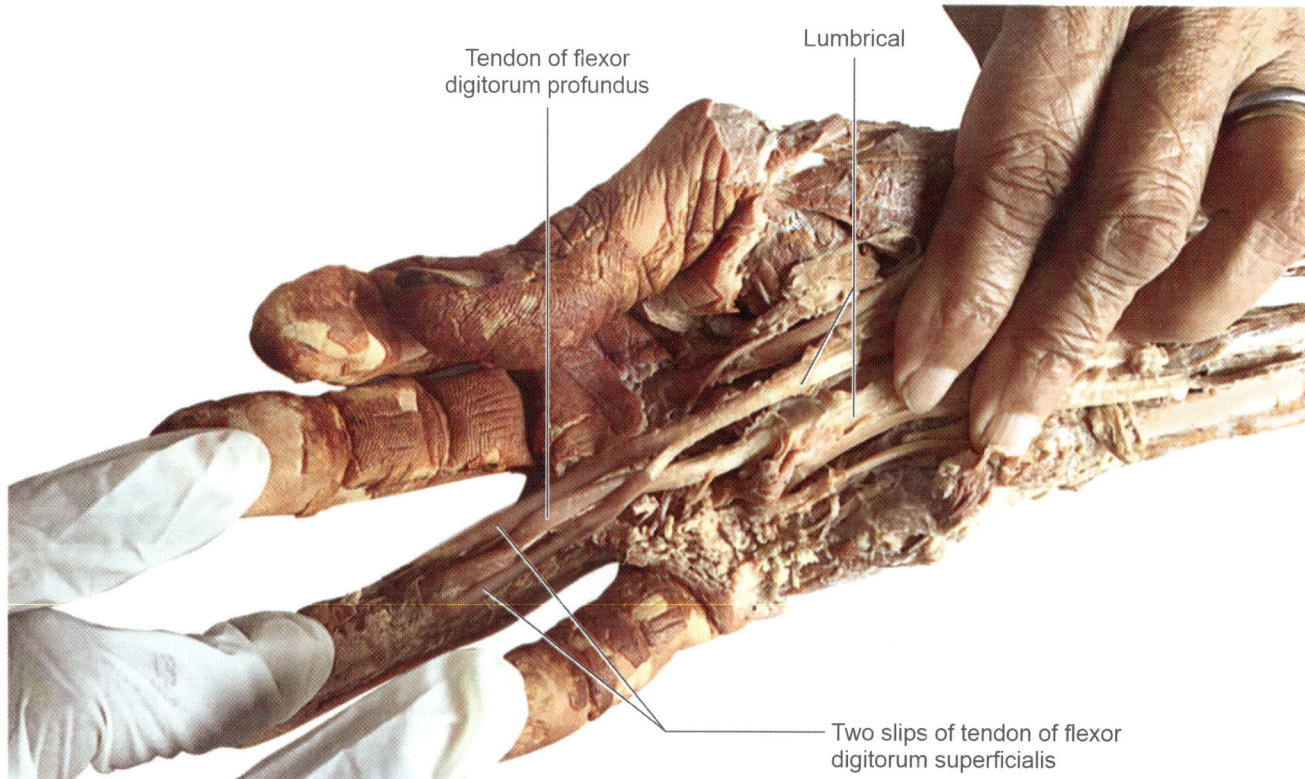

Tendon of flexor digitorum profundus

Lumbrical

Two slips of tendon of flexor digitorum superficialis

Fig. 7.8a: Tendon of flexor digitorum profundus passing between two slips of tendon of flexor digitorum superficialis

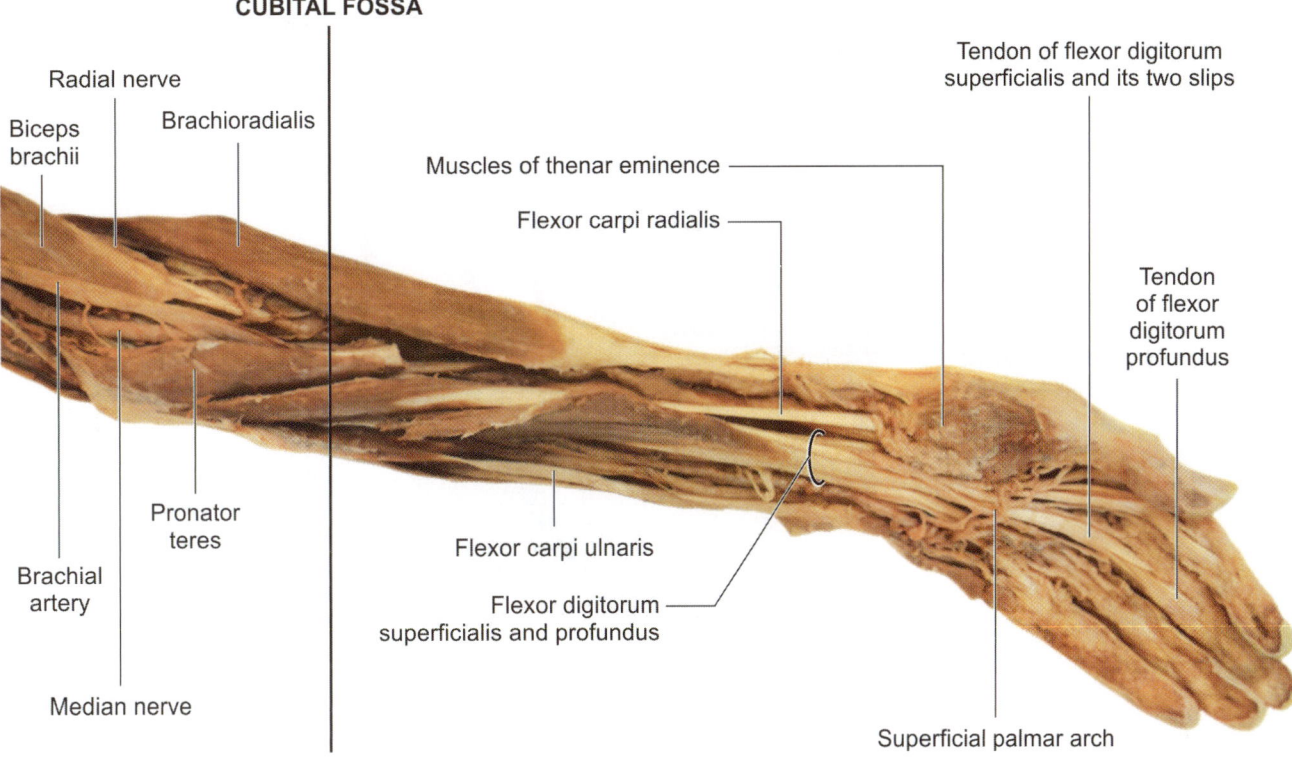

CUBITAL FOSSA

Radial nerve

Biceps brachii

Brachioradialis

Tendon of flexor digitorum superficialis and its two slips

Muscles of thenar eminence

Flexor carpi radialis

Tendon of flexor digitorum profundus

Pronator teres

Brachial artery

Flexor carpi ulnaris

Flexor digitorum superficialis and profundus

Median nerve

Superficial palmar arch

Fig. 7.8b: Boundaries and contents of cubital fossa. Muscles and tendons in front of forearm and in the palm

- Trace the radial artery from anatomical snuff box to lie in between two heads of 1st dorsal interosseous and then in between the two heads of adductor pollicis to reach the palm.
- Identify digital arteries—princeps pollicis for thumb and radialis indicis for lateral side of index finger, both from the radial artery.
- Trace the radial artery curving medially to join the deep branch of ulnar artery so as to complete the deep palmar arch.
- See that the deep palmar arch lies proximal to the superficial palmar arch.
- Trace the branches of deep palmar arch which join the common digital arteries of superficial palmar arch.
- Identify and clean deep branch of ulnar nerve (Fig. 7.10b) in the concavity of deep palmar arch. Trace its branches to:
  - Three muscles of hypothenar eminence
  - 4th and 3rd lumbricals
  - All four palmar interossei

- All four dorsal interossei
- Adductor pollicis

DEEP MUSCLES OF PALM

Steps of Dissection

- Deep to the lateral two tendons of flexor digitorum profundus muscle, note an obliquely placed muscle extending from two origins, i.e. from the shaft of the third metacarpal bone and the bases of 2nd and 3rd metacarpal bones and adjacent carpal bones to the base of proximal phalanx of the thumb. This is adductor pollicis. Reflect the adductor pollicis muscle from its origin towards its insertion.
- Identify the deeply placed interossei muscles. Identify the radial artery entering the palm between two heads of first dorsal interosseous muscle and then between two heads of adductor pollicis muscle turning medially to join the deep branch of ulnar artery to complete the deep palmar arch. Identify the deep branch of ulnar nerve lying in its

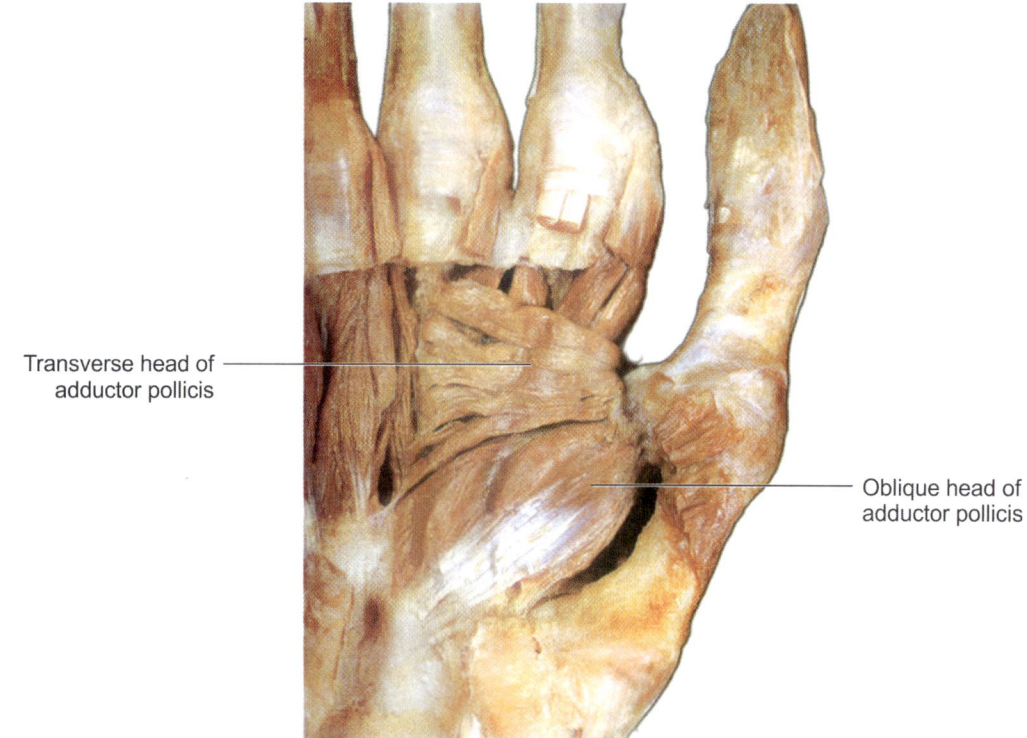

Transverse head of
adductor pollicis

Oblique head of
adductor pollicis

Fig. 7.9: Oblique and transverse heads of adductor pollicis muscle

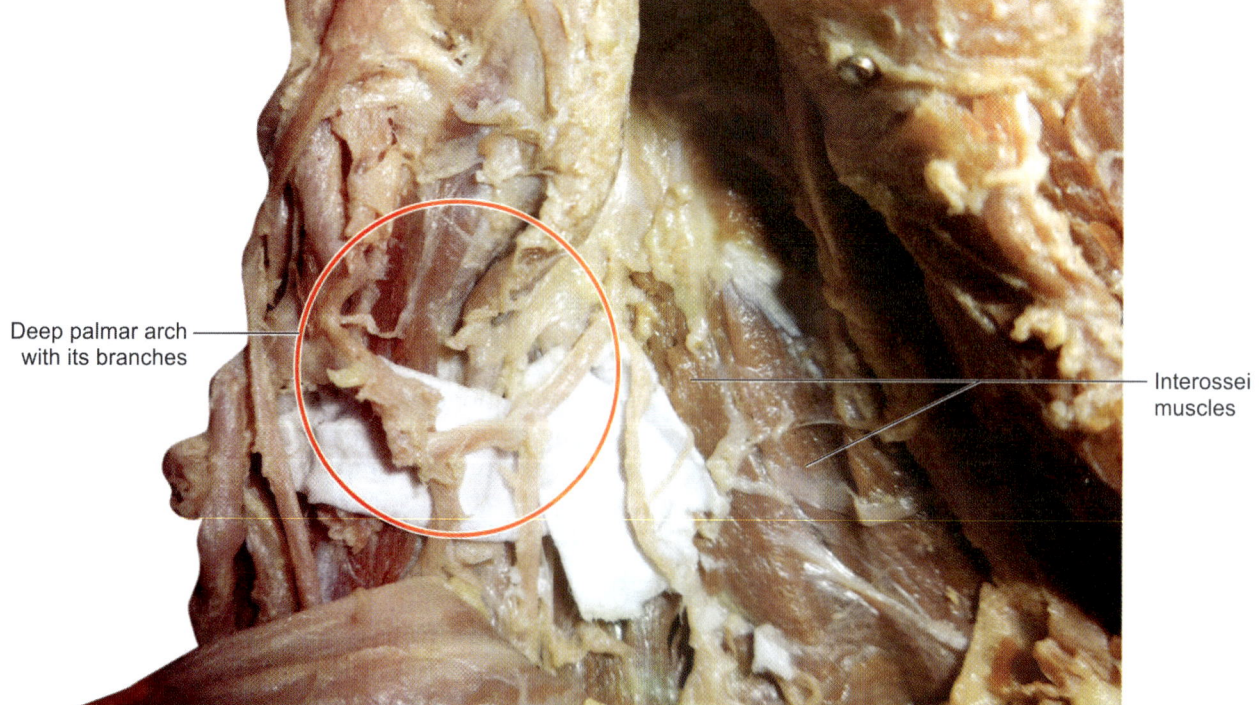

Deep palmar arch
with its branches

Interossei
muscles

Fig. 7.10a: Deep palmar arch lying on interossei muscles

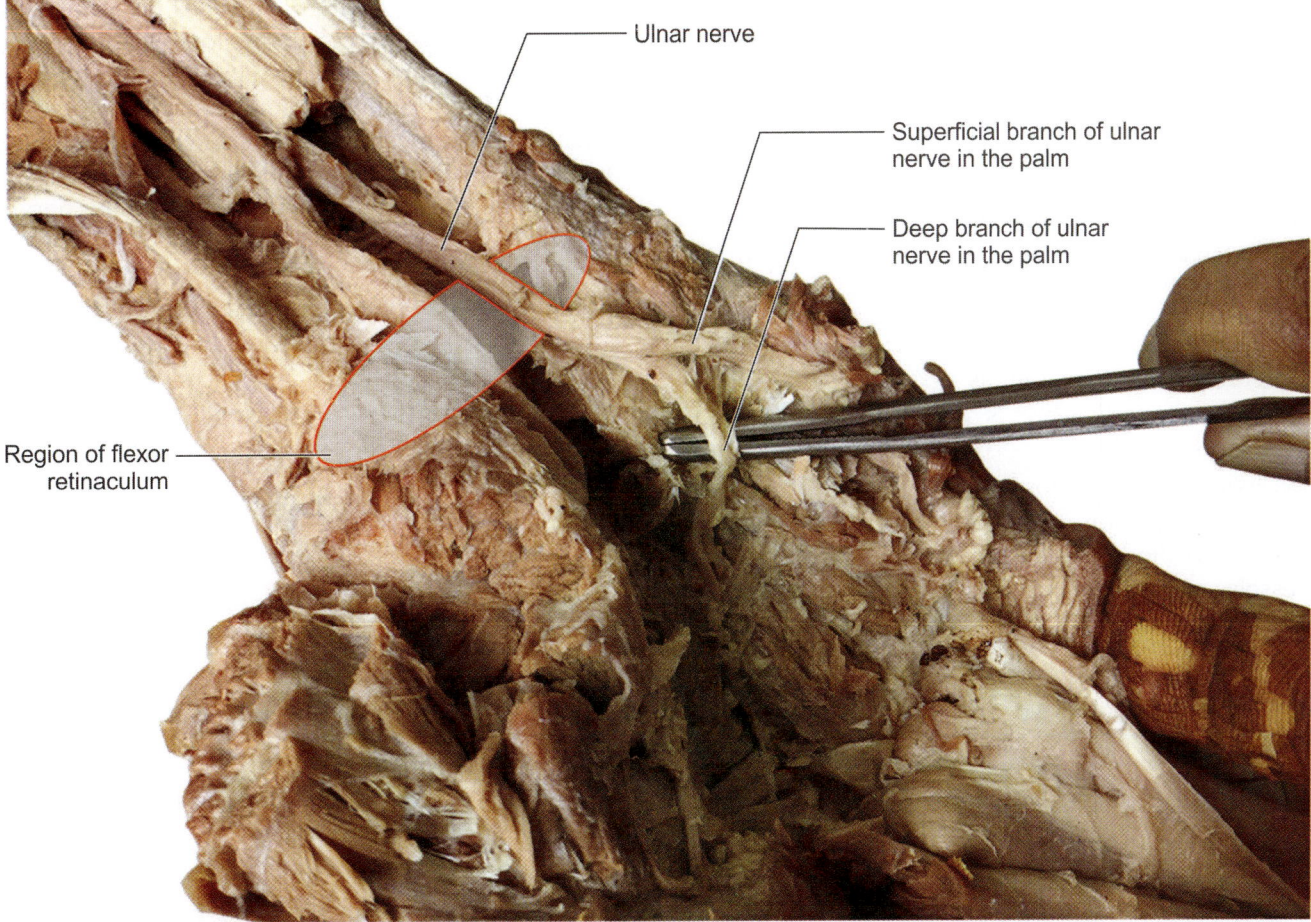

Fig. 7.10b: Ulnar nerve lying superficial to flexor retinaculum to enter the palm where it divides into a superficial and a deep branch

concavity. Carefully preserve it, including its multiple branches. Deep branch of ulnar nerve ends by supplying the adductor pollicis muscle. It may supply deep head of flexor pollicis brevis also.

- Lastly, define four small palmar interossei and four relatively bigger dorsal interossei muscles.

Interossei Muscles

- Look for four unipennate palmar interossei placed superficially. See four bipennate dorsal interossei muscles on a deeper plane (Fig. 7.10a).
- 1st palmar interosseous is a very thin muscle and is attached to the base of proximal phalanx of thumb. Note that no palmar interosseous is attached to the middle finger. 2nd, 3rd and 4th palmar interossei are inserted into dorsal digital expansion of index, ring and little fingers. Palmar

interossei are adductors towards the axial line passing through the centre of middle finger (PAD).

- The dorsal interossei are bigger and fill up the gaps between adjacent metacarpal bones. Dorsal interossei are four, out of which two are inserted into middle finger and one each into index and ring fingers. Dorsal interossei are abductors away from the axial line passing through the centre of middle finger (DAB).

POSTERIOR REGION OF FOREARM AND DORSUM OF HAND

Overview

The posterior or extensor region forearm contains muscles disposed in two layers.

Superficial layer

  i. Anconeus
 ii. Brachioradialis
iii. Extensor carpi radialis longus
 iv. Extensor carpi radialis brevis
  v. Extensor digitorum
 vi. Extensor digiti minimi
vii. Extensor carpi ulnaris

Deep layer

  i. Supinator
 ii. Abductor pollicis longus
iii. Extensor pollicis brevis
 iv. Extensor indicis
  v. Extensor pollicis longus

Nerve of this compartment is posterior interosseous nerve and blood vessels are posterior interosseous vessels.

> **Competency achievement:** The student should be able to:
>
> **AN 12.11** Identify, describe and demonstrate important muscle groups of dorsal forearm with attachments, nerve supply and actions.

Steps of Dissection

- Put the detached limb in a way that back of its forearm and hand are visible.
- Make the incision in the centre of dorsum of hand. Reflect the skin of dorsum of hand till the respective borders. Reflect the skin of dorsum of middle finger on each side. Look for nerves on the back of forearm and hand. These are superficial branch of radial nerve and dorsal branch of ulnar nerve.
- The dorsal venous network is the most prominent component of the superficial fascia of dorsum of hand. (Identify the beginning of cephalic and basilic veins by tying a tourniquet on the forearm and exercising the closed fist on oneself.)
- The deep fascia at the back of wrist is thickened to form extensor retinaculum. Define its margins and attachments. Identify the structures traversing its six compartments.
- Clear the deep fascia over the back of forearm. Define the attachment of triceps brachii muscle on the olecranon process of ulna. Define the attachments of the seven superficial muscles of the back of the forearm.

- Separate the anterolateral muscles, i.e. brachioradialis, extensor carpi radialis longus and brevis from the extensor digitorum lying in the centre and extensor digiti minimi and extensor carpi ulnaris situated on the medial aspect of the wrist. Anconeus is situated on the posterolateral aspect of the elbow joint. Dissect all these muscles and trace their nerve supply.

SUPERFICIAL MUSCLES OF BACK OF FOREARM

There are seven superficial muscles on the back of forearm. They are:

1. Anconeus
2. Brachioradialis
3. Extensor carpi radialis longus
4. Extensor carpi radialis brevis
5. Extensor digitorum
6. Extensor digiti minimi
7. Extensor carpi ulnaris (Fig. 7.11)

- Identify brachioradialis extending from upper 2/3rd of lateral supracondylar ridge of humerus to styloid process of radius.
- Medial to brachioradialis, identify extensor carpi radialis longus from lower 1/3rd of lateral supracondylar ridge to base of 2nd metacarpal.
- Now see extensor carpi radialis brevis, extensor digitorum, extensor digiti minimi and extensor carpi ulnaris attached to lateral epicondyle of humerus as common extensor origin (Fig. 7.11).
- Extensor carpi radialis brevis is attached to base of 3rd metacarpal.
- See the extensor digitorum dividing on the back of wrist into four tendons. These form part of extensor expansion on the proximal phalanx of medial four digits. The other muscles in the extensor expansion are interossei and lumbricals.
- Learn the tendons inserted into extensor expansion of digits 2–5.
- Identify the synovial sheaths covering these tendons as they pass through the tunnels under the extensor retinaculum.

DEEP MUSCLES OF THE BACK

Deep muscles are five in number. These are:
1. Supinator

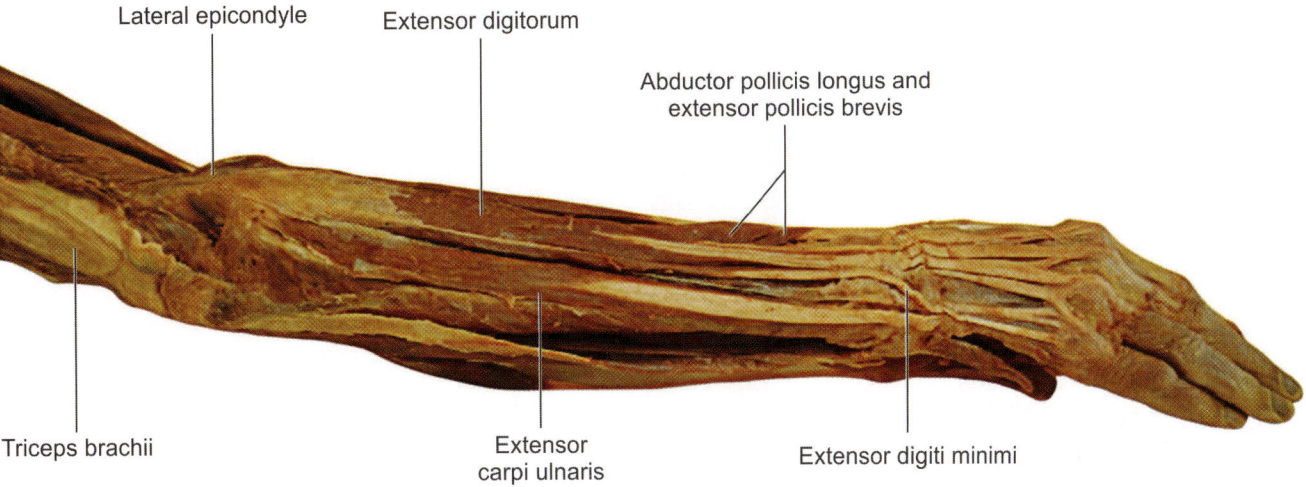

Labels on figure:
Lateral epicondyle   Extensor digitorum
Abductor pollicis longus and extensor pollicis brevis
Triceps brachii   Extensor carpi ulnaris   Extensor digiti minimi

Fig. 7.11: Superficial of back of forearm

2. Abductor pollicis longus
3. Extensor pollicis brevis
4. Extensor pollicis longus
5. Extensor indicis (Fig. 7.12)

Steps of Dissection

- Separate extensor carpi radials brevis from extensor digitorum and identify deeply placed supinator muscle.
- Just distal to supinator is abductor pollicis longus. Other three muscles: Extensor pollicis longus, extensor pollicis brevis and extensor indicis are present distal to abductor pollicis longus. Identify them all.
- Identify the supinator which is confined to the upper 1/3rd of radius.
- Identify abductor pollicis longus and extensor pollicis brevis as they arise from the back of forearm bones, curve laterally to pass through 1st compartment under extensor retinaculum (between lower sharp anterior border of radius and lateral surface of radius), to be inserted into bones of thumb.
- Extensor indicis forms part of extensor expansion of index finger.
- Extensor pollicis longus passes under extensor retinaculum to base of distal phalanx of thumb.

Competency achievement: The student should be able to:

AN 12.12 Identify and describe origin, course, relations, branches (or tributaries), termination of important nerves and vessels of back of forearm.

- Identify deep branch of radial nerve (posterior interosseous nerve) at the distal border of supinator muscle (Fig. 7.13).
- Trace the branches of the nerve supplying the extensor digitorum, extensor digiti minimi, extensor carpi ulnaris, abductor pollicis longus, extensor pollicis brevis, extensor pollicis longus and extensor indicis in the back of forearm (Fig. 7.13).
- See the posterior interosseous nerve descending to the 4th compartment and ending in a pseudoganglion which gives branches to the various neighbouring joints.
- See that the nerve is accompanied by a posterior interosseous artery in proximal part of forearm and by anterior interosseous artery in the distal part.
- Look for a foramen in the lower part of interosseous membrane for the passage of terminal part of anterior interosseous artery. Remember both posterior interosseous and anterior interosseous arteries are branches of common interosseous artery, a branch of ulnar artery.

Anatomical Snuff Box

- Identify anatomical snuff box just distal to most lateral side of extensor retinaculum. It is bounded by tendons of 1st and 3rd compartments passing under extensor retinaculum.
- *Laterally*—abductor pollicis longus, extensor pollicis brevis (Fig. 7.14a and b)
- *Medially*—extensor pollicis longus

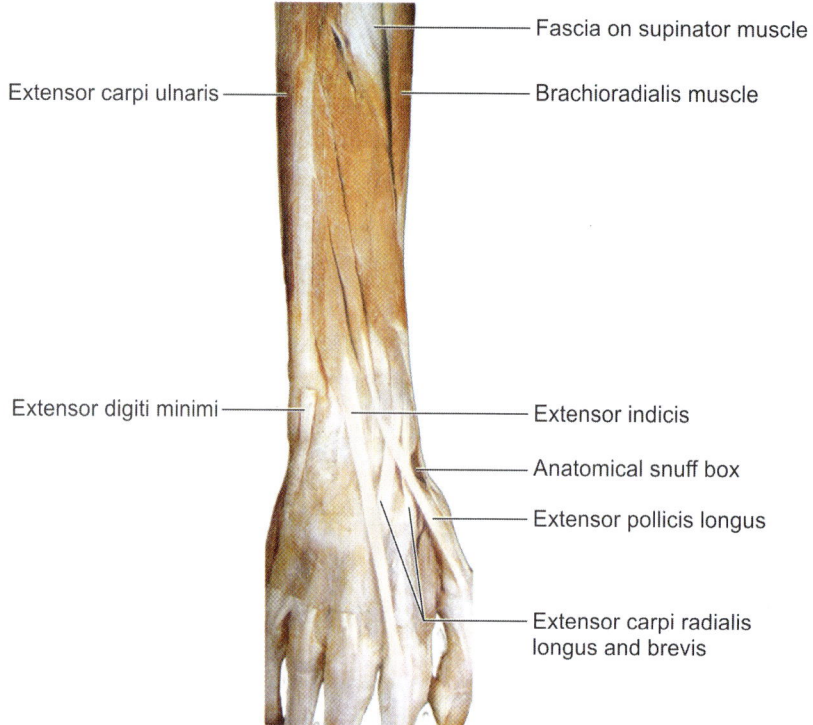

Fascia on supinator muscle

Extensor carpi ulnaris

Brachioradialis muscle

Extensor digiti minimi

Extensor indicis

Anatomical snuff box

Extensor pollicis longus

Extensor carpi radialis longus and brevis

Fig. 7.12: Some muscles of back of frearm

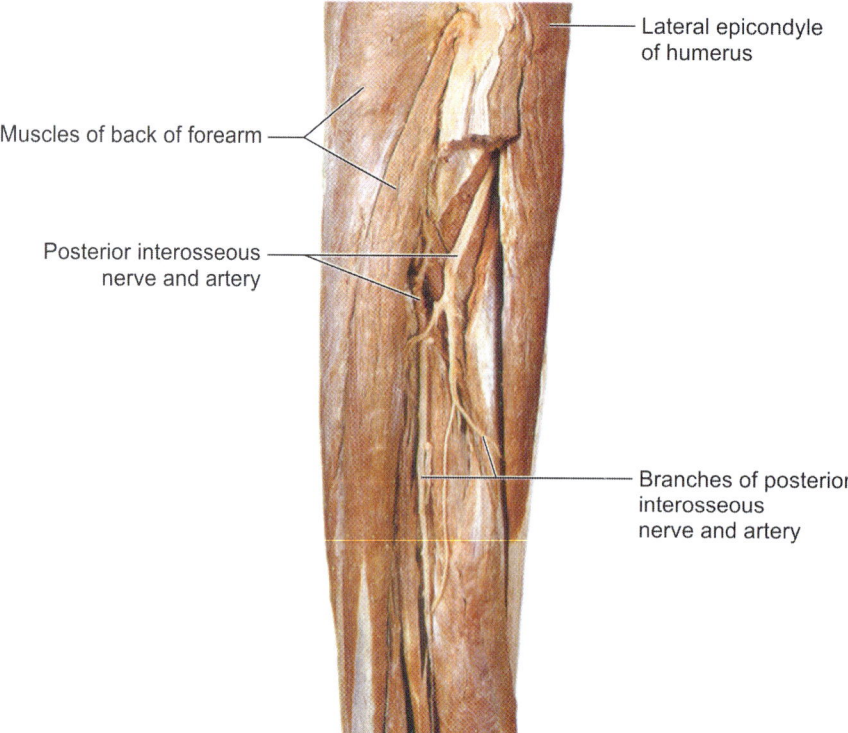

Lateral epicondyle of humerus

Muscles of back of forearm

Posterior interosseous nerve and artery

Branches of posterior interosseous nerve and artery

Fig. 7.13: Course and branches of posterior interosseous nerve and artery

- *Floor*—scaphoid and trapezium
- Contents
  - Radial artery before it enters into the palm
  - Branches of superficial division of radial nerve
  - Cephalic vein (*see* Fig. 5.2)

> *Competency achievement:* The student should be able to:
> **AN 12.14** Identify and describe compartments deep to extensor retinaculum.

EXTENSOR RETINACULUM

- Identify the long thickening of deep fascia at back of wrist known as extensor retinaculum (Fig. 7.15).

- See its attachments laterally to sharp crest like anterior border of radius and medially to styloid process of ulna, pisiform and triquetral bones. Look for its direction—downwards and medially.
- See the six compartments under extensor retinaculum. Study the lower end of dried radius and ulna bone to appreciate the compartments.
  - 1st compartment between crest like anterior border of radius and styloid process contains tendons of abductor pollicis longus and extensor pollicis brevis.
  - 2nd compartment between styloid process and dorsal tubercle contains tendons of extensor carpi

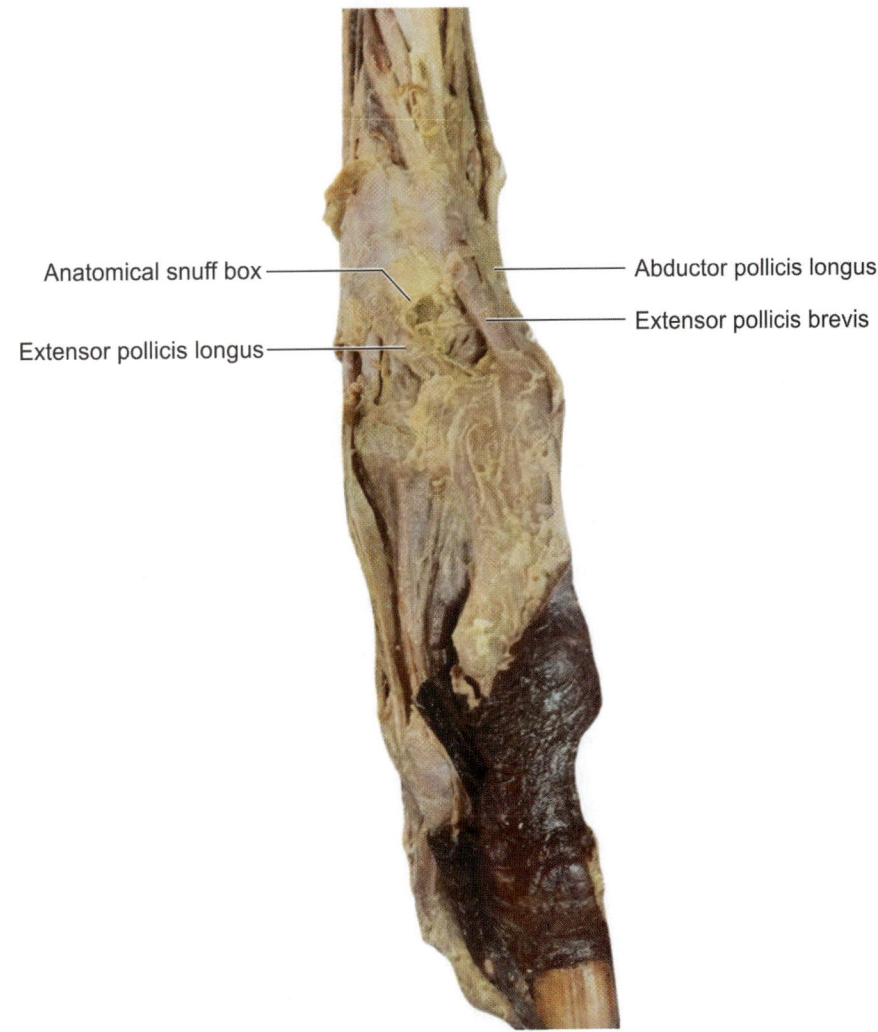

Anatomical snuff box

Extensor pollicis longus

Abductor pollicis longus

Extensor pollicis brevis

Fig. 7.14a: Boundaries of anatomical snuff box as a content

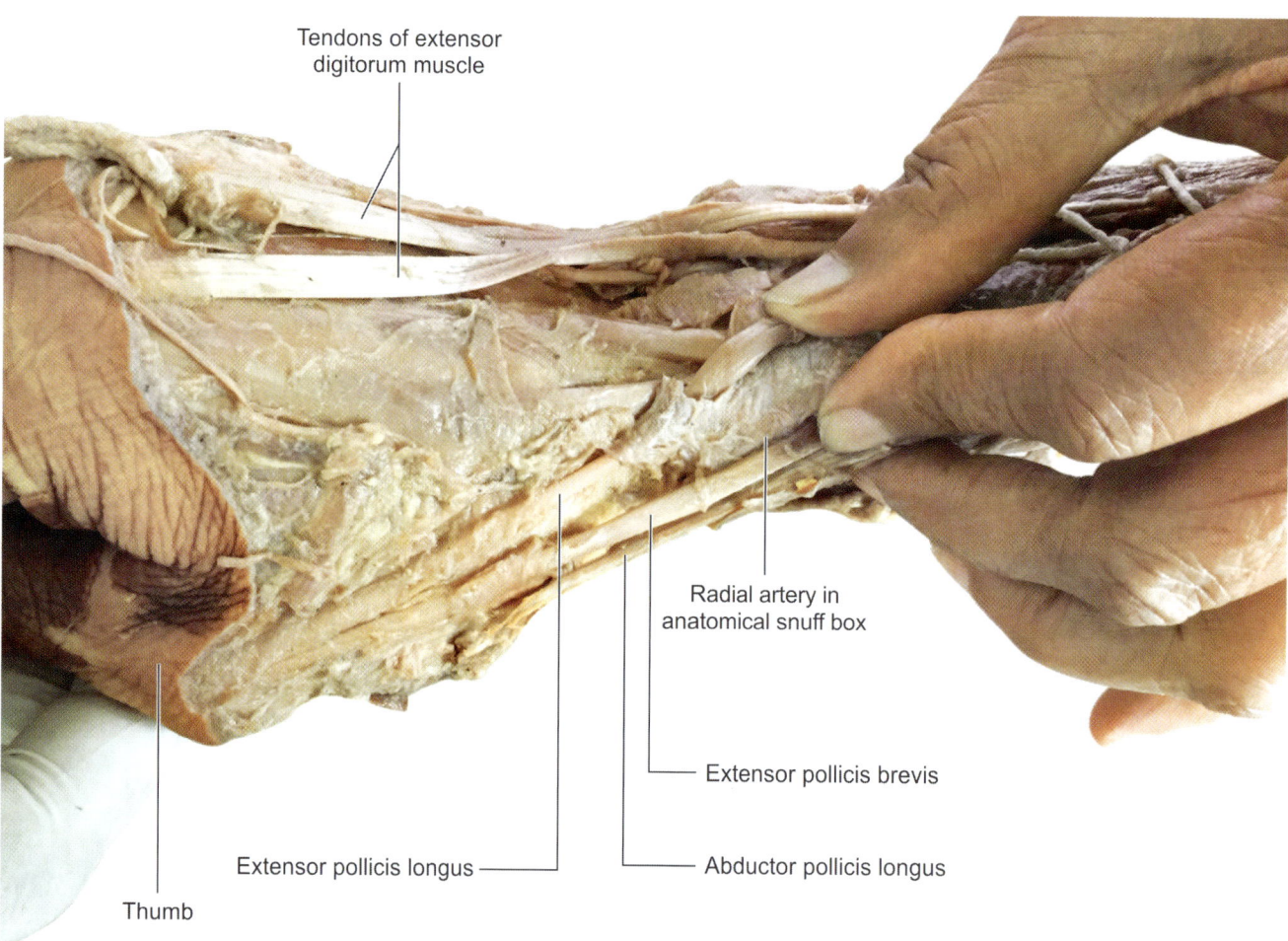

Tendons of extensor digitorum muscle

Radial artery in anatomical snuff box

Extensor pollicis brevis

Extensor pollicis longus

Abductor pollicis longus

Thumb

Fig. 7.14b: Boundaries of anatomical snuff box with radial artery as a content (magnified)

radialis longus (laterally) and extensor carpi radialis brevis (medially).

– 3rd compartment is a groove medial to dorsal tubercle and contains tendon of extensor pollicis longus.

– 4th compartment lies between the groove and the medial border of radius for passage of tendons of extensor digitorum, extensor indicis, posterior interosseous nerve and anterior interosseous artery.

– 5th compartment lies at the junction of lower end of radius and ulna and gives passage to tendon of extensor digiti minimi.

– 6th compartment between the head and styloid process of ulna gives passage to tendon of extensor carpi ulnaris.

– Note that all the tendons are covered by synovial sheaths.

Steps of Dissection

Deep terminal branch of radial nerve/posterior interosseous nerve and posterior interosseous artery:

• Identify the posterior interosseous nerve at the distal border of exposed supinator muscle. Trace its branches to the various muscles.

• Look for the radial nerve in the lower lateral part of front of arm between the brachioradialis, extensor carpi radialis longus laterally and brachialis muscle medially. Trace the two divisions of this nerve in the lateral part of the cubital fossa. The deep branch (posterior interosseous nerve) traverses between the two planes of supinator

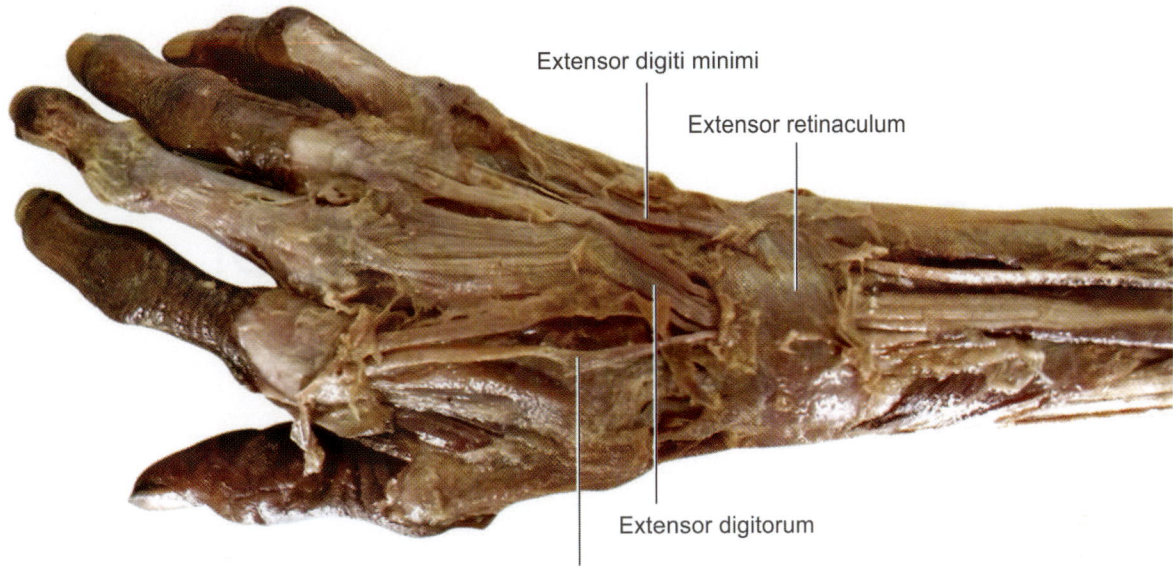

Extensor digiti minimi

Extensor retinaculum

Extensor digitorum

Extensor indicis

Fig. 7.15: Extensor retinaculum with few tendons passing beneath it

muscle and reaches the back of the forearm where it is already identified.
- The nerve runs amongst the muscles of the back of the forearm, and ends at the level of the wrist in a pseudoganglion.
- This nerve is accompanied by posterior interosseous artery distal to the supinator muscle. This artery is supplemented by anterior interosseous artery in lower one-fourth of the forearm.

DORSUM OF HAND

- Look for the dorsal venous plexus formed by metacarpal veins. Its two ends form beginning of cephalic vein on lateral side and beginning of basilic vein on medial side (*see* Figs 5.1 and 5.2).

- Identify the cutaneous nerves. These are:
  – Branches of radial in lateral ½
  – Branches of ulnar in medial ½
  – Branches of median for lateral 3½ nail beds and distal phalanx
  – Branches of ulnar for medial 1½ nail beds and distal phalanx
- Dorsal carpal arch formed by carpal branches of the radial and ulnar arteries.
- Identify its digital and metacarpal arteries
- Identify the four tendons of extensor digitorum, one tendon each of extensor indicis (Fig. 7.15) and extensor carpi ulnaris. These are united by intertendinous connections.

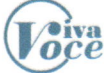

- Name the superficial muscles of front of forearm. Name their nerve supply.
- How many deep muscles are there in front of forearm? Which nerve innervates them?
- Where is the origin of lumbrical muscles? How many are unipennate and how many are bipennate muscles? How are the lumbricals innervated?
- Which is the most important nerve of the front of forearm?

- Which nerve supplies maximum muscles in the palm? Name these muscles.
- Why does 'carpal tunnel syndrome' occur and what are its symptoms?
- What are the attachments of flexor retinaculum? Name structures passing superficial to the retinaculum.
- Name the boundaries and contents of 'anatomical snuff box'.

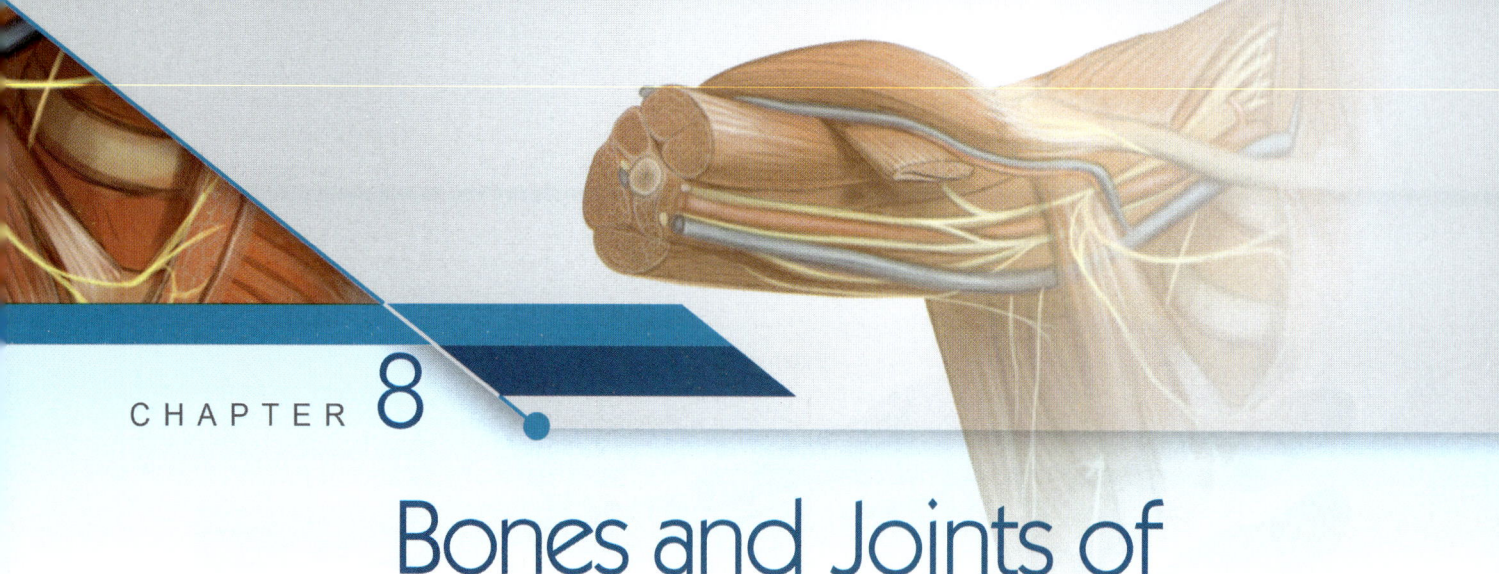

CHAPTER 8

Bones and Joints of Upper Limb

Learning Objectives

One should be able to

1. Palpate sternoclavicular and acromioclavicular joints. Name the movements which occur at these joints. List the muscles responsible for these movements.
2. Draw a diagram showing the relations of shoulder joint.
3. Name the muscles which cause abduction and over head abduction of shoulder joint. Mention their nerve supply
4. Enumerate the muscles which move the elbow joint. Give their nerve supply also.
5. What types of joints are the three radioulnar joints. Name the supinators of radioulnar joints with their nerve supply.
6. Enumerate the movements taking place at first carpometacarpal joint. What type of joint is this?
7. What type of joint is metacarpophalangeal joint. Name the movements which occur here.
8. Name the muscle responsible for flexion of distal interphalangeal joint of 4th and 5th digits. What nerve supplies this muscle.

OVERVIEW

The joints of upper limb are:

- Sternoclavicular ⎱
- Acromioclavicular ⎰ Joints of shoulder girdle
- Shoulder joint
- Elbow joint
- Proximal, middle and distal radioulnar joints
- Wrist joint, midcarpal joint
- Intercarpal and carpometacarpal joints
- Proximal and distal interphalangeal joints

All the synovial joints permit various types of movements. The articular cartilages cover. The articular ends of bones.

STERNOCLAVICULAR JOINT

See an articulated skeleton to identify the medial expanded end of clavicle and the shallow clavicular notch of manubrium sterni and upper surface of 1st costal cartilage (Fig. 8.1).

Identify sternocleidomastoid muscle arising from manubrium sterni and clavicle. Detach the parts and reflect them upwards.

Competency achievement: The student should be able to:

AN 13.4 Describe sternoclavicular joint, acromioclavicular joint, Carpometacarpa joints and Metacarpophalangeal joint.

Steps of Dissection

- Remove the subclavius muscle from first rib at its attachment with its costal cartilage. Identify the sternoclavicular ligament.
- Identify the bones forming the sternoclavicular joint. These are:
  - Medial end of clavicle
  - Notch on the manubriun sterni
  - Medial end of 1st costal cartilage (Fig. 8.1)

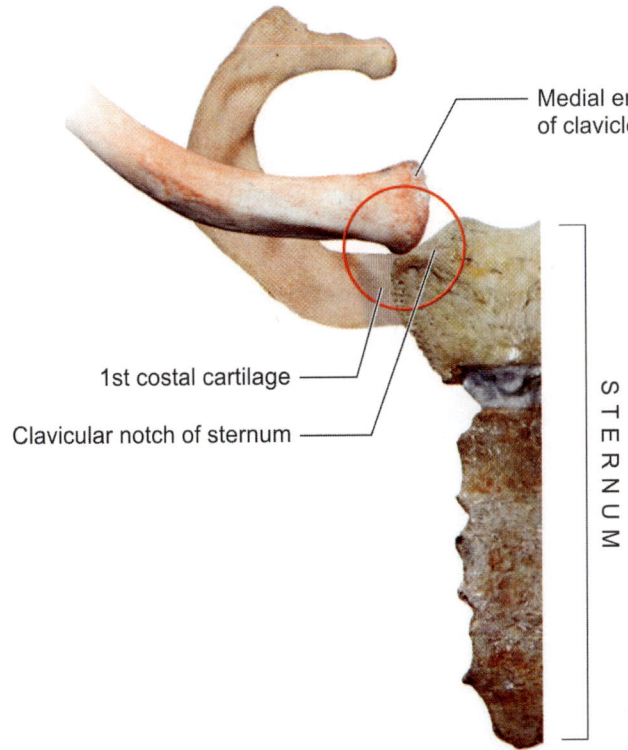

Fig. 8.1: Sternoclavicular joint

- Observe anterior sternoclavicular ligament binding the clavicle with the sternum. Incise the ligament and identify the fibrocartilaginous intra-articular disc between 1st costal cartilage and clavicle. This disc divides the joint cavity into a superomedial and an inferolateral compartment.
- Identify costoclavicular ligament between 1st costal cartilage and undersurface of clavicle near its medial end. Incise this ligament as well.
- Palpate the movements of the joint on yourself while doing the movements of shoulder girdle.

ACROMIOCLAVICULAR JOINT

Identify the bones forming acromioclavicular joint on an articulated skeleton (Fig. 8.2). These are:
- Acromion process of scapula
- Lateral end of clavicle

Steps of Dissection

- Remove the muscles attached to the lateral end of clavicle and acromion process of scapula. Define the articular capsule surrounding the joint. Cut

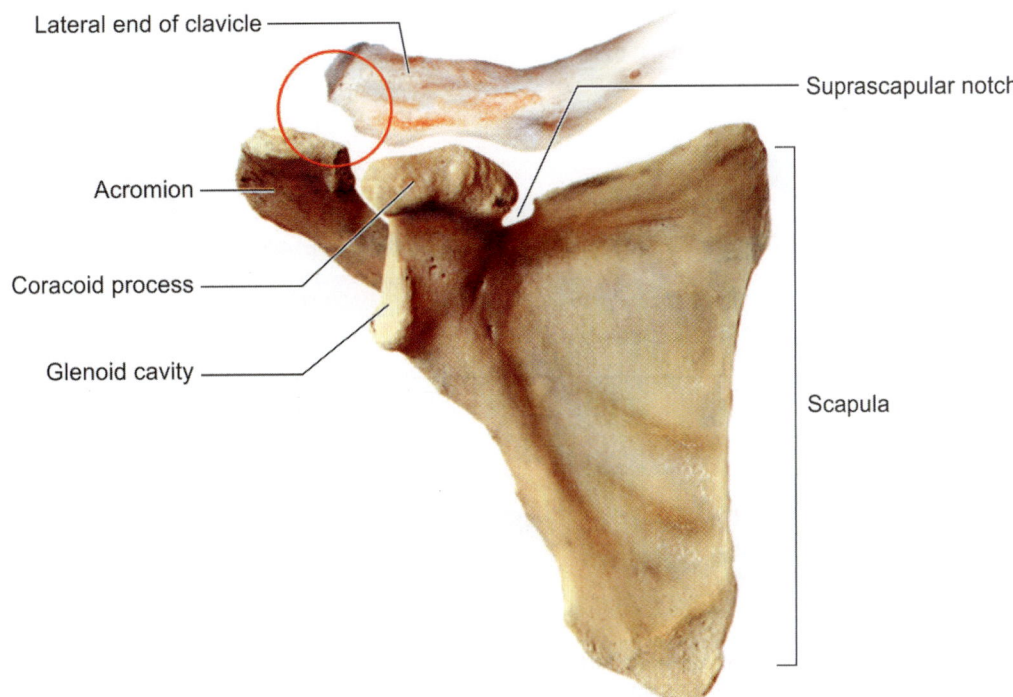

Fig. 8.2: Acromioclavicular joint

through the capsule to identify the intra-articular disc. Look for the strong coracoclavicular ligament.
- Detach the trapezius muscle from lateral end of clavicle, acromion process and spine of scapula.
- Separate short head of biceps brachii and coracobrachialis from tip of coracoid process.
- Identify and clean conoid and trapezoid parts of coracoclavicular ligament. Conoid is cord like while trapezoid is somewhat rectangular in shape.

- Incise the capsule of the joint and see the articulating surfaces covered by hyaline cartilage. The articular disc may also be seen.
- Movements of this joint occur simultaneously with movements of sternoclavicular joint.

Movements of sternoclavicular and acromio-clavicular joints (shoulder girdle) are shown in Table 8.1.

Attachments on the bones are shown in Figs 8.3 to 8.5.

Table 8.1: Showing movements at shoulder girdle with their muscles and nerve supply		
Movement	*Main muscle*	*Nerve supply*
Elevation of scapula	Upper fibres of trapezius	Spinal root of accessory (XI) nerve
	Levator scapulae	Dorsal scapular nerve
Depression of scapula	Lower fibres of serratus anterior	Long thoracic nerve
	Pectoralis minor	Medial and lateral pectoral nerves
Protraction of scapula	Serratus anterior	Long thoracic nerve
	Pectoralis minor	Medial and lateral pectoral nerves
Retraction of scapula	Rhomboid major	Dorsal scapular nerve
	Rhomboid minor	Dorsal scapular nerve
	Middle fibres of trapezius	Spinal root of XI nerve
Forward rotation of scapula	Upper and lower fibres of trapezius	Spinal root of XI nerve
	Lower fibres of serratus anterior	Long thoracic nerve
Backward rotation of scapula	Levator scapulae	Dorsal scapular nerve
	Rhomboid minor	Dorsal scapular nerve
	Rhomboid major	Dorsal scapular nerve

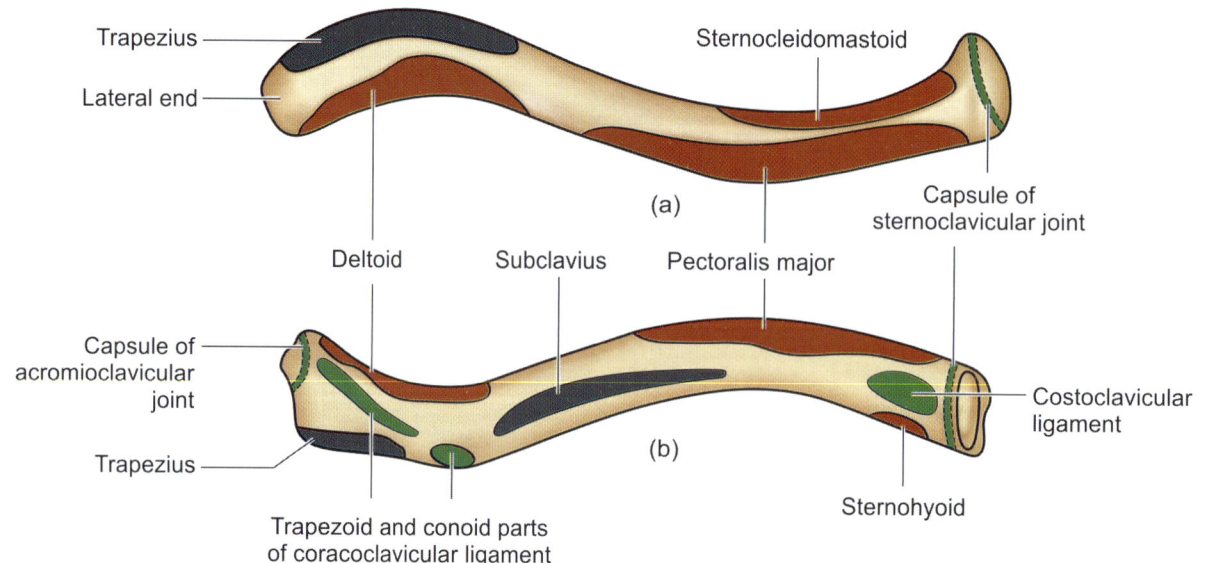

Fig. 8.3: Attachments of right clavicle: (a) Superior aspect, and (b) inferior aspect

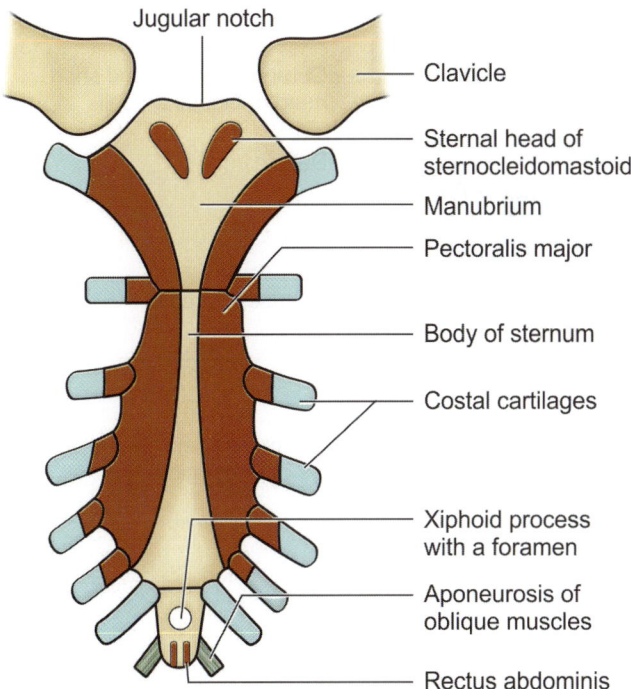

Fig. 8.4: Ther sternum: Anterior aspect, with muscle attachment

Jugular notch

Clavicle

Sternal head of sternocleidomastoid

Manubrium

Pectoralis major

Body of sternum

Costal cartilages

Xiphoid process with a foramen

Aponeurosis of oblique muscles

Rectus abdominis

Competency achievement: The student should be able to:

AN 10.12 Describe and demonstrate shoulder joint for type, artcular surfaces, capsule, synovial membrane, ligaments, relations, movements, muscles involved, blood supply and applied anatomy.

SHOULDER JOINT

Shoulder joint is a highly mobile ball and socket type of synovial joint. Identify the shallow glenoid cavity and almost round head of humerus in the articulated skeleton (Fig. 8.6a). The mobility of the joint is at the cost of its stability.

- Having studied all the muscles at the upper end of the scapula, it is wise to open and peep into the most mobile shoulder joint.
- Identify the muscles attached to the greater and lesser tubercles of humerus. Deep to the acromion process look for the subacromial bursa.
- Identify coracoid process, acromion process and triangular coracoacromial arch binding these two bones together

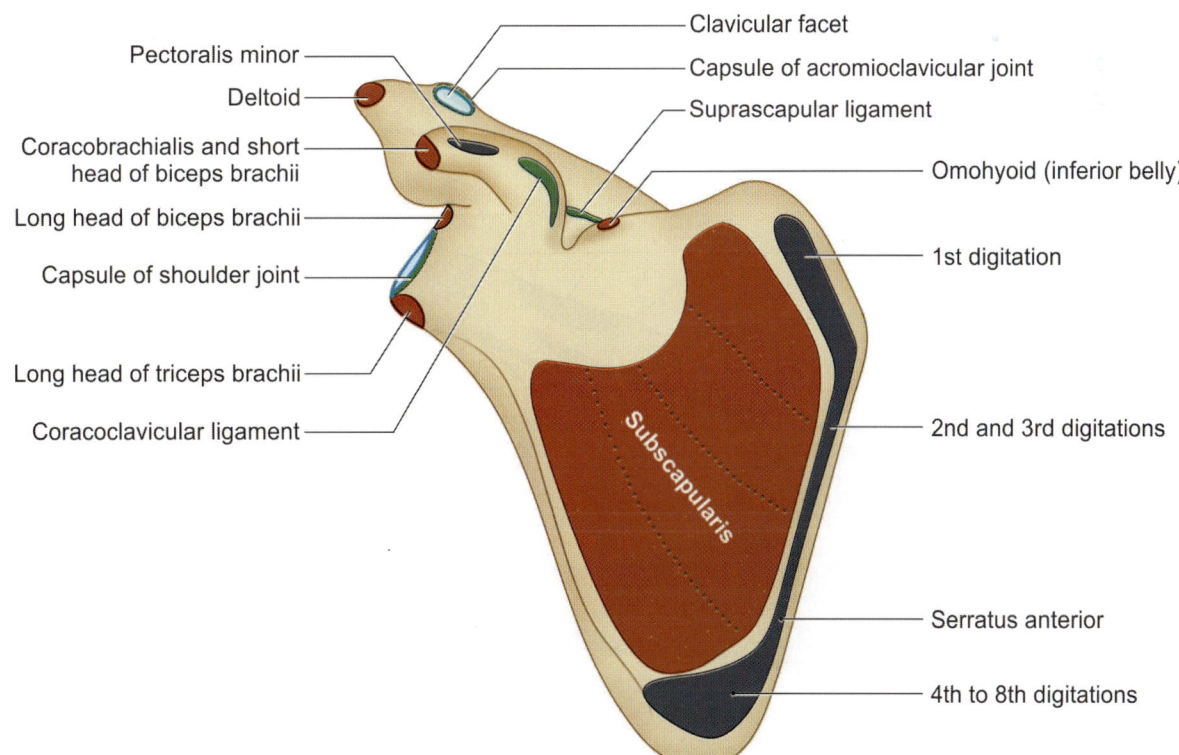

Pectoralis minor

Deltoid

Coracobrachialis and short head of biceps brachii

Long head of biceps brachii

Capsule of shoulder joint

Long head of triceps brachii

Coracoclavicular ligament

Clavicular facet

Capsule of acromioclavicular joint

Suprascapular ligament

Omohyoid (inferior belly)

1st digitation

Subscapularis

2nd and 3rd digitations

Serratus anterior

4th to 8th digitations

Fig. 8.5a: Attachments of right scapula: Costal aspect

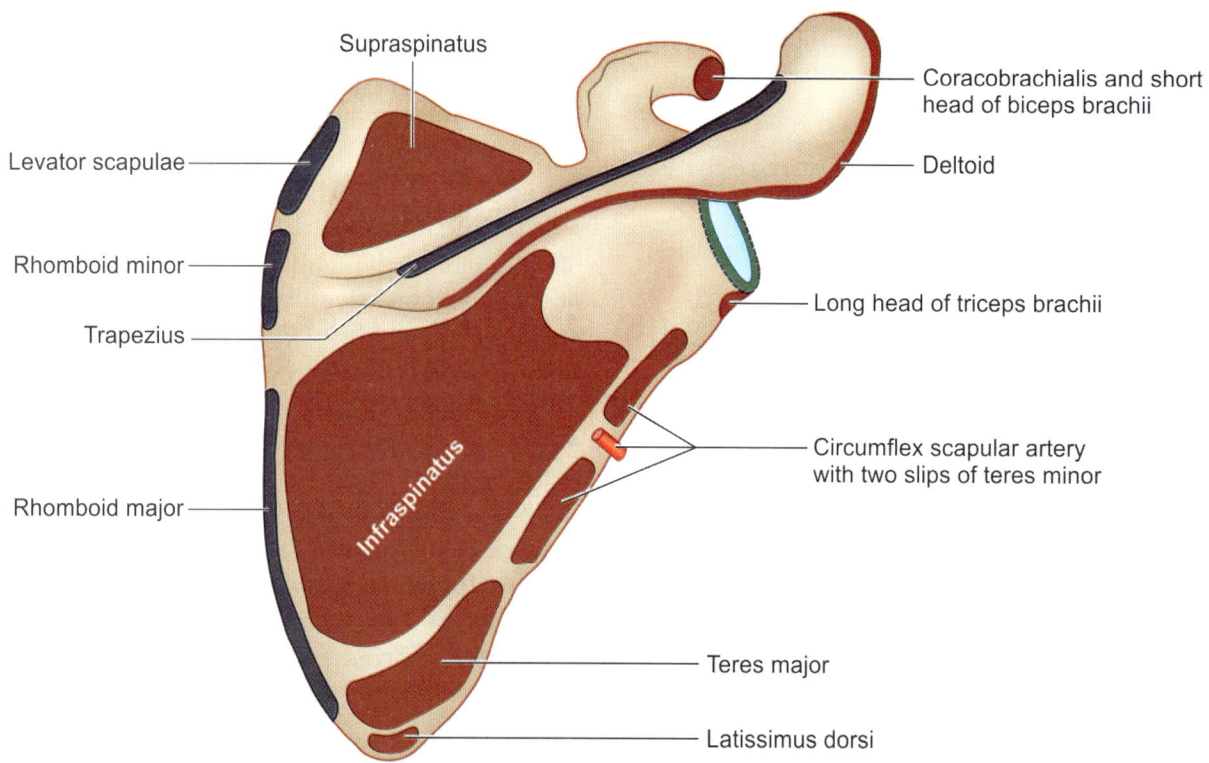

Fig. 8.5b: Attachments of right scapula: Dorsal aspect

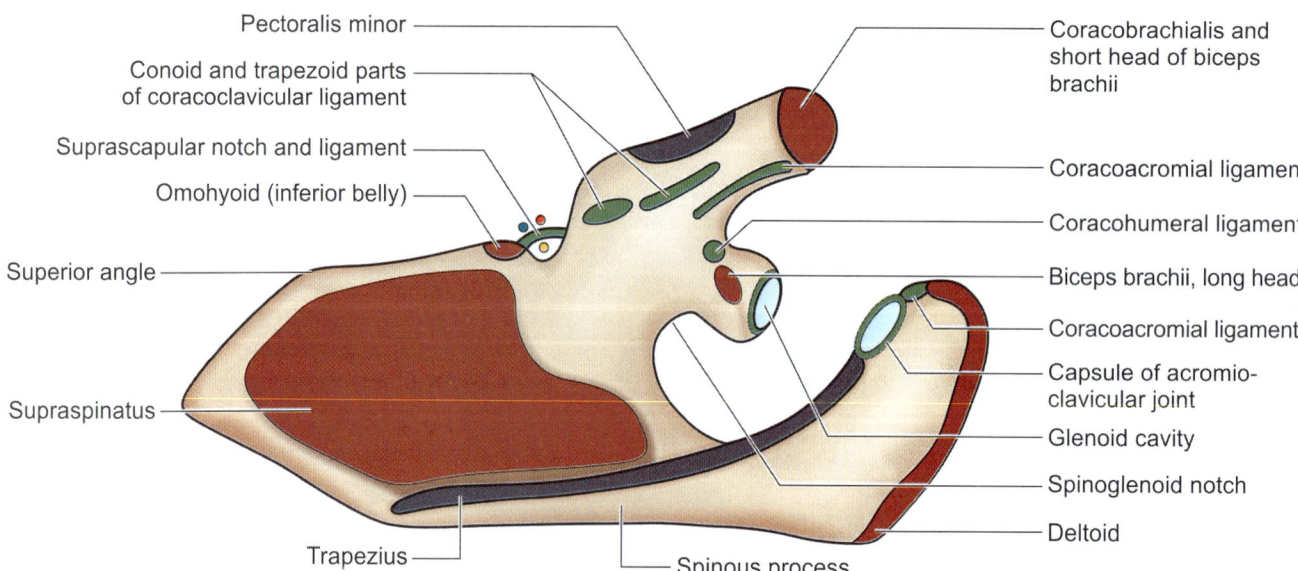

Fig. 8.5c: Attachments of right scapula: Superior aspect

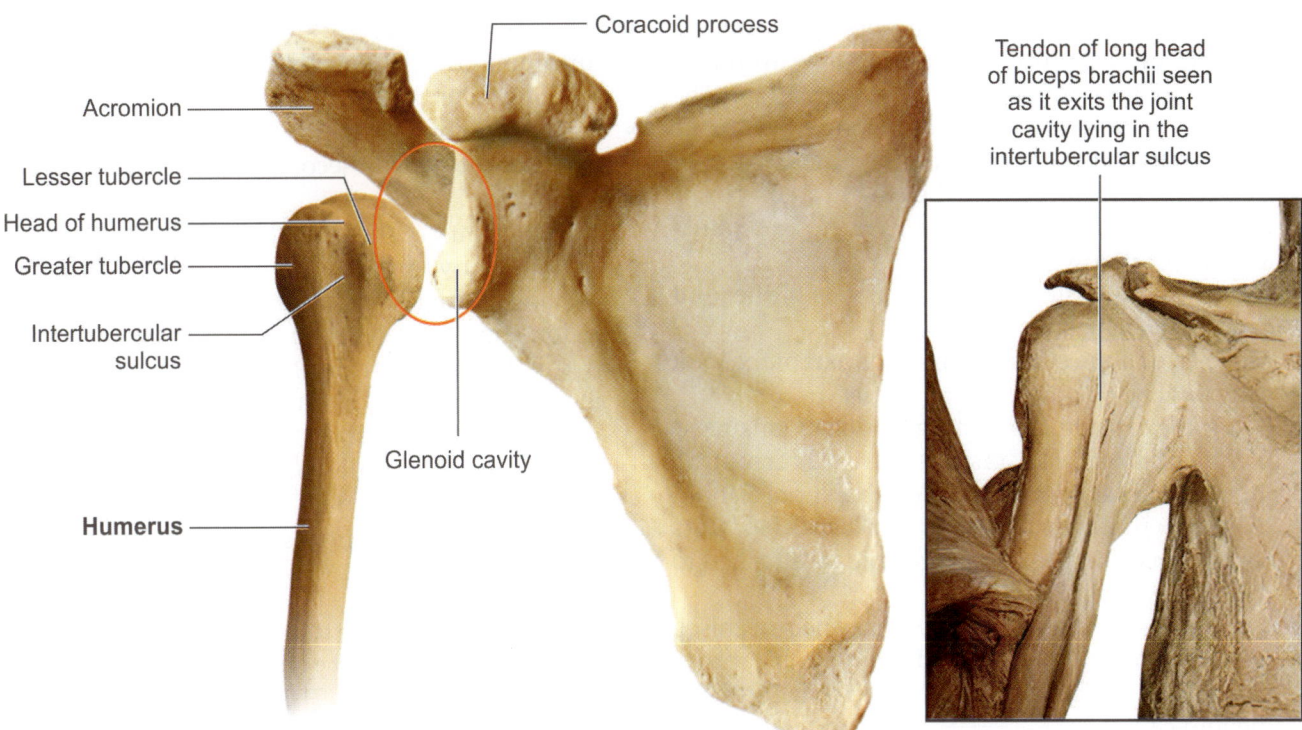

Coracoid process

Acromion

Lesser tubercle

Head of humerus

Greater tubercle

Intertubercular sulcus

Glenoid cavity

Humerus

Tendon of long head of biceps brachii seen as it exits the joint cavity lying in the intertubercular sulcus

Fig. 8.6a: Glenohumeral/shoulder joint

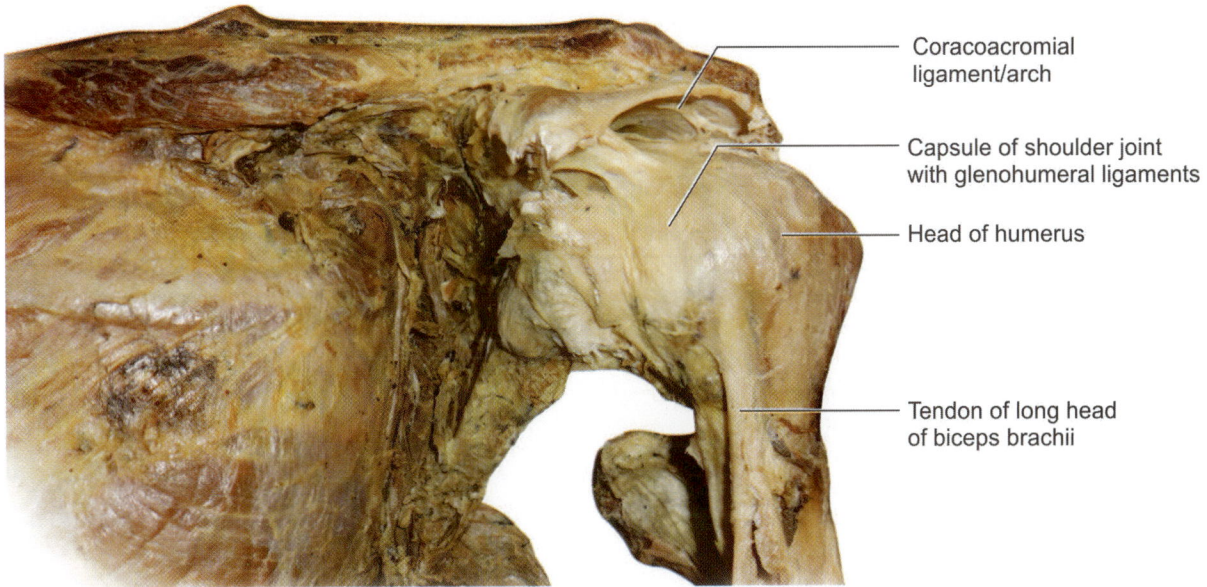

Coracoacromial ligament/arch

Capsule of shoulder joint with glenohumeral ligaments

Head of humerus

Tendon of long head of biceps brachii

Fig. 8.6b: Capsule of shoulder joint

- Trace and remove all the muscles covering the capsule of the joint. These are subscapularis, supraspinatous, infraspinatus and teres minor. The tendons of these four muscles blend with capsule of shoulder joint to form a rotator cuff.
- Inferiorly, trace and incise the long head of triceps brachii from the infraglenoid tubercle of scapula and reflect it downwards.
- Cut open the posterior part of capsule of the joint by a vertical incision.
- Make an oblique cut in the anterior part of the joint capsule (Fig. 8.6b).
- Inside the capsule, the shining tendon of long head of biceps brachii is visible as it traverses the intertubercular sulcus to reach the supraglenoid tubercle of scapula. This tendon also gets continuous with the labrum glenoidale attached to the rim of glenoid cavity.
- Remove the head of humerus with the help of chisel.
- Identify the shallow glenoid cavity and labrum glenoidale-cartilaginous rim to deepen the shallow glenoid cavity.
- Identify the tendon of long head of biceps brachii arising from supraglenoid tubercle of humerus. It traverses the glenoid cavity and intertubercular sulcus of humerus to reach the front of arm. Appreciate the tubular synovial membrane enclosing the tendon.

- Identify the three glenohumeral ligaments supplementing the anterior part of capsule of shoulder joint.
- Identify the coracoacromial ligament above the joint (Fig. 8.6b). It acts as a secondary socket for the head of humerus.
- Palpate your own shoulder joint while doing various movements. Appreciate the muscles responsible for the movement when the movement is done against resistance. Movements permitted at this joint are flexion, extension, adduction, abduction including overhead abduction, medial and lateral rotation and circumduction.

Muscles responsible for these movements at shoulder joint are shown in Table 8.2.

Attachments on the bones are shown in Figs 8.5 and 8.7.

> *Competency achievement:* The student should be able to:
>
> **AN 13.3** Identify and describe the type, articular surfaces, capsule, synovial membrane, ligaments, relations, movements, blood and nerve supply of elbow joint, proximal and distal radioulnar joints, wrist joint and first carpometacarpal joint.

ELBOW JOINT INCLUDING PROXIMAL RADIOULNAR JOINT

Identify the bones taking part in these joints in an articulated skeleton (Fig. 8.8). These are:

Table 8.2: Showing movement at shoulder joint with their muscles and nerve supply

Movement	Muscles	Nerve supply
Flexion	Clavicular head of pectoralis major	Lateral pectoral nerve
	Anterior fibres of deltoid	Axillary nerve
Extension	Posterior fibres of deltoid	Axillary nerve
	Latissimus dorsi	Thoracodorsal nerve
Adduction	Pectoralis major	Medial and lateral pectoral nerves
Abduction	Supraspinatus	Suprascapular nerve
0° to 90°	Middle fibres of deltoid	Axillary nerve
90° to 180°	Serratus anterior	Long thoracic nerve
	Upper and lower fibres of trapezius	Spinal root of XI nerve
Medial rotation	Pectoralis major	Medial and lateral pectoral nerves
	Anterior fibres of deltoid	Axillary nerve
	Latissimus dorsi	Thoracodorsal nerve
	Teres major	Lower subscapular nerve
Lateral rotation	Posterior fibres of deltoid	Axillary nerve
	Infraspinatus	Suprascapular nerve
	Teres minor	Axillary nerve

Circumduction: A movement involving above movements in a sequence.

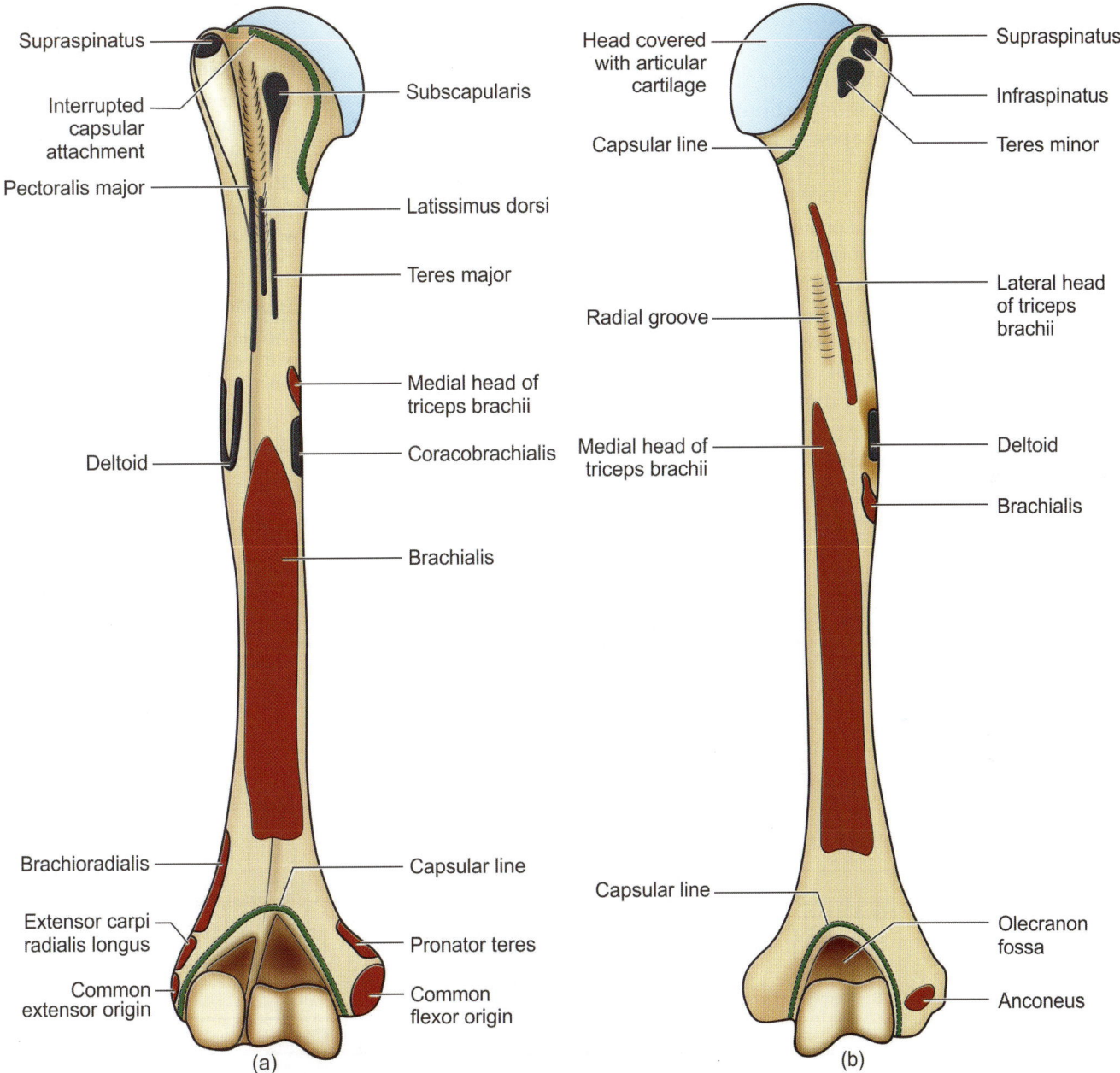

Fig. 8.7: Attachments of right humerus: (a) Anterior view, and (b) posterior view

- Trochlea of humerus
- Trochlear notch of ulna
- Capitulum of humerus
- Head of radius
- Radial notch of ulna

Elbow joint is a hinge variety of synovial joint. In recent state it is covered by muscles on anterior and posterior aspects.

- Detach brachialis from humerus and reflect it downwards.
- Detach triceps brachii from back of humerus and reflect it downwards.
- Identify the thin capsule of elbow joint both anteriorly (Fig. 8.9) and posteriorly.
- Detach the common flexor origin from medial epicondyle of humerus.

- Detach common extensor origin from lateral epicondyle of humerus.
- Identify ulnar collateral/medial ligament, comprising strong anterior portion and fan-shaped posterior portion. Its apex is attached to medial epicondyle of humerus and its base to coronoid process and olecranon process of ulna.
- Identify and clean radial collateral/lateral ligament from lateral epicondyle of humerus to lateral part of head of radius and to annular ligament.
- Observe annular ligament of superior radioulnar joint attached to anterior border of radial notch of ulna, around the head of radius to the posterior border of radial notch of ulna.

Movements at elbow joint are flexion and extension. Muscles responsible for these movements at elbow joint are shown in Table 8.3.

Attachments on the bones are shown in Figs 8.7 and 8.10.

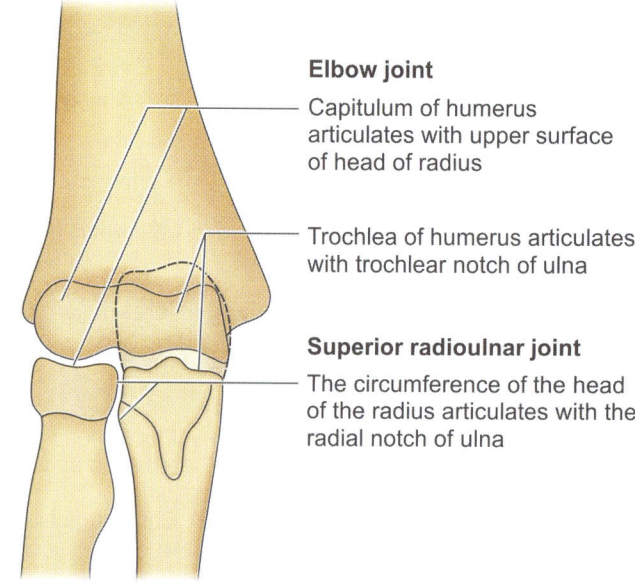

Elbow joint
Capitulum of humerus articulates with upper surface of head of radius

Trochlea of humerus articulates with trochlear notch of ulna

Superior radioulnar joint
The circumference of the head of the radius articulates with the radial notch of ulna

Fig. 8.8: The cubital articulations, including the elbow and superior radioulnar joints

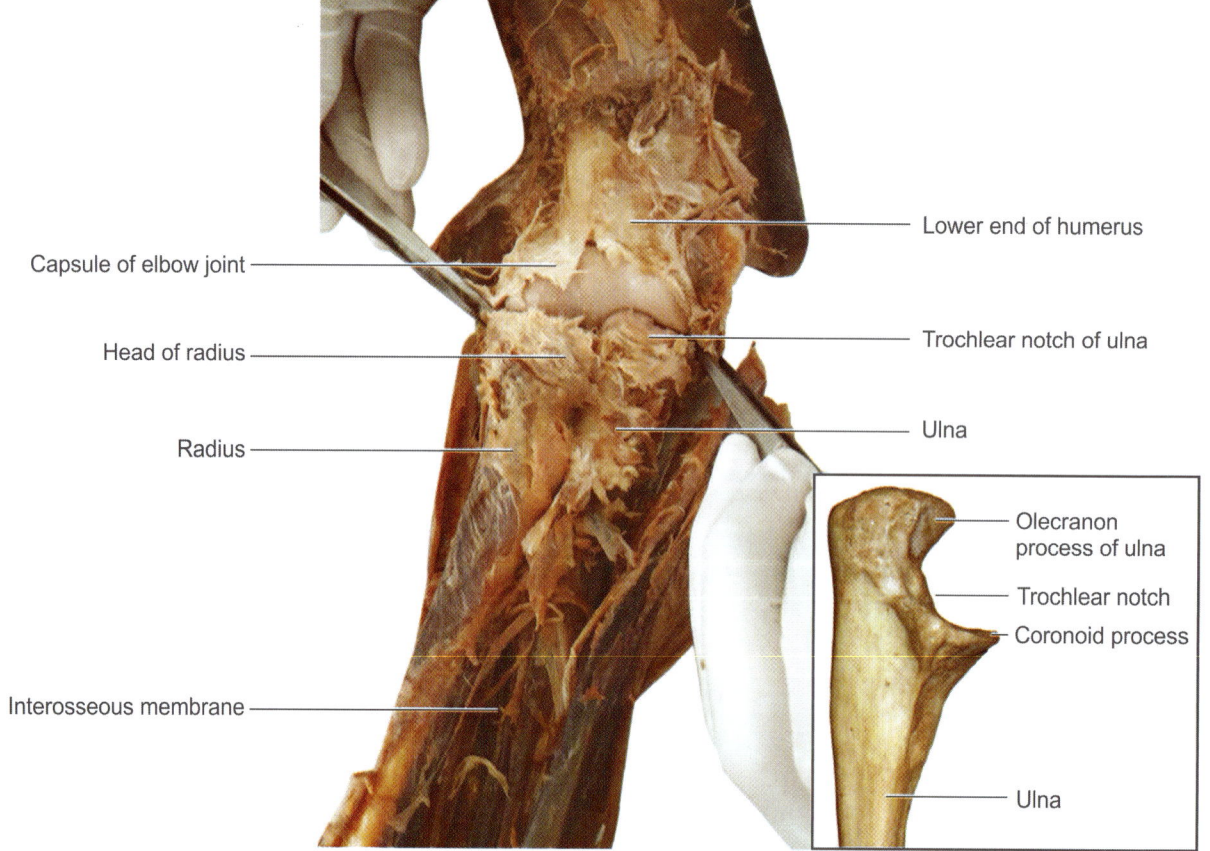

Capsule of elbow joint
Head of radius
Radius
Interosseous membrane

Lower end of humerus
Trochlear notch of ulna
Ulna

Olecranon process of ulna
Trochlear notch
Coronoid process
Ulna

Fig. 8.9: Elbow joint with interosseous membrane

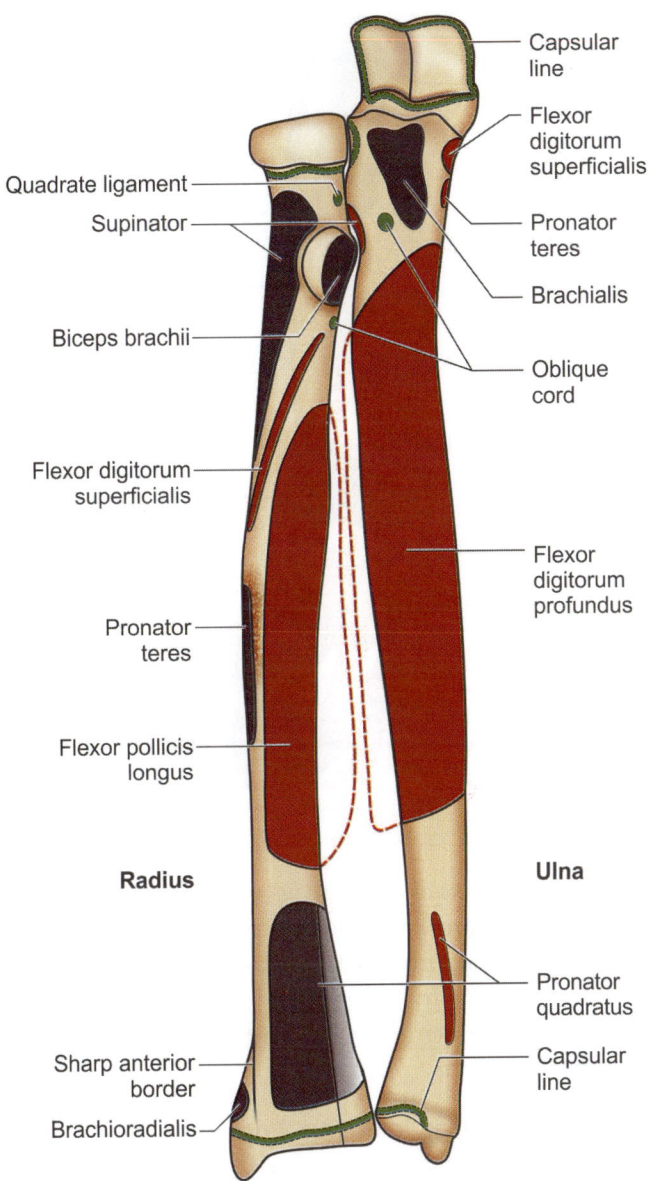

Fig. 8.10a: Attachments of right radius and ulna: Anterior aspect

Fig. 8.10b: Attachments of right radius and ulna: Posterior aspect

Table 8.3: Showing movements at elbow joint with their muscles and nerve supply

Movement	Main muscle	Nerve supply
Flexion	Brachialis	Musculocutaneous nerve
	Biceps brachii	Musculocutaneous nerve
	Brachioradialis	Radial nerve
Extension	Triceps brachii	Radial nerve
	Anconeus	Radial nerve
	Gravity	—

RADIOULNAR JOINTS

There are three radioulnar joints viz. superior, middle and inferior (Fig. 8.11).

Superior Proximal Radioulnar Joint

Superior radioulnar joint is a synovial joint of pivot variety (Fig. 8.12).

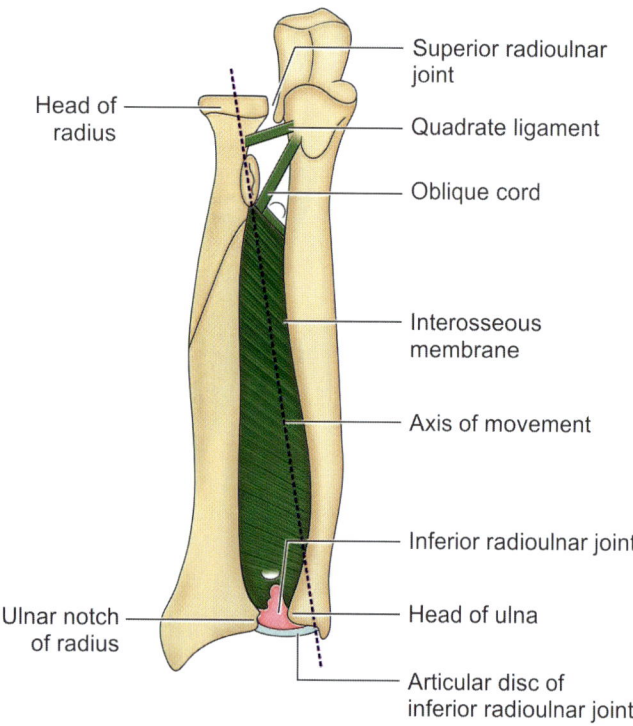

Fig. 8.11: Radioulnar joints

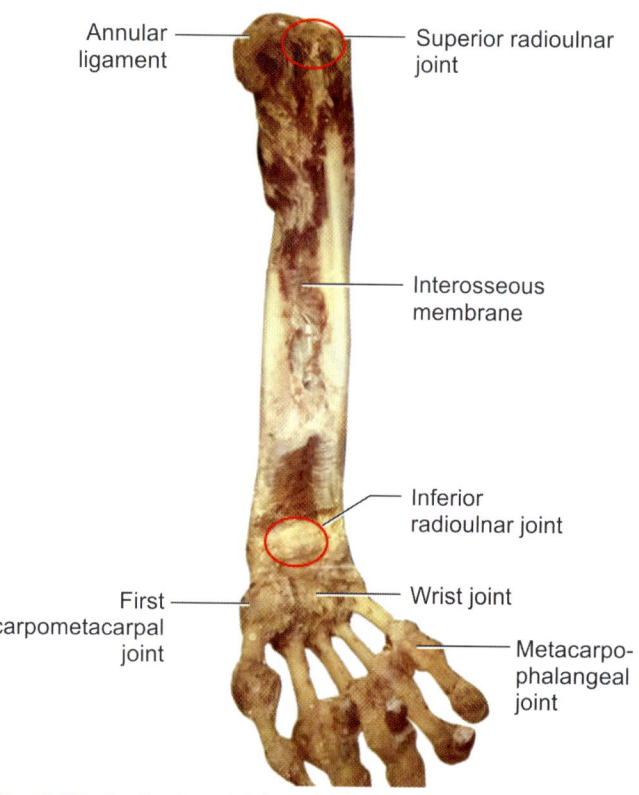

Fig. 8.12: Radioulnar joints, wrist joint, 1st carpometacarpal joint and metacarpophalangeal joints

- Incise the anterior and posterior aspects of the capsule to peep inside the joints and see the synovial membrane.
- Do the movements of flexion and extension on elbow joint and movements of pronation and supination for radioulnar joint. Feel the muscles responsible for all these movements.

Middle Radioulnar Joint

This joint is a fibrous/syndesmosis type of joint between the interosseous borders of radius and ulna. The interosseous membrane joins the two borders (Figs 8.9, 8.11 and 8.12).

- Identify a foramen at the upper end of membrane for the passage of posterior interosseous artery to reach the posterior compartment of forearm.
- Identify another foramen at the lower end of membrane for passage of anterior interosseous artery to reach into posterior compartment of forearm.
- See the attachment of interosseous membrane on posterior border of triangular area on lowest part of medial surface of radius.

Recollect functions of interosseous membrane
1. Keeps the bones together at appropriate distance
2. Transfers the force from radius towards ulna
3. Gives passage for vessels
4. Increases surface area for the attachment of muscles on both aspects.

Inferior Radioulnar Joint and Wrist Joint

Inferior radioulnar joint is a joint between head of ulna and ulnar notch of radius (Fig. 8.12). It is also a pivot joint of synovial variety.

Movements and muscles involved at superior and inferior radioulnar joints are pronation and supination. These are shown in Table 8.4.

Attachments on the bones are shown in Fig. 8.10.

WRIST JOINT

Wrist joint is formed by distal end of radius including the intra-articular disc of inferior radioulnar joint and two carpal bones, i.e. scaphoid and lunate. It is an ellipsoid joint of synovial variety (Fig. 8.13).

Table 8.4: Showing movements at superior and inferior radioulnar joints with their muscles and nerve supply

Movement	Main muscle	Nerve supply
Pronation	Pronator quadratus	Anterior interosseous nerve
	Pronator teres	Median nerve
½ pronation	Brachioradialis	Radial nerve
Supination	Biceps brachii	Musculocutaneous nerve
	Supinator	Posterior interosseous nerve
½ supination	Brachioradialis	Radial nerve

Remove all the tendons from the anterior and posterior aspects of inferior radioulnar joint and wrist joints.

Cut through the capsule of inferior radioulnar joint to locate the intra-articular fibrocartilagenous disc in inferior radioulnar joint. The movement of pronation and supination occur at this joint along with same movement at superior radioulnar joint.

Steps of Dissection

- Cut through the thenar and hypothenar muscles from their origins and reflect them distally.
- Separate the flexor and extensor retinacula of the wrist from the bones.
- Cut through flexor and extensor tendons (if not already done) and reflect them distally.
- Define the capsular attachments and ligaments and relations of the wrist joint.
- Identify the capsule surrounding the wrist joint.
- Identify palmar radiocarpal and palmar ulnocarpal ligaments.

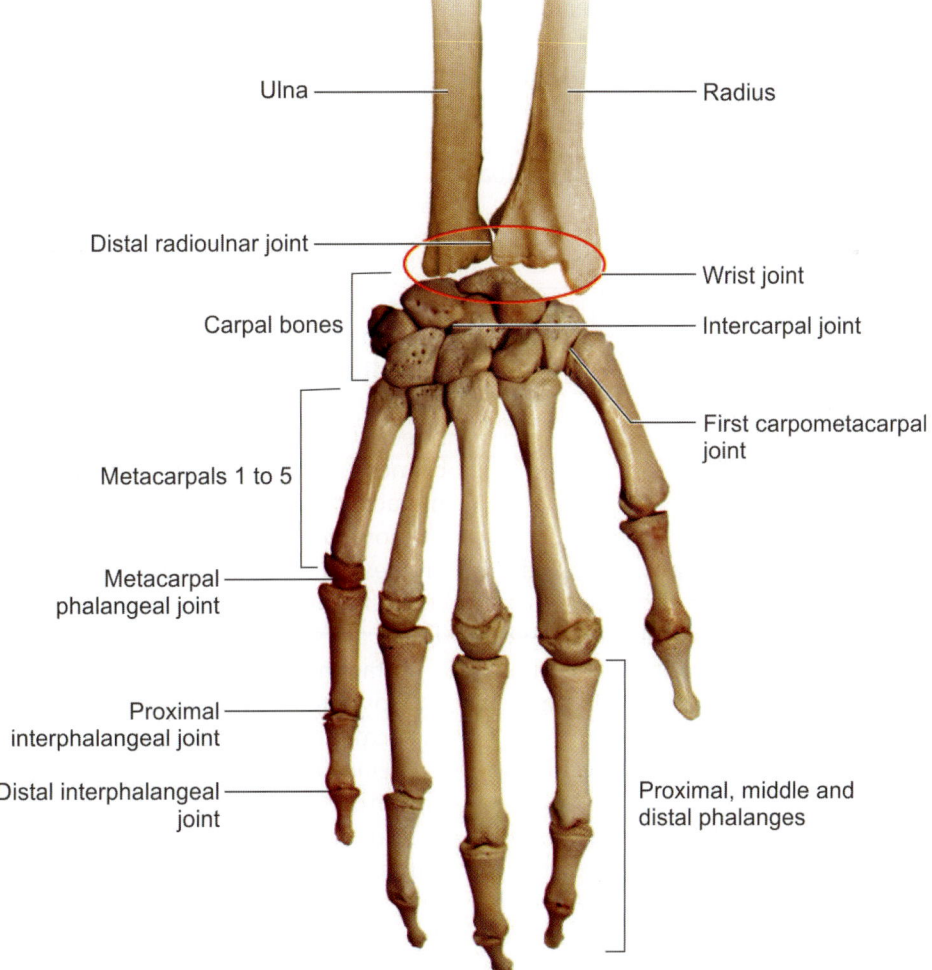

Fig. 8.13: Lower ends of radius, ulna, carpals, metacarpals and phalanges with their joints

Table 8.5: Showing movements at wrist joint, intercarpal and 2nd–5th carpometacarpal joints with their muscles and nerve supply

Movement	Main muscles	Nerve supply
Flexion	Flexor carpi radialis	Median nerve
	Flexor carpi ulnaris	Ulnar nerve
	Palmaris longus	Median nerve
Extension	Extensor carpi radialis longus	Posterior interosseous nerve
	Extensor carpi radialis brevis	Posterior interosseous nerve
	Extensor carpi ulnaris	Posterior interosseous nerve
Abduction	Flexor carpi radialis	Median nerve
	Extensor carpi radialis longus	Posterior interosseous nerve
	Extensor carpi radialis brevis	Posterior interosseous nerve
	Abductor pollicis longus	Posterior interosseous nerve
Adduction	Flexor carpi ulnaris	Ulnar nerve
	Extensor carpi ulnaris	Posterior interosseous nerve

Circumduction: A movement involving above movements in a sequence.

- On the back of the wrist look for weaker dorsal radiocarpal ligament.
- Movements of flexion, extension, abduction, adduction and circumduction take place at wrist joint. These are shown in Table 8.5.

Attachments on the bones are shown in Figs 8.10a and b and 8.15a and b.

JOINTS OF HAND

The joints of hand include:

- Intercarpal
- Carpometacarpal
- Metacarpophalangeal
- Interphalangeal joints (Fig. 8.13)

Steps of Dissection

- Out of these, the most important joint with a separate joint cavity is the first carpometacarpal joint. This is the joint of the thumb and a wide variety of functionally useful movements take place here. Identify the distal surface of trapezium and base of first metacarpal bone.
- Define the metacarpophalangeal and interphalangeal joints.
- For their dissection, remove all the muscles and tendons from the anterior and posterior aspects of any two metacarpophalangeal joints. Define the articular capsule and ligaments. Do the same for proximal and distal interphalangeal joints of one of the fingers and define the ligaments.

Intercarpal joint chiefly lies between proximal and distal rows of carpal bones. The synovial cavity to all the intercarpal joints is common. Only two bones triquetral and pisiform have a separate synovial cavity (Fig. 8.14).

Carpometacarpal joints are present between distal row of carpal bones and the bases of metacarpal bones cavity (Fig. 8.14).

The joint cavity is common to all joints. Only the cavity of distal surface of trapezium and base of first metacarpal, i.e. 1st carpometacarpal joint is separate. Thus the intercarpal and carpometacarpal joints have one big synovial cavity except two separate cavities, one between triquetral and pisiform (at upper medial corner) and other one between trapezium and 1st metacarpal (at lower lateral corner).

Movements permitted at first carpometacarpal joint are flexion with medial rotation, extension with lateral rotation, abduction, adduction and circumduction. These are shown in Table 8.6.

Attachments on the bones are shown in Fig. 8.15.

Movements at intercarpal joints are assisting in the movement at the wrist joint.

Metacarpophalangeal joint of thumb: For movements and muscles involved at this joint Table 8.7.

2nd–5th metacarpophalangeal joints are ellipsoid joints of synovial variety. Take the index finger as a sample.

- Remove tendons of long flexor muscles (flexor digitorum profundus and flexor digitorum superficialis).

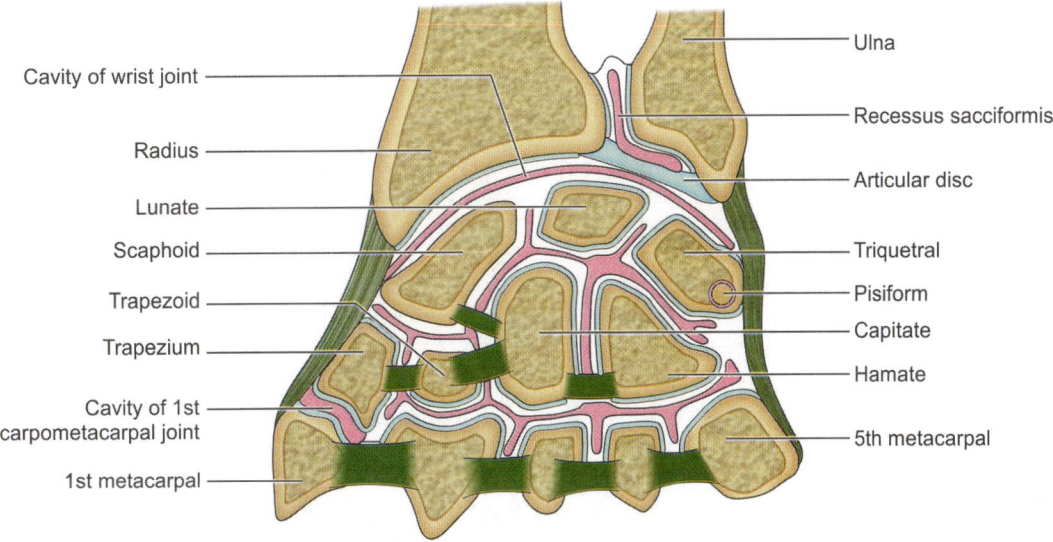

Fig. 8.14: Cavity of wrist, inferior radioulnar, intercarpal and 1st carpometacarpal joints

Table 8.6: Showing movements at 1st carpometacarpal joint with their muscles and nerve supply

Movement	Main muscles	Nerve supply
Flexion	Flexor pollicis brevis	Median nerve
	Opponens pollicis	Median nerve
Extension	Extensor pollicis brevis	Posterior interosseous nerve
	Extensor pollicis longus	Posterior interosseous nerve
Abduction	Abductor pollicis brevis	Median nerve
	Abductor pollicis longus	Posterior interosseous nerve
Adduction	Adductor pollicis	Ulnar nerve
Opposition	Opponens pollicis	Median nerve

Circumduction: A movement involving above movements in a sequence.

Table 8.7: Showing movements at 1st metacarpophalangeal joint with their muscles and nerve supply

Movement	Main muscles	Nerve supply
Flexion	Flexor pollicis brevis	Median nerve
Extension	Extensor pollicis brevis	Posterior interosseous nerve
Abduction	Abductor pollicis brevis	Median nerve
Adduction	Adductor pollicis	Deep branch of ulnar nerve

Circumduction: A movement involving above movements in a sequence.

- Remove the interossei, lumbricals, extensor digitorum and extensor indicis tendons.
- See the capsule is thin on anterior and posterior aspects
- Identify and clean the collateral ligaments on each side.
- These joints permit flexion, extension, abduction, adduction and circumduction movements. These with the muscles involved are shown in Table 8.8. Attachments on the bones are shown in Fig. 8.15.

Interphalangeal joint of thumb. For movements with muscles at this joint (Table 8.9).

Interphalangeal joints are synovial joints of hinge variety allowing movements of flexion and extension only. The joint capsule is supplemented by strong collateral ligaments.

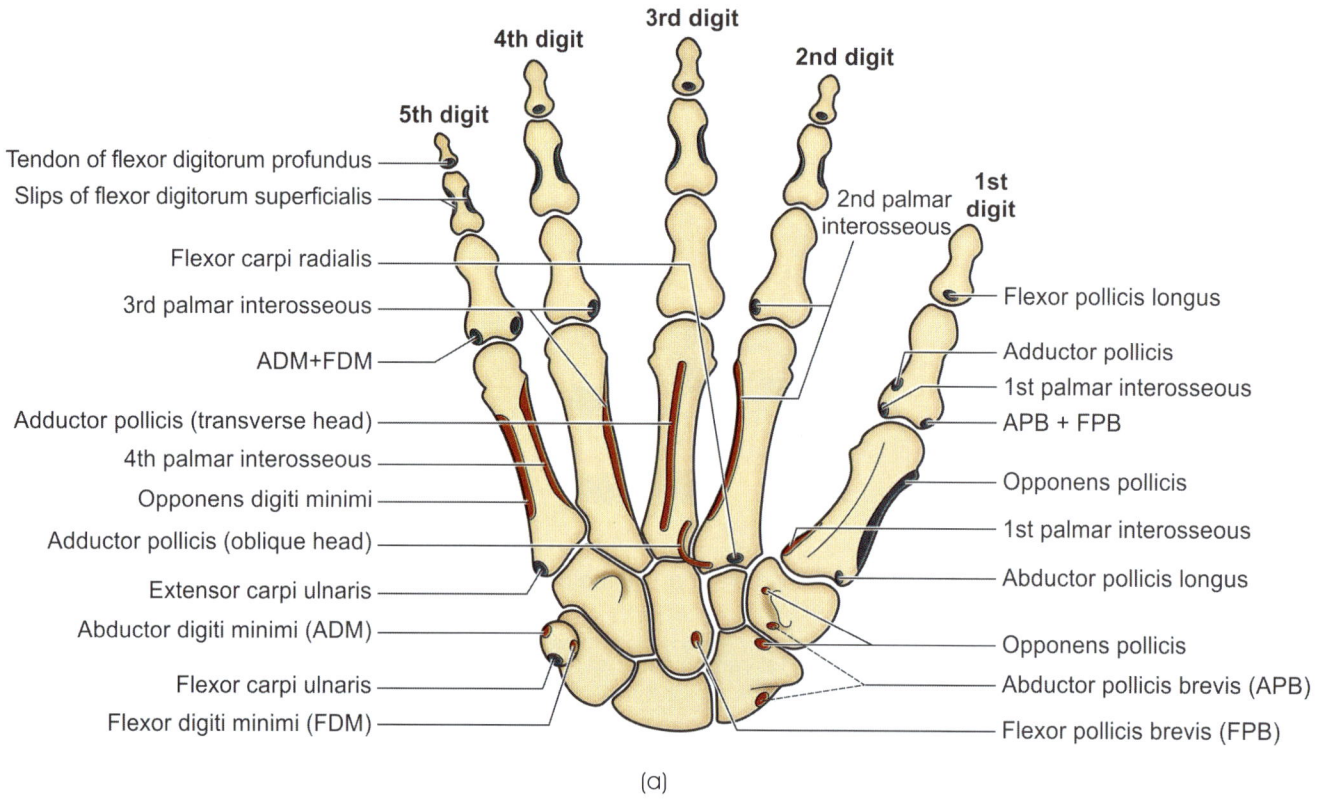

4th digit

3rd digit

2nd digit

5th digit

Tendon of flexor digitorum profundus
Slips of flexor digitorum superficialis

2nd palmar interosseous

1st digit

Flexor carpi radialis

3rd palmar interosseous

Flexor pollicis longus

ADM+FDM

Adductor pollicis
1st palmar interosseous
APB + FPB

Adductor pollicis (transverse head)
4th palmar interosseous
Opponens digiti minimi
Adductor pollicis (oblique head)
Extensor carpi ulnaris
Abductor digiti minimi (ADM)
Flexor carpi ulnaris
Flexor digiti minimi (FDM)

Opponens pollicis
1st palmar interosseous
Abductor pollicis longus
Opponens pollicis
Abductor pollicis brevis (APB)
Flexor pollicis brevis (FPB)

(a)

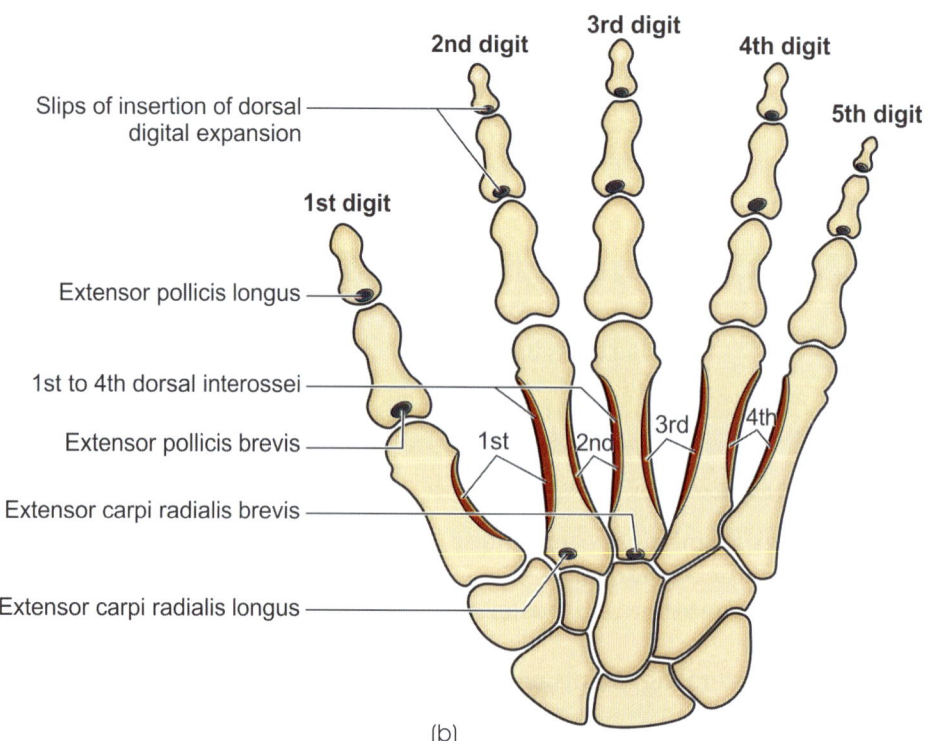

3rd digit

2nd digit

4th digit

5th digit

Slips of insertion of dorsal digital expansion

1st digit

Extensor pollicis longus

1st to 4th dorsal interossei

Extensor pollicis brevis

1st   2nd   3rd   4th

Extensor carpi radialis brevis

Extensor carpi radialis longus

(b)

Fig. 8.15: Attachments on the skeleton of hand: (a) Anterior aspect, and (b) posterior aspect

Table 8.8: Showing movements at 2nd to 5th metacarpophalangeal joints with their muscles and nerve supply

Movement	Main muscles	Nerve supply
Flexion	Flexor digitorum superficialis	Median nerve
	Flexor digitorum profundus	Median for tendons of 2nd and 3rd digits, ulnar for tendons of 4th and 5th digits
Extension	Extensor digitorum	Posterior interosseous
Abduction	Dorsal interossei	Deep branch of ulnar nerve
Adduction	Palmar interossei	Deep branch of ulnar nerve

Circumduction: A movement involving above movements in a sequence.

Table 8.9: Showing movements at interphalangeal joint of thumb/1st digit with their muscles and nerve supply

Movement	Main muscles	Nerve supply
Flexion	Flexor pollicis longus	Anterior interosseous nerve
Extension	Extensor pollicis longus	Posterior interosseous nerve

Table 8.10: Proximal interphalangeal joints of 2nd–5th digits

Movement	Main muscles	Nerve supply
Flexion	Flexor digitorum superficialis	Median nerve
	Flexor digitorum profundus	Anterior interosseous nerve for tendons of 2nd, 3rd digits, and ulnar nerve for tendons of 4th, 5th digits
Extension	Lumbricals (1–4)	Median nerve for 1st and 2nd, and ulnar nerve for 3rd and 4th lumbricals
	Interossei—4 palmar and 4 dorsal	Deep branch of ulnar nerve

Table 8.11: Showing movements at distal interphalangeal joints of 2nd–5th digits with their muscles and nerve supply

Movement	Main muscles	Nerve supply
Flexion	Flexor digitorum profundus	Anterior interosseous nerve for 2nd, 3rd digits, and ulnar nerve for 4th, 5th digits
Extension	Lumbricals (1–4)	Median nerve for 1st and 2nd, ulnar nerve for 3rd and 4th
	Interossei	Deep branch of ulnar nerve

The first digit/thumb contains only one interphalangeal joint.

2nd–5th digits contain proximal and distal interphalangeal joints.

Movements with muscles of the proximal interphalangeal joints are shown in Table 8.10. Movements with muscles of distal interphalangeal joints are shown in Table 8.11.

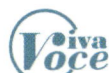

Viva Voce

- What type of joint is sternoclavicular joint?
- Name the movements of shoulder girdle.
- Which tendon is intracapsular in the shoulder joint?
- What types of joints are superior and inferior radio-ulnar joints?
- Name the functions of interosseous membrane.
- Name the bones participating in 1st carpometacarpal joint. Show the movements of this joint.
- Which is the only muscle causing flexion of distal interphalangeal joints of the fingers?

1. a. Identify the condition given in figure.
    b. When does it occur?

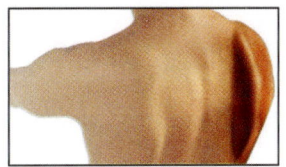

2. a. Name the nerves in given figure.
    b. What is the effect of paralysis of nerve lying behind medial epicondyle of humerus?

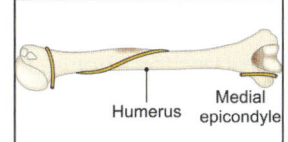

3. a. Identify the structure shown in figure.
    b. Where does it drain?

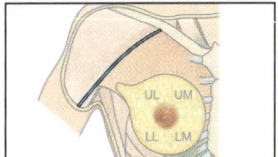

4. a. Identify the structures shown in figure.
    b. Where does the nerve arise from?

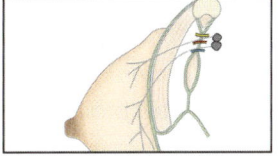

5. a. Identify the nerve in the centre of figure.
    b. What syndrome is associated with this nerve?

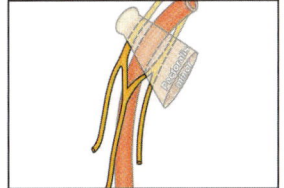

6. a. Identify the point in given figure.
    b. Name the nerves related to this point?

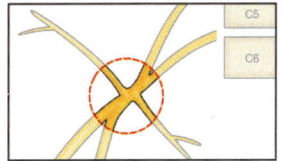

7. a. Identify the nerve in the figure.
    b. Name the muscles supplied by it.

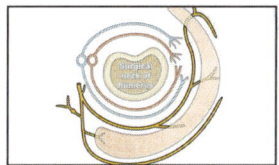

8. a. Identify the space in the given figure.
    b. What are its contents?

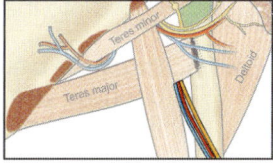

9. a. Identify the septum in given figure.
    b. Name structures piercing the septum.

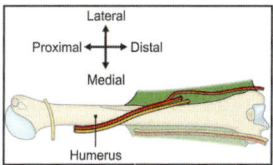

10. a. What does the given picture show?
    b. What nerve innervates this muscle?

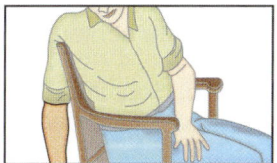

11. a. Name these 4 muscles shown in figure.
    b. Which nerves innervate these muscles?

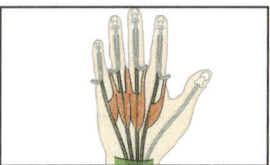

12. a. Which test is shown in the figure?
    b. For which syndrome is this test done?

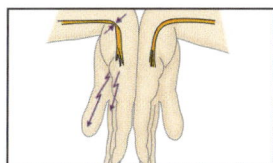

ANSWERS: SPOTS ON UPPER LIMB

1. a. Winging of the scapula.
    b. Occurs when nerve to serratus anterior/long thoracic nerve is injured.

2. a. The nerves are axillary, radial and ulnar.
    b. Paralysis of ulnar nerve leads to partial clawing of the hand, atrophy of most intrinsic muscles with gutters in the hand.

3. a. Cephalic vein running in deltopectoral groove.
    b. Drains into the axillary vein.

4. a. Structures piercing the clavipectoral fascia are lateral pectoral nerve, thoracoacromial artery and cephalic vein.
    b. The lateral pectoral nerve is a branch of lateral cord of brachial plexus.

5. a. Nerve in the centre is the median nerve.
    b. Carpal tunnel syndrome.

6. a. The point is Erb's point.
    b. Nerves here are ventral rami of C5, C6 to form upper trunk; nerve to subclavius, suprascapular nerve, and terior and posterior divisions of the upper trunk. Thus there are 6 nerves at Erb's point.

7. a. Nerve is axillary/circumflex nerve.
    b. Its muscular branches are given to deltoid and teres minor muscles.

8. a. The space is lower triangular space.
    b. Its contents are profunda brachii vessels and radial nerve.

9. a. Septum is lateral intermuscular septum.
    b. It is pierced by radial nerve and anterior branch of profunda brachii artery.

10. a. Saturday night palsy due to paralysis of triceps brachii muscle.
    b. Radial nerve innervates this muscles.

11. a. These muscles are 4 lumbrical muscles.
    b. The lateral 2 lumbricals are innervated by median nerve. Medial 2 lumbricals get innervated by deep branch of ulnar nerve.

12. a. The test shown is Phalen's test.
    b. It is positive in carpal tunnel syndrome.

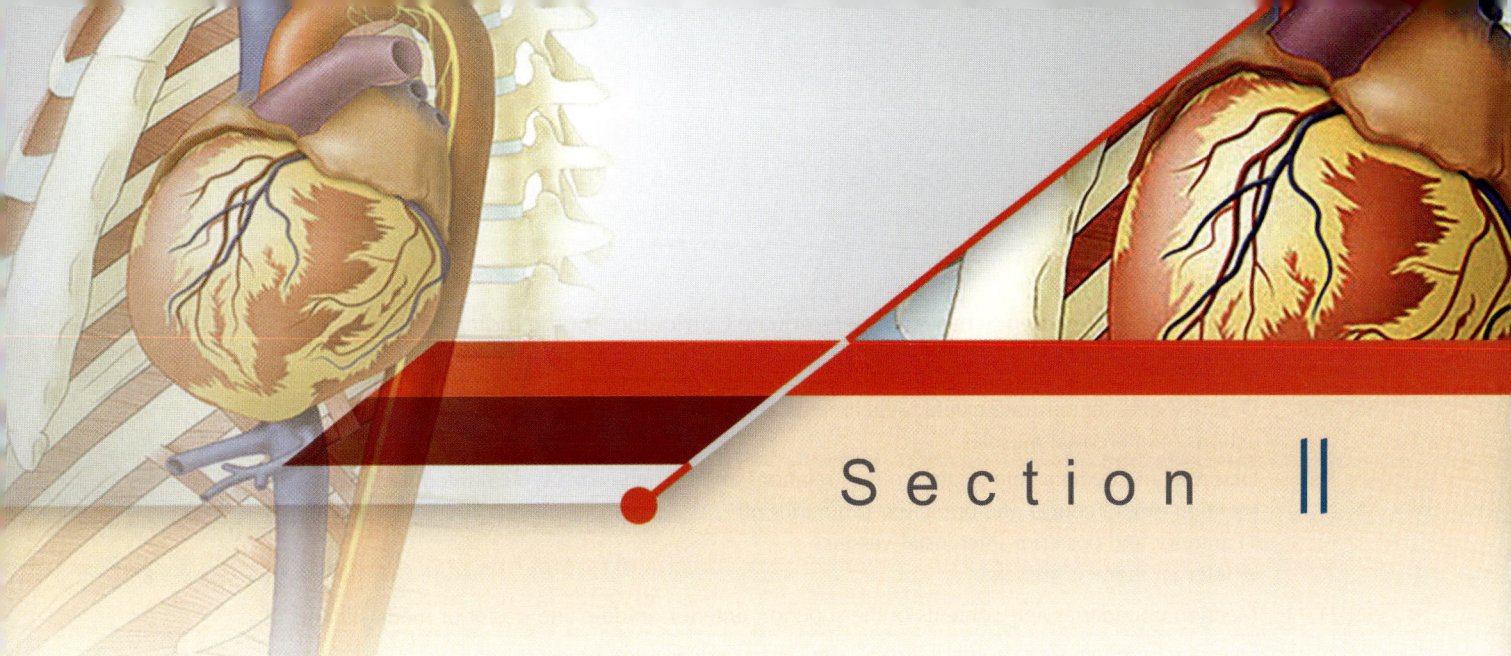

Section II

Thorax

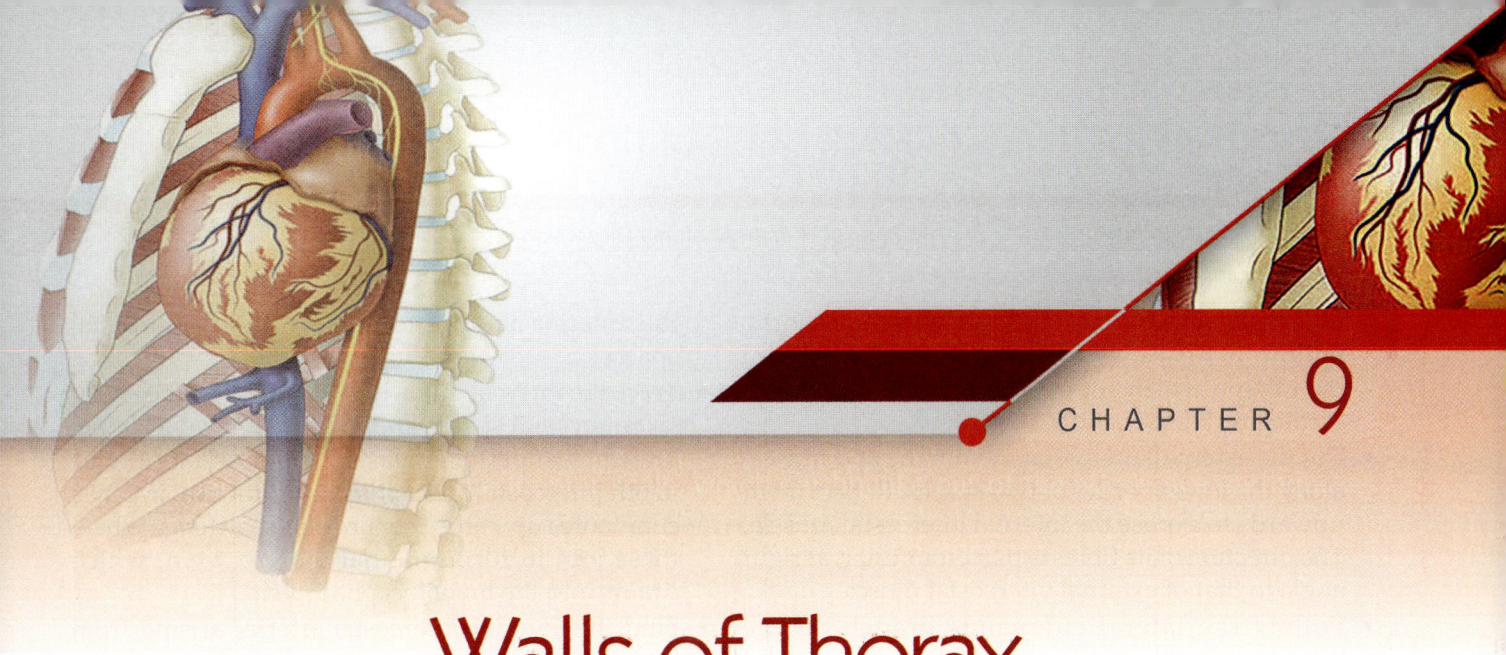

CHAPTER 9

Walls of Thorax

Learning Objectives

One should be able to

1. Correlate the direction of fibres of external and internal intercostal muscles with their actions.
2. Name the three subdivisions of the innermost intercostal muscle.
3. Name the arteries which provide branches as anterior intercostal and posterior intercostal arteries for the thoracic wall?
4. Enumerate the veins which carry venous blood from various intercostal spaces?

OVERVIEW

Thorax is covered by muscles of thorax. In addition the wall is covered by muscles of upper limb, e.g. pectoralis major in front, serratus anterior laterally and latissimus dorsi, trapezius, etc. posteriorly.

The muscular wall of thorax comprises external intercostal, internal intercostal and innermost intercostal muscles. Their main actions are to maintain integrity of the thoracic wall. External intercostal prevents indrawing of thoracic wall during inspiration. Internal intercostal prevents outward bulging of the wall during expiration. The neurovascular bundle lies between internal intercostal and interrupted innermost intercostal muscle.

Blood supply is from internal thoracic artery. The nerves are upper and lower intercostal nerves. The upper intercostal nerves not only supply these muscles, but also supply parietal pleura, periosteum of the ribs and skin overlying these intercostal spaces. The lower intercostal nerves supply in addition to the above structures, the parietal peritoneum of abdominal cavity. Since there are twelve ribs and intercostal space is below respective rib, there are eleven intercostal nerves and the 12th nerve is called subcostal nerve.

Each intercostal space contains three sets of muscles. In addition, it contains two arteries and veins coming from posterior aspect and two from anterior aspect which anastomose with each other.

Thorax also contains the sympathetic trunks which give branches for the thoracic viscera and splanchnic branches for abdominal and pelvic viscera.

> *Competency achievement:* The student should be able to:
>
> **AN 21.4** Describe and demonstrate extent, attachments, direction of fibres, nerve supply and actions of intercostal muscles.
>
> **AN 21.5** Describe and demonstrate origin, course, relations and branches of a typical intercostal nerve.
>
> **AN 21.6** Mention origin, course and branches/ tributaries of:
> 1. Anterior and posterior intercostal vessels
> 2. Internal thoracic vessels.

STEPS OF DISSECTION

- Detach the serratus anterior and the pectoralis major muscles from the upper ribs. Note the external intercostal muscle in the second and third intercostal spaces. Its fibres run anteroinferiorly. Follow it forwards to the external intercostal membrane which replaces it between the costal cartilages (Figs 9.1 and 9.2).

- Cut the external intercostal membrane and muscle along the lower border of two spaces. Reflect them upwards to expose the internal intercostal muscle. The direction of its fibres is posteroinferior, at right angle to that of external intercostal muscle.

- Follow the lateral cutaneous branch of one intercostal nerve to its trunk deep to internal intercostal muscle. Trace the nerve and accompanying vessels round the thoracic wall. Note their collateral branches lying along the upper margin of the rib below. Trace the muscular branches of the trunk of intercostal nerve and its collateral branch. Trace the anterior cutaneous nerve as well.

- Identify the deepest muscle in the intercostal space, the innermost intercostal muscle (Fig. 9.3). This muscle does not form a continuous sheet. It is seen to consist of three parts—sternocostalis, intercostalis intimi and subcostalis. This muscle is deficient in

the anterior and posterior ends of the intercostal spaces.

- Trace the internal thoracic artery through the upper six intercostal spaces and identify its two terminal branches, superior epigastric and musculophrenic in 6th intercostal space (Fig. 9.4). Trace their venae comitantes upwards till third costal cartilage where these join to form internal thoracic vein, which drains into the brachiocephalic vein.

- Find the anterior intercostal arteries arising from internal thoracic artery.

- Incise the periosteum of the fifth rib longitudinally along its length. Divide the rib at posterior axillary line and at the costochondral junction. Take the rib out leaving the periosteum. This way one can visualise intercostal vessels and intercostal nerve in the costal groove.

- Identify the main intercostal nerve (Fig. 9.5) and trace its collateral, lateral cutaneous, muscular, periosteal and anterior cutaneous branches. Its collateral branch runs along the upper border of the rib below along with collateral branch of posterior intercostal artery and its accompanying

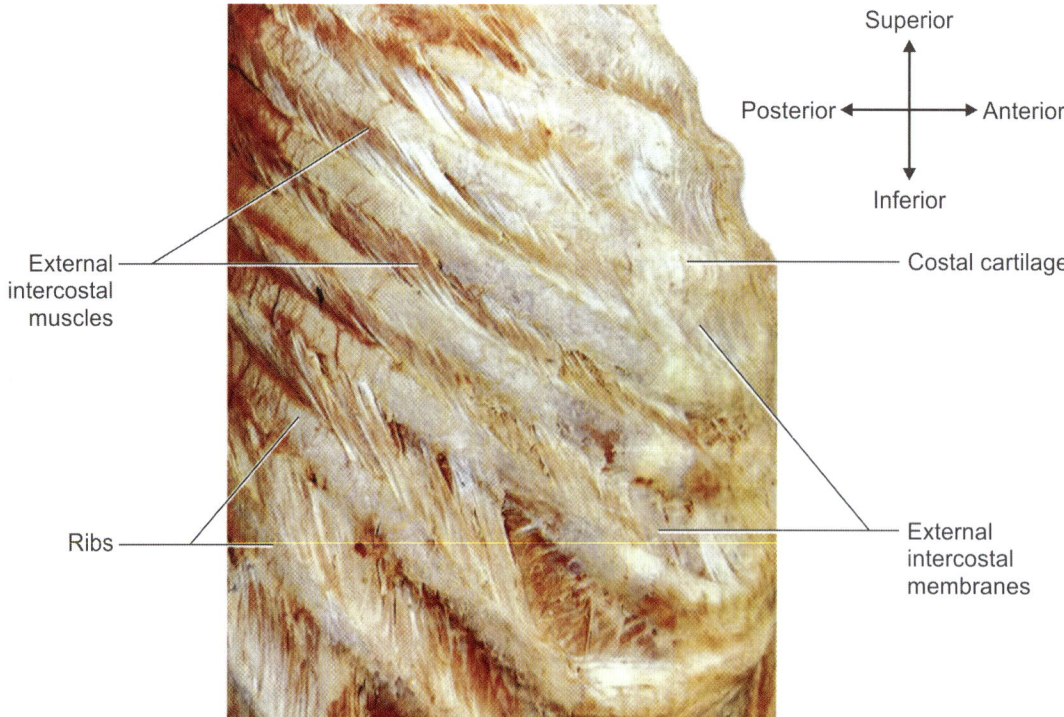

Fig. 9.1: External intercostal muscles and membranes

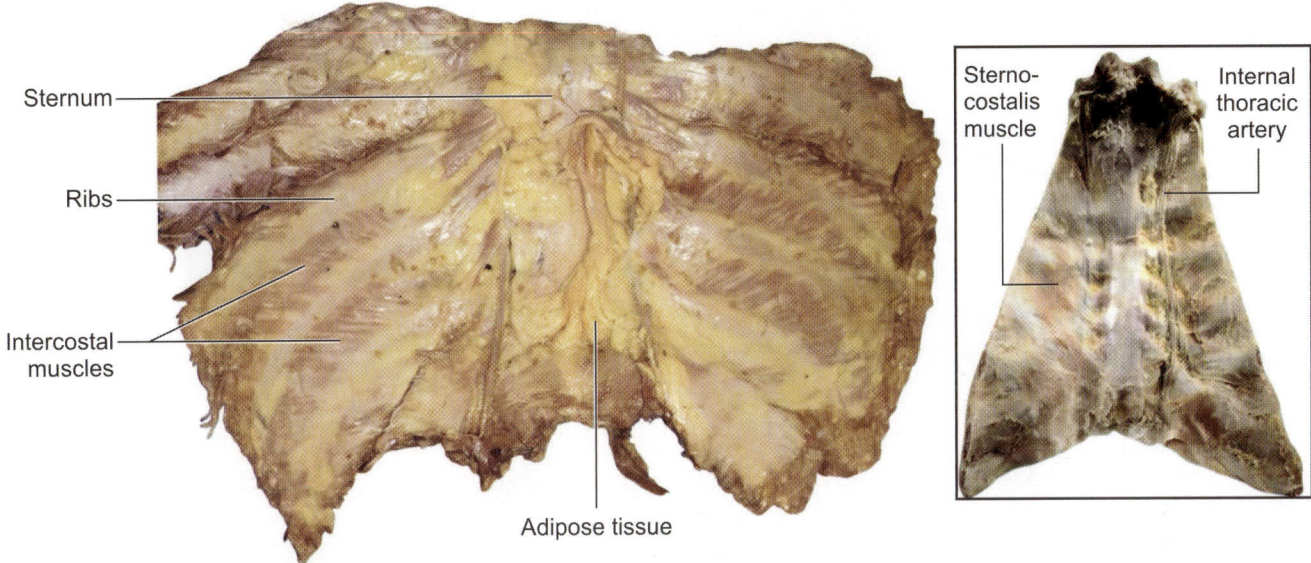

Fig. 9.2: Posterior aspect of sternum and intercostal spaces with muscles and artery

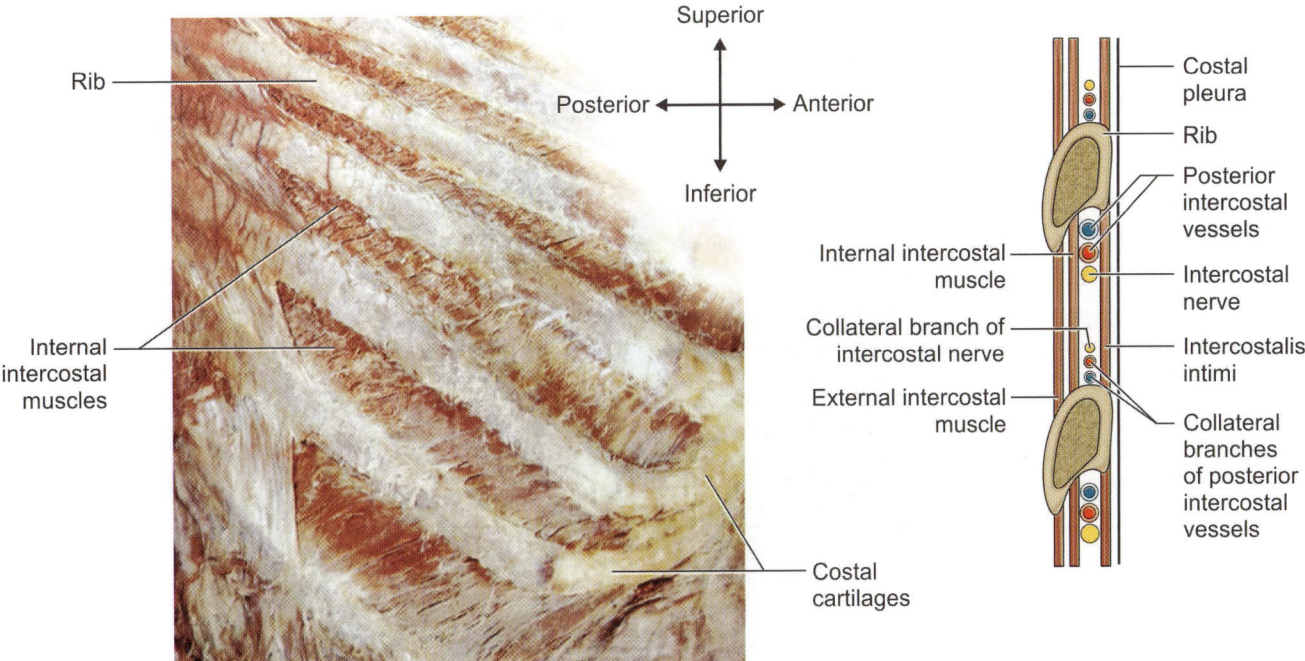

Fig. 9.3: Internal intercostal muscles

vein. Appreciate the order of structures as posterior intercostal **v**ein, posterior intercostal **a**rtery and intercostal **n**erve (VAN). The posterior intercostal artery and its collateral branch anastomose with two small anterior intercostal branches of internal thoracic artery.

• See that the neurovascular plane lies between internal intercostal and innermost intercostal muscles.

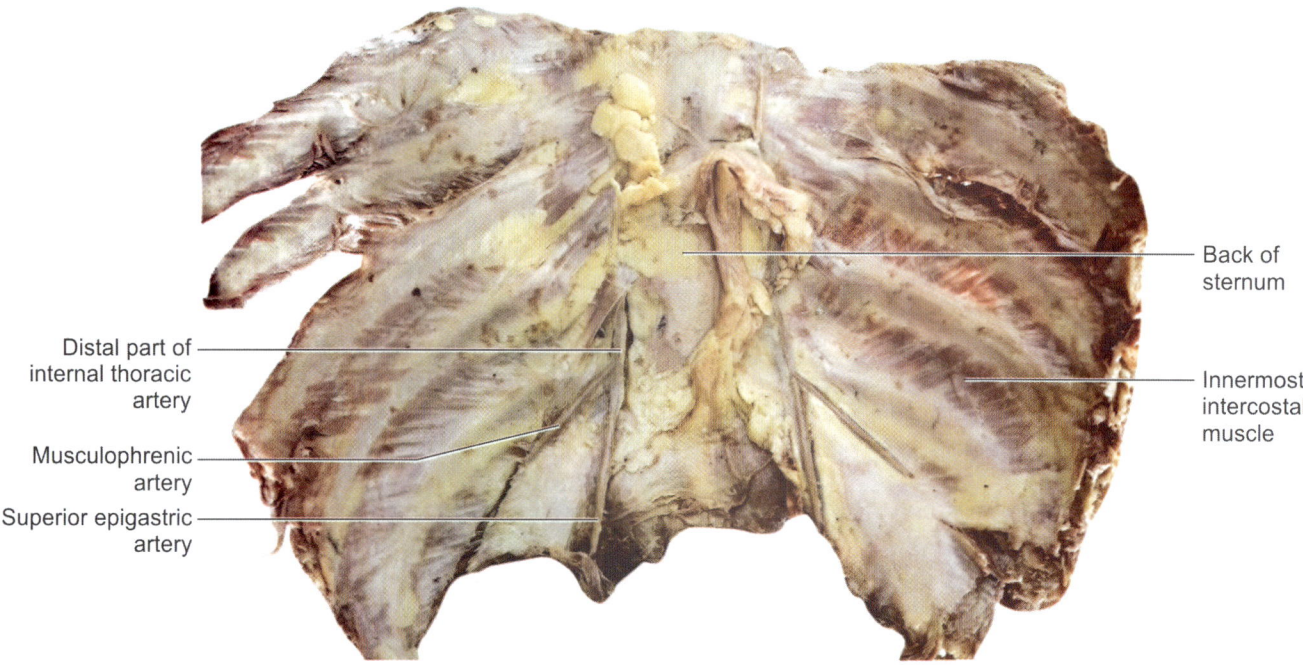

Distal part of internal thoracic artery

Musculophrenic artery

Superior epigastric artery

Back of sternum

Innermost intercostal muscle

Fig. 9.4: Internal thoracic artery with its two terminal branches

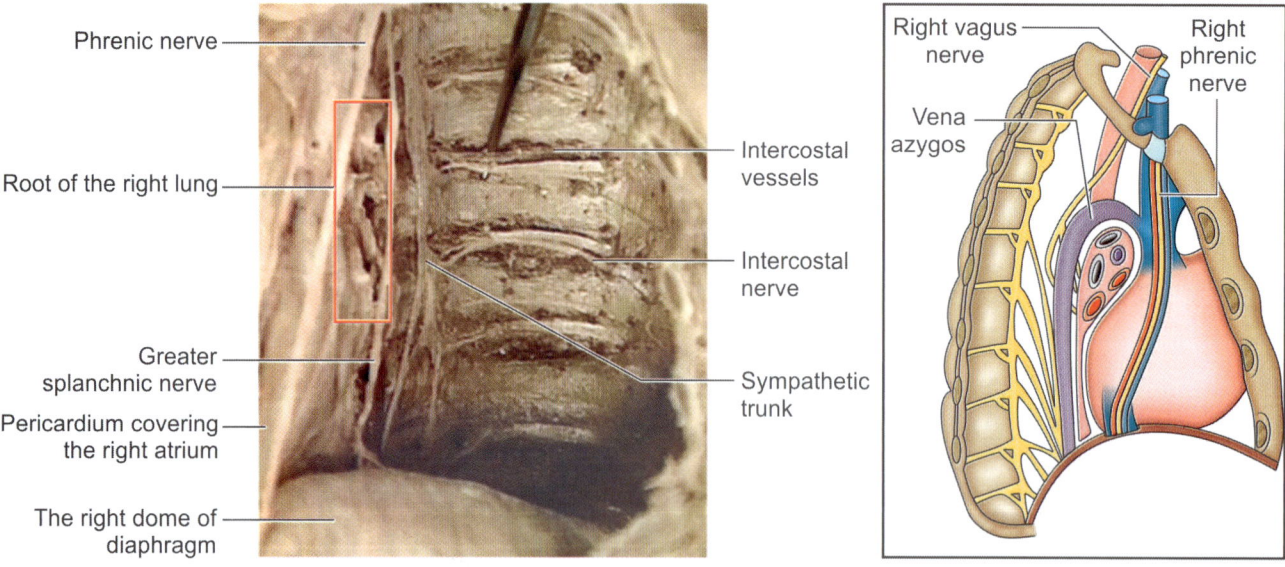

Phrenic nerve

Root of the right lung

Greater splanchnic nerve

Pericardium covering the right atrium

The right dome of diaphragm

Intercostal vessels

Intercostal nerve

Sympathetic trunk

Right vagus nerve

Right phrenic nerve

Vena azygos

Fig. 9.5: Structures in the mediastinum as seen from right side

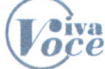

- Name the layers of intercostal muscles.
- Where does the neurovascular plane lie?
- How many intercostal spaces are on the anterior aspect of thorax?
- Name the structures in order in the costal groove.

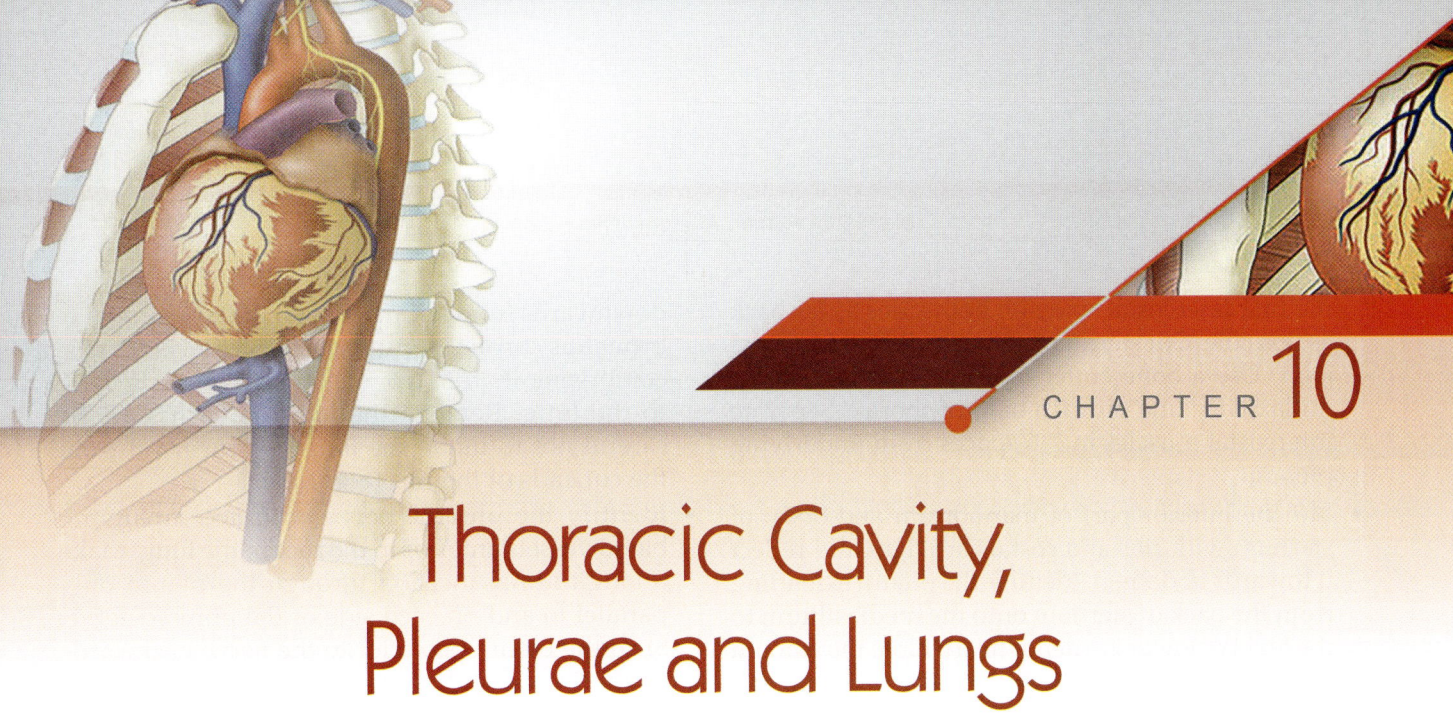

CHAPTER 10

Thoracic Cavity, Pleurae and Lungs

Learning Objectives

One should be able to

1. Do the surface marking of the parietal pleura.
2. Compare the visceral and parietal pleurae.
3. Enumerate the nerve supply of various parts of parietal pleura.
4. Explain the anatomical basis of paracentesis thoracis.

5. Compare the structures at the hila of the right and left lung.
6. Enumerate differences in the bronchopulmonary segments of right and left lungs.
7. Enumerate the differences between the right and left lungs.

OVERVIEW

Most of the thoracic cavity is occupied by the right and left pleural cavities. These cavities contain the lung and a small amount of pleural fluid between the visceral and parietal layers. The parietal layer of pleura behaves like the parieties whereas visceral layer behaves like the lungs as far as the nerve supply and vascular supply is concerned. The differences between the two layers should be read from BD Chaurasia's *Human Anatomy*. Parietal pleura extends into the neck above the clavicles and below the necks of 12th ribs posteriorly on both sides and only into the right xiphicostal angle. These are five areas where parietal pleura goes beyond the costal margin. Injury in these areas can cause lots of complications.

On the left side, close to the left margin of sternum, between 4th and 6th intercostal spaces an enlarged space called left costomediastinal recess. It lies between visceral and parietal layers of pleurae. Similarly on each side of the thorax there are costodiaphragmatic recesses. Into these three spaces the lungs expand during inspiration.

Parietal pleura is innervated by thoracic nerves and phrenic nerve.

Visceral pleura gets sympathetic nerve supply from T2–T5 ganglia and parasympathetic from vagi.

The clinical conditions associated with pleura are pleural effusion, pneumothorax, hemothorax, etc.

The two lungs occupy most of the thoracic cavity leaving little space for the heart. Heart excavates more into the left lung, leaving it longer, thinner and lighter than the right lung.

Competency achievement: The student should be able to:

AN 24.1 Mention the blood supply, lymphatic drainage and nerve supply of pleura, extent of pleura and describe the pleural recesses and their applied anatomy.

AN 24.2 Identify side, external features and relations of structures which form root of lung and bronchial tree and their clinical correlate.

STEPS OF DISSECTION

- Divide the manubrium sterni transversely immediately inferior to its junction with the first costal cartilage. Cut through the parietal pleura in the first intercostal space on both sides as far back as possible. Cut sternum at the level of xiphisternal joint. Use a bone cutter to cut 2nd to 7th ribs in midaxillary line on each side of thorax. Separate intercostal muscles in 1–6 spaces from underlying pleura.

- Lift the inferior part of manubrium and body of sternum with ribs and costal cartilages and reflect it towards abdomen. Identify the pleura extending from the back of sternum onto the mediastinum to the level of lower border of heart. Note the smooth surface of pleura where it lines the thoracic wall and covers the lateral aspects of mediastinum. Trace the surface marking of parietal pleura on the skeleton.

- Remove the pleura and the endothoracic fascia from the back of sternum and costal cartilages which is reflected towards abdomen. Identify the transversus thoracis muscle and internal thoracic vessels (*see* Fig 9.4).

- Examine the lower limits of the lungs. These limits are two ribs above the parietal pleura at midclavicular, midaxillary and paravertebral lines (Fig 10.1). These are 6th, 8th and 10th ribs, respectively.

- Pull the lung laterally from the mediastinum and find its root with the pulmonary ligament extending downwards from it. Cut through the structures, i.e. bronchus/bronchi, pulmonary vessels, nerves, comprising its root from above downwards close to the lung. Remove the lung on each side. Be careful not to injure the lung or your hand from the cut ends of the ribs (Fig. 10.2).

- Identify the phrenic nerve with accompanying blood vessels anterior to the root of the lung. Make a longitudinal incision through the pleura only parallel to and on each side of the phrenic nerve. Strip the pleura posterior to the nerve backwards to the intercostal spaces. Pull the anterior flap forwards to reveal part of the pericardium with the heart. Identify the following structures seen through the pleura.

Right side

1. Bulge of the heart and pericardium anteroinferior to the root of the lung.
2. A longitudinal ridge formed by right brachiocephalic vein down to first costal cartilage and by superior vena cava up to the bulge of the heart.
3. A smaller longitudinal ridge formed by inferior vena cava formed between the heart and the diaphragm.
4. Phrenic nerve with accompanying vessels forming a vertical ridge on these two venae cavae passing anterior to root of the lung (*see* Fig 9.5).

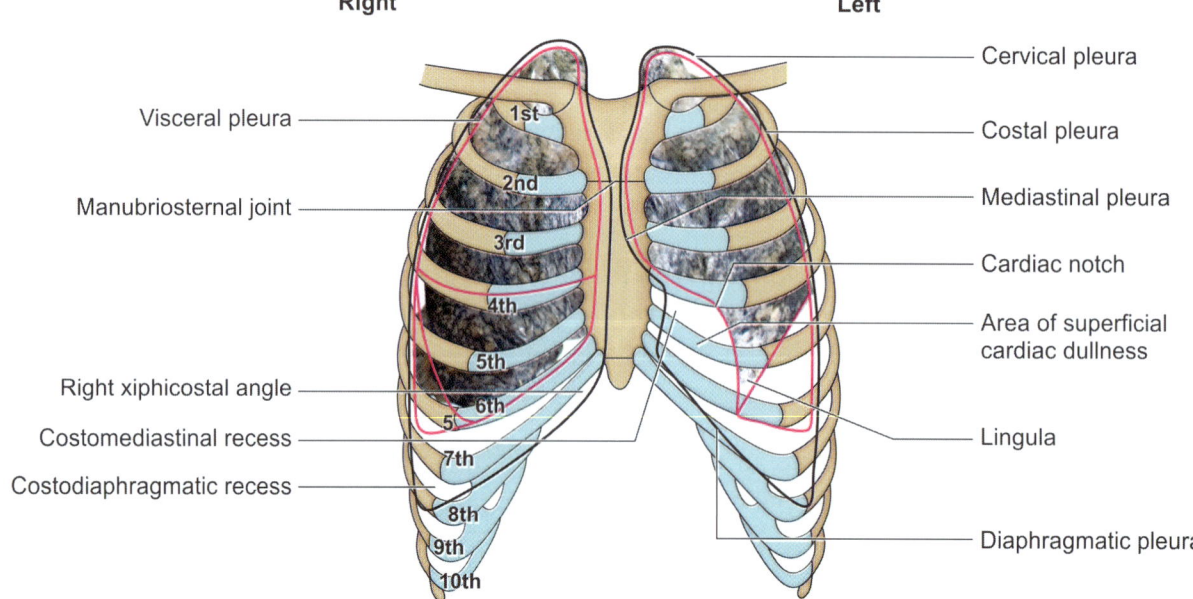

Fig. 10.1: Surface projection of parietal pleura (black): visceral pleura and lung (pink) on the front of thorax

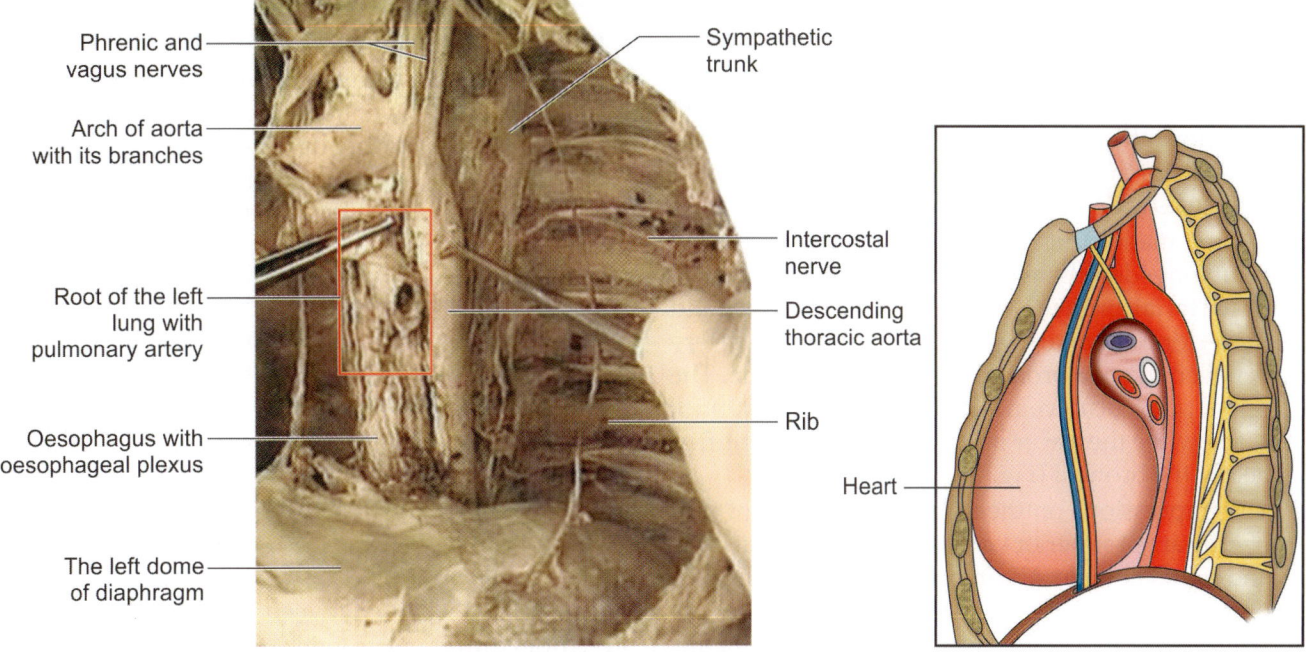

Fig. 10.2: Structures in the mediastinum as seen from left side

5. Vena azygos arching over root of the lung to enter the superior vena cava (*see* Fig. 9.5).
6. Trachea and oesophagus posterior to the phrenic nerve and superior vena cava.
7. Right vagus nerve descending posteroinferiorly across the trachea, behind the root of the lung.
8. Bodies of the thoracic vertebrae behind oesophagus with posterior intercostal vessels and azygos vein lying over them.
9. Sympathetic trunk on the heads of the upper ribs and on the sides of the vertebral bodies below this, anterior to the posterior intercostal vessels and intercostal nerves.

Left side
1. Bulge of the heart.
2. Root of lung posterosuperior to it.
3. Descending aorta between (1) and (2) in front and vertebral column behind (Fig. 10.2).
4. Arch of aorta over the root of the lung.
5. Left common carotid and left subclavian arteries passing superiorly from the arch of aorta.
6. Phrenic and vagus nerves descending between these vessels and the lateral surface of the aortic arch (Fig. 10.2).
7. Sympathetic trunk same as on right side.

• Identify longitudinally running sympathetic trunk on the posterior part of thoracic cavity. Find delicate greater and lesser splanchnic nerves arising from the trunk on the medial side. Look carefully for grey and white rami communicantes between the intercostal nerve and the ganglia on the sympathetic trunk.
• Trace the intercostal vessels above the intercostal nerve. The order being **v**ein, **a**rtery and **n**erve (VAN).
• On the right side, identify and follow one of the divisions of trachea to the lung root and the superior and inferior venae cavae till the pericardium.
• On the left side of thoracic cavity, dissect the arch of aorta. Identify the superior cervical cardiac branch of the left sympathetic trunk and the inferior cervical cardiac branch of the left vagus on the arch of the aorta between the vagus nerve posteriorly and phrenic nerve anteriorly (cardiac nerves).
• The cavity of the thorax contains the right and left pleural cavities which are completely invaginated and occupied by the lungs. The right and left pleural cavities are separated by a thick median partition called mediastinum. The heart lies in the mediastinum (Fig. 10.2).

- Identify the lungs by the thin anterior border, thick posterior border, conical apex, wider base, medial surface with hilum and costal surface with impressions of the ribs and intercostal spaces. In addition, the right lung is distinguished by the presence of three lobes, whereas left lung comprises two lobes only (Figs 10.3 and 10.4).
- On the mediastinal part of the medial surface of right lung identify two bronchi—the eparterial and hyparterial bronchi, with bronchial vessels and posterior pulmonary plexus, the pulmonary artery between the two bronchi on an anterior plane. The upper pulmonary vein is situated still on an anterior plane while the lower pulmonary vein is identified below the bronchi (Fig. 10.5a).
- The impressions on the right lung in front of root of lung are of superior vena cava, inferior vena cava, and right ventricle. The impressions behind the root of lung are those of vena azygos and oesophagus.
- Hilum of the left lung shows the single bronchus situated posteriorly, with bronchial vessels and posterior pulmonary plexus. The pulmonary artery lies above the bronchus. Anterior to the bronchus is the upper pulmonary vein, while the lower vein lies below the bronchus (Fig. 10.5b).
- The mediastinal surface of left lung has the impression of left ventricle, ascending aorta. Behind the root of the left lung are the impressions of descending thoracic aorta while oesophagus leaves an impression in the lower part only (Fig. 10.5b).

RIGHT LUNG

The right lung is heavier and broader than the left lung. It has an oblique and horizontal fissures. The horizontal fissure extends from the middle of oblique fissure forwards till the anterior border. Thus the right lung comprises upper, middle and lower lobes (Fig. 10.4a).

The structures at the hilum (from posterior to anterior aspect) are:

  i. Eparterial and hyparterial bronchi (Fig. 10.5a)
 ii. Pulmonary artery between two bronchi
iii. Upper pulmonary vein anterior to pulmonary artery
 iv. Lower pulmonary vein below the pulmonary artery

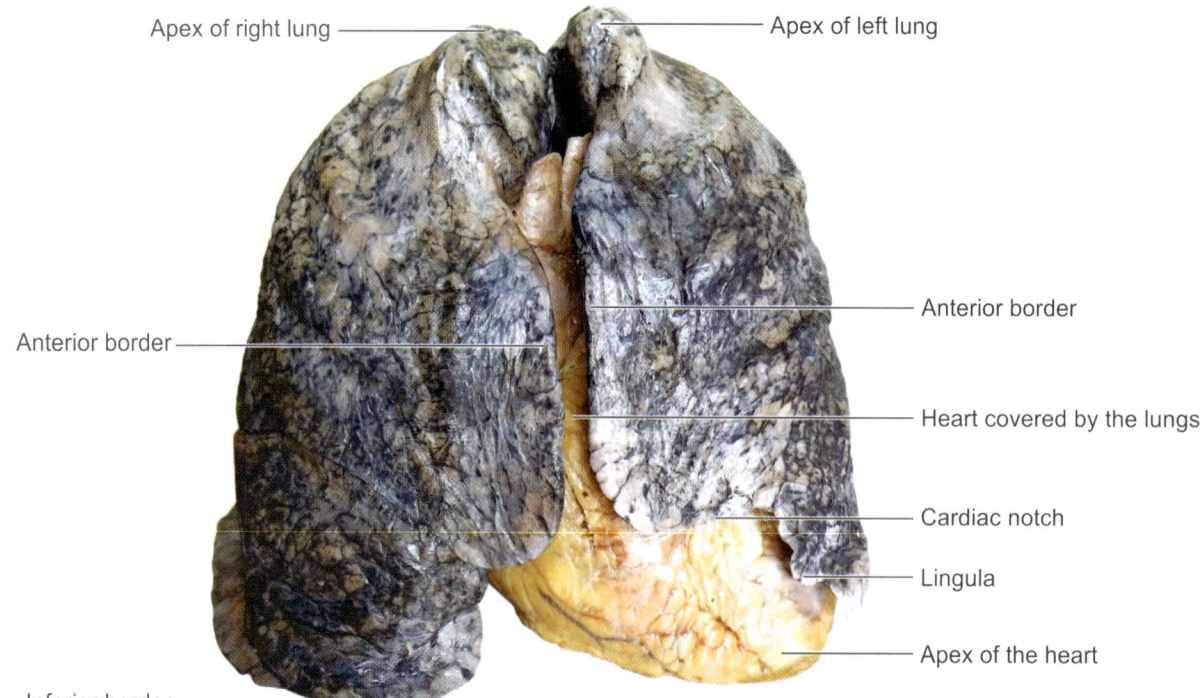

Fig. 10.3: Gross anatomy of the lungs

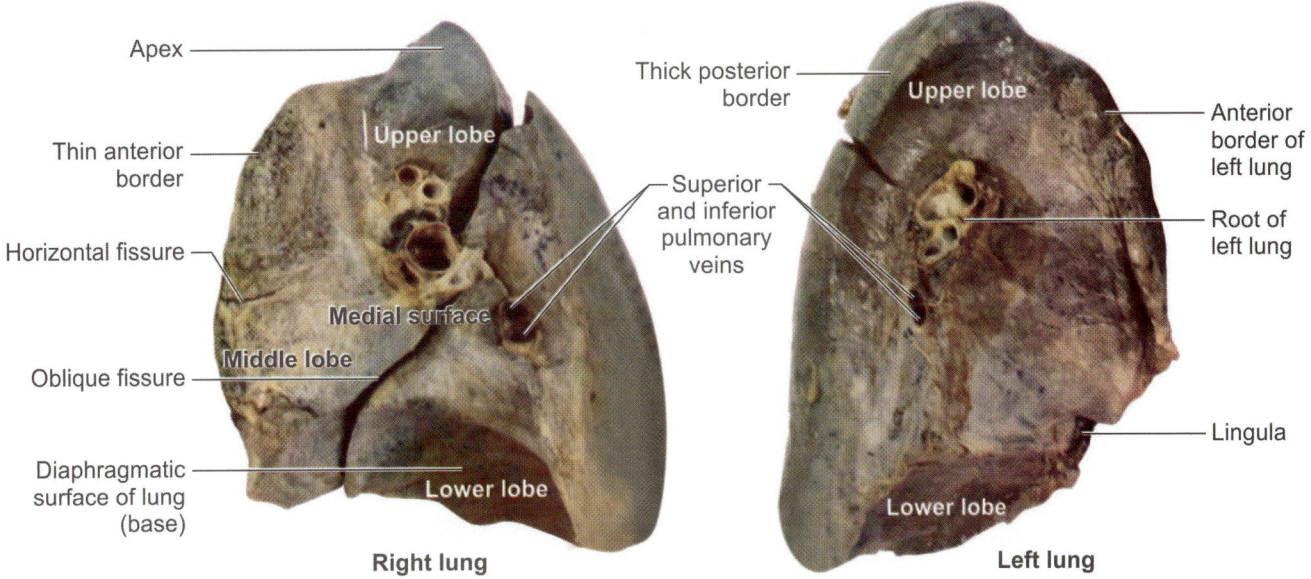

Fig. 10.4: Mediastinal surfaces of the lungs

Apex

Thin anterior border

Horizontal fissure

Oblique fissure

Diaphragmatic surface of lung (base)

Upper lobe

Medial surface

Middle lobe

Lower lobe

Right lung

Thick posterior border

Upper lobe

Superior and inferior pulmonary veins

Anterior border of left lung

Root of left lung

Lingula

Lower lobe

Left lung

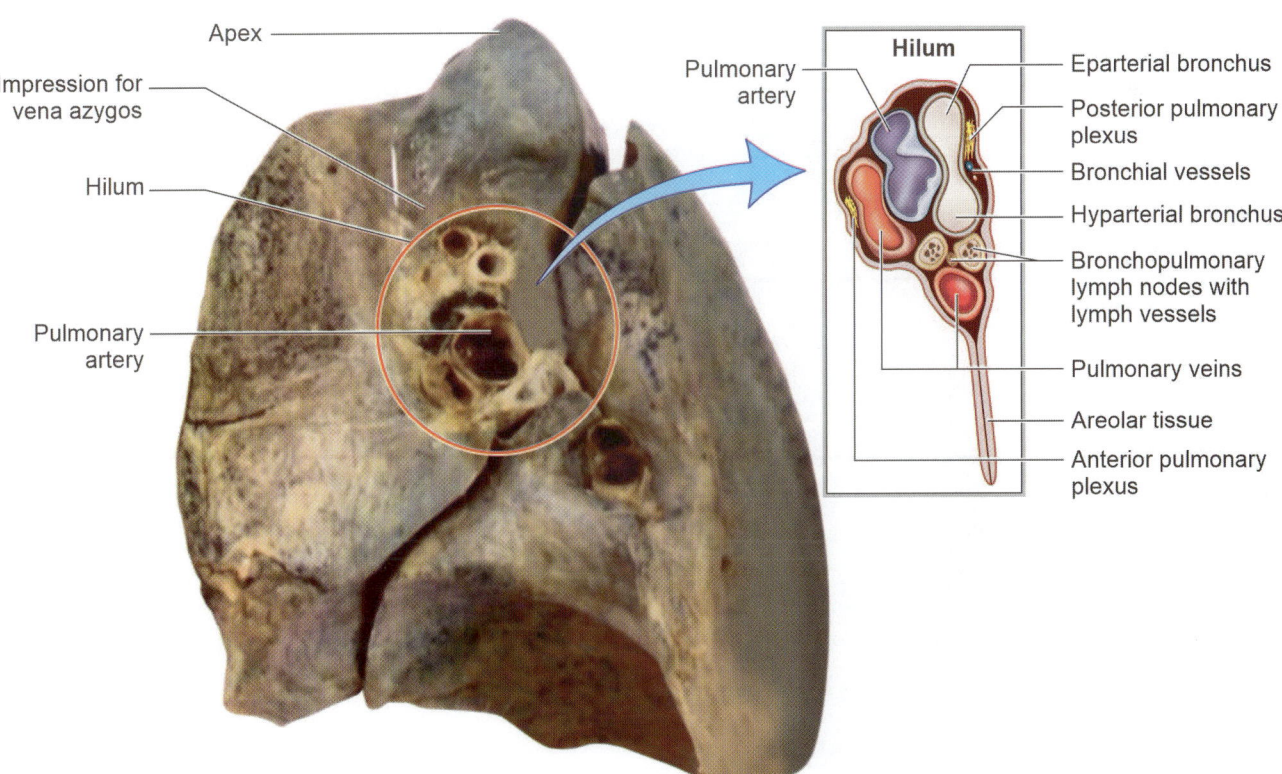

Fig. 10.5a: Impressions on the mediastinal surfaces of lung (right lung)

Apex

Impression for vena azygos

Hilum

Pulmonary artery

Pulmonary artery

Hilum

Eparterial bronchus

Posterior pulmonary plexus

Bronchial vessels

Hyparterial bronchus

Bronchopulmonary lymph nodes with lymph vessels

Pulmonary veins

Areolar tissue

Anterior pulmonary plexus

Mediastinal Surface

i. Impression for the heart (Fig. 10.5a).

ii. Groove for the vena azygos.

iii. Oesophagus behind hilum of the lung.

iv. Groove for inferior vena cava below hilum anterior to the pulmonary ligament.

LEFT LUNG

The anterior border of the left lung is thin. It shows the cardiac notch along the lower part of the anterior border of the left lung. In this part the left pleura passes laterally between 4th and 6th costal cartilages.

Oblique fissure is seen in the lung extending from posterior border above to inferior border below. A small tongue like process of upper lobe, the lingula, is identifiable between the cardiac notch and oblique fissure (Figs 10.3 and 10.4).

Hilum is a depressed area of lung where the root (number of structures) enters/leaves the lung. It comprises one bronchus, pulmonary artery above the bronchus, upper pulmonary vein anterior to bronchus

and second lower pulmonary vein below the bronchus.

Mediastinal Surface

Anterior to hilum is:

i. Cardiac impression (Fig. 10.5b).

ii. Above and behind is the impression for arch of aorta and descending thoracic aorta respectively.

iii. Near the apex is groove for left subclavian artery.

iv. Below the left subclavian artery is the groove for left common carotid artery.

Competency achievement: The student should be able to:

AN 24.3 Describe a bronchopulmonary segment.

BRONCHIAL TREE

- Dissect the principal bronchus into the left lung. Remove the pulmonary tissue and follow the main bronchus till it is seen to divide into two lobar bronchi. Try to dissect till these divide into the segmental bronchi.

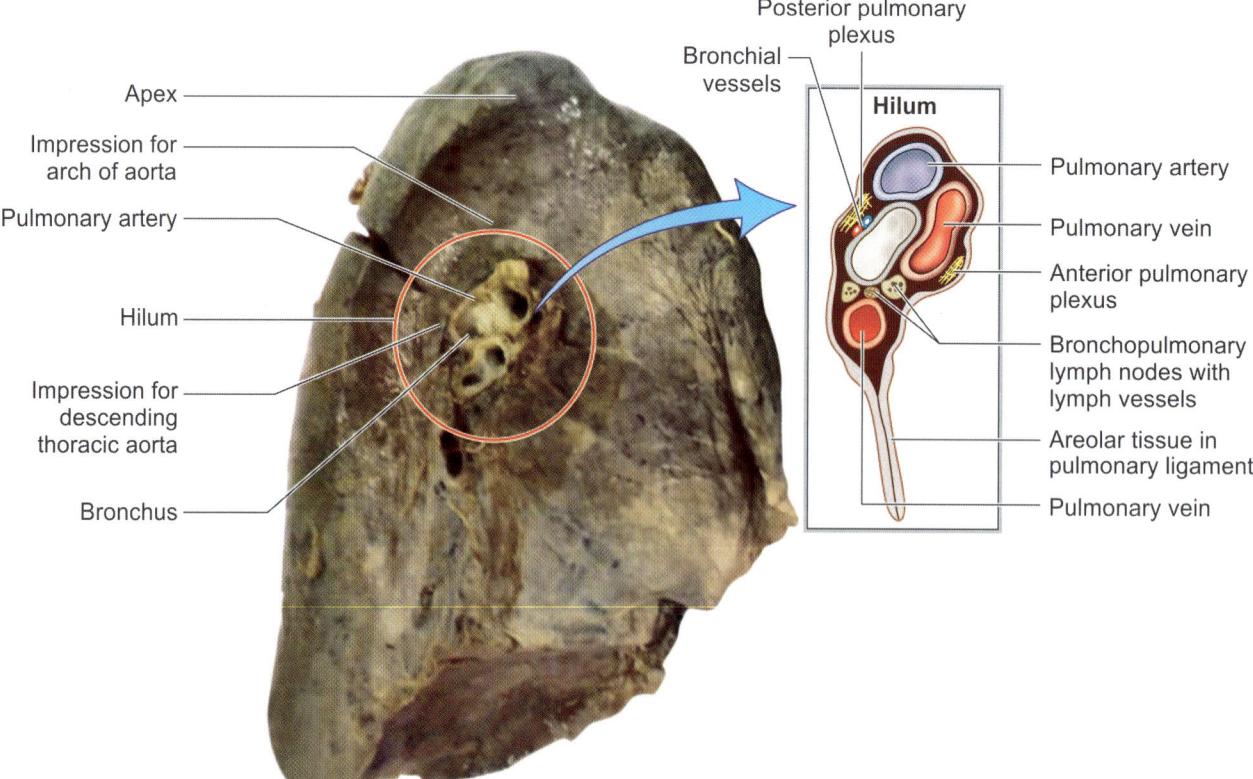

Fig. 10.5b: Impressions on the mediastinal surface of lung (left lung)

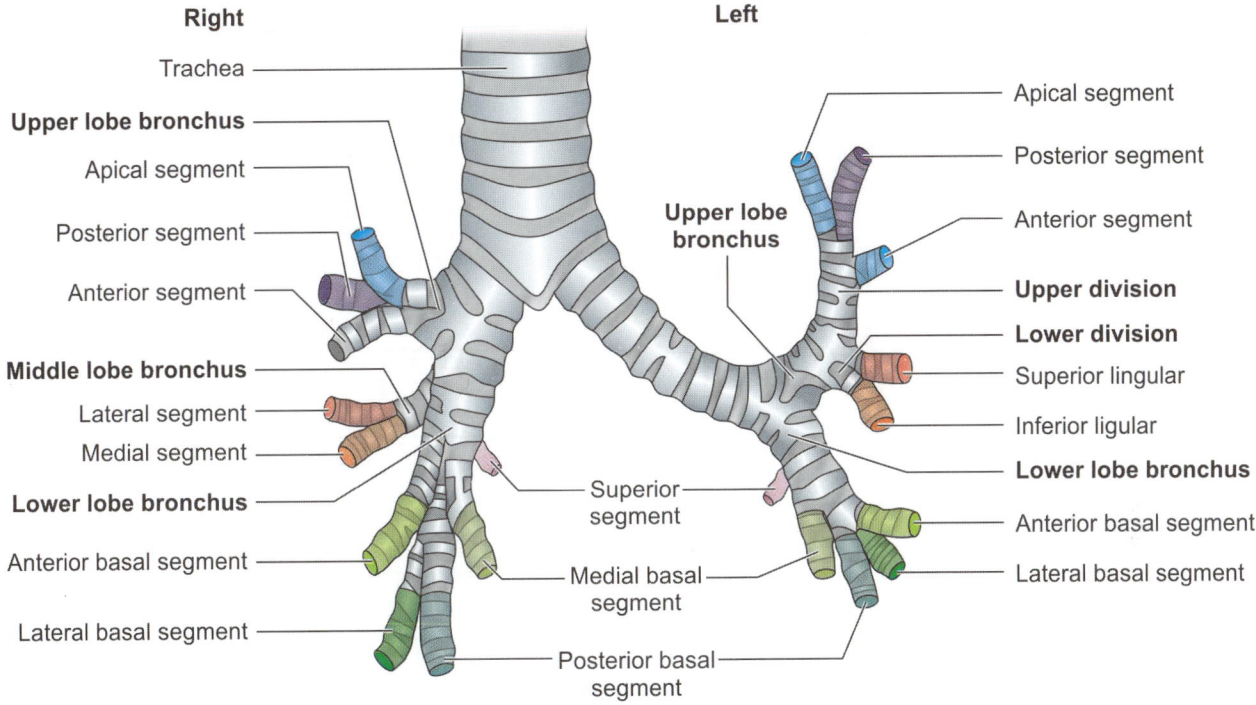

Right

Trachea

Upper lobe bronchus

Apical segment

Posterior segment

Anterior segment

Middle lobe bronchus

Lateral segment

Medial segment

Lower lobe bronchus

Anterior basal segment

Lateral basal segment

Left

Apical segment

Posterior segment

Anterior segment

Upper lobe bronchus

Upper division

Lower division

Superior lingular

Inferior ligular

Lower lobe bronchus

Anterior basal segment

Lateral basal segment

Superior segment

Medial basal segment

Posterior basal segment

Fig. 10.6: Bronchopulmonary segments of right and left lungs

- Dissect the principal bronchus into the right lung. Remove the pulmonary tissue and follow the main bronchus till it is seen to divide into three lobar bronchi. Try to dissect till these divide into segmental bronchi.
- Trachea is seen to divide into two primary bronchi, the right and the left (Fig. 10.6).
- Trace the right primary bronchus dividing into the upper, middle and lower lobe bronchi.
- The left primary bronchus divides into only two secondary bronchi.
- Identify the grey to black lymph nodes in relation to the hilum.
- Try and look for bronchial arteries and trace them along with bronchi for some distance. Single right

bronchial artery arises from 3rd posterior intercostal artery. The two left bronchial arteries arise from the descending thoracic aorta.

- Dissect one of the secondary bronchi into the lung and trace its subdivision—the segmental/tertiary bronchi.
- Trace the segmental bronchus into a pyramidal shaped segment of lung, known as bronchopulmonary segment.
- Identify the branch of pulmonary artery (deoxygenated blood) accompanying the segmental bronchus. Look for the corresponding vein present in between the segmental bronchi.
- Try and dissect the ten bronchopulmonary segments in each right and left lungs.

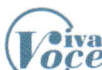

Viva Voce

- Name the borders and surfaces of lung.
- Name the structures present in the hilum of right lung.
- What is the function of pulmonary ligament?
- Define a bronchopulmonary segment.
- Why does the foreign body mostly enter through the right bronchus?
- What is postural drainage?

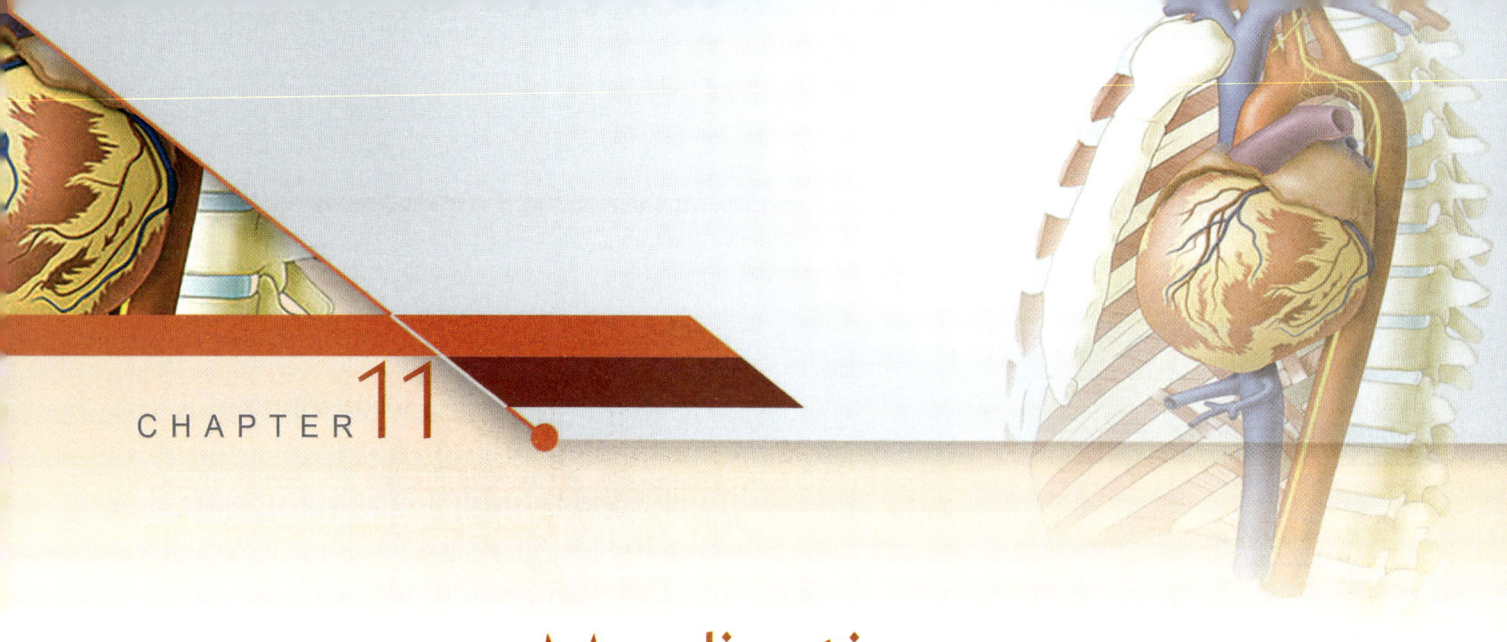

CHAPTER 11

Mediastinum

Learning Objectives

One should be able to
1. Mark the position of the line demarcating the superior and inferior mediastina.
2. Enumerate boundaries and contents of superior mediastinum
3. Enumerate boundaries and contents of middle and posterior mediastina.

OVERVIEW

Mediastinum (middle space) is the little space between right and left pleural cavities.

The mediastinum is divided into superior and inferior mediastina by an imaginary line passing through manubriosternal angle anteriorly till lower border of T4 vertebra posteriorly.

The superior mediastinum contains the arch of aorta and its three main branches.

The inferior mediastinum is subdivided into:
i. A thin anterior mediastinum
ii. A big middle mediastinum with heart with its pericardium and roots of big vessels
iii. A longitudinal posterior mediastinum

The anterior mediastinum contains only few blood vessels and ligaments. Posterior mediastinum contains the longitudinal structures like descending thoracic aorta and oesophagus.

Competency achievement: The student should be able to:

AN 21.11 Mention boundaries, and contents of superior, anterior, middle and posterior mediastina.

AN 24.4 Identify phrenic nerve and describe its formation and distribution.

STEPS OF DISSECTION

- Reflect the upper half of manubrium sterni upwards and study the boundaries and contents of superior and three divisions of the inferior mediastinum.
- Try to identify contents of superior mediastinum:
  - Bilobed thymus gland—hardly seen in adult cadavers. It is seen only till puberty.
  - Left brachiocephalic vein, which passes across back of manubrium sterni till lower border of 1st costal cartilage, where it joins the right brachiocephalic vein to form the second largest vein of the body—the superior vena cava.
  - Superior vena cava extends from the 1st costal cartilage till 3rd right costal cartilage (Fig. 11.1). At the level of 2nd right costal cartilage, vena azygos joins the superior vena cava.
- Trace and clean the three branches of arch of aorta (Fig. 11.2).
- Trace the right and left phrenic nerves.

The right phrenic nerve lies lateral to right brachiocephalic vein and superior vena cava (*see* Fig. 9.5). The left phrenic nerve runs between left common carotid artery and left subclavian artery to

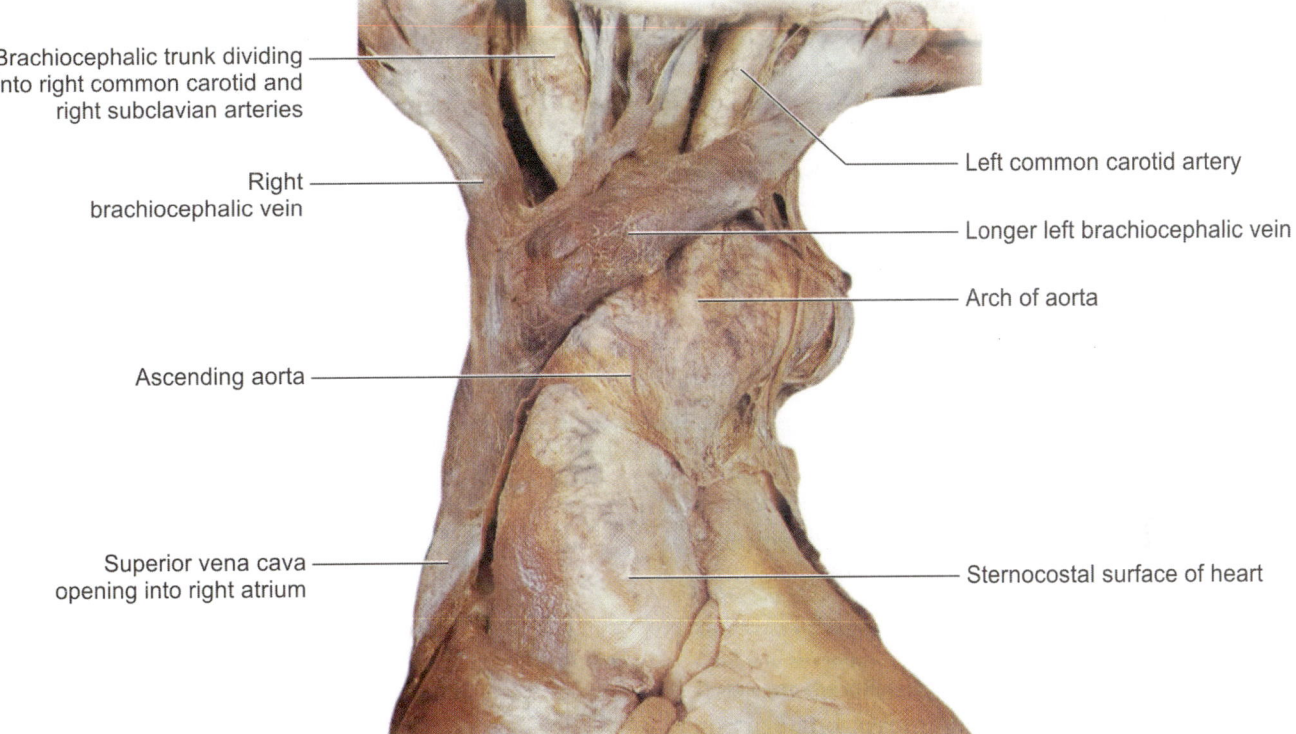

Brachiocephalic trunk dividing into right common carotid and right subclavian arteries

Right brachiocephalic vein

Ascending aorta

Superior vena cava opening into right atrium

Left common carotid artery

Longer left brachiocephalic vein

Arch of aorta

Sternocostal surface of heart

Fig. 11.1: Formation and termination of superior vena cava

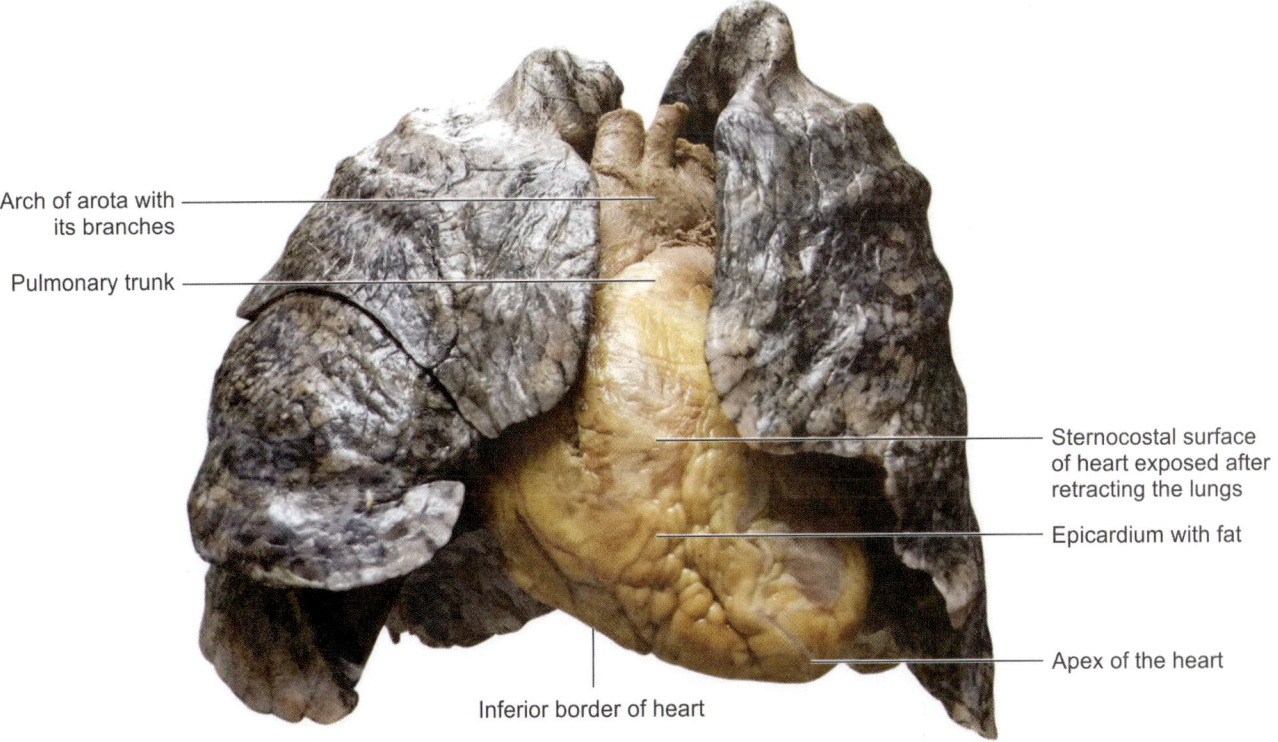

Arch of arota with its branches

Pulmonary trunk

Sternocostal surface of heart exposed after retracting the lungs

Epicardium with fat

Apex of the heart

Inferior border of heart

Fig. 11.2: Arch of aorta with its three branches

descend on arch of aorta. Behind phrenic nerve lies left vagus on arch of aorta.

Left vagus as it lies on the arch of aorta gives left recurrent laryngeal nerve. This left recurrent laryngeal nerve hooks under the arch and ligamentum arteriosum to ascend in the interval between the trachea anteriorly and oesophagus posteriorly.

- Identify and trace left superior intercostal vein running between left phrenic and left vagus nerves to end into left brachiocephalic vein.

- Trace the right vagus nerve from right carotid sheath onto the superficial aspect of subclavian artery to enter the inlet of thorax. Then it passes posterior to the root of lung to form posterior pulmonary plexus.

Besides these, the superior mediastinum also contains trachea, oesophagus, and thoracic duct. Trachea divides into right and left bronchi. Right bronchus is vertical and left one is more horizontal. The deep cervical plexus lies in front of the tracheal bifurcation.

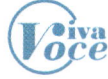

- Name the boundaries of superior mediastinum.
- What are the contents of middle mediastinum?
- What are the contents of posterior mediastinum?

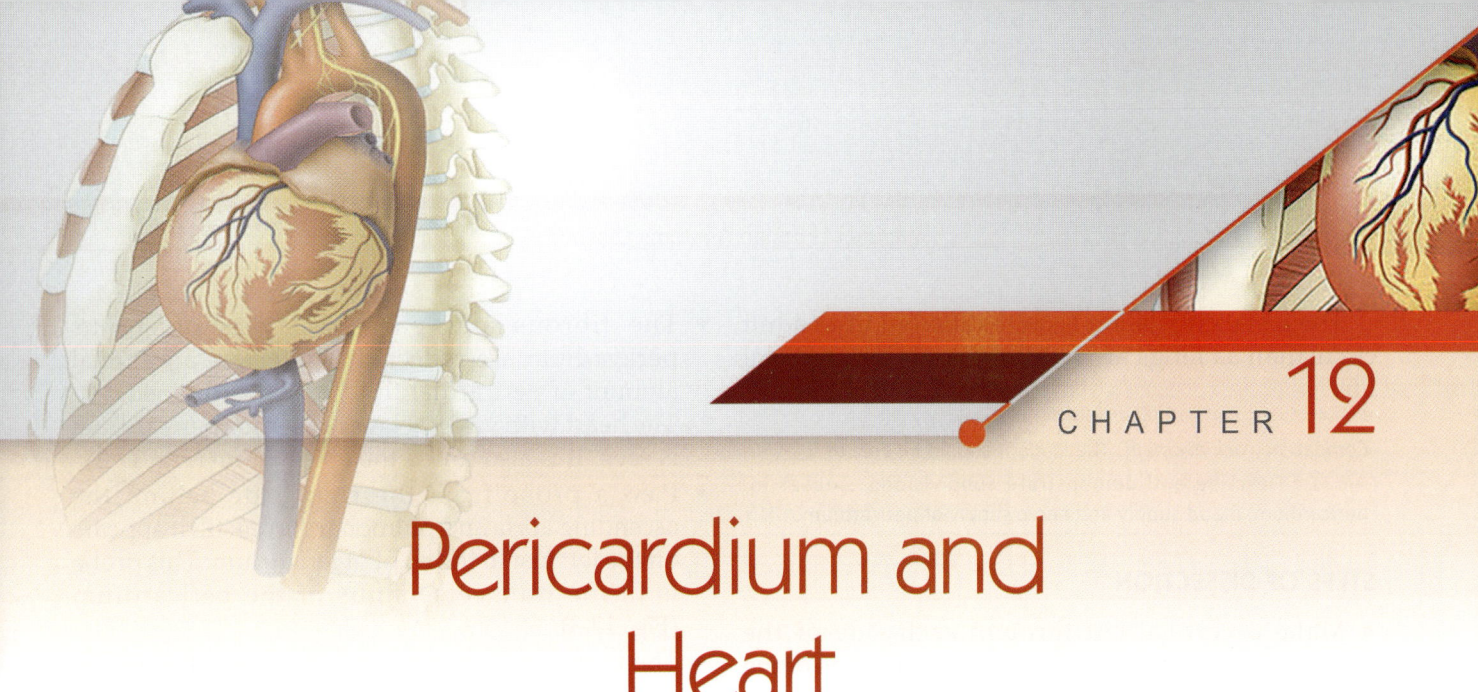

CHAPTER 12

Pericardium and Heart

Learning Objectives

One should be able to

1. Explain the increased thickness of myocardium of the left ventricle.
2. Explain the differences between the systemic/caval and pulmonary circulations.
3. Enumerate differences between left and right atria.
4. Enumerate differences between right and left ventricles

OVERVIEW

Heart, a vital organ lies in the middle mediastinum of thoracic cavity. It is enclosed by one layer of fibrous and two layers of serous pericardia. There are two sinuses—the transverse and oblique sinus in relation to the serous pericardium. The serous pericardium comprises an outer parietal and an inner visceral layer with pericardial fluid in between its two layers. Pericardial effusion if occurs has to be drained.

Heart has six entry channels and two exit channels. The entry channels are two venae cavae and four pulmonary veins while the exit channels are ascending aorta and the pulmonary trunk.

Heart comprises an apex pulsating in left 5th intercostal space, 9 cm lateral to midsternal line and a posteriorly placed base. Heart has a sternocostal/ anterior surface and an inferior/diaphragmatic surface. Its borders are right, inferior, left and superior/upper.

Heart comprises right and left atria and right and left ventricles. Each of these four chambers have entry and exit channels. Entry channels are on a posterior plane compared to the exit channels. Left side of heart is arterial while the right side of heart (both atrium and ventricle) is venous in nature. The atrioventricular valves and semilunar valves permit unidirectional flow of blood through the heart under normal circumstances.

Heart consists of an inner endocardium, middle myocardium and an outer epicardium (visceral layer of serous pericardium). The myocardium of left ventricle is thickest as it needs to pump the blood to the whole body. The myocardium of right ventricle is one-third the thickness of left ventricle as it pumps the blood only till the lungs. The muscle of the atria are still thinner.

Heart is supplied by two functional end arteries- the right and left coronary arteries. There is little collateral circulation between the coronary arteries and the extracardiac arteries. Veins run along with the arteries but their names are different from those of the arteries.

Heart is innervated by autonomic nerves from three cervical and 1–5 thoracic sympathetic ganglia and by branches of vagus nerve.

The foetal circulation is quite different from adult circulation as lungs are not functional during foetal life.

Competency achievement: The student should be able to:

AN 22.1 Describe and demonstrate subdivisions, sinuses in pericardium, blood supply and nerve supply of pericardium.

STEPS OF DISSECTION

• Make a vertical cut through each side of the pericardium immediately anterior to the line of the phrenic nerve. Join the lower ends of these two incisions by a transverse cut approximately 1 cm above the diaphragm (Fig. 12.1). Turn the flap of pericardium upwards and sideways to examine the pericardial cavity. See that the turned flap comprises fibrous and parietal layer of serous pericardium. The pericardium enclosing the heart is its visceral layer.

• The fibrous and parietal layers of serous pericardium are reflected. There was a minimal amount of pericardial fluid which is drained out. The heart with visceral layer of serous pericardium is seen. It is also called the epicardium (Fig. 12.2).

• Pass a probe from the right side behind the ascending aorta and pulmonary trunk till it appears on the left just to the right of left atrium. This probe is in the transverse sinus of the pericardium (Fig. 12.3).

• The transverse sinus is a gap between the arterial and venous ends of the heart tube (Fig. 12.4). Its appearance is due to changes appearing in the heart during its development.

• Lift the apex of the heart upwards. Put a finger behind the left atrium into a cul-de-sac, bounded to the right and below by inferior vena cava and above and to left by lower left pulmonary vein. This is the oblique sinus of pericardium (Fig. 12.4).

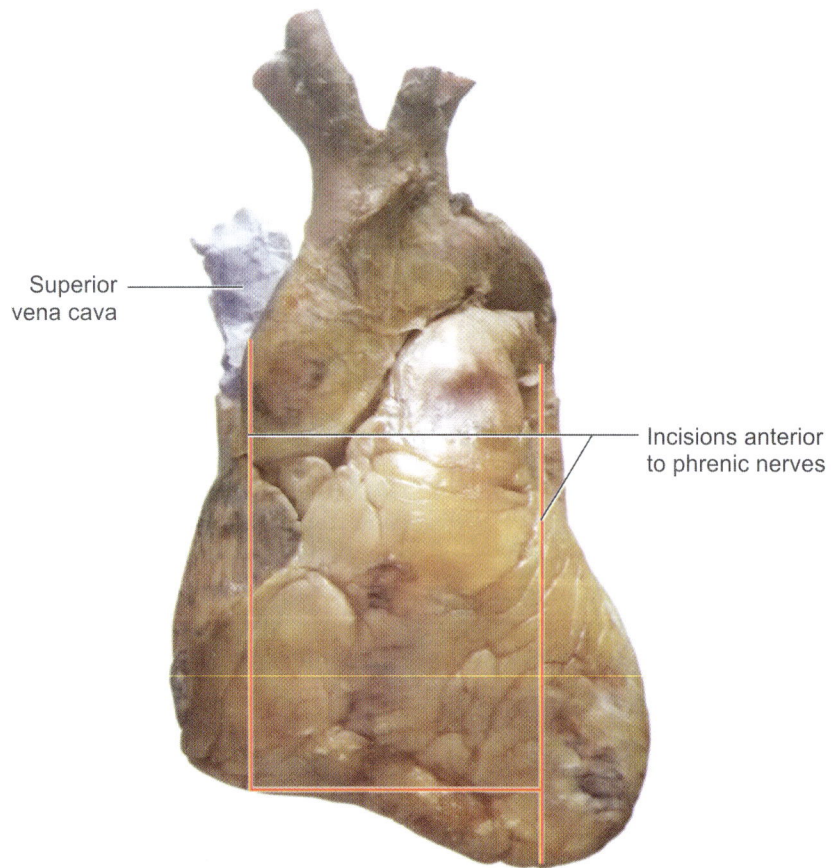

Superior vena cava

Incisions anterior to phrenic nerves

Fig. 12.1: Lines of incision

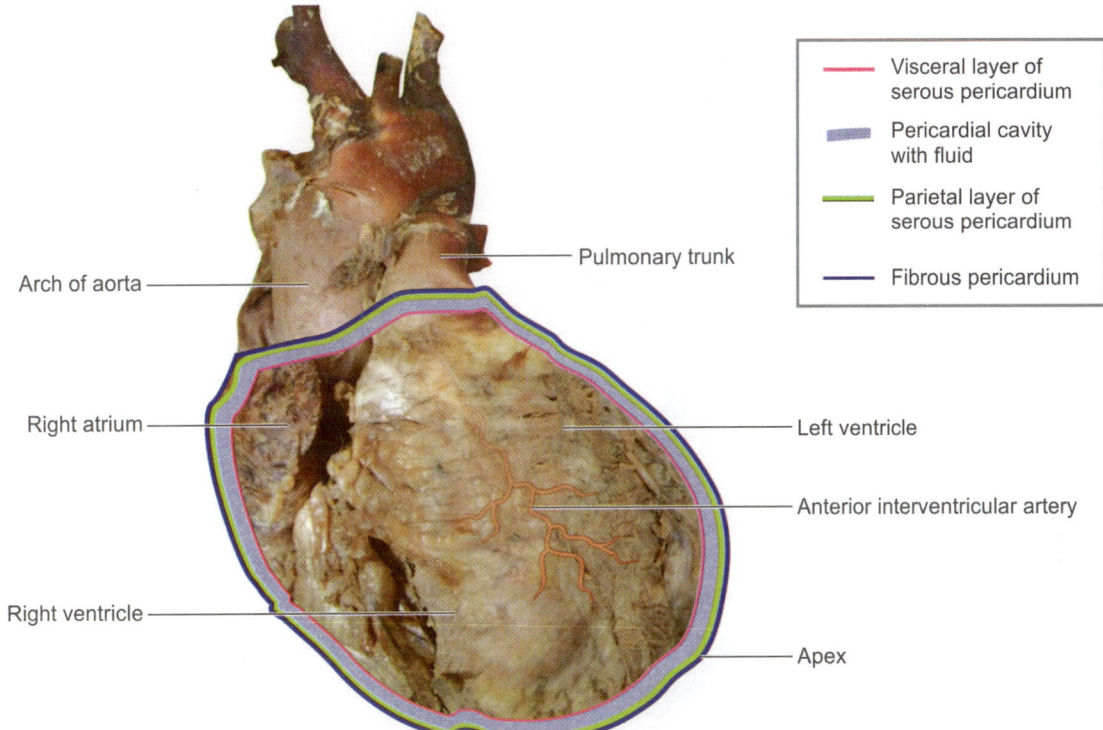

Arch of aorta

Pulmonary trunk

Right atrium

Left ventricle

Anterior interventricular artery

Right ventricle

Apex

Visceral layer of serous pericardium

Pericardial cavity with fluid

Parietal layer of serous pericardium

Fibrous pericardium

Fig. 12.2: Layers of pericardium

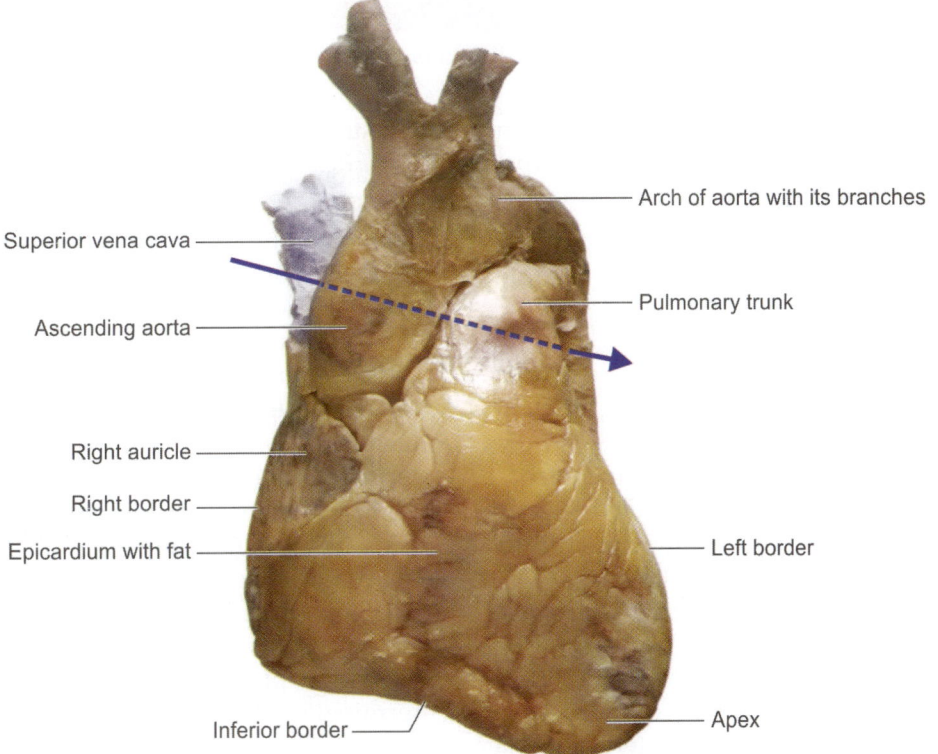

Arch of aorta with its branches

Superior vena cava

Pulmonary trunk

Ascending aorta

Right auricle

Right border

Epicardium with fat

Left border

Inferior border

Apex

Fig. 12.3: Transverse sinus of pericardium shown with black line

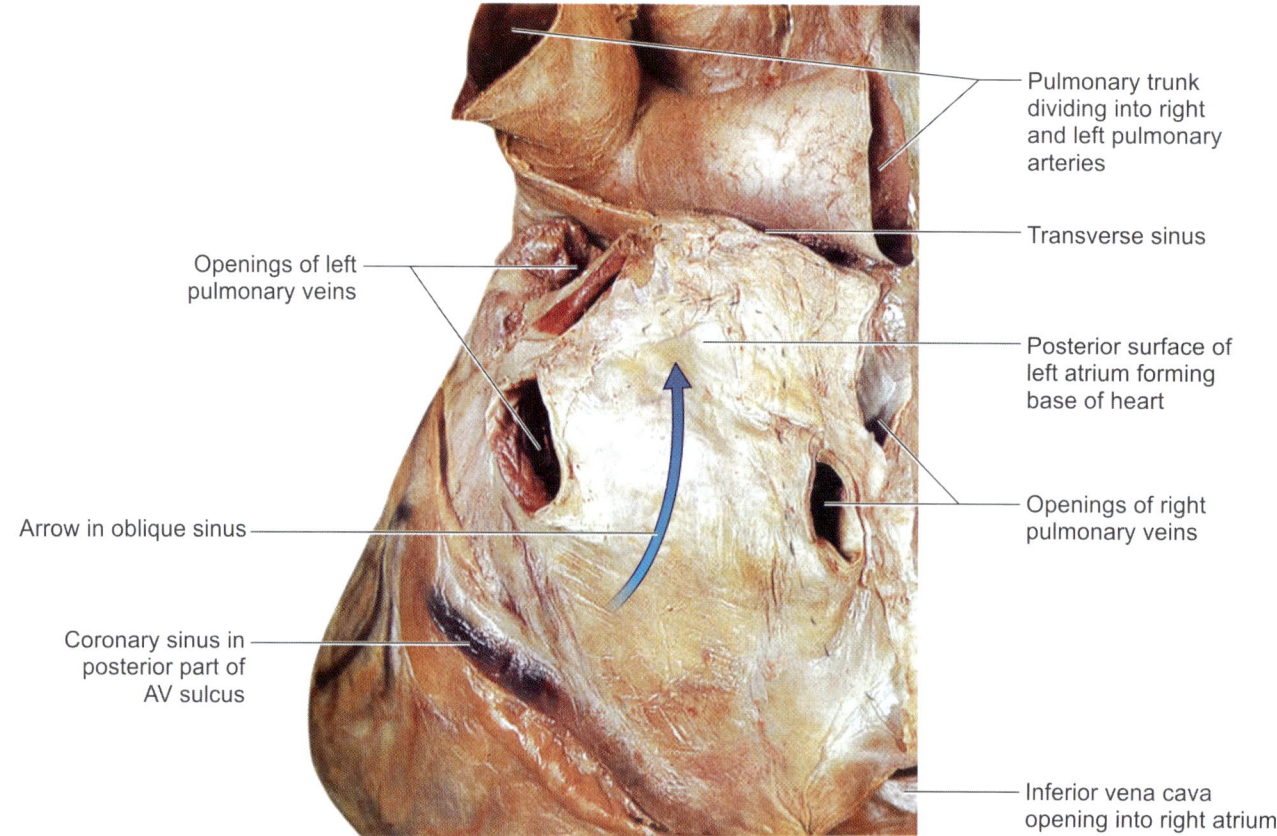

Pulmonary trunk
dividing into right
and left pulmonary
arteries

Transverse sinus

Posterior surface of
left atrium forming
base of heart

Openings of right
pulmonary veins

Inferior vena cava
opening into right atrium

Openings of left
pulmonary veins

Arrow in oblique sinus

Coronary sinus in
posterior part of
AV sulcus

Fig. 12.4: Transverse and oblique sinuses of pericardium

The oblique sinus is a space situated between the visceral and parietal pericardia behind the left atrium with the oesophagus posterior to it. This space gets obliterated in cases of mitral stenosis.

Competency achievement: The student should be able to:

AN 22.2 Describe and demonstrate external and internal features of each chamber of heart.

GROSS ANATOMY OF HEART

Borders of heart are right, inferior, left and superior. Base is formed mainly by left atrium. It is also called posterior surface. Apex is pulsating all the time. It is formed exclusively by left ventricle (Figs 12.3, 12.5a and b).

Sternocostal and diaphragmatic surfaces are mainly formed by right and left ventricles (Fig. 12.6). Right ventricle forms 2/3rd of sternocostal and 1/3rd of diaphragmatic surface. There are coronary sulci, anterior interventricular and posterior interventricular grooves (Fig. 12.5a).

Right Atrium

- Cut along the upper edge of the right auricle by an incision from the anterior end of the superior vena caval opening to the left side. Similarly cut along its lower edge by an incision extending from the anterior end of the inferior vena caval opening to the left side. Incise the anterior wall of the right atrium near its left margin and reflect the flap to the right (Fig. 12.7a, position 1-1-1).

- On its internal surface, see the vertical crista terminalis and horizontal pectinate muscles.

Right atrium receives the venous blood of the whole body including the heart (Fig. 12.6). A groove seen on the external surface of heart between the openings of superior vena cava and inferior vena cava is sulcus terminalis. Its upper part contains SA node. Opposite this sulcus is a ridge called crista terminalis. The musculi pectinati are transverse muscular ridges in the rough anterior part of right atrium.

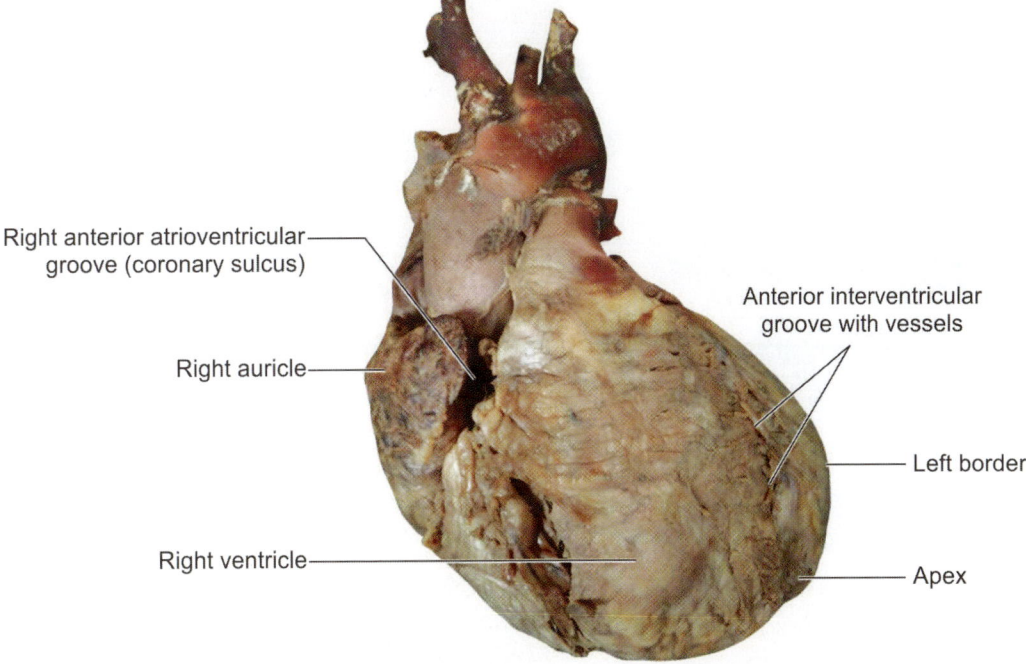

Right anterior atrioventricular groove (coronary sulcus)

Right auricle

Right ventricle

Anterior interventricular groove with vessels

Left border

Apex

Fig. 12.5a: Gross anatomy of heart

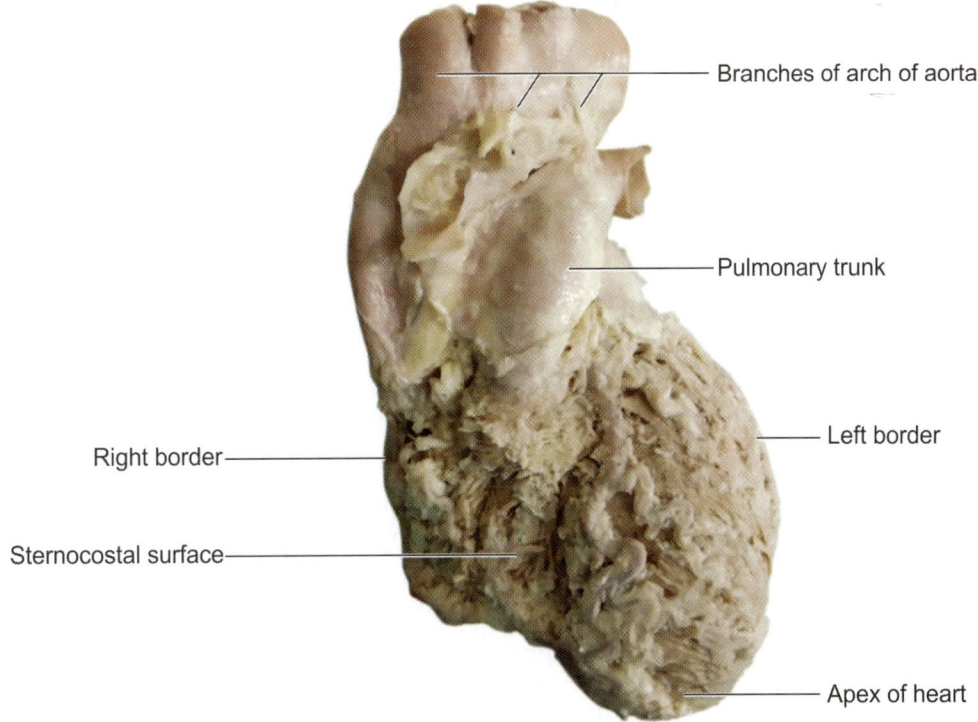

Branches of arch of aorta

Pulmonary trunk

Left border

Right border

Sternocostal surface

Apex of heart

Fig. 12.5b: Whole heart

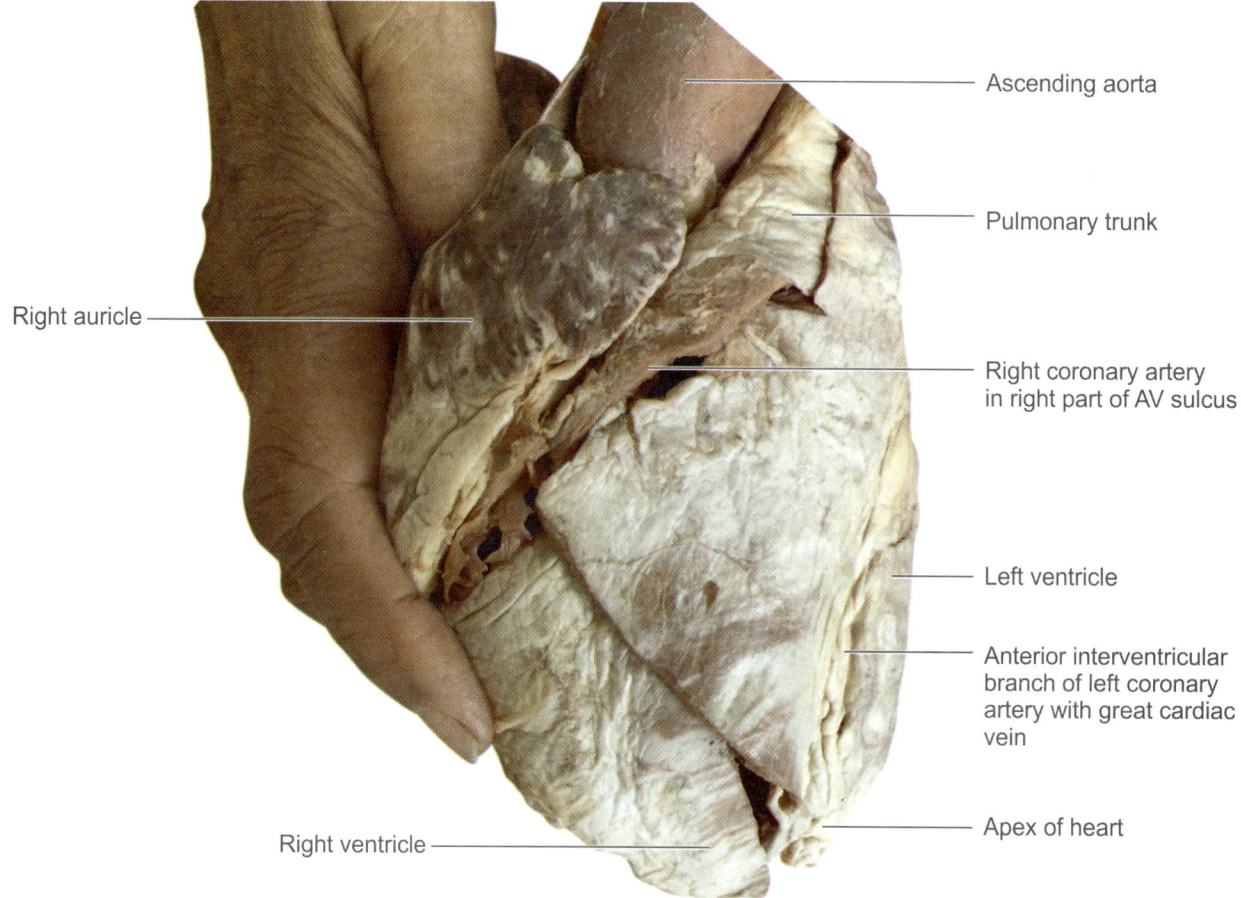

Right auricle

Ascending aorta

Pulmonary trunk

Right coronary artery in right part of AV sulcus

Left ventricle

Anterior interventricular branch of left coronary artery with great cardiac vein

Apex of heart

Right ventricle

Fig. 12.6: Sternocostal surface of heart

- The fossa ovalis is on the interatrial septum and the opening of the coronary sinus is to the left of the inferior vena caval opening.
- Define the three cusps of tricuspid valve (Fig. 12.7b). The exposed interatrial septum separating the right and left atria reveals an annulus fossa ovalis, a curved prominent margin around a shallow depression, the fossa ovalis. Between the annulus and the fossa there may be remnant of a foramen— the foramen ovale functioning during foetal life.
- Define three cusps of tricuspid valve (Fig. 12.8a). Tricuspid valve lies between right atrium and right ventricle
- Tricuspid valve between right atrium and right ventricle comprises an anterior, a posterior and septal cusps lying against the three walls of the right ventricle.

Right Ventricle

- Incise along the ventricular aspect of right AV groove, till you reach the inferior border. Continue to incise along the inferior border till the inferior end of anterior interventricular groove. Next cut along the infundibulum (Fig. 12.7a, position 2-2-2). Now the anterior wall of right ventricle is reflected to the left to study its interior (Fig. 12.8a).
- Right ventricle pumps venous blood to the lungs for oxygenation. Identify its inflowing rough part and its outflowing smooth infundibular part (Fig. 12.8a and b).
- See the tricuspid valve between right atrium and ventricle (Fig. 12.8a).
- Identify the three cusps of pulmonary semilunar valve between right ventricle and pulmonary trunk

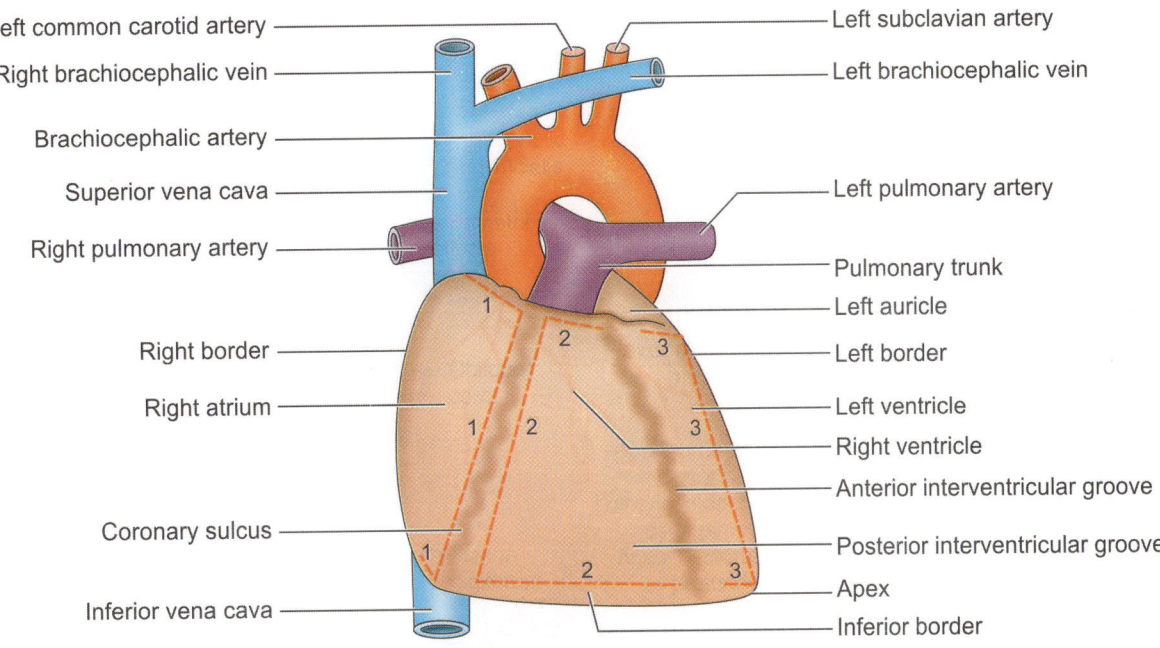

Left common carotid artery

Right brachiocephalic vein

Brachiocephalic artery

Superior vena cava

Right pulmonary artery

Right border

Right atrium

Coronary sulcus

Inferior vena cava

Left subclavian artery

Left brachiocephalic vein

Left pulmonary artery

Pulmonary trunk

Left auricle

Left border

Left ventricle

Right ventricle

Anterior interventricular groove

Posterior interventricular groove

Apex

Inferior border

Fig. 12.7a: Lines of incision for right atrium, right ventricle and left ventricle

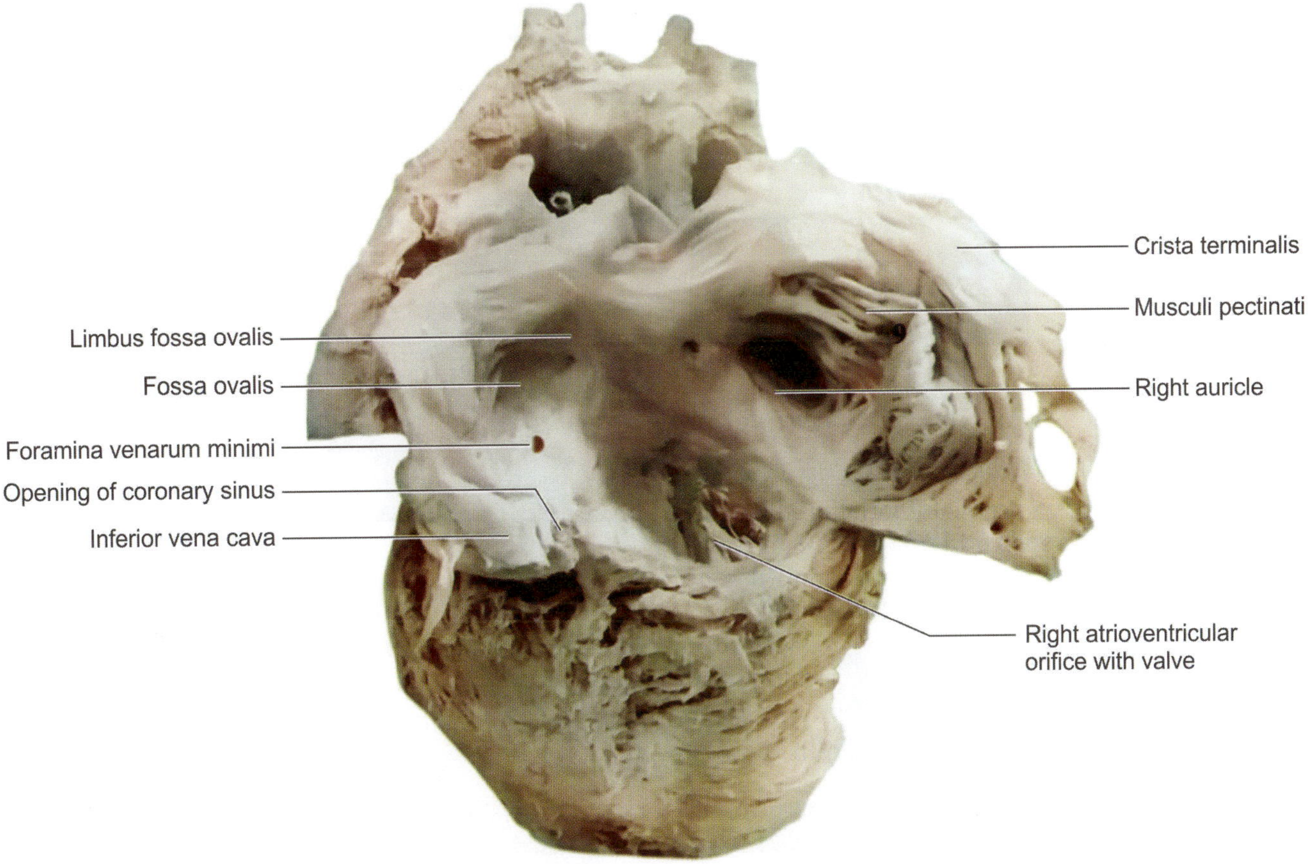

Crista terminalis

Musculi pectinati

Right auricle

Limbus fossa ovalis

Fossa ovalis

Foramina venarum minimi

Opening of coronary sinus

Inferior vena cava

Right atrioventricular orifice with valve

Fig. 12.7b: Interior of right atrium

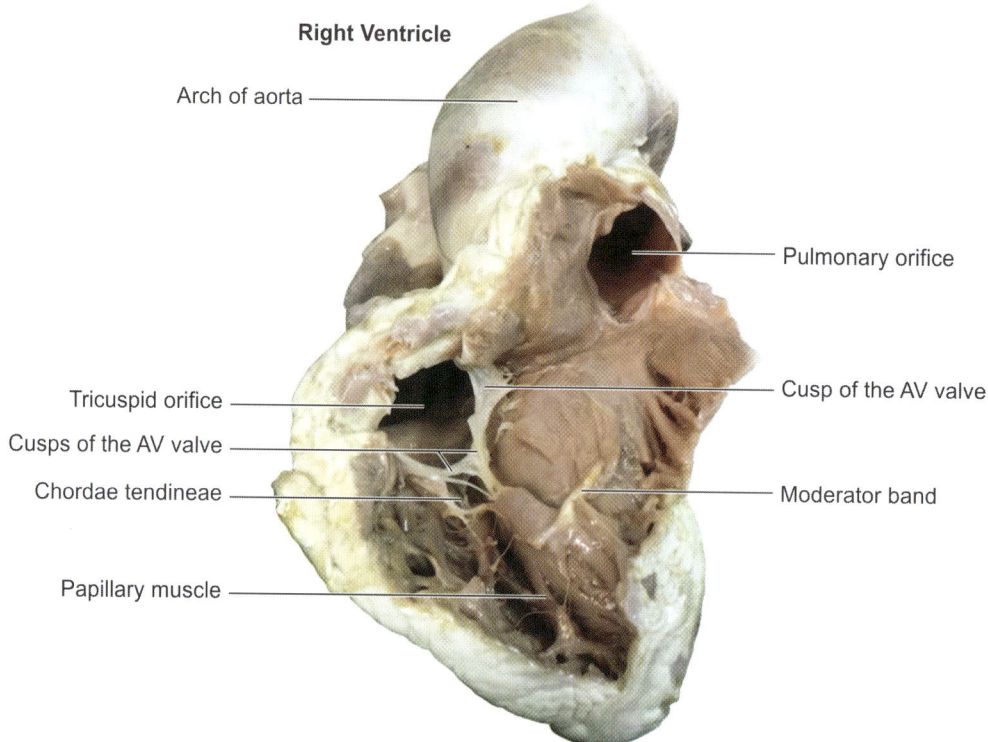

Right Ventricle

Arch of aorta ——————————

—————— Pulmonary orifice

—————— Cusp of the AV valve

Tricuspid orifice ——————

Cusps of the AV valve ——————

Chordae tendineae ——————

—————— Moderator band

Papillary muscle ——————

Fig. 12.8a: Tricuspid orifice and pulmonary orifice of the right ventricle

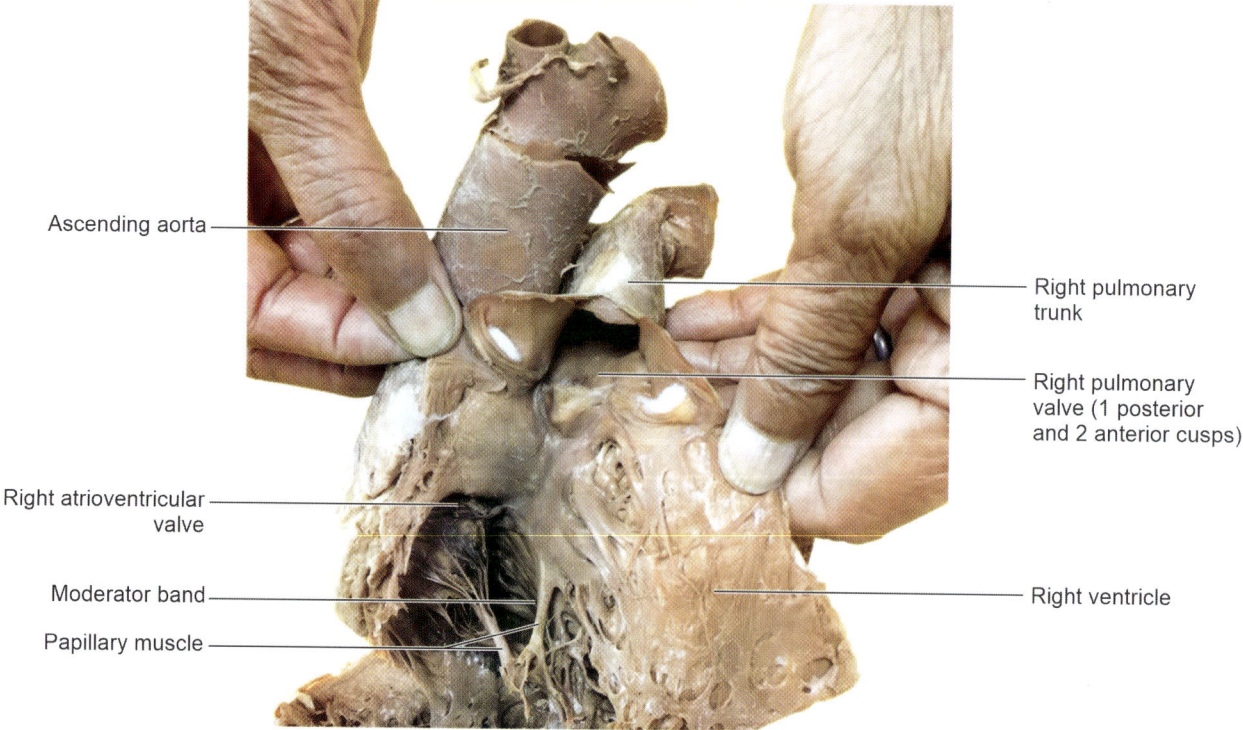

Ascending aorta ——————

—————— Right pulmonary trunk

—————— Right pulmonary valve (1 posterior and 2 anterior cusps)

Right atrioventricular valve ——————

—————— Right ventricle

Moderator band ——————

Papillary muscle ——————

Fig. 12.8b: Right atrioventicular and right pulmonary valve

(Fig. 12.8b). The cusps are posterior, right anterior and left anterior.

- Appreciate the rough part of right ventricle formed by three types of muscles, i.e. ridges, bridges and papillary muscles. One end of papillary muscle is attached to ventricular wall and the other end is connected to the cusps of tricuspid valve by thin chordae tendineae (Fig. 12.8a and b).
- Wash and clean the ventricle so that one is able to see the septomarginal trabecula/moderator band containing right branch of AV bundle.
- Clean the obliquely placed interventricular septum separating right ventricle from left ventricle (Fig. 12.9).

- Identify its lower thick muscular part and an uppermost thin membranous part. Trace the circulation through the right heart.

Left Atrium

- Cut off the pulmonary trunk and ascending aorta, immediately above the three cusps of the pulmonary and aortic valves. Remove the upper part of the left atrium to visualise its interior. See the upper surface of the cusps of the mitral valve. Revise the fact that left atrium forms the anterior wall of the oblique sinus of the pericardium (Fig. 12.4).
- Left atrium forms the base/posterior surface of the heart.

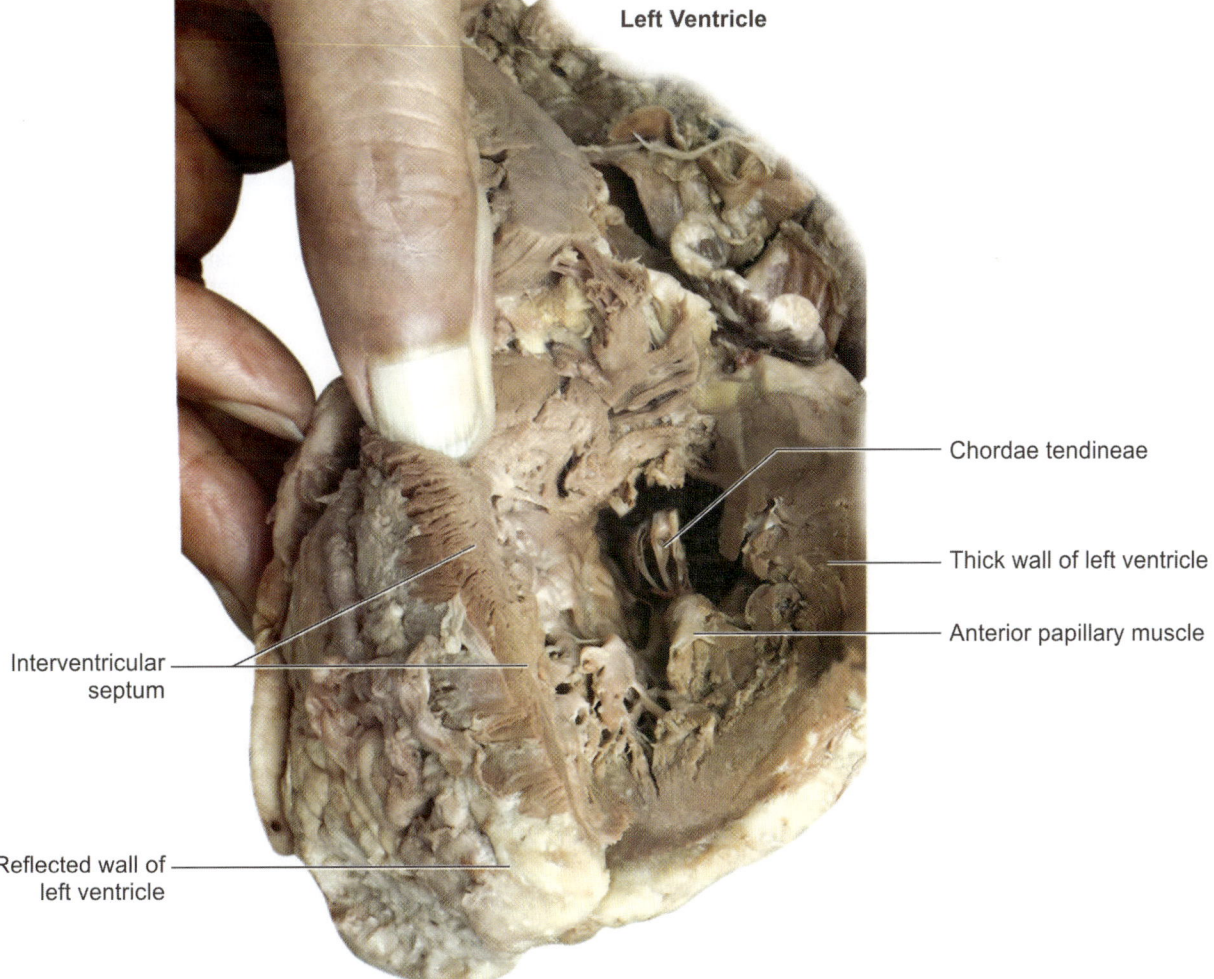

Fig. 12.9: Interventricular septum

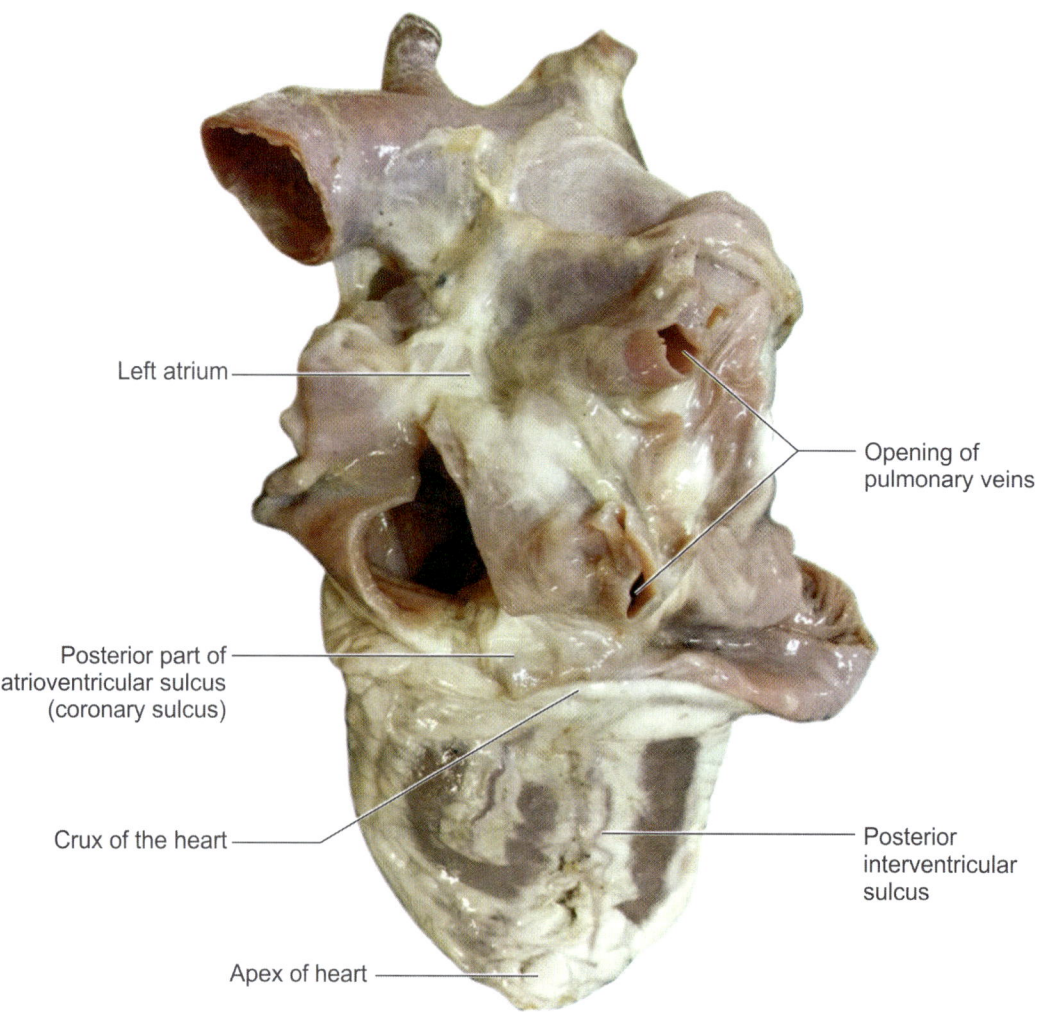

Left atrium

Opening of pulmonary veins

Posterior part of atrioventricular sulcus (coronary sulcus)

Crux of the heart

Posterior interventricular sulcus

Apex of heart

Fig. 12.10: Left atrium

- See the openings of four pulmonary veins in the left atrium, two veins each bring oxygenated blood from right and left lungs (Fig. 12.10).
- See the smooth part where pulmonary veins open and a small rough part called auricle.
- The interatrial septum from left side shows fossa lunata corresponding to fossa ovalis of the right atrium.

Left Ventricle

- Open the left ventricle by making a bold incision on the ventricular aspect of atrioventricular groove below left auricle and along whole thickness of left ventricle from above downwards till its apex. Curve the incision towards right till the inferior end of anterior interventricular groove. Reflect the flap to the right and clean the atrioventricular and aortic valves (Fig. 12.7a, position 3-3-3).
- See that the left ventricle is the thickest chamber (Fig. 12.11).
- Wash and clean its interior
- See the two strong cusps of the bicuspid valve—the anterior and the posterior (Fig. 12.13a). Their margins give attachment to the chordae tendineae which are attached inferiorly to the strong anterior and posterior papillary muscle of the wall of left ventricle (Fig. 12.12).
- See the three cusps of aortic semilunar valve/aortic valve. The cusps are 2 posterior (right and left) and one anterior. It permits unidirectional flow of blood from left ventricle into ascending aorta (Fig. 12.13b).

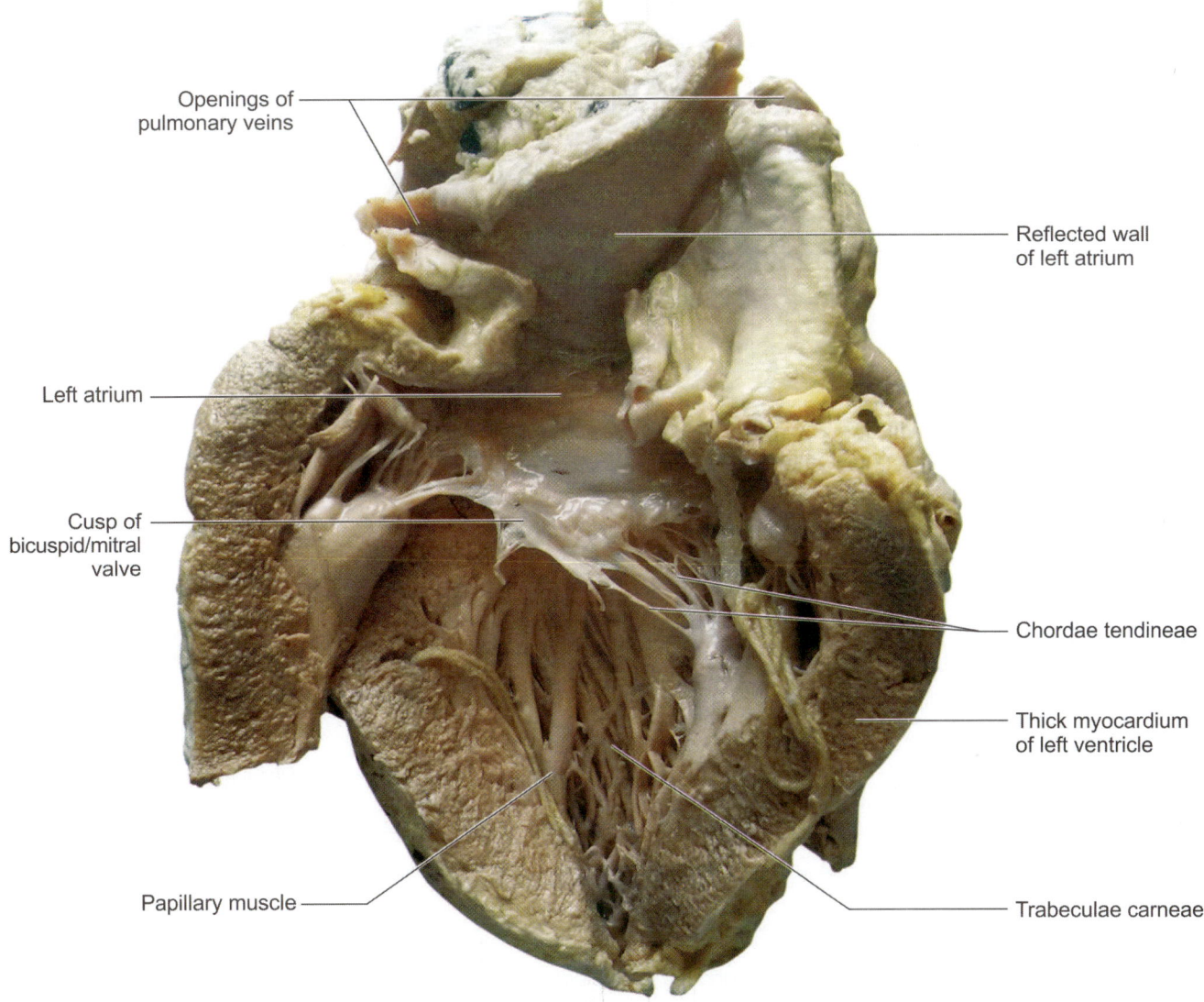

Openings of pulmonary veins

Reflected wall of left atrium

Left atrium

Cusp of bicuspid/mitral valve

Chordae tendineae

Thick myocardium of left ventricle

Papillary muscle

Trabeculae carneae

Fig. 12.11: Thick left ventricular wall

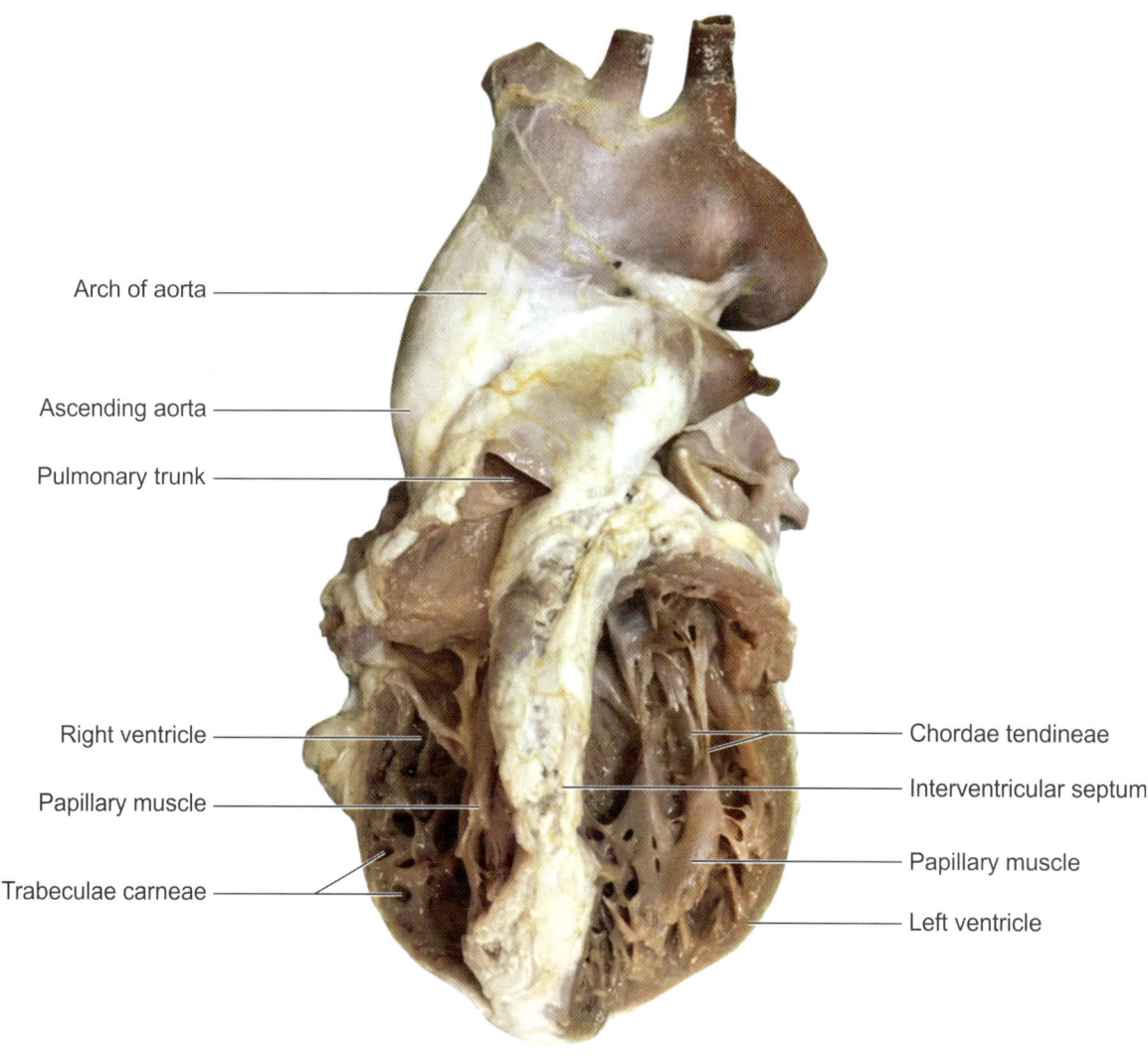

Arch of aorta

Ascending aorta

Pulmonary trunk

Right ventricle

Papillary muscle

Trabeculae carneae

Chordae tendineae

Interventricular septum

Papillary muscle

Left ventricle

Fig. 12.12a: Right and left ventricles with interventicular septum

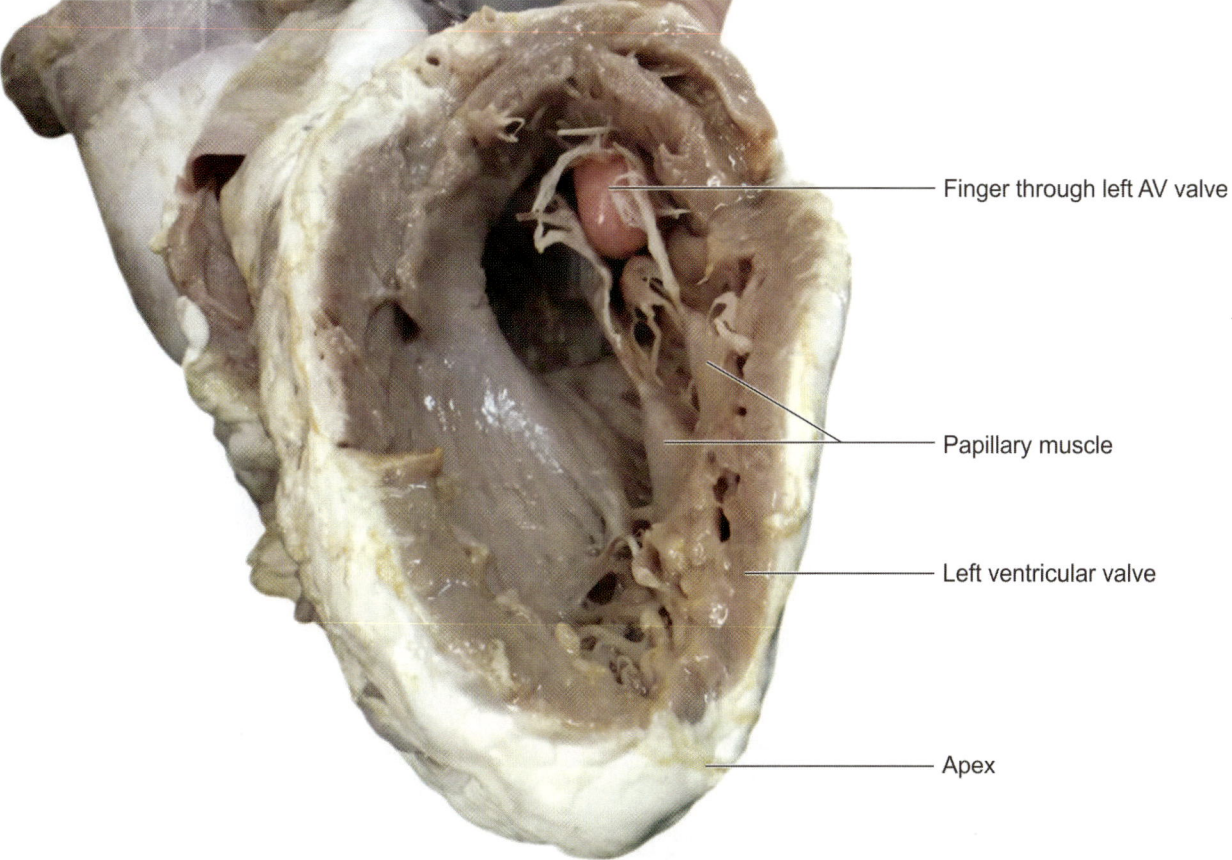

Fig. 12.12b: Section through left ventricle

Labels on figure:
- Finger through left AV valve
- Papillary muscle
- Left ventricular valve
- Apex

Competency achievement: The student should be able to:

AN 22.3 Describe and demonstrate origin, course and branches of coronary arteries.

AN 22.5 Describe and demonstrate the formation, course, tributaries and termination of coronary sinus.

Right Coronary Artery

- Carefully remove the fat from the coronary sulcus. Identify the right coronary artery in the depth of the right part of the atrioventricular sulcus (Figs 12.14 and 12.15).

- Trace the right coronary artery superiorly to its origin from the anterior aortic sinus and inferiorly till it turns onto the posterior surface of the heart to lie in its atrioventricular sulcus. It gives off the right marginal artery lying along inferior border and posterior interventricular branch which is seen in posterior interventricular groove.

- The right coronary artery ends by anastomosing with the circumflex branch of left coronary artery or by dipping itself deep in the myocardium there.

- Right coronary artery is the artery mainly supplying the right side of the heart (Figs 12.6 and 12.14).

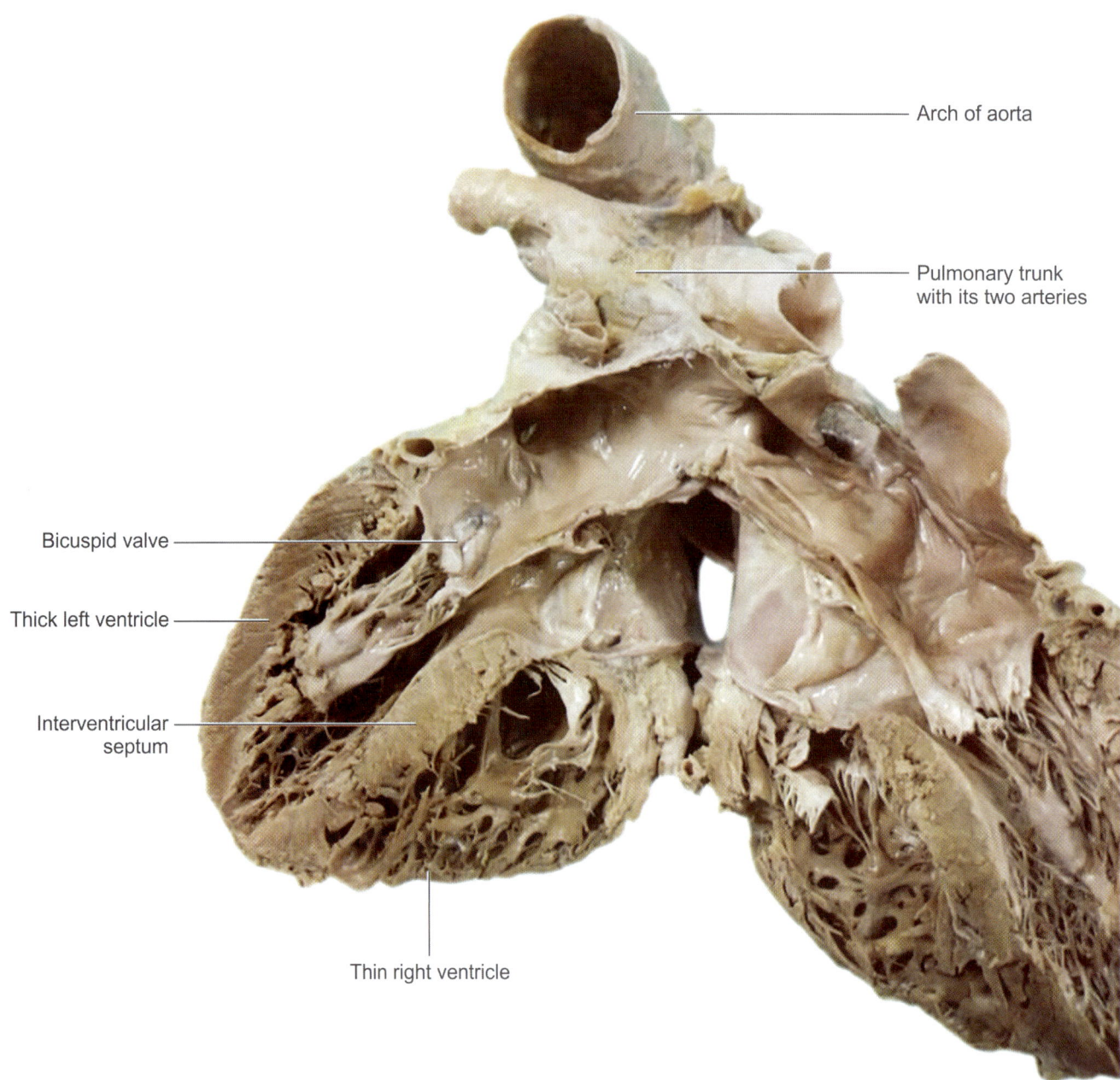

Arch of aorta

Pulmonary trunk with its two arteries

Bicuspid valve

Thick left ventricle

Interventricular septum

Thin right ventricle

Fig. 12.13a: Full cut section of heart

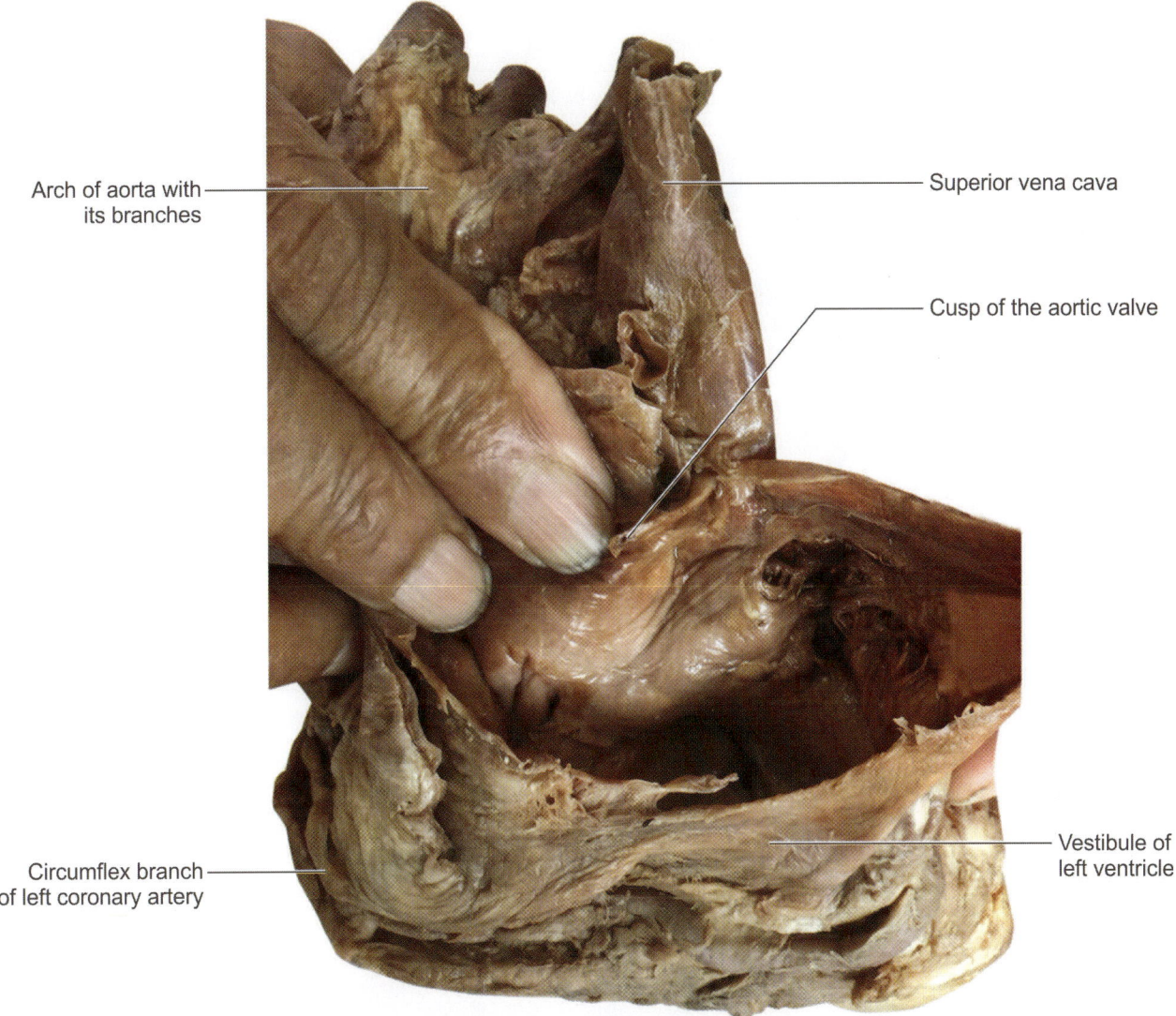

Arch of aorta with its branches

Superior vena cava

Cusp of the aortic valve

Circumflex branch of left coronary artery

Vestibule of left ventricle

Fig. 12.13b: *Aortic valve of left ventricle*

- Trace the origin, course, termination of this artery.
- See its multiple branches.

Left Coronary Artery

The artery arises from left posterior aortic sinus
- Strip the visceral pericardium from the sternocostal surface of the heart. Expose the anterior inter-ventricular branch of the left coronary artery and the great cardiac vein by carefully removing the fat

from the anterior interventricular sulcus (Figs 12.5a and 12.6). Note the branches of the artery to both ventricles and to the interventricular septum which lies deep to it. Trace the artery inferiorly to the diaphragmatic surface and superiorly to the left of the pulmonary trunk.

- Identify and trace the origin, course and termination of left coronary artery. See its multiple branches to left side of heart (Fig. 12.15).

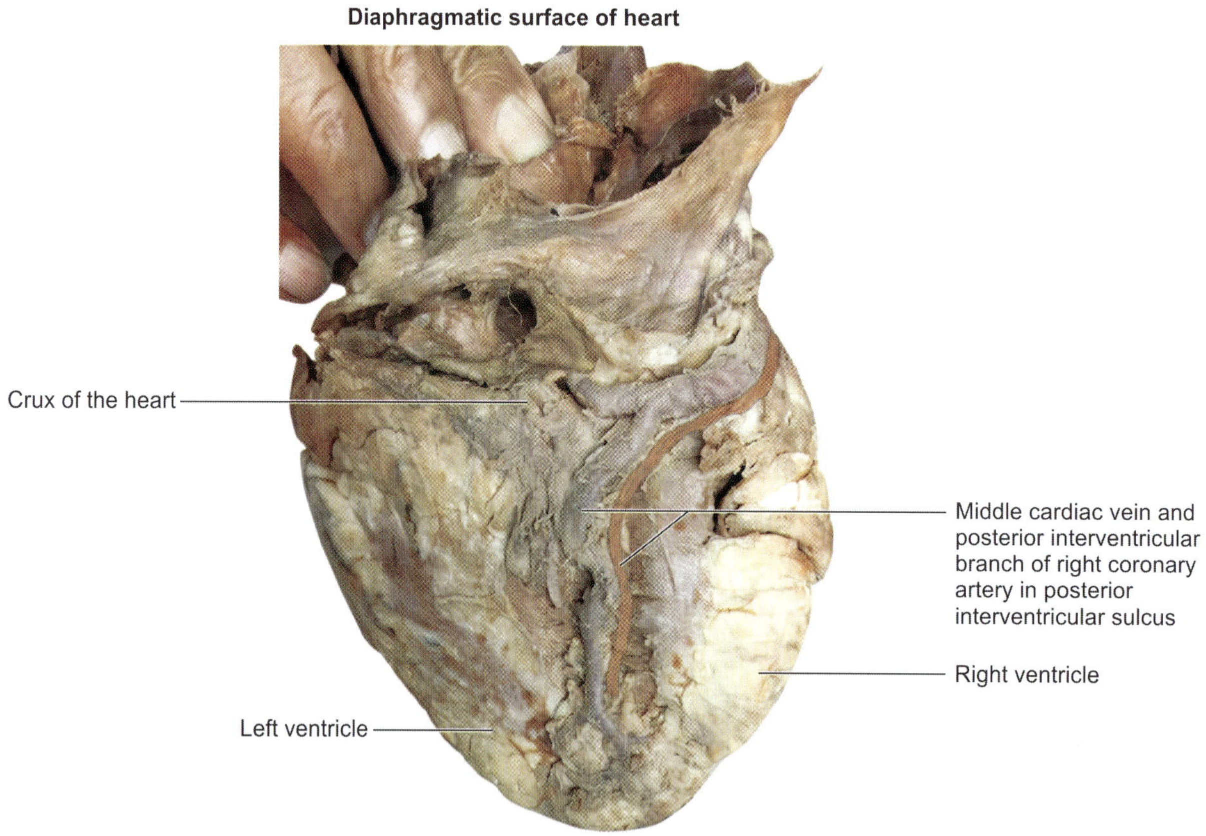

Diaphragmatic surface of heart

Crux of the heart

Middle cardiac vein and posterior interventricular branch of right coronary artery in posterior interventricular sulcus

Right ventricle

Left ventricle

Fig. 12.14: Course of right coronary artery and middle cardiac vein

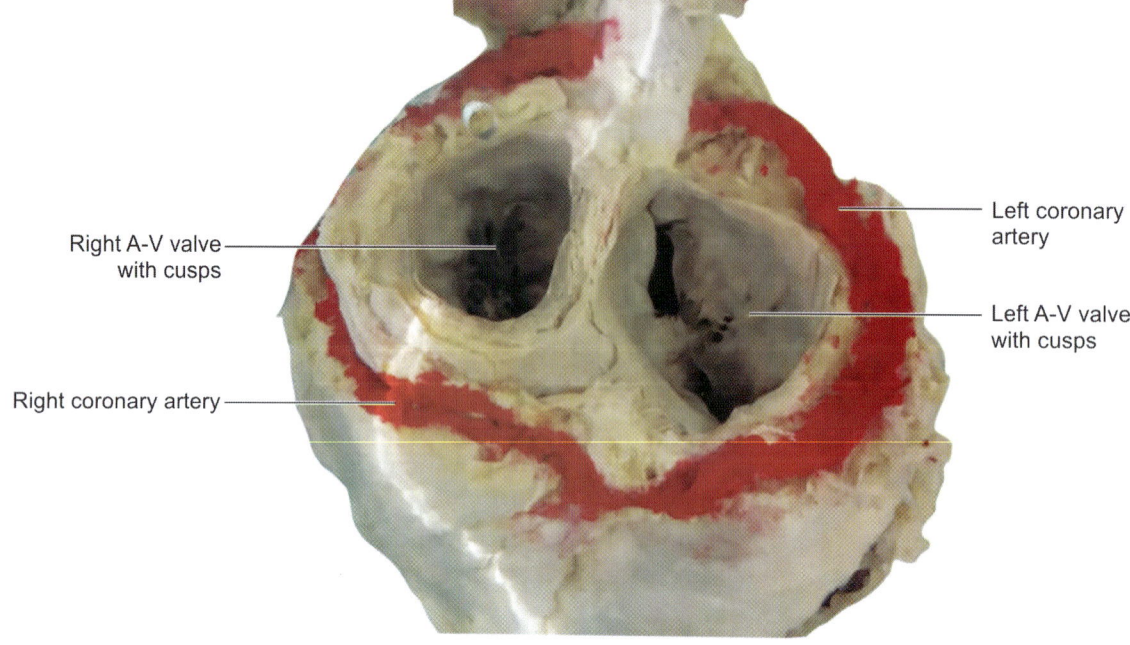

Right A-V valve with cusps

Left coronary artery

Left A-V valve with cusps

Right coronary artery

Fig. 12.15: Right and left coronary arteries

- Trace the circumflex branch of left coronary artery on the left border of heart into the posterior part of the sulcus, where it may end by anastomosing with the right coronary artery or by dipping into the myocardium.
- Try to dissect and identify the anastomosis between right coronary artery and circumflex branch of left coronary artery in the posterior part of coronary sulcus.
- Try to dissect and identify the anastomosis between anterior interventricular artery and posterior interventricular artery near the apex of heart.
- Follow the veins which run with the coronary arteries and their branches:

i. Great cardiac vein accompanies anterior interventricular branch and then circumflex artery.

ii. Middle cardiac vein accompanies posterior interventricular branch (Fig. 12.14)

iii. Small cardiac vein accompanies the right coronary artery.

iv. Right marginal vein accompanies right marginal artery.

All the cardiac veins end in the coronary sinus.

- See the opening of coronary sinus into the cavity of right atrium between the opening of inferior vena cava and right atrioventricular orifice (Fig. 12.7b).

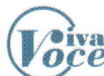

- What are the boundaries of transverse sinus of the pericardium?
- Name the boundaries of oblique sinus of the pericardium.
- Name the veins opening in right atrium and in left atrium.

- Why is left ventricle the thickest chamber of the heart?
- Name the cusps of the aortic and pulmonary valve.
- Trace the course of right coronary artery.
- Trace the course of left coronary artery.
- What is cardiac dominance?

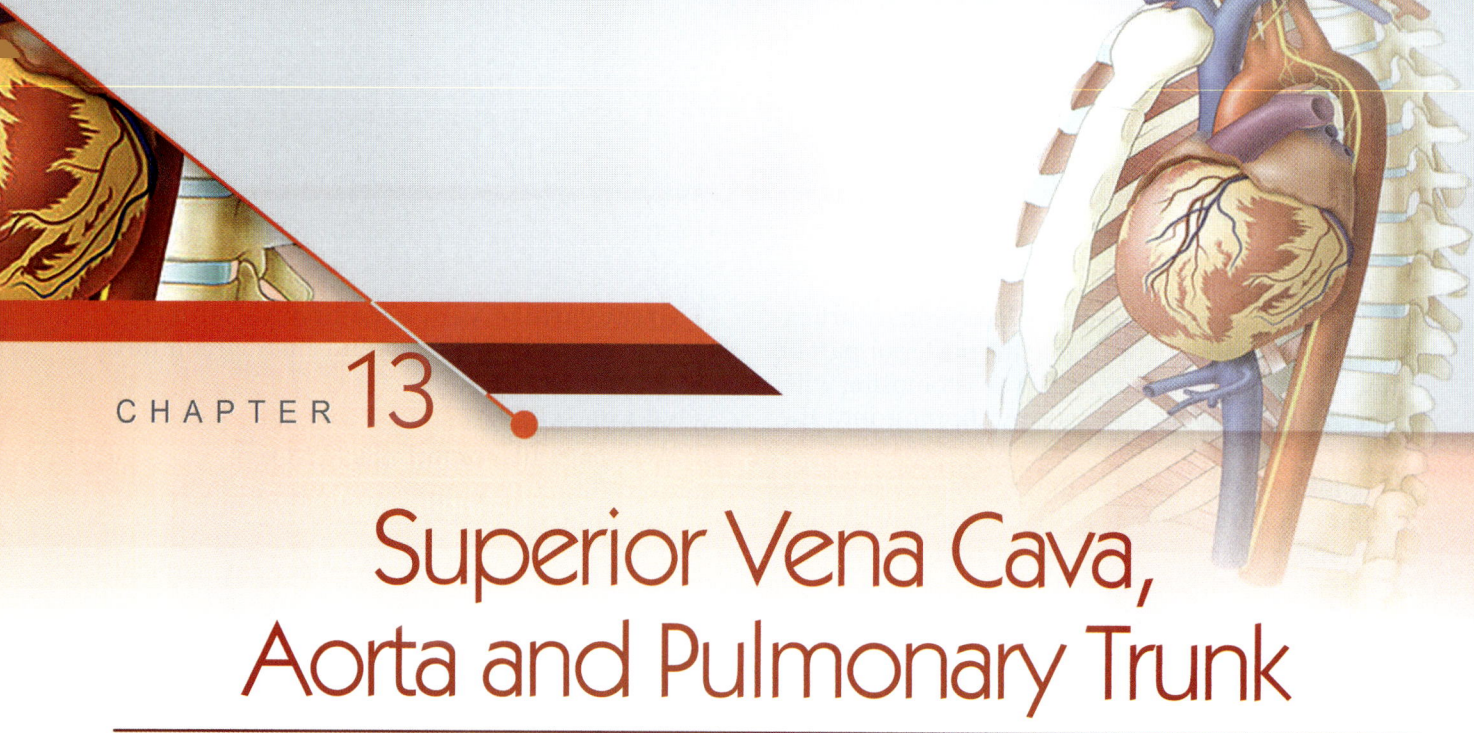

CHAPTER 13

Superior Vena Cava, Aorta and Pulmonary Trunk

Learning Objectives

One should be able to

1. Enumerate the tributaries of brachiocephalic vein
2. Name the branches of ascending aorta.
3. Name the branches of arch of aorta.

OVERVIEW

Superior vena cava brings deoxygenated blood from the brain, head, neck, upper limb and thorax into the right atrium. It is the 2nd largest vein of the body present along the upper border of the heart. Vena azygos draining from the thoracic wall ends in the superior vena cava at the level of 2nd costal cartilage. Aorta, the largest artery, arises from the vestibular region of left ventricle. It comprises three parts—the ascending aorta, arch of aorta and descending aorta, which is subdivided into thoracic part and an abdominal part. Ascending aorta is enclosed in the pericardium. It gives origin to the right and left coronary arteries.

Ascending aorta continues as arch of aorta at the sternal end of upper border of the 2nd right costal cartilage. Arch of aorta lies behind lower half of manubrium sterni. It passes downwards on left side of 4th thoracic vertebra to continue as descending thoracic aorta.

Three branches arise from arch of aorta which supply head, neck and upper limbs.

Descending thoracic aorta is situated in the posterior mediastinum. It passes through the median arcuate ligament of thoracoabdominal diaphragm to continue as abdominal aorta. The branches of thoracic aorta are mainly posterior intercostal arteries.

Pulmonary trunk arises from the infundibulum of right ventricle and soon divides into right and left pulmonary arteries. It carries deoxygenated blood from right ventricle to both the lungs for oxygenation of blood. The left pulmonary artery is connected to inferior aspect of arch of aorta via the ligamentum arteriosum. This ligament is a remnant of ductus arteriosus which takes an important part in foetal circulation.

Competency achievement: The student should be able to:

AN 23.3 Describe and demonstrate origin, course, relations, tributaries and termination of superior vena cava, azygos, hemiazygos and accessory hemiazygos veins.

STEPS OF DISSECTION

- Trace superior vena cava from level of first right costal cartilage where it is formed by union of left and right brachiocephalic veins till the third costal cartilage where it opens into right atrium.
- Superior vena cava is formed by union of right and left brachiocephalic or innominate veins behind the

114

- lower border of 1st right costal cartilage close to the sternum (*see* Fig. 11.1).
- Medial to superior vena cava are the ascending aorta and pulmonary trunk (*see* Fig. 12.3).
- Identify the trachea and vagus nerve posteromedial to the upper part superior vena cava.
- See and trace right phrenic nerve lateral to superior vena cava. See the nerve coursing down anterior to the root of right lung.
- Trace the left recurrent laryngeal nerve to the medial aspect of arch of aorta.

- Lift the side of oesophagus forwards to expose the anterior surface of the descending aorta.
- Lift the diaphragm forwards and expose the descending thoracic aorta in the inferior part of the posterior mediastinum.

Competency achievement: The student should be able to:

AN 23.4 Mention the extent, branches and relations of arch of aorta and descending thoracic aorta.

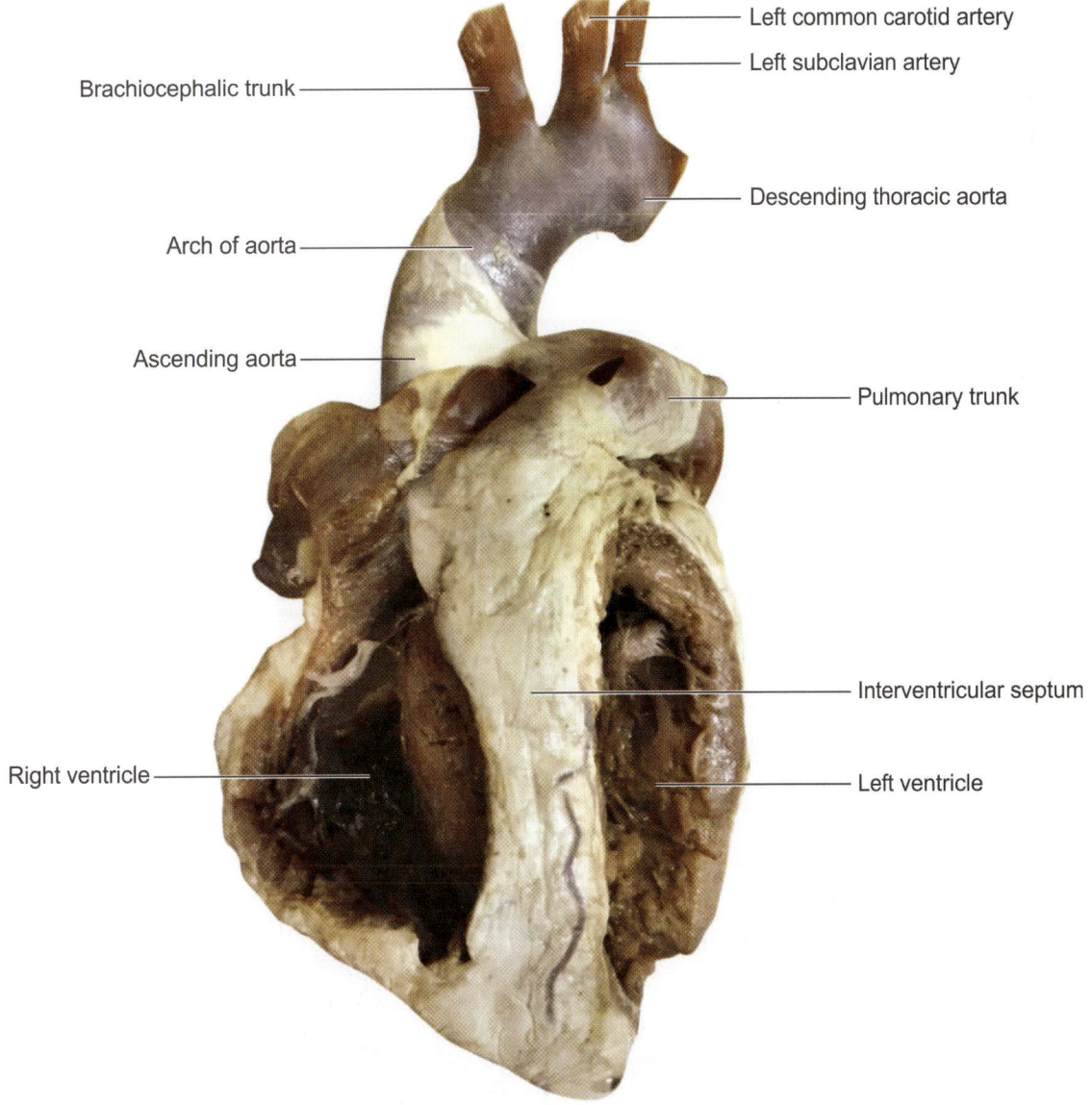

Fig. 13.1: Interventricular septum with pulmonary trunk and arch of aorta

Aorta is the largest artery of the body comprising an ascending part, arch part and a descending thoracic part.

Ascending aorta lies in between superior vena cava and pulmonary trunk. The transverse sinus of pericardium lies posterior to ascending aorta.

- See and trace relations of arch of aorta.
- Trace the phrenic and vagus nerves lying anterior and to the left of arch of aorta.
- Left phrenic nerve passes anterior to the root of left lung while left vagus nerve lies posterior to it where the nerve forms the pulmonary plexus.
- Trace the thin left superior intercostal vein lying behind phrenic nerve and anterior to vagus nerve.
- See trachea and oesophagus posterior and to right of arch of aorta. Identify important recurrent laryngeal nerve in the tracheo-oesophageal groove. This nerve ascends up to supply most of the muscles of larynx.
- Identify three branches of arch of aorta above it (Fig. 13.1).

These are:

  i. Brachiocephalic trunk which divides into right common carotid and right subclavian artery.

 ii. Left common carotid artery

iii. Left subclavian artery

- Look for bifurcation of pulmonary trunk in the concavity of arch of aorta.
- Trace left recurrent laryngeal nerve hooking inferior to the arch of aorta and then ascending up in the tracheo-oesophageal groove (Fig. 13.2).
- Look for ligamentum arteriosum—a remnant of ductus arteriosus.
- Descending thoracic aorta starts at T4 and ends at T12 vertebra to continue as descending abdominal aorta. Its branches are 3rd–11th right intercostal arteries and few other branches.
- Trace pulmonary trunk arising from the summit of infundibulum of right ventricle. Pulmonary trunk runs to the left to lie in the concavity of arch of aorta,

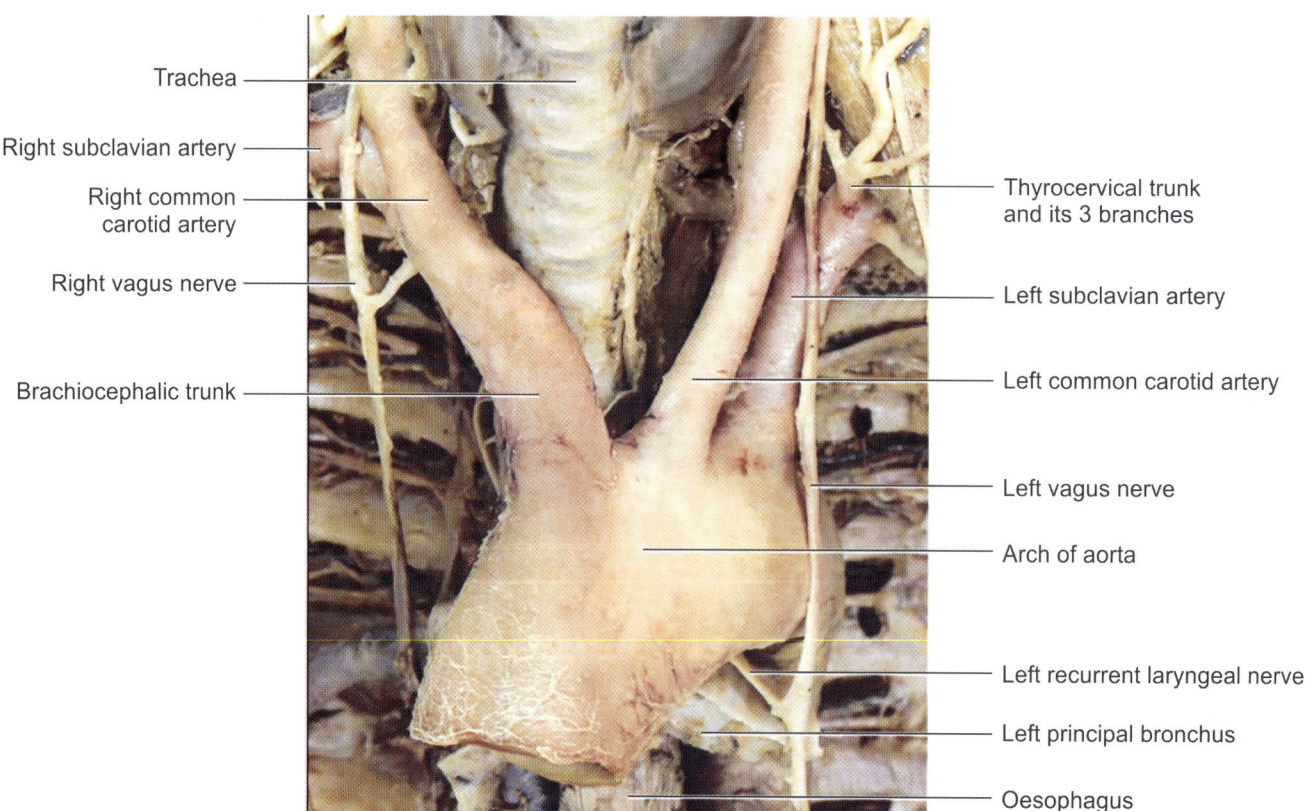

Fig. 13.2: Arch of aorta and its branches

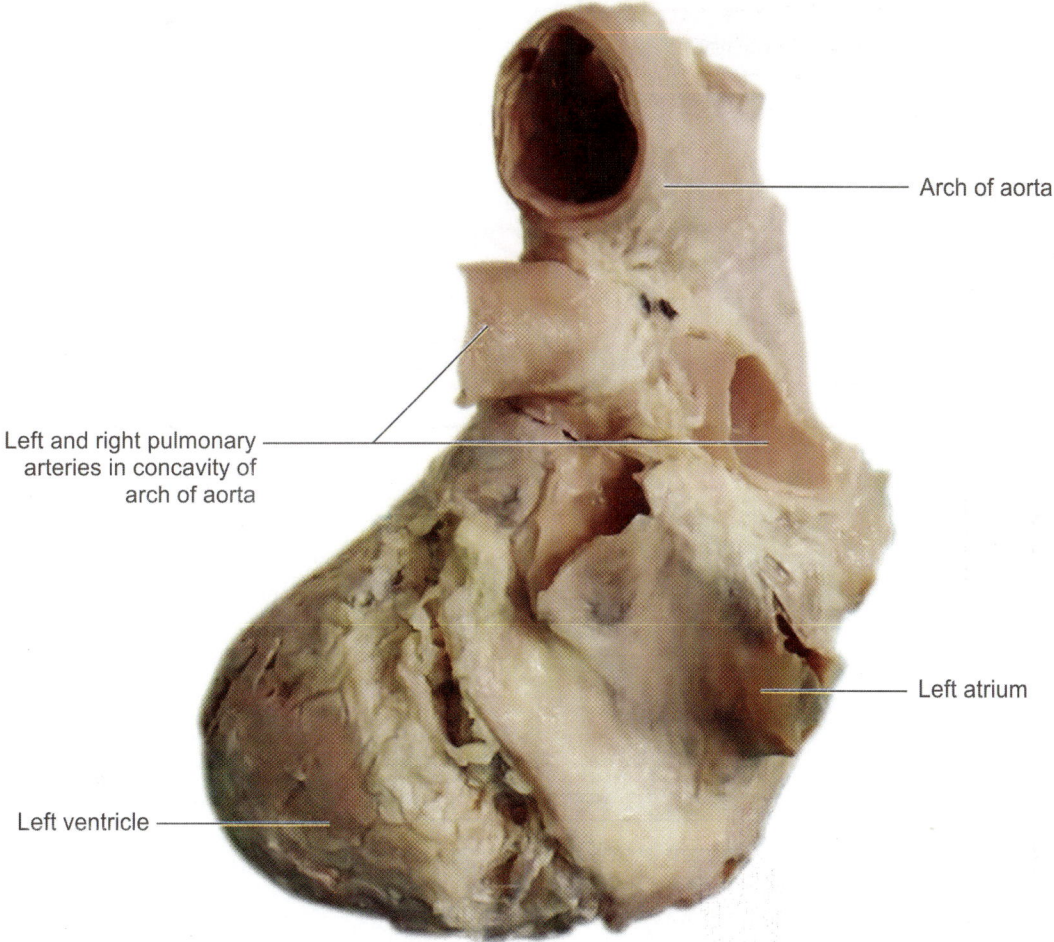

Arch of aorta

Left and right pulmonary
arteries in concavity of
arch of aorta

Left atrium

Left ventricle

Fig. 13.3: Pulmonary trunk dividing into right and left arteries in concavity of aortic arch

where it divides into right and left pulmonary arteries for each of the two lungs (Fig. 13.3).

- See the right pulmonary artery passing behind the ascending aorta, superior vena cava, anterior to oesophagus to reach the root of right lung.
- See the left pulmonary artery passing to left, anterior to descending thoracic aorta to reach root of left lung.

- Appreciate the triple relationship between pulmonary trunk and ascending aorta. Close to heart, pulmonary trunk lies anterior to ascending aorta. At upper border of heart, pulmonary trunk lies to the left of ascending aorta. A little above this, right pulmonary artery lies posterior to the ascending aorta.

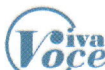

- What are the parts of aorta?
- Name the branches of ascending aorta.
- Name the branches of arch of aorta.

- Name the branches of descending thoracic aorta.
- What is the triple relation between pulmonary trunk and ascending aorta?

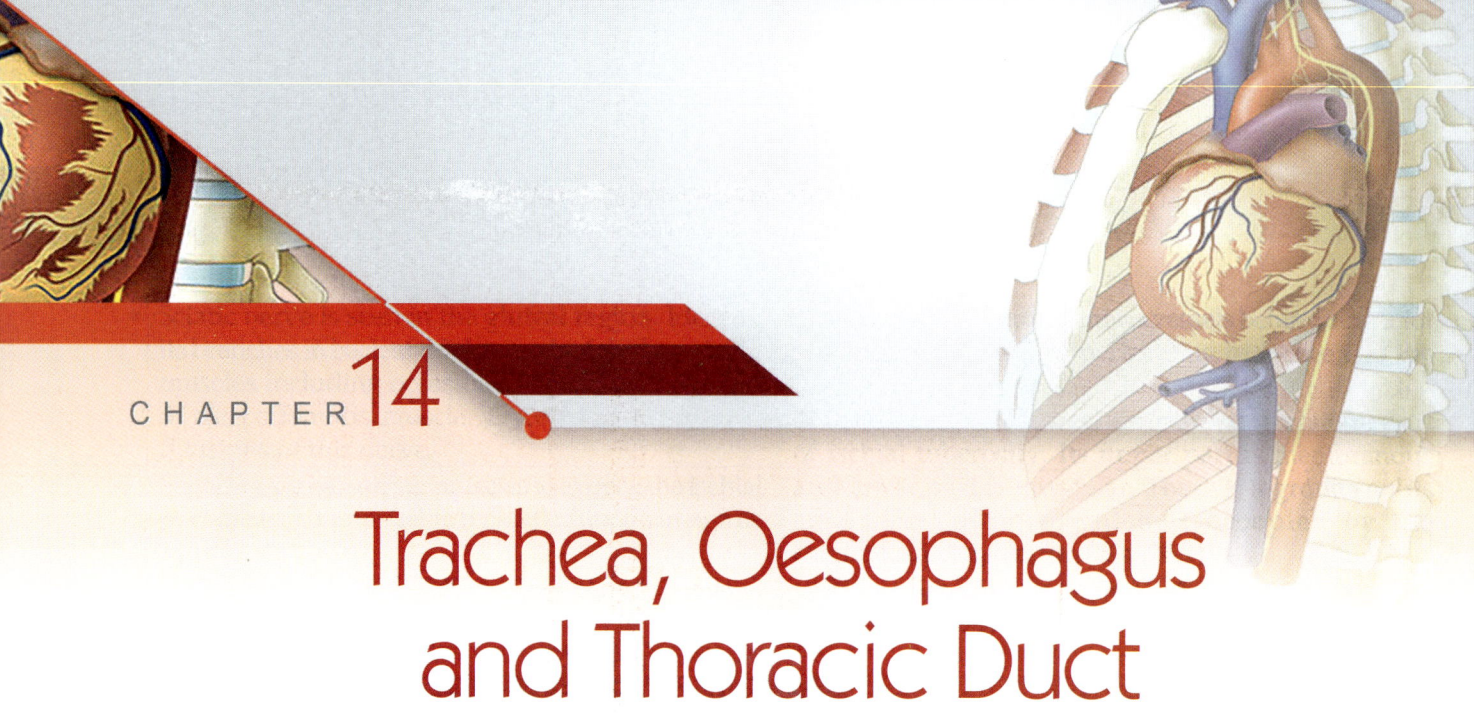

CHAPTER 14

Trachea, Oesophagus and Thoracic Duct

Learning Objectives

One should be able to

1. Explain why is the posterior aspect of trachea deficient in cartilage.
2. Name the regions of the body through which the oesophagus courses.
3. Enumerate the sites of normal constrictions of oesophagus and their clinical importance.
4. Name the lymph duct which drains right upper limb, right side of head and neck and right side of thorax. Where does this duct drain?

OVERVIEW

Trachea is a patent wide tube carrying air to and fro between the upper nasal passages and the lungs. It starts from C6 vertebra, lies partly in neck region and partly in thoracic region. It divides at the level of lower border of T4 vertebra into right and left bronchi. Trachea contains 'C' shaped hyaline cartilages to keep it patent. Posteriorly, the cartilage is absent where it is related to the oesophagus.

Oesophagus or food pipe lies posterior to trachea in superior mediastinum. Then it courses through posterior mediastinum of thorax and through thoraco-abdominal diaphragm to reach the abdominal cavity. It lies behind the left atrium in the upper part of posterior mediastinum. In its lower part, oesophagus lies anterior to descending thoracic aorta. The oesophagus shows four normal constrictions at various levels. These have to be kept in mind while passing nasogastric tube for feeding the patient or for getting samples of gastric juice. The lowest end of oesophagus in the abdomen is a site of portosystemic anastomoses.

Thoracic duct is the largest lymphatic duct in the body. It courses through the abdomen, posterior mediastinum, superior mediastinum of thorax and finally enters the neck region. In the neck it ends at the angle between left subclavian and left internal jugular veins.

Thoracic duct receives lymph from both the lower limbs, abdomen and pelvis, left half of thorax, left upper limb and left side of head and neck.

Competency achievement: The student should be able to:

AN 23.1 Describe and demonstrate the external appearance, relations, blood supply, nerve supply, lymphatic drainage and applied anatomy of oesophagus.

AN 23.2 Describe and demonstrate the extent, relations tributaries of thoracic duct and enumerate its applied anatomy.

AN 24.6 Describe the extent, length, relations, blood supply, lymphatic drainage and nerve supply of trachea.

STEPS OF DISSECTION

- Clean the trachea from its beginning till the level of manubriosternal angle (Fig. 14.1). Remove the lobes of thyroid gland if present.
- Remove the posterior surface of the parietal pericardium between the right and left pulmonary veins.

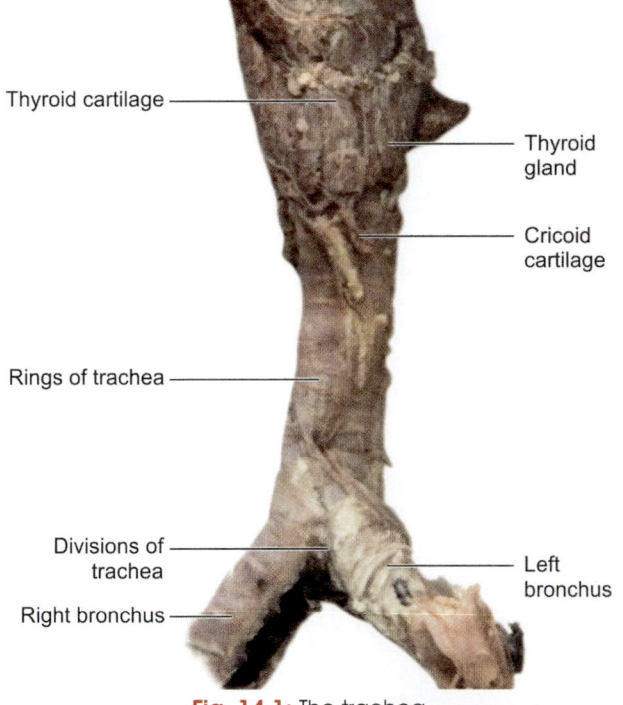

Fig. 14.1: The trachea

Thyroid cartilage

Thyroid gland

Cricoid cartilage

Rings of trachea

Divisions of trachea

Right bronchus

Left bronchus

- Clean the oesophagus from its beginning in the neck.
- Trace it down into superior mediastinum where it lies posterior to trachea.
- Trace it further into the posterior mediastinum posterior to the parietal layer of serous pericardium and fibrous pericardium. Lower down it lies anterior to the descending thoracic aorta (Fig. 14.2).
- See the oesophagus piercing the thoracoabdominal diaphragm at the level of T10 vertebra and surrounded by right crus of the diaphragm. Trace the arteries supplying the oesophagus.
- Thoracic duct drains most of the lymph of the body into the veins of neck.
- Look for cisterna chyli at level of 2nd lumbar vertebrae (Fig. 14.2). It continues as thoracic duct and enters the thorax via the aortic opening.
- Identify the structures passing through the aortic opening. These are:
  - i. Descending thoracic aorta
  - ii. Vena azygos to the right of aorta

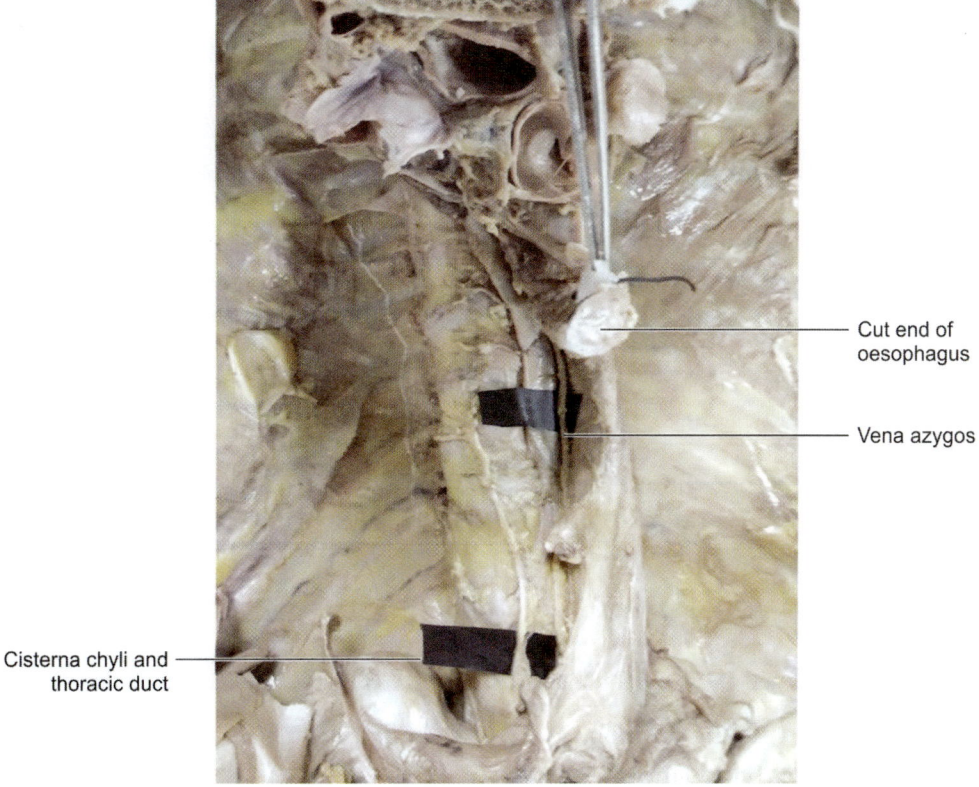

Cut end of oesophagus

Vena azygos

Cisterna chyli and thoracic duct

Fig. 14.2: Oesophagus and thoracic duct

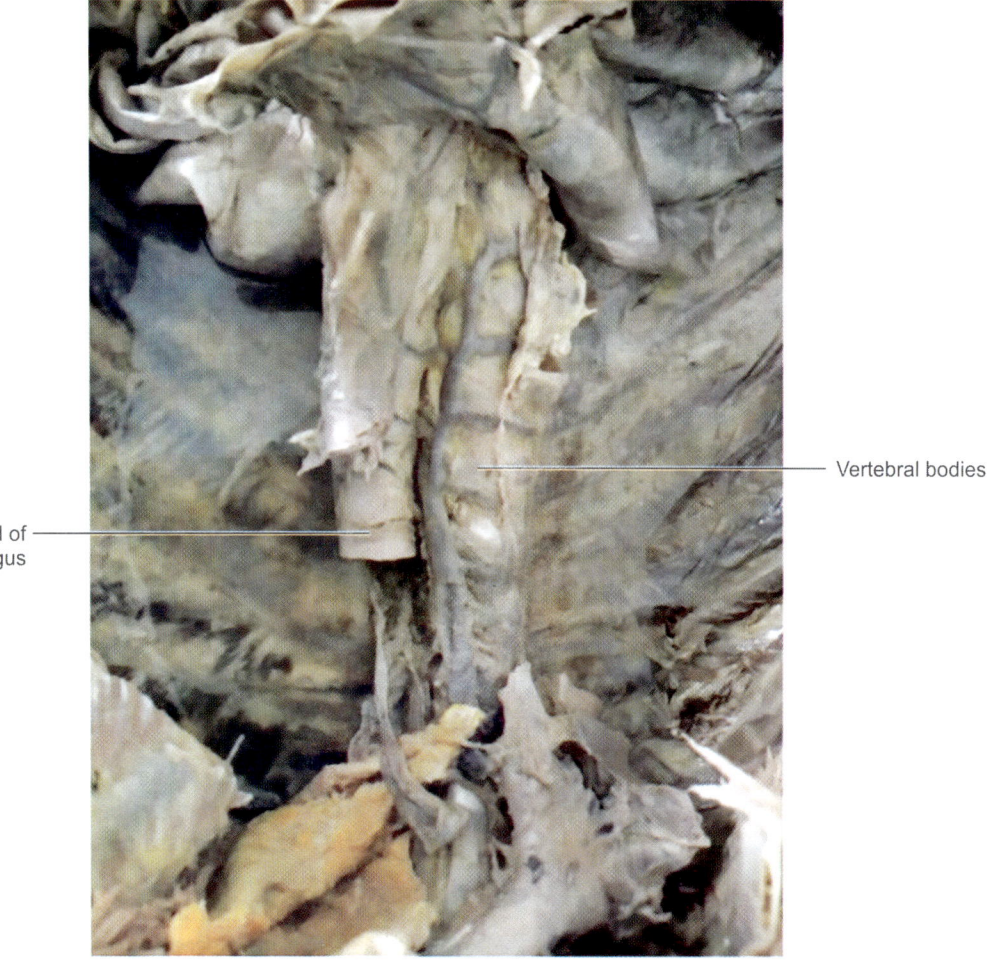

Cut end of oesophagus

Vertebral bodies

Fig. 14.3: Part of oesophagus

iii. Thoracic duct between the vena azygos and the aorta.

• Trace the thoracic duct ascending through posterior mediastinum till 5th thoracic vertebra.

• See the thoracic duct passing across 5th thoracic vertebra from right to left side. Trace the duct along the left margin of oesophagus where it courses through superior mediastinum to reach the neck.

In the neck the thoracic duct opens at the angle of junction between left subclavian and left internal jugular veins.

• See a corresponding duct—the right lymphatic duct draining right side of head and neck, right upper limb and right thorax and drains into the angle of junction between right subclavian and right internal jugular veins.

• What is extent of trachea in supine position?
• What type of cartilage is present in trachea and bronchi?

• Name the sites of anatomical constrictions in the course of oesophagus.
• Where does thoracic duct start?

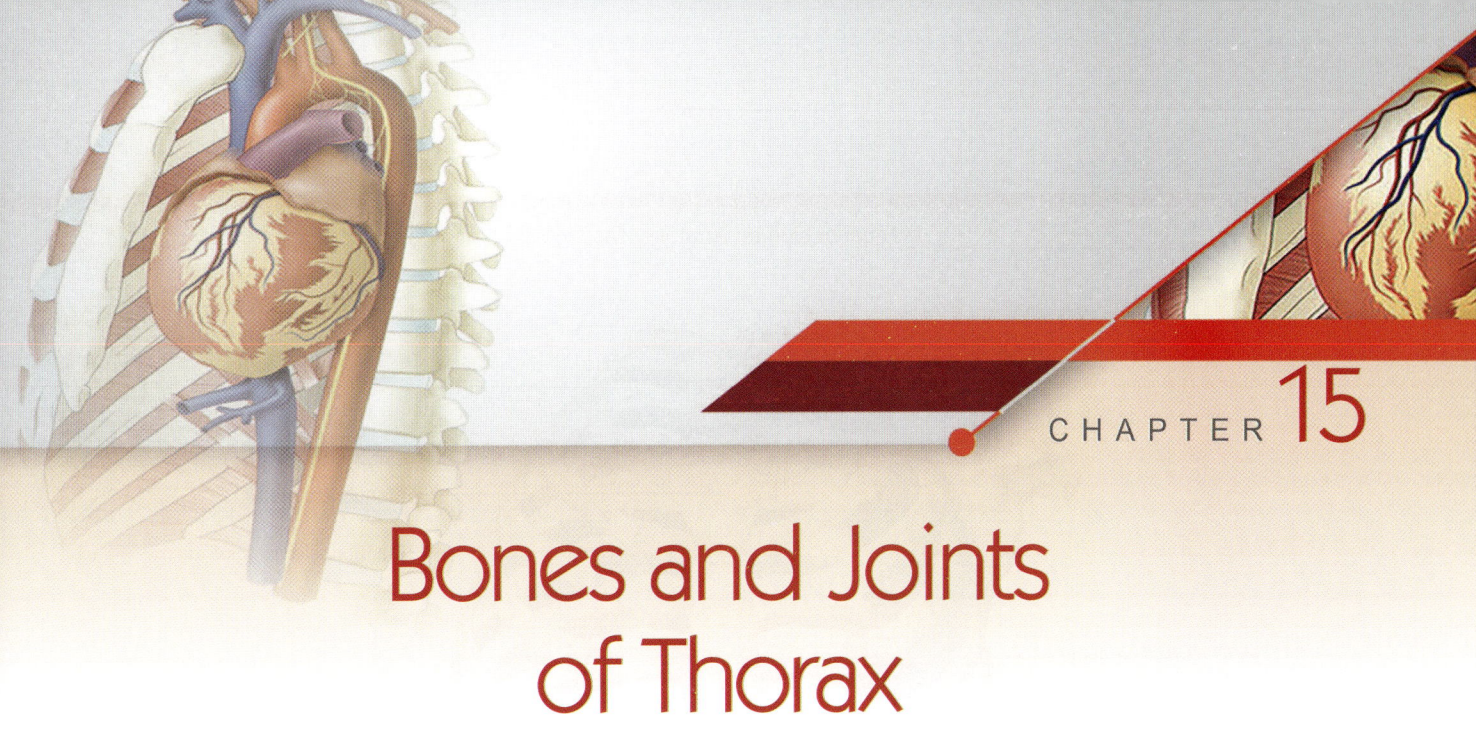

Bones and Joints of Thorax

Bones of thorax form thoracic cage seen from anterior aspect and posterior aspect (Figs 15.1 and 15.2). These are:

i. Single sternum ventrally (Fig 15.1)
ii. 12 thoracic vertebrae dorsally and laterally (Figs 15.2a and b)
iii. 12 pairs of arched ribs with costal cartilages (Fig. 15.3)
   a. 1–7 pairs are vertebrosternal ribs (true ribs)
   b. 8–10 pairs are vertebrochondral ribs (false ribs)
   c. 11 and 12 pairs are vertebral ribs (floating ribs)

The inner aspect of lower 6 costal cartilages give origin to thoracoabdominal diaphragm (Fig. 15.4). Its digitations interdigitate with fibres of transversus abdominis muscle.

These bones form numerous joints. Sternum articulates with:

i. Right and left clavicles above (Fig. 15.1)
ii. Right and left upper 7 costal cartilages (Fig. 15.1)
iii. Costal cartilages of 8th ribs articulate with costal cartilages of the 7th ribs and similarly the costal cartilages of the 9th and 10th ribs articulate with the costal cartilages of the rib above.

Thus the 1st–10th pairs of ribs articulate through the costal cartilages with sternum, 1–7 directly and 8–10 indirectly. 11th and 12th ribs tipped with costal cartilages have free ends.

One important joint in sternum is manubriosternal joint, a secondary cartilaginous joint. This acts as a hinge in raising the body of sternum upwards and forwards (by upper ribs) thus increasing antero-posterior diameter of thorax (Fig. 15.1).

Posterior end of rib comprises head, neck and an articular and non-articular parts of tubercle (Fig. 15.3).

3rd rib to 9th rib, i.e. 7 ribs are typical ribs, rest 5 ribs, i.e. 1st, 2nd, 10th–12th ribs are atypical (Fig. 15.1).

Typical rib forms costovertebral joint with two adjacent vertebrae and intervening intervertebral disc (Fig. 15.2b).

Tubercle of rib forms costotransverse joint with facet on the transverse process of the corresponding thoracic vertebra (Fig. 15.5).

3rd to 6th transverse processes have concave facets. These form concavo-convex joints with the tubercle of rib facets. 7th to 9th transverse processes have flattened facets. They form plane joints with tubercles of respective ribs (Fig. 15.6).

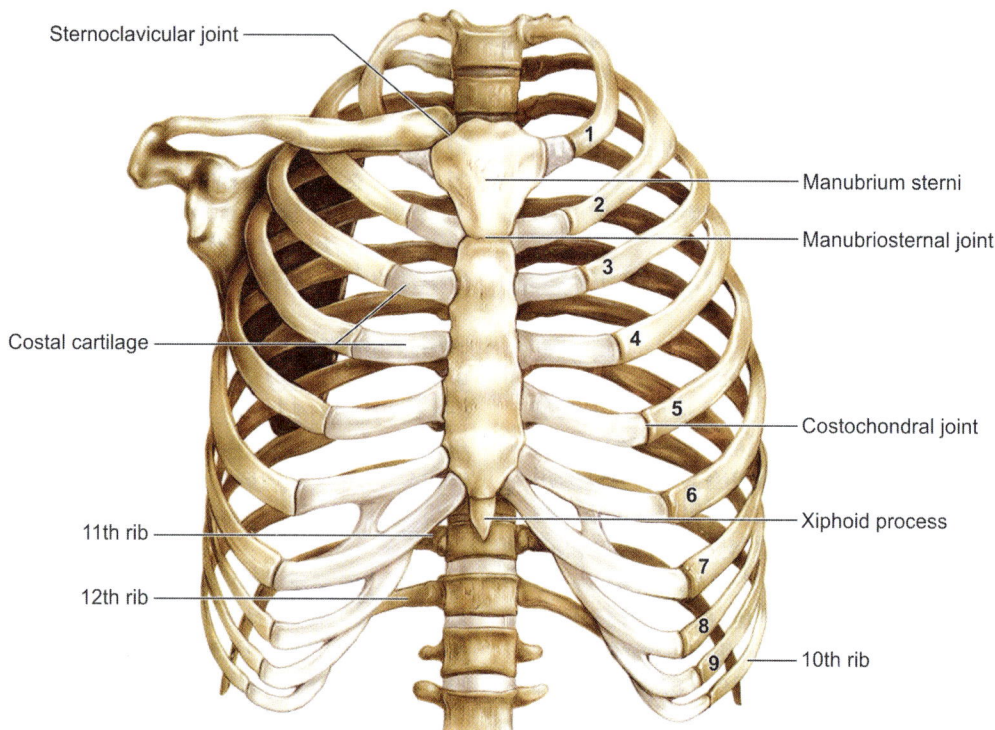

Sternoclavicular joint

Manubrium sterni

Manubriosternal joint

Costal cartilage

Costochondral joint

11th rib

Xiphoid process

12th rib

10th rib

1 2 3 4 5 6 7 8 9

Fig. 15.1: Bones of thoracic cage seen from anterior aspect

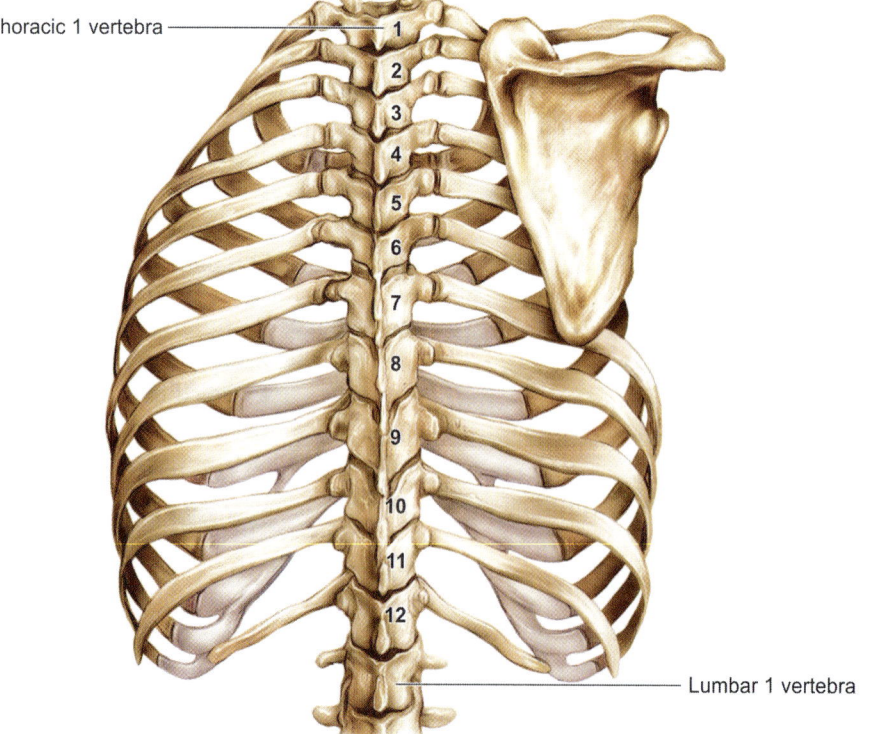

Thoracic 1 vertebra

Lumbar 1 vertebra

1 2 3 4 5 6 7 8 9 10 11 12

Fig. 15.2a: Bones of thoracic cage seen from posterior aspect

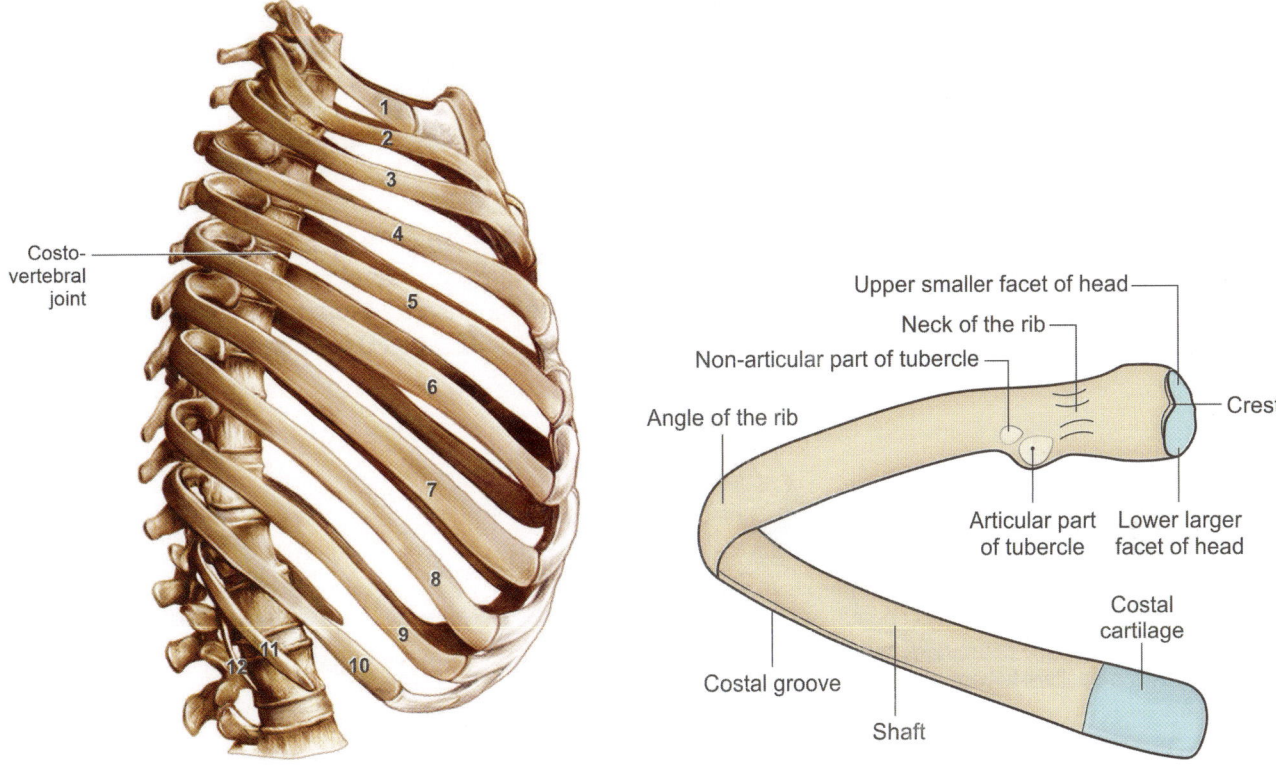

Fig. 15.2b: Bones of thoracic seen from lateral aspect

Costo-vertebral joint

1
2
3
4
5
6
7
8
9
10
11
12

Fig. 15.3: Parts of a typical rib

Upper smaller facet of head

Neck of the rib

Non-articular part of tubercle

Angle of the rib

Crest

Articular part of tubercle

Lower larger facet of head

Costal cartilage

Costal groove

Shaft

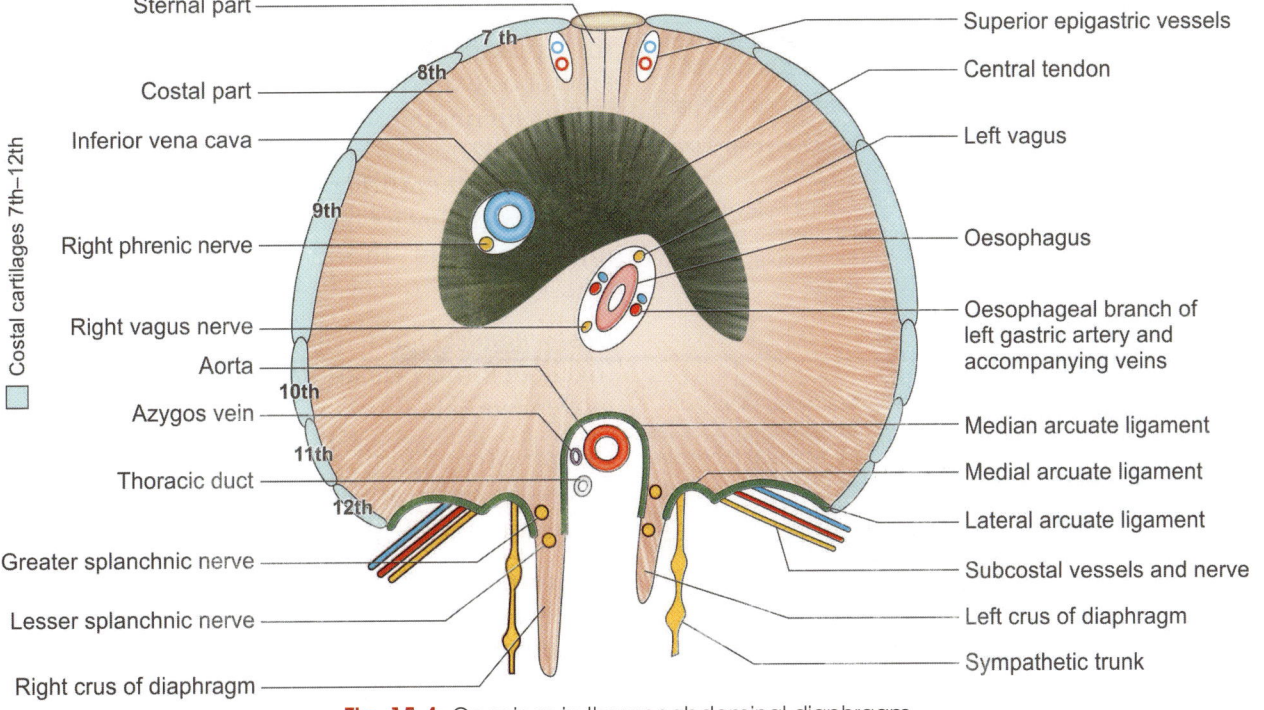

Sternal part

Costal part

Inferior vena cava

Costal cartilages 7th–12th

Right phrenic nerve

Right vagus nerve

Aorta

Azygos vein

Thoracic duct

Greater splanchnic nerve

Lesser splanchnic nerve

Right crus of diaphragm

7 th
8th
9th
10th
11th
12th

Superior epigastric vessels

Central tendon

Left vagus

Oesophagus

Oesophageal branch of left gastric artery and accompanying veins

Median arcuate ligament

Medial arcuate ligament

Lateral arcuate ligament

Subcostal vessels and nerve

Left crus of diaphragm

Sympathetic trunk

Fig. 15.4: Openings in thoracoabdominal diaphragm

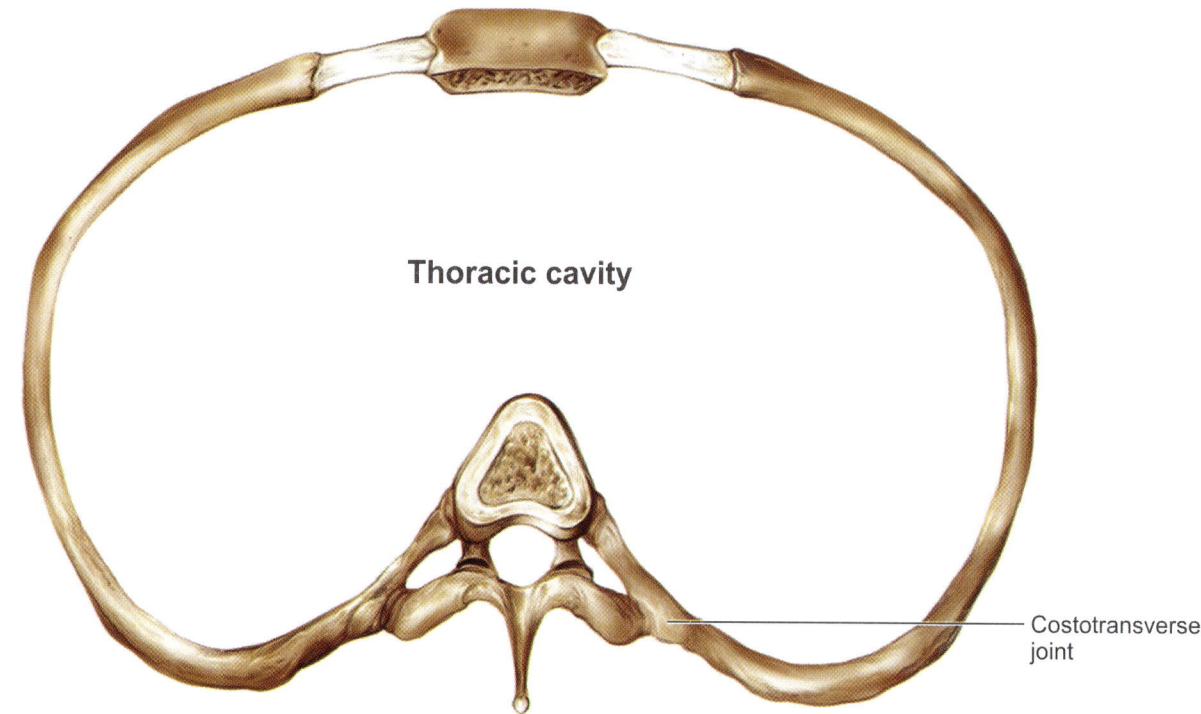

Fig. 15.5: Thoracic cavity

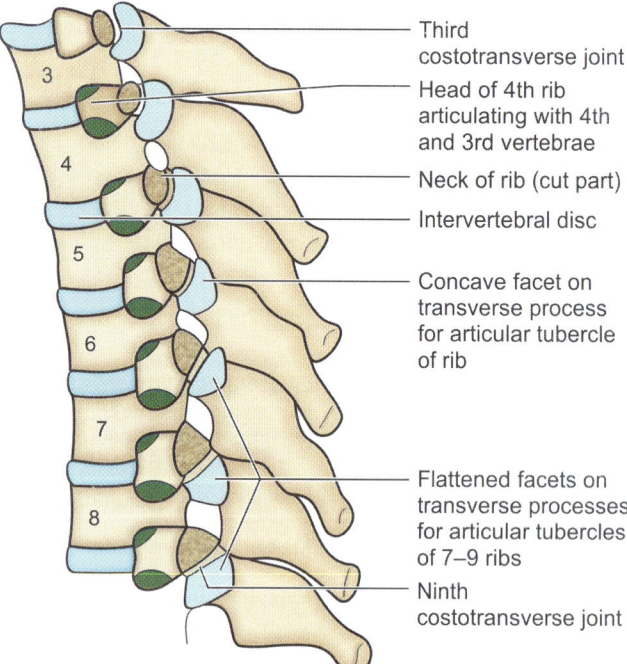

Fig. 15.6: A section through the costotransverse joints from the third to the ninth inclusive. Contrast the concave facets on the upper with the flattened facets on the lower transverse processes

Thus upper ribs permit rotation of the neck of rib for "pump handle movement" increasing the anteroposterior diameter of thorax (Fig. 15.7).

7th–9th ribs permit gliding movements or "bucket handle movements" resulting in increase in transverse diameter of thorax (Fig. 15.8).

Vertical diameter of thorax is increased by piston movements of thoracoabdominal diaphragm (Fig. 15.9).

Costochondral joint: Each rib with its costal cartilage (hyaline) forms primary cartilaginous joint with 'No movement' (Fig. 15.5).

Chondrosternal joint
- 1st—primary cartilaginous joint
- 2nd–7th—plane synovial joints

Intervertebral joints, e.g. between 5th and 6th thoracic vertebrae are three viz, one between body of the 5th and 6th and two other between inferior articular processes of 5th and superior articular processes of 6th on the right side and left side.

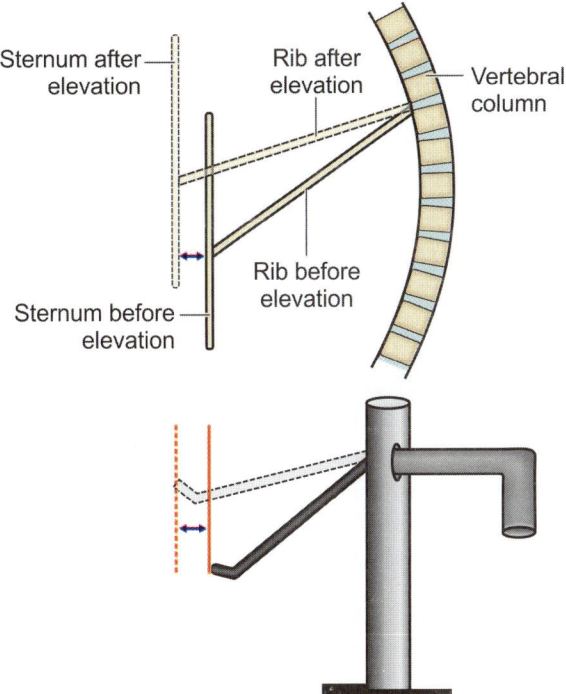

Sternum after elevation

Rib after elevation

Vertebral column

Rib before elevation

Sternum before elevation

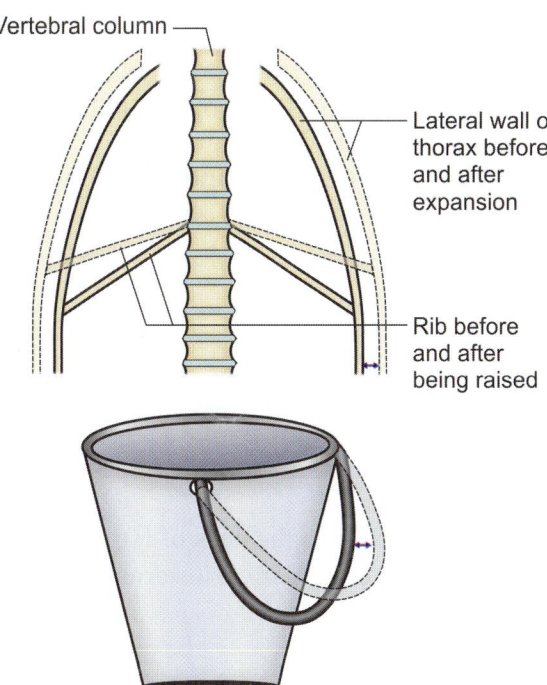

Vertebral column

Lateral wall of thorax before and after expansion

Rib before and after being raised

Fig. 15.7: Diagram showing how 'pump-handle' movements of the sternum bring about an increase in the anteroposterior diameter of the thorax

Fig. 15.8: Showing how 'bucket-handle' movements of the vertebrochondral ribs bring about an increase in the transverse diameter of the thorax

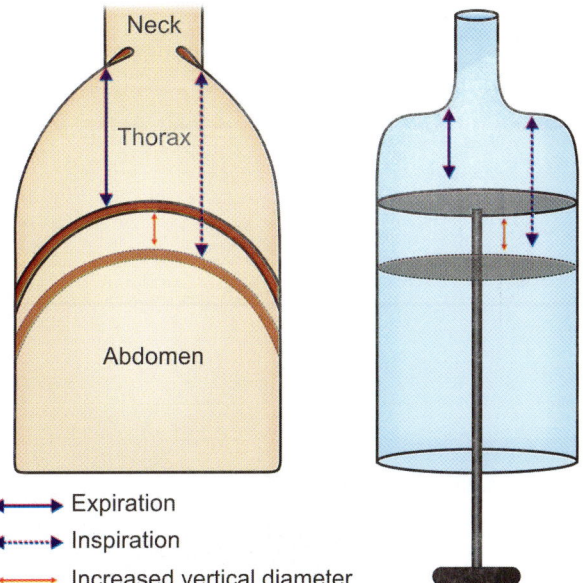

Neck

Thorax

Abdomen

→ Expiration

┅→ Inspiration

→ Increased vertical diameter

Fig. 15.9: Showing how piston movements of thoracoabdominal diaphragm bring about an increase in the vertical diameter of the thorax

Respiratory Movements

Quiet inspiration

i. Inspiration is chiefly brought about by the thoracoabdominal diaphragm.

ii. The external intercostal, interchondral part of internal intercostal may elevate rib during inspiration.

Deep inspiration

i. Movements of quiet inspiration get increased.

ii. Erector spinae and pectoral muscles increase size of thoracic cavity

Quiet expiration: This is a passive process by elastic recoil of thoracic wall and pulmonary alveoli.

Deep expiration: This is done by contraction of anterolateral muscles of abdominal wall.

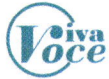 **Viva Voce**

- Name the vertebrae with which head of 4th rib articulates.
- What structures lie at the neck of 1st rib?
- What type of joint is manubriosternal joint?
- What is sternal puncture? Where is it done and why?
- Which are the primary and secondary curvatures of the vertebral column?
- What are pump-handle and bucket-handle movements?

1. a. Identify the angle.
    b. What is its clinical importance?

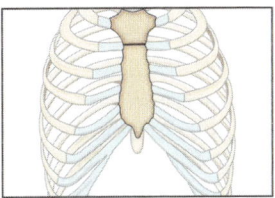

2. a. Identify the upper most ribs.
    b. What symptoms arise from such a rib?

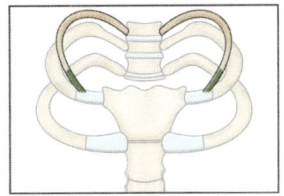

3. a. Name the groove.
    b. What structures lie in the groove in order?

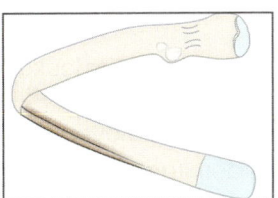

4. a. What puncture is shown here?
    b. Why is it done?

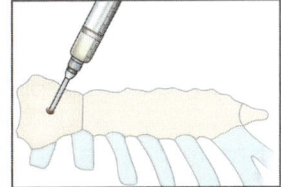

5. a. Name the joint along which the rib moves.
    b. Which diameter of thoracic cage increases?

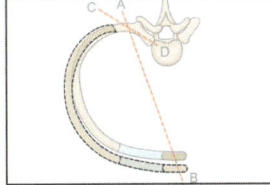

6. a. How can one recognise the thoracic vertebra from cervical and
    b. Lumbar vertebrae?

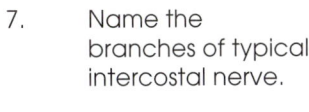

7. Name the branches of typical intercostal nerve.

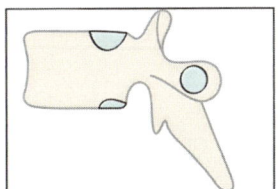

8. a. How many posterior intercostal and subcostal arteries are there?
    b. How many arise from descending thoracic aorta?

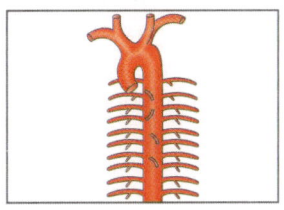

9. a. Identify the artery.
    b. Name all branches of this artery.

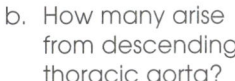
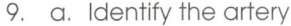

10. a. Name all the parts of parietal pleura.
    b. Name their nerve supply.

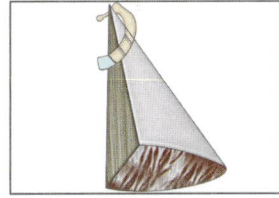

11. a. How much is the angle between trachea and right principal bronchus?
    b. What is its importance?

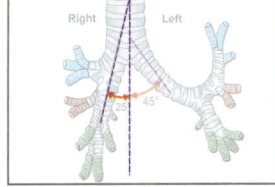

12. a. Name the cusps of the aortic valve.
    b. Which aortic sinuses give rise to the right and left coronary arteries?

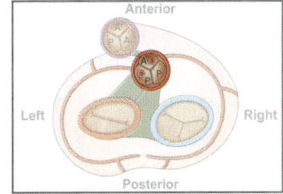

13. a. Which vein joins lateral thoracic and superficial epigastric veins?
    b. What is its importance?

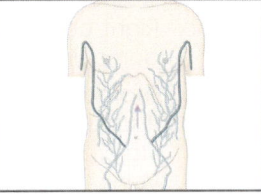

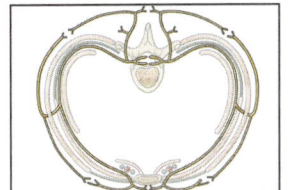

ANSWERS: SPOTS ON THORAX

1   a. The angle is manubriosternal angle.
      b. It is the junction of manubrium sterni with the body of sternum.
- 2nd costal cartilages are attached to this prominent angle on each side.
- Below this costal cartilage is 2nd intercostal space followed by 3rd costal cartilage and 3rd rib. This angle is used for counting the ribs.
- Arch of aorta starts and ends also at this level.
- This angle lies at level of T4 vertebra—the plane between superior and posterior mediastina.

2   a. The uppermost ribs are cervical ribs present bilaterally.
      b. The rib may stretch the lower trunk of brachial lexus and/or subclavian artery. There may be neural or vascular symptoms or both.

3   a. The groove is costal groove.
      b. Posterior intercostal vein, posterior intercostal artery and intercostal nerve lie in this groove from above downwards.

4   a. Sternal puncture is shown in this figure.
      b. It is done to withdraw bone marrow to confirm type of anemia or leukemia sterni.

5   a. Ribs move along costovertebral joints.
      b. Anteroposterior diameter of thoracic cage increases by this movement.

6   a. Thoracic vertebra is recognised by the presence of demifacets along the upper and lower borders of the body on both sides.
- This vertebra also shows facets on its transverse processes for articulation with the tubercles of the right and left ribs.
- Cervical vertebra contains foramen tansversarium.

      b. The lumbar vertebrae are large, massive with broad body and small spine.

7. Muscular for 3 intercostal muscles.
Cutaneous, lateral cutaneous nerve, anterior cutaneous nerve, also pleural branches and periosteal branches.

8. a. There are 11 pairs of posterior intercostal and one pair of subcostal arteries.
      b. Lower 9 pairs of posterior intercostal and 1 pair of subcostal arteries arise from descending thoracic aorta.

9. a. The artery is anterior thoracic.
      b. Its branches:
- 2 anterior intercostal arteries each in 1st–6th intercostal spaces.
- Pericardiacophrenic and muscular branches
- Superior epigastric artery and musculophrenic artery as terminal branches.

10. a. The parts of parietal pleura are cervical, costal, mediastinal and diaphragmatic.
      b. Mediastinal and central part of diphragmatic pleurae by phrenic nercve. Rest by intercostal nerves.

11. a. The angle is 25°. It is more in line with trachea.
      b. Foreign bodies if any, tend to pass in right bronchus.

12. a. Cusps are anterior, right posterior and left posterior.
      b. Right coronary artery arises from anterior aortic sinus and left coronary artery arises from left posterior aortic sinus.

13. a. Thoracoepigastric vein joins lateral thoracic vein and superficial epigiastric vein.
      b. If superior vena cava gets blocked below the entry of vena azygos, the flow of venous blood is returned via brachiocephalic vein → axillary lateral thoracic vein → thoracoepigastric vein → superficial epigastric vein → long saphenous vein → femoral vein → external iliac vein → common iliac vein → inferior vena cava heart.

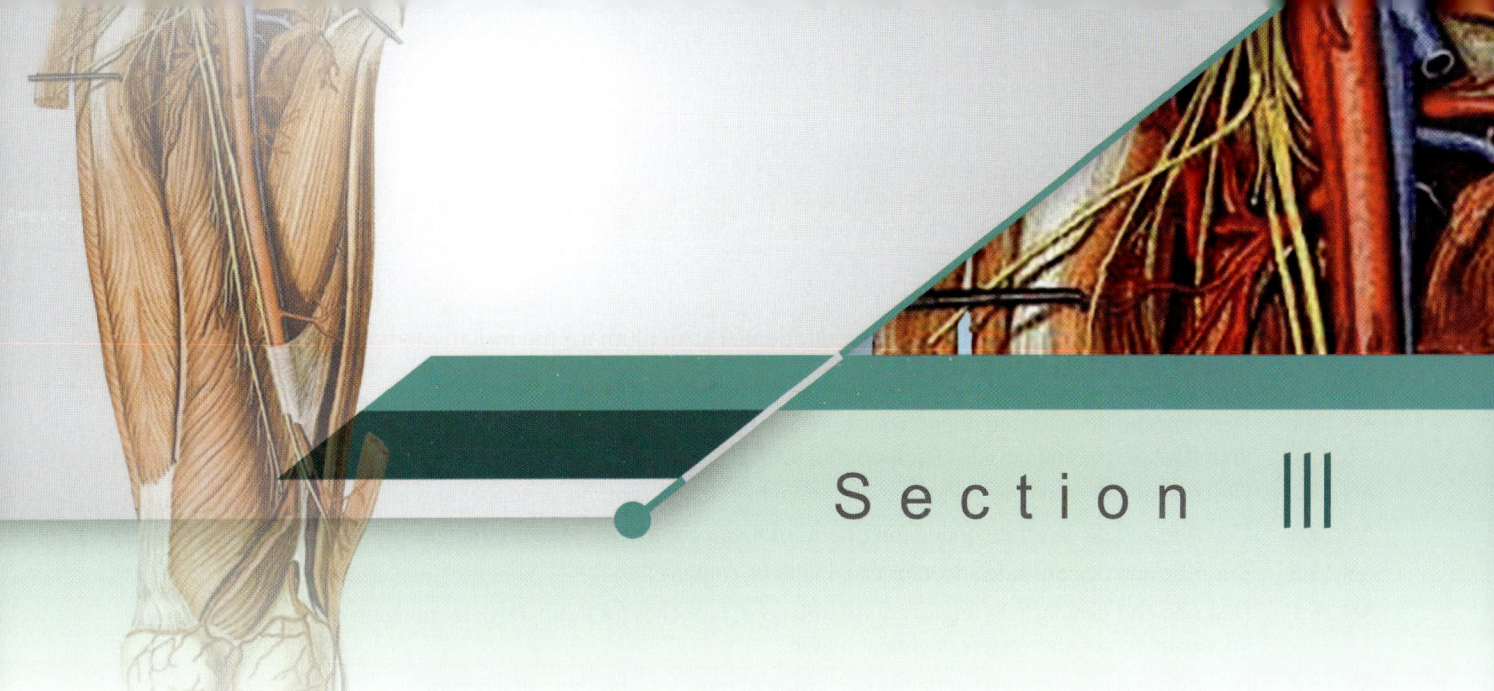

Section III

Lower Limb

Index of Competencies (Competency based Undergraduate Curriculum for the Indian Medical Graduate 2018;1:44–80)

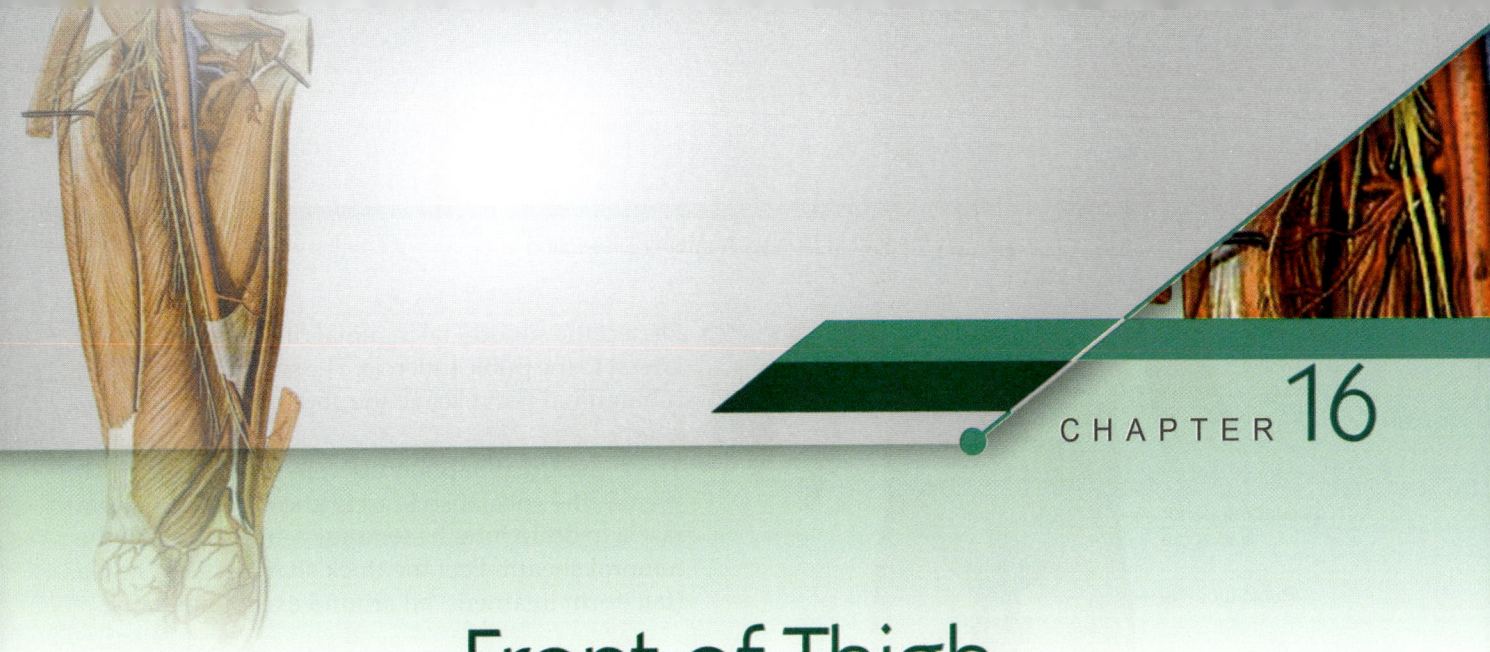

CHAPTER 16

Front of Thigh

Learning Objectives

One should be able to

1. Name the cutaneous nerves in the superficial fascia.
2. Trace the course of great saphenous vein draining into femoral vein through saphenous opening.
3. Enumerate boundaries and contents of femoral triangle.
4. How is the femoral sheath formed?
5. Enumerate the boundaries and contents of adductor/subsartorial canal.
6. Name the parts of the quadriceps femoris muscle.
7. Name the areas draining into superficial and deep inguinal lymph nodes.

OVERVIEW

Front of thigh extends from inguinal ligament to the knee joint. The neurovascular bundle, i.e. femoral artery, femoral vein and femoral nerve located in the femoral triangle are the most important structures in this region. This region contains the longest muscle viz. sartorius, part of the longest vein viz. the long saphenous and part of the longest cutaneous nerve viz. the saphenous nerve. It also houses the four headed quadriceps femoris muscle. Its upper medial region is also a site for femoral hernia. Femoral vessels course through the adductor canal to be able to reach the popliteal fossa.

Competency achievement: The student should be able to:

AN 15.1 Describe and demonstrate origin, course, relations, branches (or tributaries), termination of important nerves and vessels of anterior thigh.

STEPS OF DISSECTION

- Make a curved incision from anterior superior iliac spine to the pubic tubercle (Fig. 16.1).

- Give a curved incision around the scrotum/pudendal cleft towards upper medial side of thigh. Extend it vertically down below the medial condyle of tibia till the level of tibial tuberosity.
- Make a horizontal incision below the tibial tuberosity till the lateral side of leg.
- Reflect the skin laterally, exposing the superficial fatty and deeper membranous layers of superficial fascia. Remove the fatty layer.
- Look for cutaneous nerves, e.g.
  i. Lateral cutaneous nerve of thigh
  ii. Femoral branch of genitofemoral nerve
  iii. Intermediate cutaneous nerve of thigh
  iv. Medial cutaneous nerve of thigh
  v. Femoral branch of genitofemoral nerve
- Identify the great saphenous vein in the medial part of anterior surface of thigh. Draining into its upper part are its three superficial tributaries, namely superficial circumflex iliac, superficial epigastric and superficial external pudendal (Fig. 16.2).
- The vertical group of superficial inguinal lymph nodes lie along the upper part of saphenous vein.

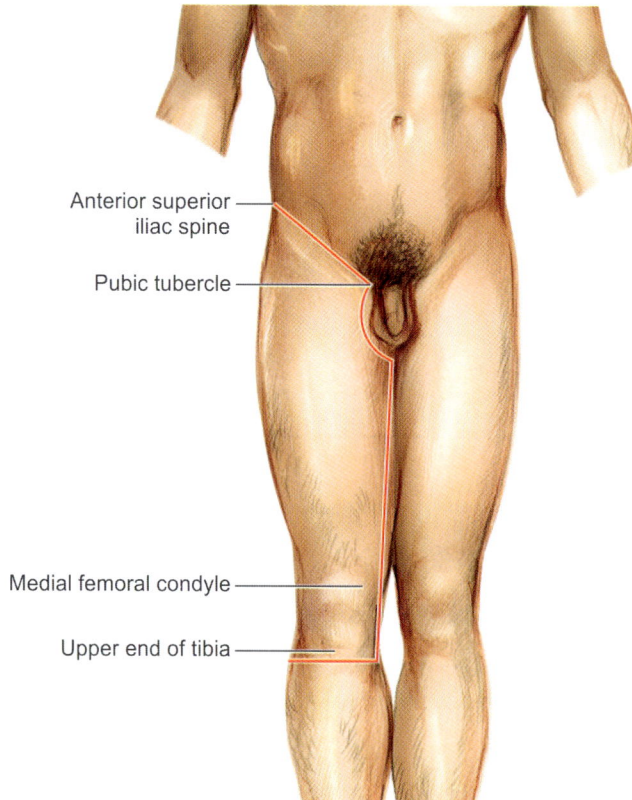

Anterior superior iliac spine

Pubic tubercle

Medial femoral condyle

Upper end of tibia

Fig .16.1: Lines of incision

- Dissect the superficial inguinal ring 1 cm above and lateral to the pubic tubercle. The spermatic cord and ilioinguinal nerve leave the abdomen through this ring.
- Trace the great saphenous vein backwards till it pierces the specialised fascia known as cribriform fascia to drain into the femoral vein enclosed in the femoral sheath. Feel the thick sharp edge of fascia (falciform ligament) all around except medially.

Competency achievement: The student should be able to:

AN 15.3 Describe and demonstrate boundaries, floor, roof and contents of femoral triangle.

DEEP FASCIA

- After the reflection of the superficial fascia, the deep fascia of thigh is visible. Study its attachments, modifications and extensions.
- Follow the great saphenous vein through the cribriform fascia and the anterior wall of femoral sheath into the femoral vein.
- Split the femoral sheath on medial and lateral sides of femoral vein. The femoral vein occupies the intermediate compartment of the femoral sheath. Medial compartment of femoral sheath is the

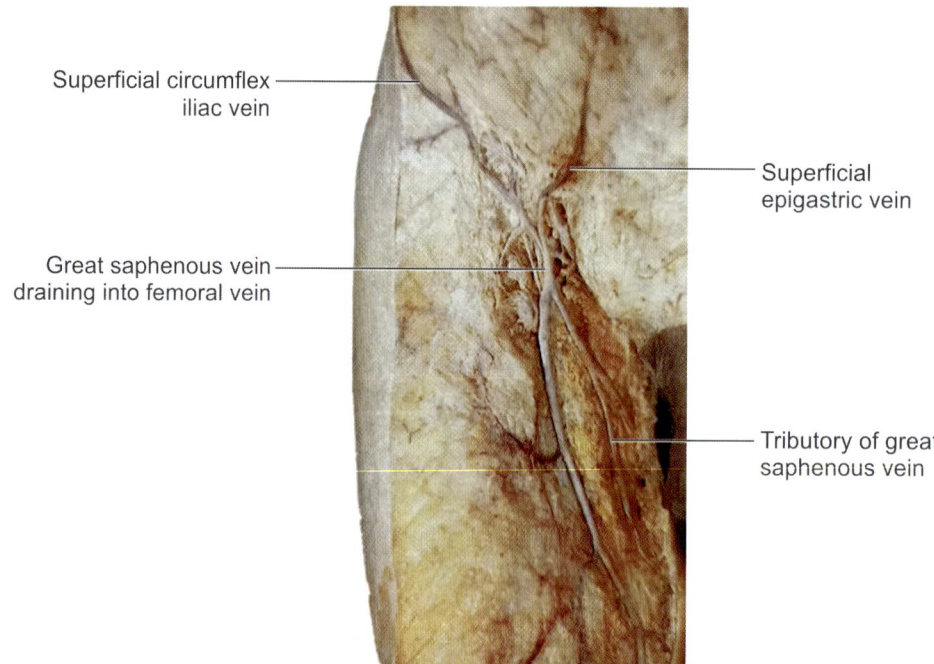

Superficial circumflex iliac vein

Superficial epigastric vein

Great saphenous vein draining into femoral vein

Tributory of great saphenous vein

Fig. 16.2: Two superficial veins draining into great saphenous vein

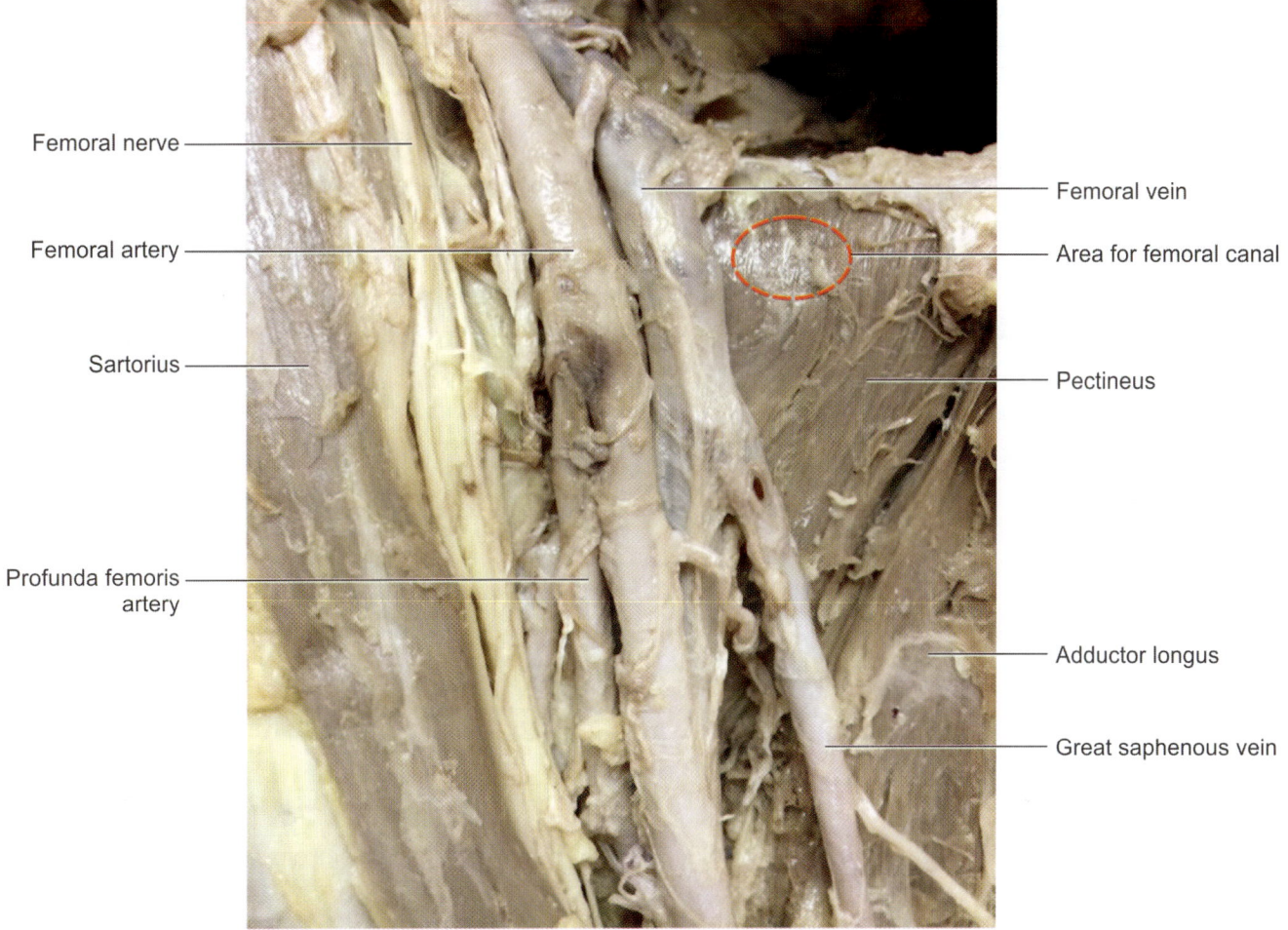

Fig. 16.3: Some contents of femoral triangle

femoral canal occupied by a lymph node while the lateral compartment is occupied by the femoral artery.

- Put a little finger in femoral canal and push the finger upwards (Fig. 16.3). Let the finger feel the peritoneum covering the abdominal aspect of the femoral canal. Feel its boundaries. These are the inguinal ligament anteriorly, free margin of lacunar ligament medially and pecten pubis posteriorly.

- Give a vertical incision in the deep fascia of thigh from tubercle of iliac crest till the lateral condyle of femur and remove the deep fascia or fascia lata in lateral part of thigh. This will expose the tensor fasciae latae muscle and gluteus maximus muscle getting attached to iliotibial tract. Identify the four heads of quadriceps femoris muscle.

- Remove the entire deep fascia from upper one-third of the front of thigh.

- Identify the sartorius muscle stretching gently across the thigh from lateral to medial side and the adductor longus muscle extending from medial side of thigh towards lateral side into the femur, being crossed by the sartorius.

- This triangular depression in the upper one-third of the thigh is the femoral triangle (Fig. 16.3).

- The medial border of sartorius forms lateral boundary and medial border of adductor longus forms medial boundary. The base of this triangle is formed by the inguinal ligament.

- Dissect its boundaries, and contents, e.g. femoral nerve, artery and vein, and accompanying structures.

- Expose the sartorius muscle till its insertion into the upper medial surface of shaft of tibia.

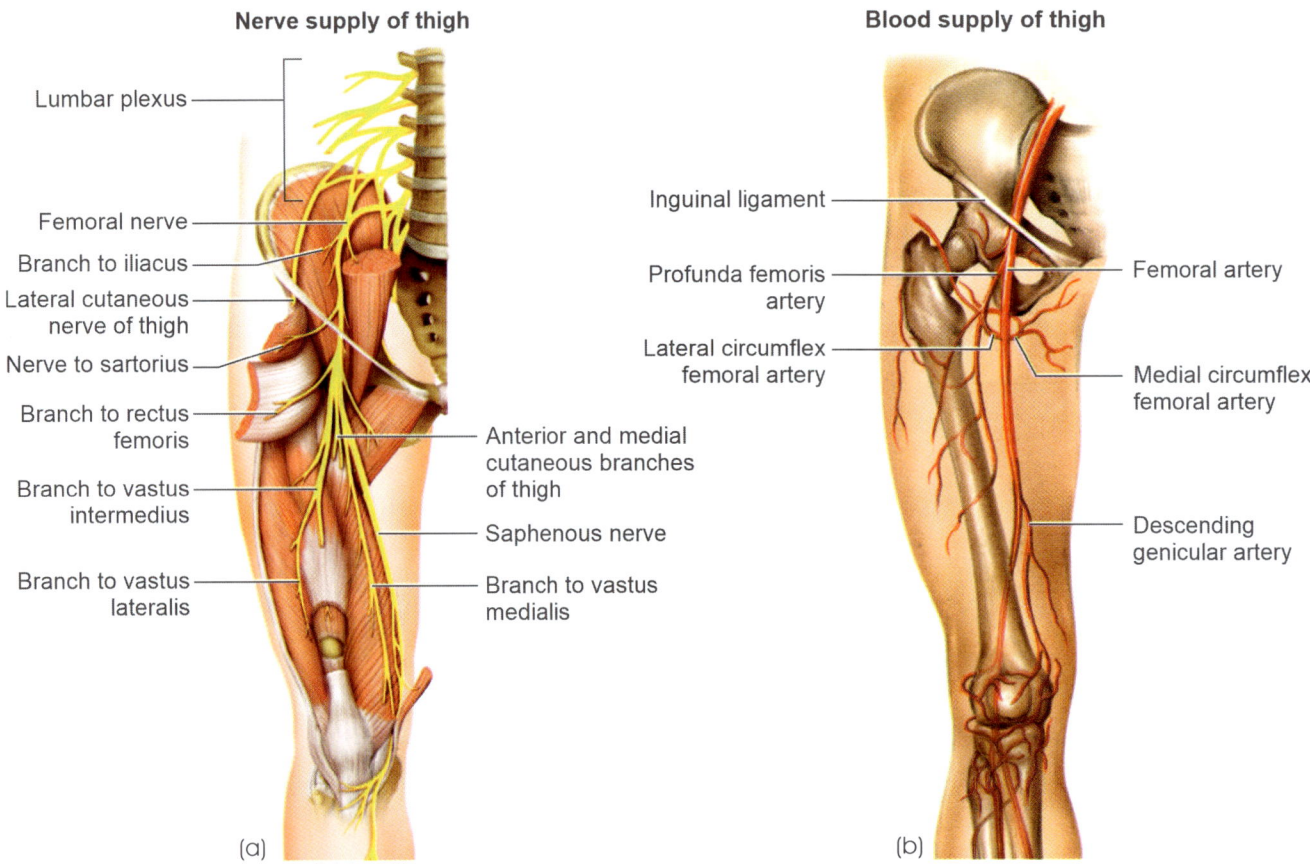

Nerve supply of thigh

Lumbar plexus

Femoral nerve

Branch to iliacus

Lateral cutaneous nerve of thigh

Nerve to sartorius

Branch to rectus femoris

Branch to vastus intermedius

Branch to vastus lateralis

Anterior and medial cutaneous branches of thigh

Saphenous nerve

Branch to vastus medialis

(a)

Blood supply of thigh

Inguinal ligament

Profunda femoris artery

Lateral circumflex femoral artery

Femoral artery

Medial circumflex femoral artery

Descending genicular artery

(b)

Fig. 16.4: Contents of femoral triangle; (a) Femoral nerve; (b) Femoral artery

- Look for femoral nerve resting lateral to femoral artery, outside femoral sheath. It lies between iliacus and psoas major muscle. About 2.5 cm below the inguinal ligament it is seen to divide into anterior and posterior divisions. Both these divisions give numerous cutaneous and muscular branches (Fig. 16.4a).

- Identify and clean femoral artery (Fig. 16.4b). Trace its three superficial branches which pierce the cribriform fascia to accompany the veins. These are superficial epigastric, towards anterior abdominal wall; superficial circumflex iliac below inguinal ligament towards iliac crest and superficial external pudendal towards external genital organs. The veins accompanying these arteries drain into great saphenous vein and do not pierce cribriform fascia.

- The important deep branch of femoral artery is profunda femoris artery (Fig. 16.3). To locate this artery, retract the femoral artery medially and look

for a big artery arising from the posterolateral aspect of femoral artery. Trace this artery with its vein till the apex of femoral triangle. At the apex of femoral triangle look for the order of structures from before backwards. These are femoral artery, femoral vein, adductor longus muscle, profunda femoris vein and profunda femoris artery.

- Arising from profunda femoris, try to locate the lateral and medial circumflex femoral branches of profunda femoris artery. Lateral circumflex femoral runs amongst the branches of femoral nerve and divides into ascending, transverse and descending branches.

- Strip the fascia between psoas major and iliacus muscles and trace tendon of psoas major till its insertion into lesser trochanter of femur. Now locate the medial circumflex femoral artery passing backwards between psoas major and pectineus muscles.

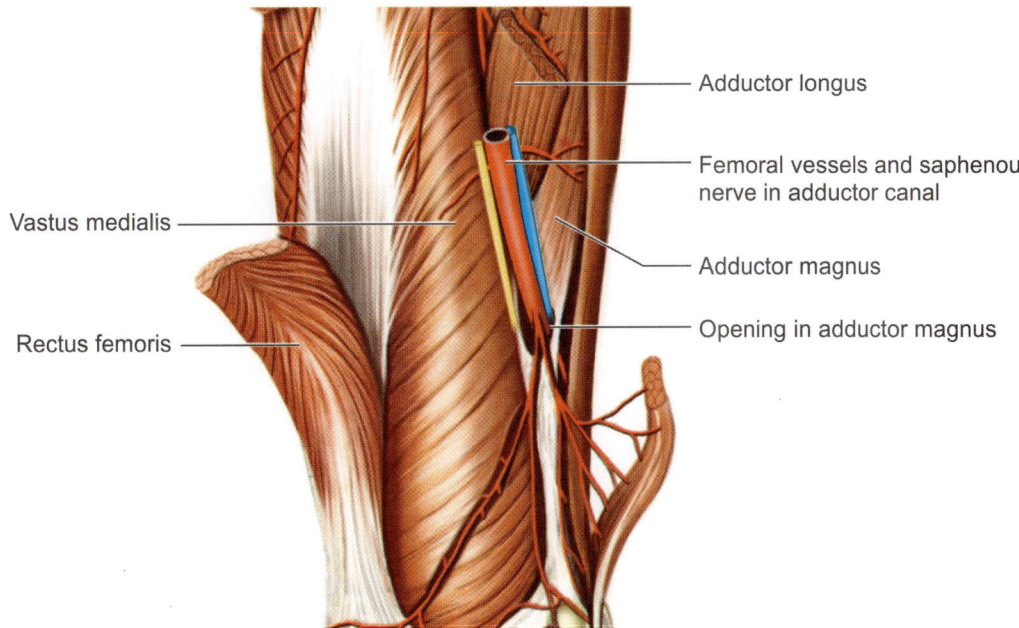

Fig. 16.5: Adductor canal: boundaries and contents

Labels: Adductor longus; Femoral vessels and saphenous nerve in adductor canal; Adductor magnus; Opening in adductor magnus; Vastus medialis; Rectus femoris

Competency achievement: The student should be able to:

AN 15.5 Describe and demonstrate adductor canal with its content.

ADDUCTOR CANAL

Steps of Dissection

- Upper one-third of sartorius forms the lateral boundary of the femoral triangle.
- On lifting the middle one-third of sartorius, a part of deep fascia stretching between vastus medialis and adductor muscles is exposed. On longitudinal division of this strong fascia, the adductor canal/subsartorial canal/Hunter's canal is visualised.
- Dissect its contents, e.g. femoral vessels, saphenous nerve and nerve to vastus medialis, and distal parts of both divisions of obturator nerve.
- Identify the femoral vein as it lies posterior to femoral artery. The femoral vessels exit the adductor canal by passing through the opening of adductor magnus to enter the popliteal fossa (Fig. 16.5).
- Identify the bipennate arrangement of muscle fibres in rectus femoris muscle (Fig. 16.5). On medial and lateral sides of the rectus femoris are the vastus medialis and vastus lateralis muscles. Identify

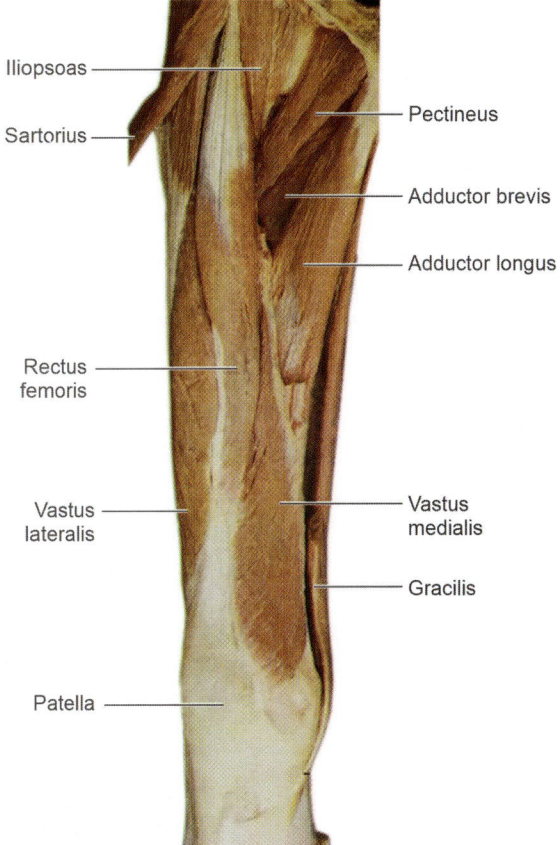

Labels: Iliopsoas; Pectineus; Sartorius; Adductor brevis; Adductor longus; Rectus femoris; Vastus lateralis; Vastus medialis; Gracilis; Patella

Fig. 16.6: Muscles of front of thigh

vastus intermedius on deep aspect of rectus femoris as it is retracted to one side. Appreciate that the tendons of these four muscles are attached to the borders of patella. From here these tendons continue as ligamentum patellae to be attached to upper half of tibial tuberosity.

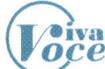

- Name the contents of three compartments of the femoral sheath.
- Name the heads of quadriceps femoris muscle. Show the action of the muscle.
- What are the boundaries of femoral triangle?
- What are the boundaries of adductor canal?
- Which is the longest cutaneous nerve in lower limb?
- Name the coverings of femoral hernia.

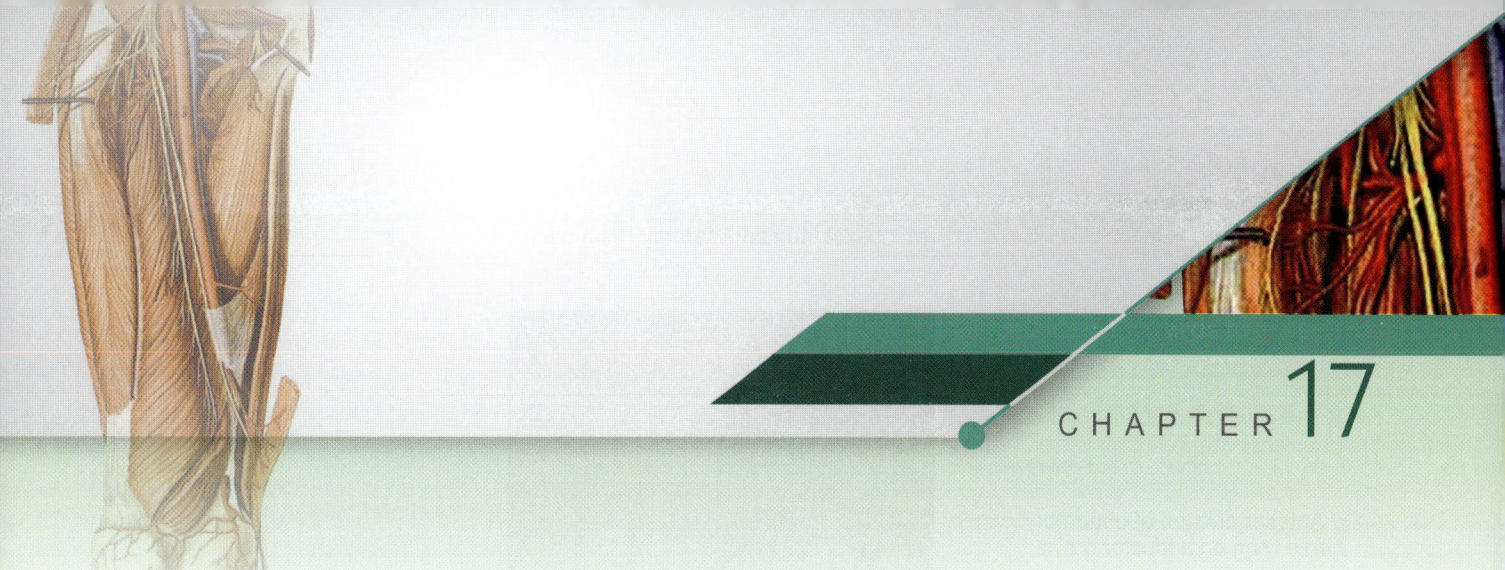

Medial Compartment of Thigh

OVERVIEW

The medial compartment is a smaller compartment of thigh. It is chiefly muscular, comprised of pectineus, adductor longus (superficial layer); adductor brevis (middle layer) and obturator externus with adductor magnus (deep layer). The most medial muscle is the thin gracilis muscle.

The nerve of this region is the obturator nerve. All the above mentioned muscles get innervated by obturator nerve.

Competency achievement: The student should be able to:

AN 15.2 Describe and demonstrate major muscles with their attachment, nerve supply and actions.

STEPS OF DISSECTION

- The triangular adductor longus was seen to form the medial boundary of femoral triangle. Cut this muscle 3 cm below its origin and reflect the distal part laterally. On its deep surface, identify the anterior division of obturator nerve which supplies both adductor longus and gracilis muscles.
- Lateral to adductor longus on the same plane is the pectineus muscle. Cut it close to its origin and reflect

it laterally, tracing the branch of anterior division of obturator nerve to this muscle. Obturator nerve is accompanied by the branches of obturator artery and medial circumflex femoral artery.

- Deeper to adductor longus and pectineus is the adductor brevis. Look for its nerve supply either from anterior/posterior division.
- Divide adductor brevis close to its origin. Deepest plane of muscles comprises adductor magnus and obturator externus, both supplied by posterior division of obturator nerve.
- Lying vertically along the medial side of thigh is the 'graceful' gracilis. Study these muscles and the course of obturator nerve.
- Look for accessory obturator nerve. If present, it supplies pectineus.
- Lastly, remove the obturator externus from its origin to expose the obturator artery and its branches.
- Adductor longus and pectineus form the superficial layer. Adductor brevis forms the intermediate layer, obturator externus and adductor magnus form the deep layer (*see* Figs 16.6).
- Gracilis lies medially to all the three layers (*see* Fig. 16.6).

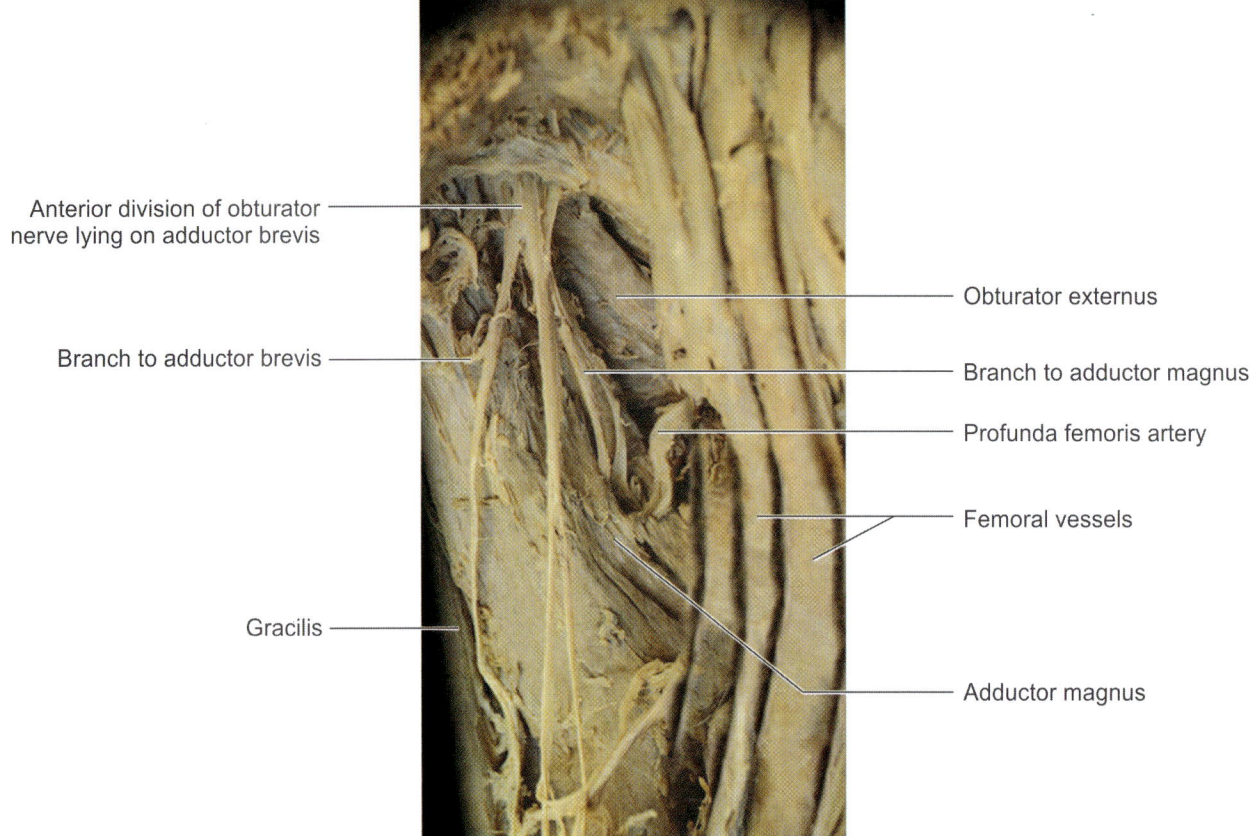

Anterior division of obturator
nerve lying on adductor brevis

Branch to adductor brevis

Gracilis

Obturator externus

Branch to adductor magnus

Profunda femoris artery

Femoral vessels

Adductor magnus

Fig. 17.1: Branches of obturator nerve

- Obturator nerve arises from ventral divisions of ventral rami of L 2, 3, 4 segments of spinal cord. It lies on the medial side of thigh. See its anterior division giving branches to pectineus, adductor longus and gracilis (Fig. 17.1). Trace its posterior division which passes through obturator externus, supplies it and descends between adductor brevis and adductor magnus supplying both these muscles. Follow the thin terminal parts of the two divisions into the adductor canal.

- Trace the branches of obturator artery and medial circumflex femoral artery accompanying the divisions of obturator nerve.

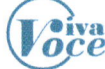

- What type of muscle is adductor magnus according to its nerve supply?
- Name the muscles supplied by posterior division of obturator nerve.

- What are the branches of medial circumflex femoral artery?
- What is the difference between root values of femoral and obturator nerves?

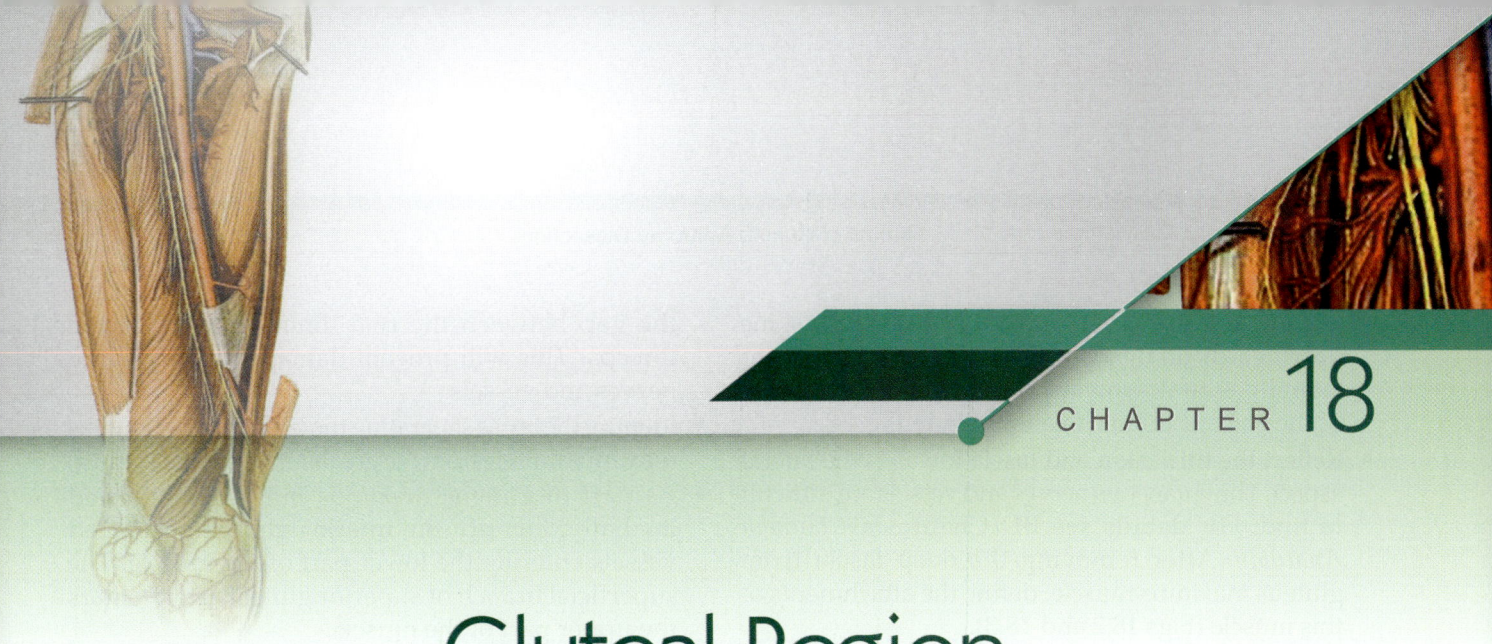

CHAPTER 18

Gluteal Region

Learning Objectives

One should be able to

1. Enumerate all the structures under cover of gluteus maximus muscle.
2. Explain actions of gluteus medius and minimus during walking.
3. Learn attachments, nerve supply and actions of the muscles of this region.

OVERVIEW

Gluteal region is an extensive region over the posterior aspect of the hip bone. The buttock is the most prominent part of the gluteal region. This region contains:

i. Three gluteal muscles, piriformis—the key muscle of this region, obturator internus with two gemelli and obturator externus. Besides these muscles, there are:

ii. The superior and inferior gluteal nerves and vessels which end in this region.

iii. The thickest nerve of the body—sciatic nerve runs across the region to enter back of thigh.

iv. Pudendal nerve and vessels which enter this region through greater sciatic foramen and exit it by passing into lesser sciatic foramen.

v. Few small branches of lumbosacral plexus.

Competency achievement: The student should be able to:

AN 16.1 Describe and demonstrate origin, course, relations, branches (or tributaries), termination of important nerves and vessels of gluteal region.

STEPS OF DISSECTION

- Put the cadaver in prone position.
- Make a curved incision from spine of second sacral vertebra (i); along the iliac crest till its tubercle (ii);

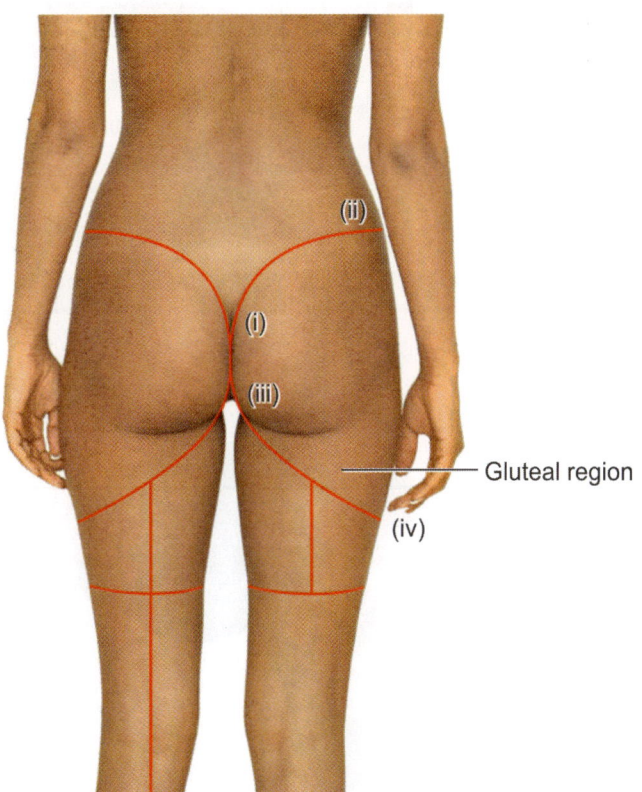

Fig. 18.1: Incision lines (i–iv) for gluteal region

Gluteal region

139

make a vertical incision from the second sacral spine downwards till the natal cleft (iii); taking it further laterally with downward convexity till the middle of the back of thigh (iv) as shown in Fig. 18.1.

- Reflect the thick skin and fascia towards the lateral aspect. The cutaneous nerves and vessels are difficult to find. For details see BD Chaurasia's *Human Anatomy*. After removing the deep fascia from gluteus maximus muscle, define the attachments of this muscle (Figs 18.2 and 18.3).
- Insert a forceps from middle of the lower border of gluteus maximus. Cut and reflect the gluteus maximus 3–4 cm medial to ischial tuberosity along the gap between the two limbs of the inserted forceps. This will prevent damage to underlying nerves and vessels.
- Identify the bursa separating the lateral part of gluteus maximus muscle from the greater trochanter of femur.
- As part of gluteus maximus muscle is reflected medially, identify the inferior gluteal nerve and vessels entering the lower part of the muscle. The superficial branch of superior gluteal artery enters the upper part of the muscle.
- Piriformis is key muscle of the region, define its margins. Identify the structures above and below this muscle, most important being the sciatic nerve.

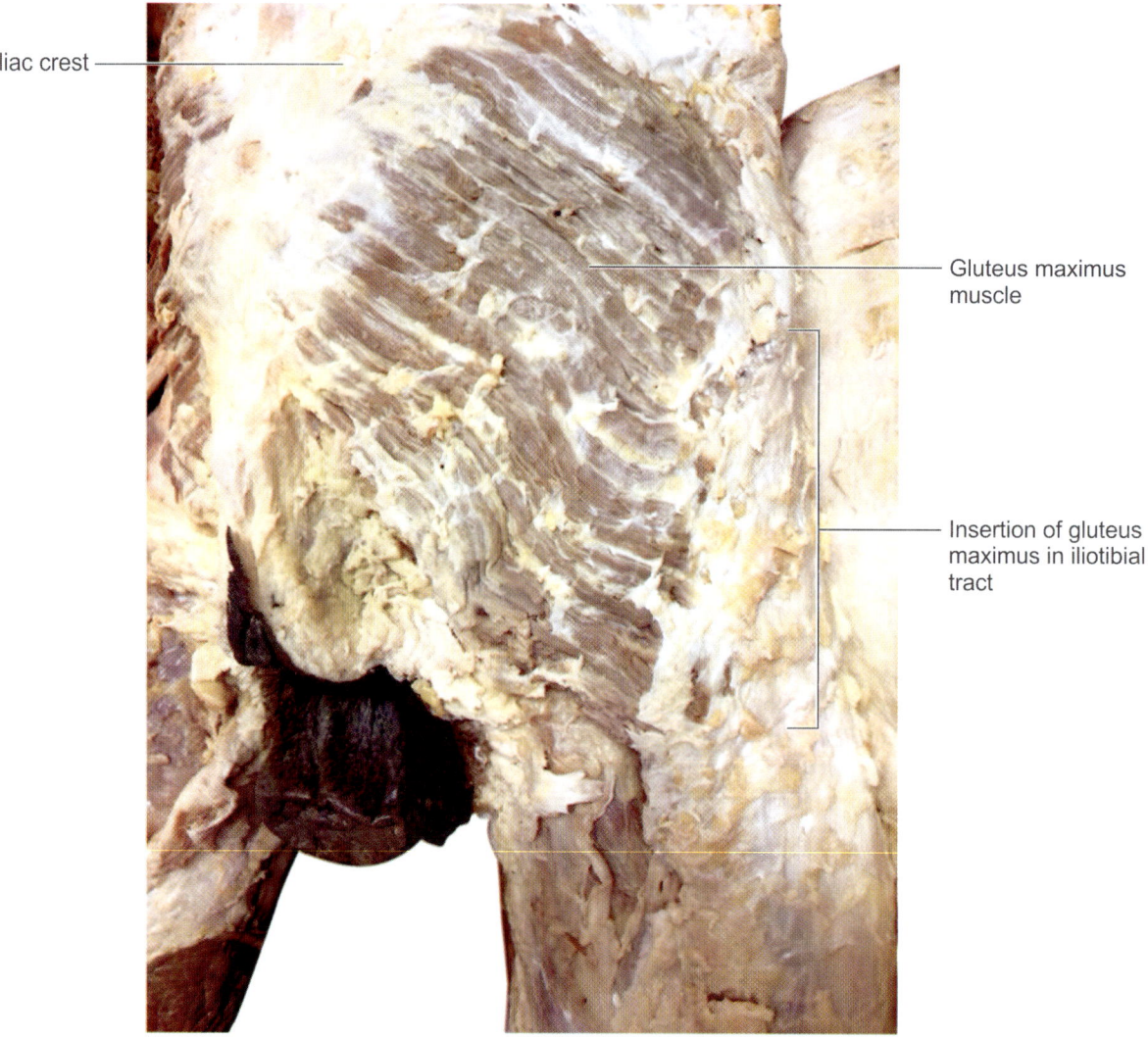

Iliac crest

Gluteus maximus muscle

Insertion of gluteus maximus in iliotibial tract

Fig. 18.2: Gluteus maximus muscle

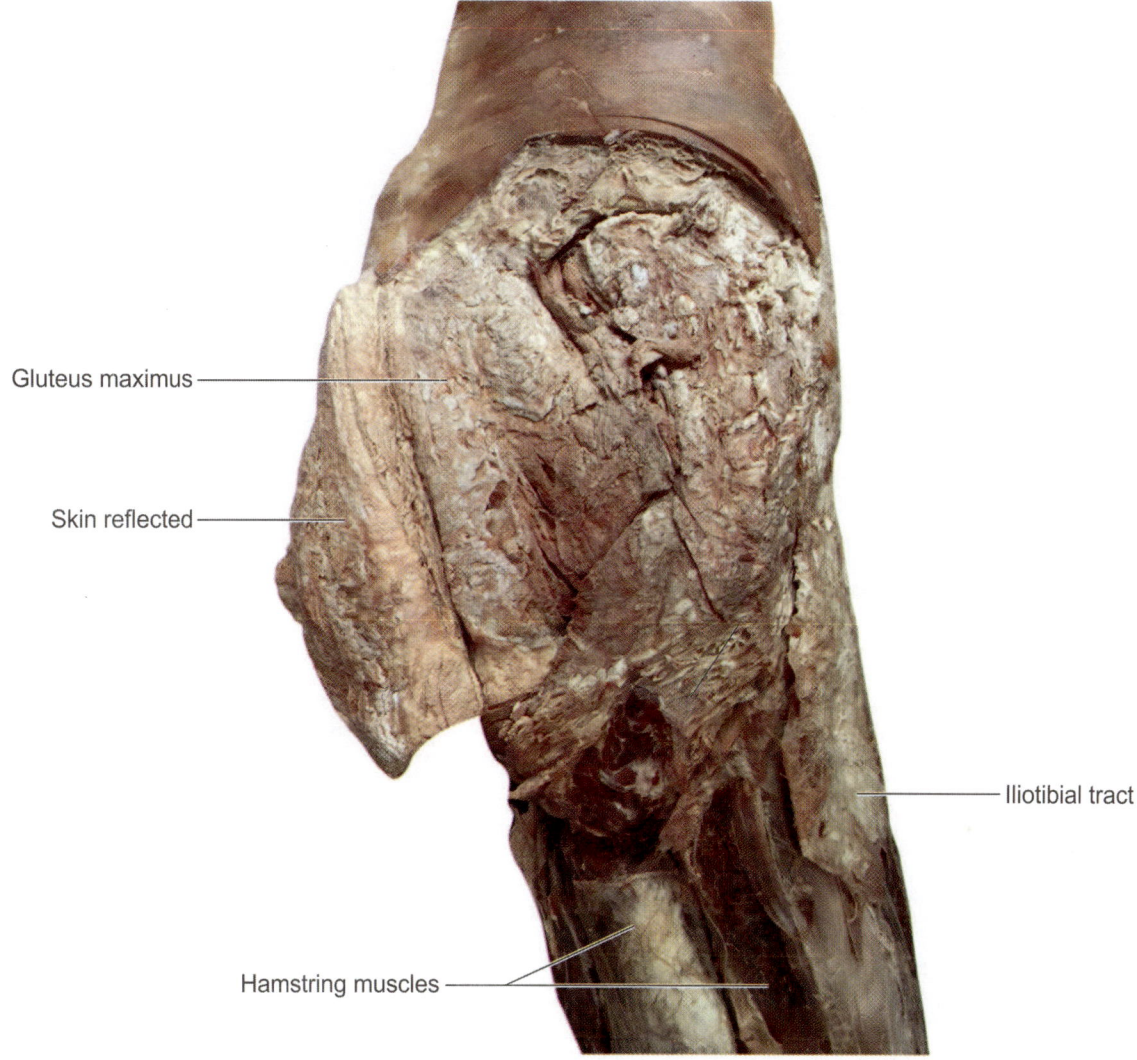

Gluteus maximus

Skin reflected

Iliotibial tract

Hamstring muscles

Fig .18.3: Gluteus maximus and hamstring muscles

Above piriformis—superior gluteal vessels and nerve. Below piriformis—inferior gluteal vessels and nerve (Figs 18.5 and 18.6).

- The thickest nerve of the body, sciatic nerve also enters the gluteal region through the greater sciatic notch below piriformis muscle (Fig. 18.4). Trace it down till the midpoint between the greater trochanter and ischial tuberosity (Fig. 18.5).

- Lift the sciatic nerve laterally and locate a delicate nerve to quadratus femoris. The nerve passes deep to the two gemelli and tendon of obturator internus to innervate the quadratus femoris muscle.

- Remove the fascia from the muscles lying anterior to sciatic nerve. These five muscles are superior gemellus, tendon of obturator internus, inferior gemellus, quadratus femoris and adductor magnus.

- Deep to the most medial part of gluteus maximus lie the pudendal nerve, internal pudendal vessels and nerve to obturator internus from medial to lateral side (Fig. 18.6). See that these four structures lie in relation to ischial spine and its attached sacrospinous ligament. These structures enter gluteal region through greater sciatic foramen and leave it via lesser sciatic foramen.

- Under the lower and medial part of the gluteus maximus muscle, ischial tuberosity is easily palpable. Separate the hamstring muscles from the ischial tuberosity.

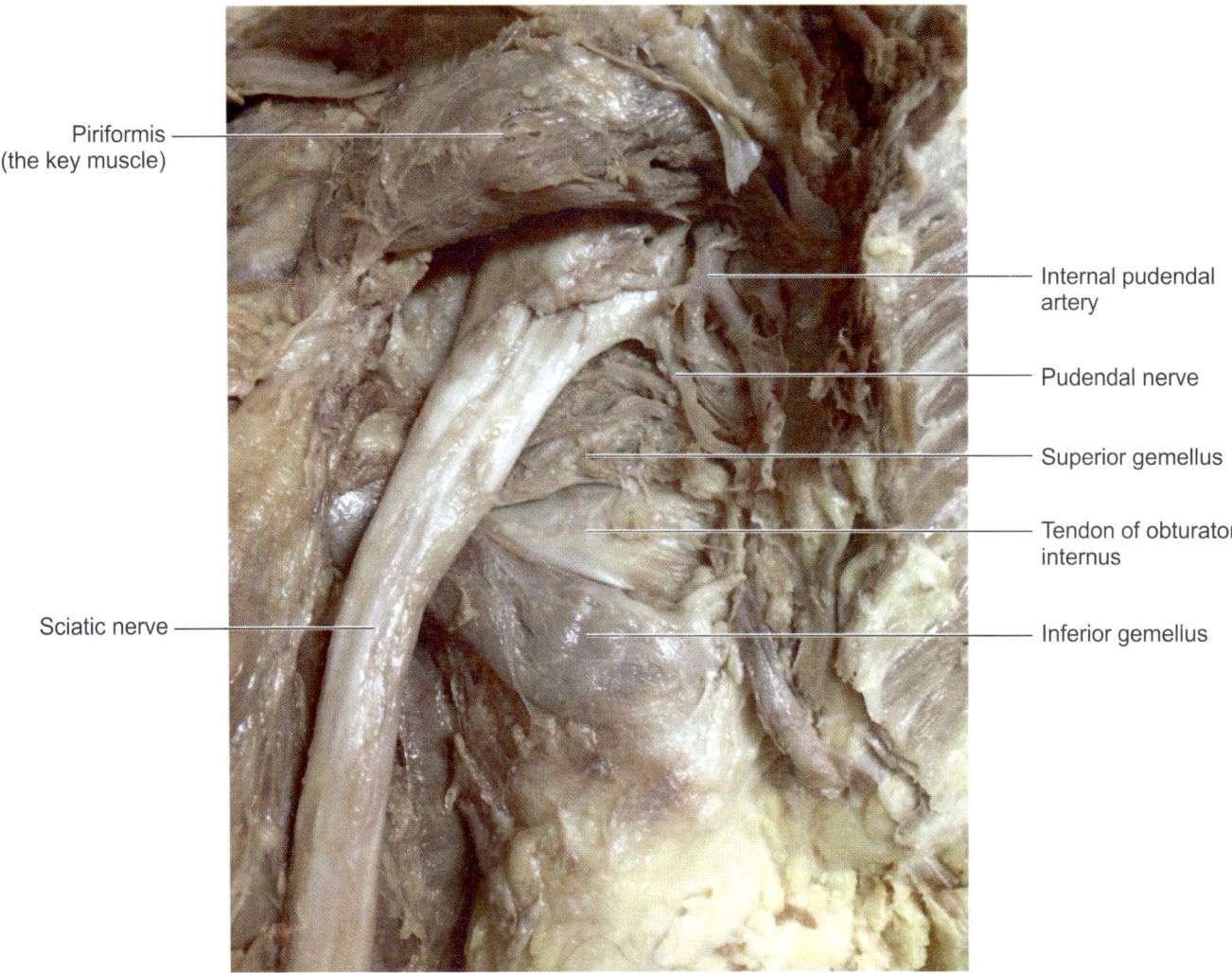

Piriformis
(the key muscle)

Internal pudendal artery

Pudendal nerve

Superior gemellus

Tendon of obturator internus

Sciatic nerve

Inferior gemellus

Fig. 18.4: Sciatic nerve entering gluteal region through greater sciatic notch

- Identify long vertical sacrotuberous ligament and smaller horizontal sacrospinous ligament to demarcate the greater and lesser sciatic foramina and structures entering and leaving them. Greater sciatic notch is the 'gateway' of the gluteal region.
- Define the borders of the gluteus medius muscle. Cut through the muscle 5 cm above its insertion into the greater trochanter of femur. The superior gluteal vessels and nerve are now exposed which are to be traced into gluteus minimus and tensor fascia latae.
- Reflect gluteus minimus from its origin towards the insertion to expose the straight and reflected heads of rectus femoris muscle and the capsule of the hip joint.
- Figure 18.7 shows early division of sciatic nerve into its two terminal branches.

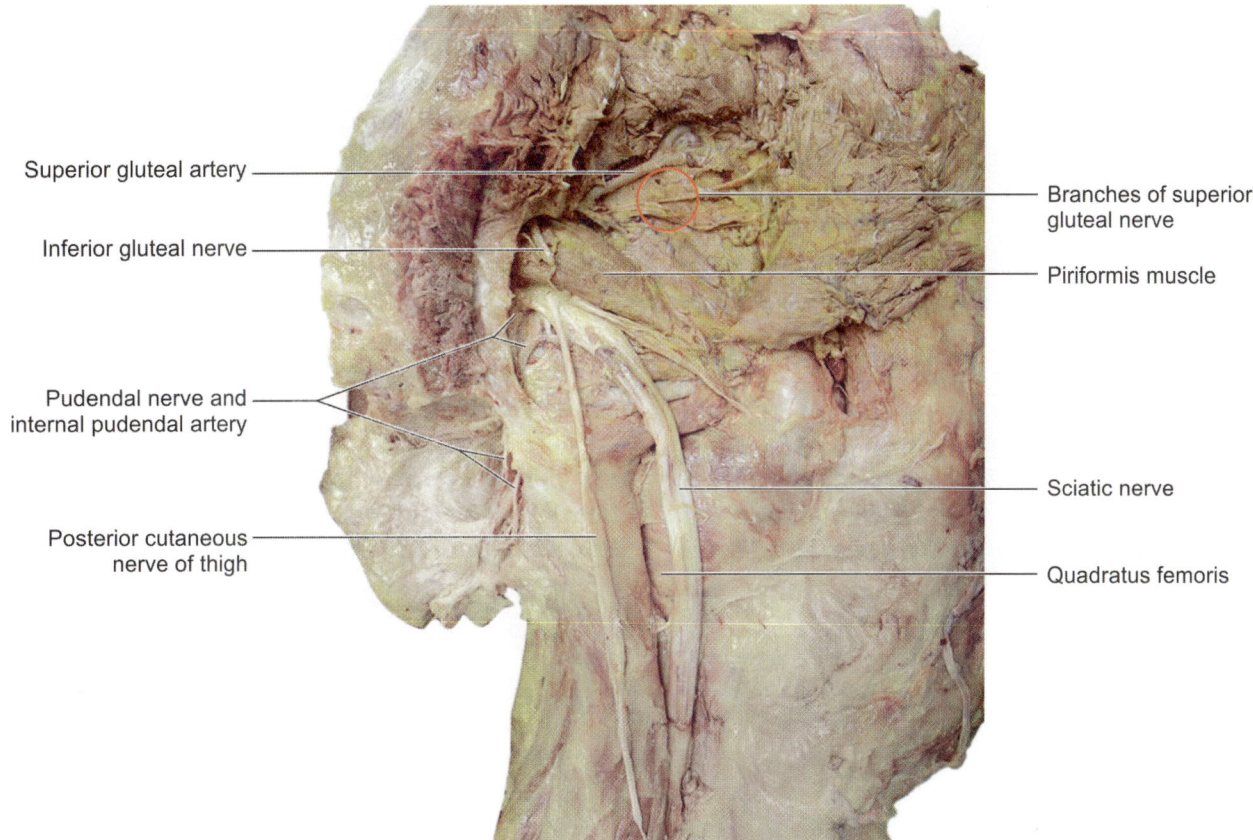

Superior gluteal artery

Inferior gluteal nerve

Pudendal nerve and
internal pudendal artery

Posterior cutaneous
nerve of thigh

Branches of superior
gluteal nerve

Piriformis muscle

Sciatic nerve

Quadratus femoris

Fig. 18.5: Structures seen in gluteal region

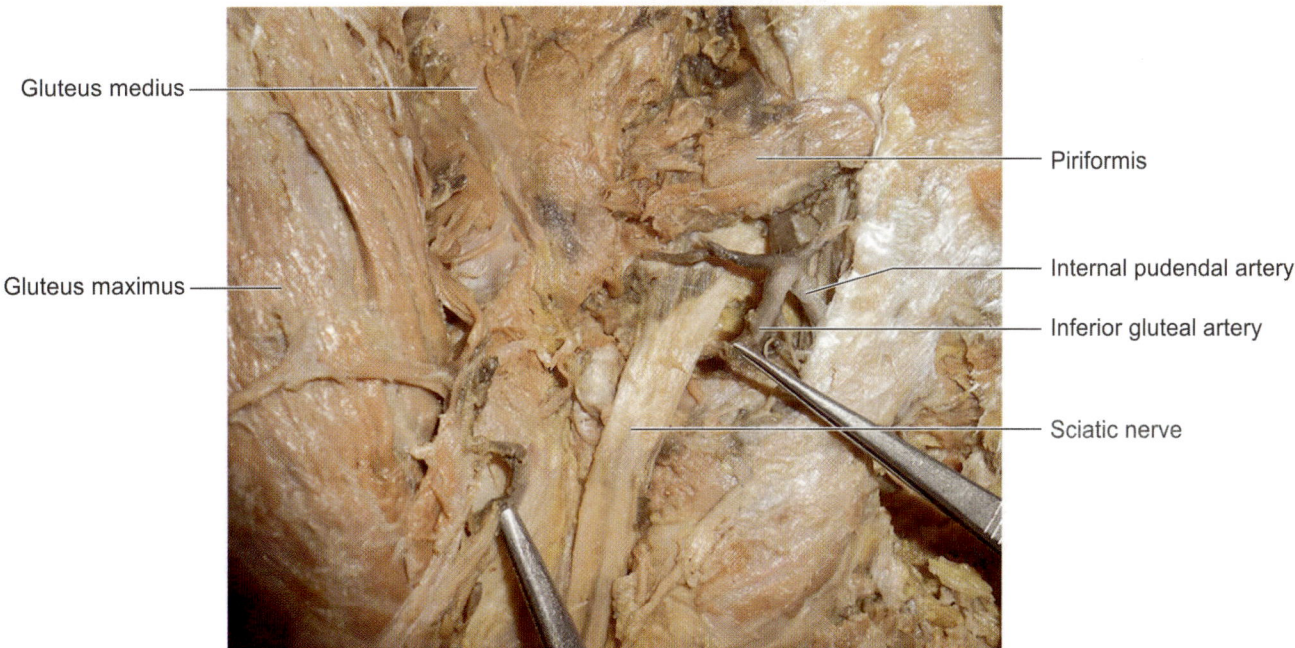

Gluteus medius

Gluteus maximus

Piriformis

Internal pudendal artery

Inferior gluteal artery

Sciatic nerve

Fig. 18.6: Structures seen in gluteal region

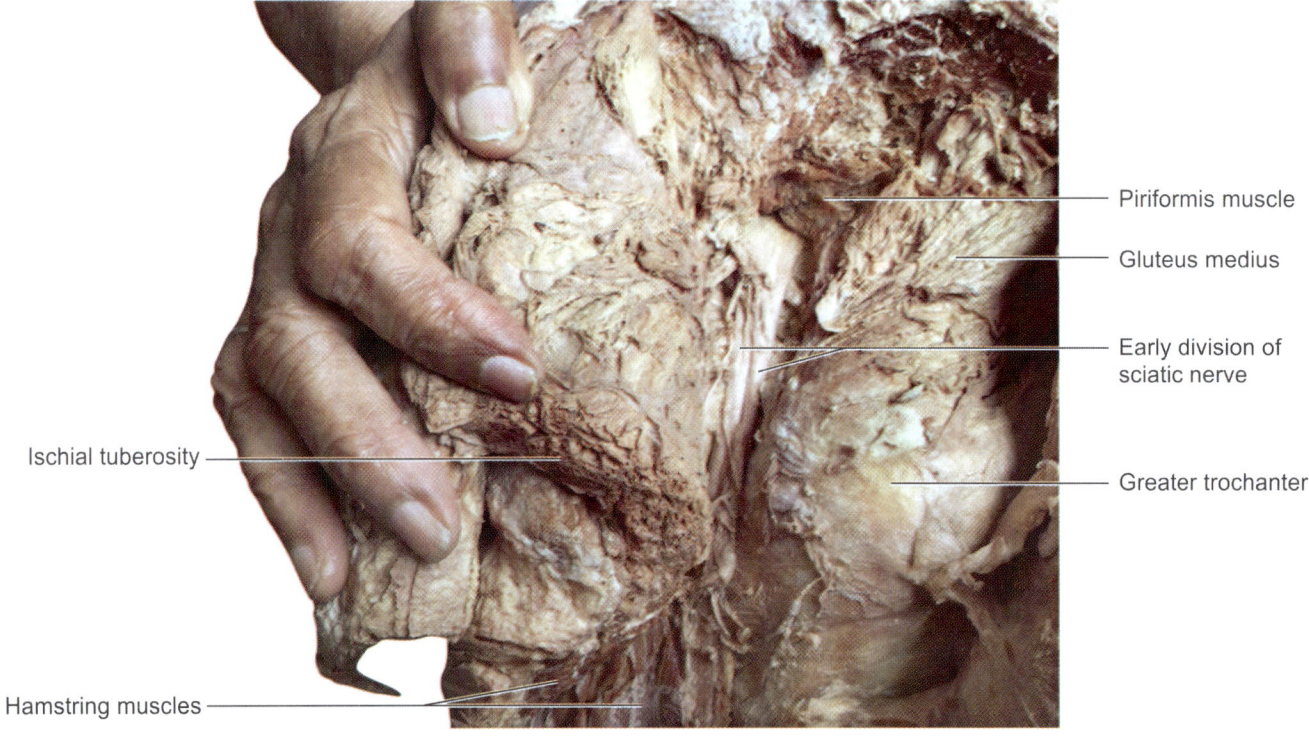

Piriformis muscle

Gluteus medius

Early division of sciatic nerve

Greater trochanter

Ischial tuberosity

Hamstring muscles

Fig. 18.7: Early division of sciatic nerve

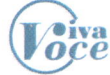

- What is the key muscle of gluteal region?
- Name structure passing above piriformis muscle.
- Name structures passing below piriformis muscle.
- How do gluteus medius and minimus help in walking?
- Where is the insertion of gluteus maximus muscle?
- What is sciatica?

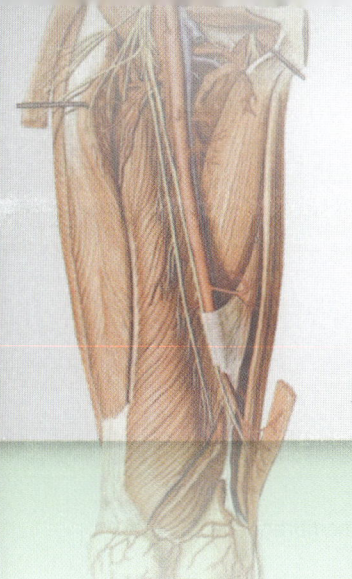

Popliteal Fossa

1. Enumerate the upper medial, upper lateral, lower medial and lower lateral boundaries of popliteal fossa.
2. Name the structures forming the roof and floor of the popliteal fossa.
3. Enumerate muscular, cutaneous, articular (genicular) branches of the popliteal artery, tibial nerve and common peroneal nerve.
4. Give clinical importance of popliteal artery.

OVERVIEW

Popliteal fossa is a diamond-shaped shallow space behind the knee joint. It is felt only in the flexed knee joint. Vessels and nerves to leg and sole pass from the thigh through the popliteal fossa. It corresponds to the cubital fossa of the forearm.

Competency achievement: The student should be able to:

AN 16.6 Describe and demonstrate the boundaries, roof, floor, contents and relations of popliteal fossa.

STEPS OF DISSECTION

- Make a horizontal incision across the back of thigh at its junction of upper two-thirds with lower one-third and another horizontal incision at the back of leg at its junction of upper one-third and lower two-thirds (v, vi) (Fig. 19.1)
- Draw a vertical incision joining the midpoints of the two horizontal incisions made (vii). Reflect the skin and fascia on either side.
- Find the cutaneous nerves, e.g. posterior cutaneous nerve of thigh, posterior division of medial

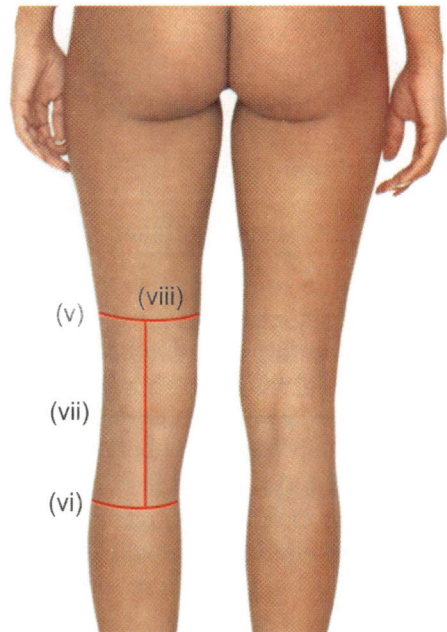

Fig. 19.1: Lines of incision

cutaneous nerve, sural communicating nerve and short saphenous vein. Cut and clean the deep fascia.

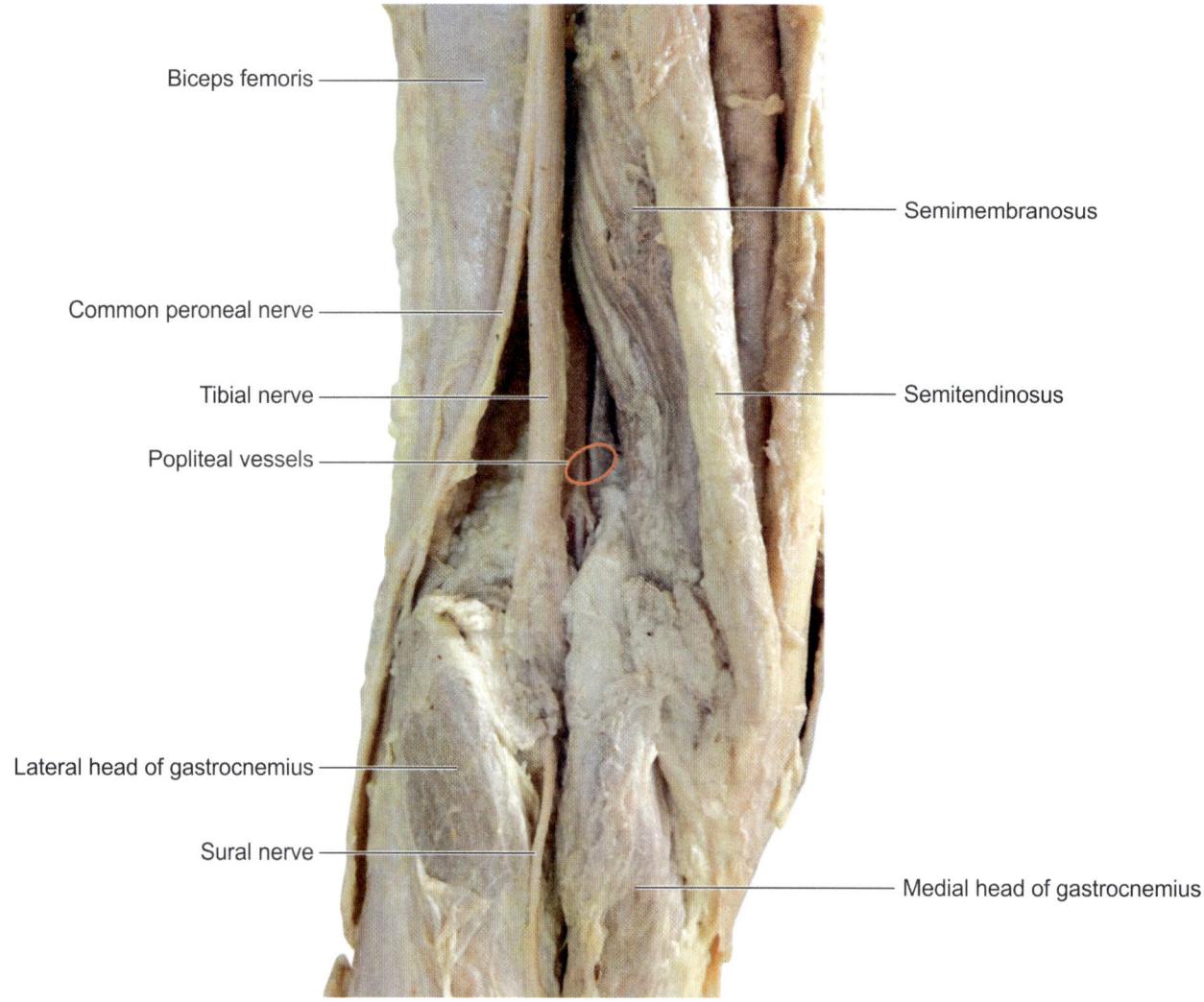

Fig. 19.2: Boundaries and contents of popliteal fossa

- Identify the boundaries and contents of popliteal fossa. Above and medially trace semimembranosus muscle (½ upper part membranous and ½ lower part muscular) from ischial tuberosity to posterior aspect of medial condyle of tibia (Figs 19.2 and 19.3).
- Identify semitendenosus lying on its superficial aspect. This tendon courses towards upper medial surface of front of tibia deep to sartorius and gracilis muscles.
- Above and laterally clean and identify the biceps femoris muscle with its two heads, viz. the long

head from ischial tuberosity and the short head from linea aspera. This muscle ends in the head of fibula in front of its apex.
- Below and laterally the muscle forming the boundary is lateral head of gastrocnemius supplemented by small plantaris muscle (Fig. 19.4). Below and medially is the medial head of gastrocnemius muscle. These three muscles descend down to the back of leg.
- Trace the tibial nerve as it courses through the centre of the popliteal fossa. Its three delicate

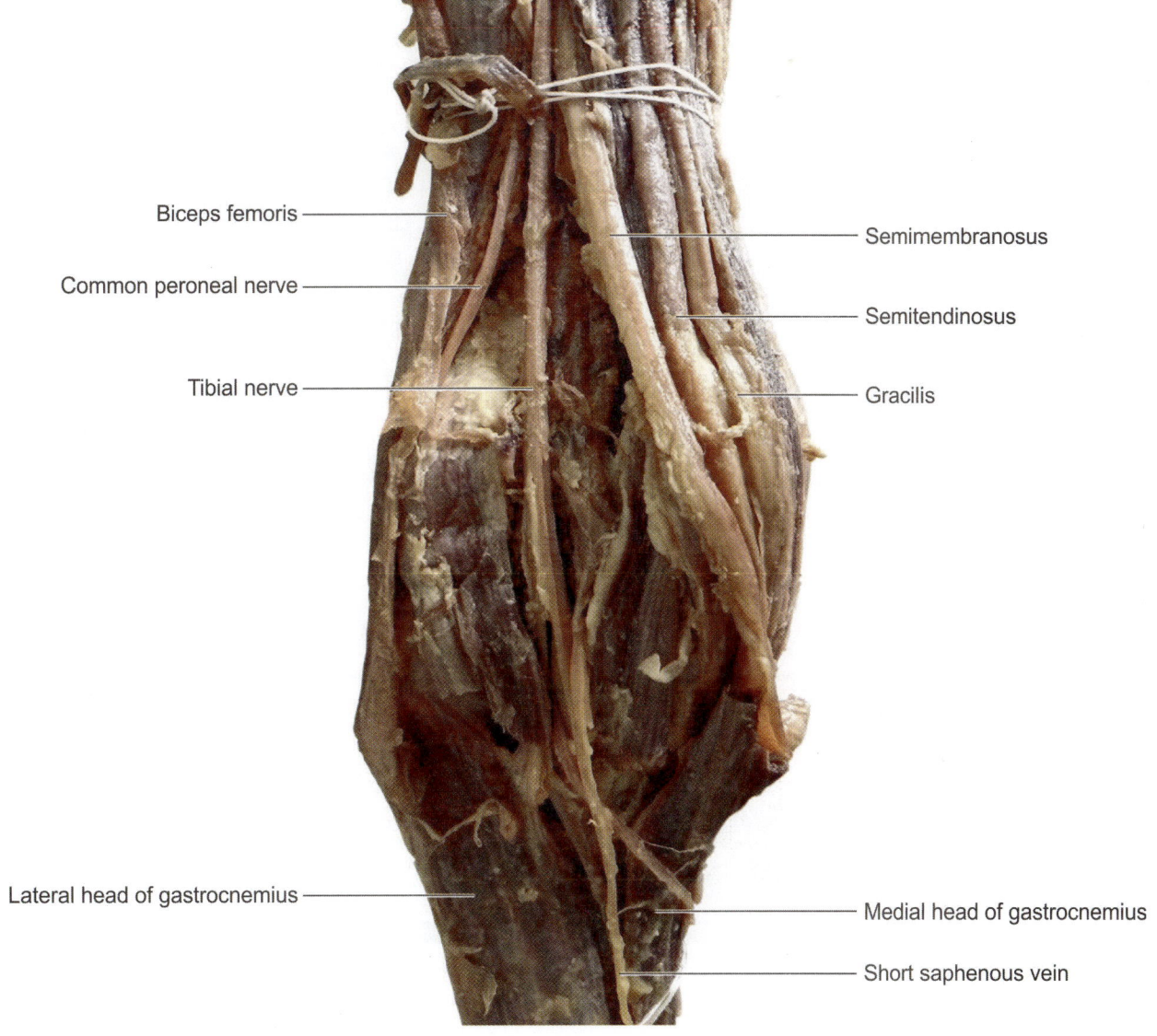

Biceps femoris

Common peroneal nerve

Tibial nerve

Semimembranosus

Semitendinosus

Gracilis

Lateral head of gastrocnemius

Medial head of gastrocnemius

Short saphenous vein

Fig. 19.3: Boundaries of popliteal fossa

articular branches are given off in the upper part of the fossa, cutaneous branch in the middle part and muscular branches in lower part of the fossa.

- Common peroneal nerve is lying just medial to the tendon of biceps femoris muscle (Fig. 19.5). Trace its branches.

- Popliteal vein is deep to tibial nerve. Identify the short saphenous vein draining into the popliteal vein.

- Popliteal artery is the deepest as seen from the back. Trace all the muscular, cutaneous, genicular and terminal branches of the popliteal artery.

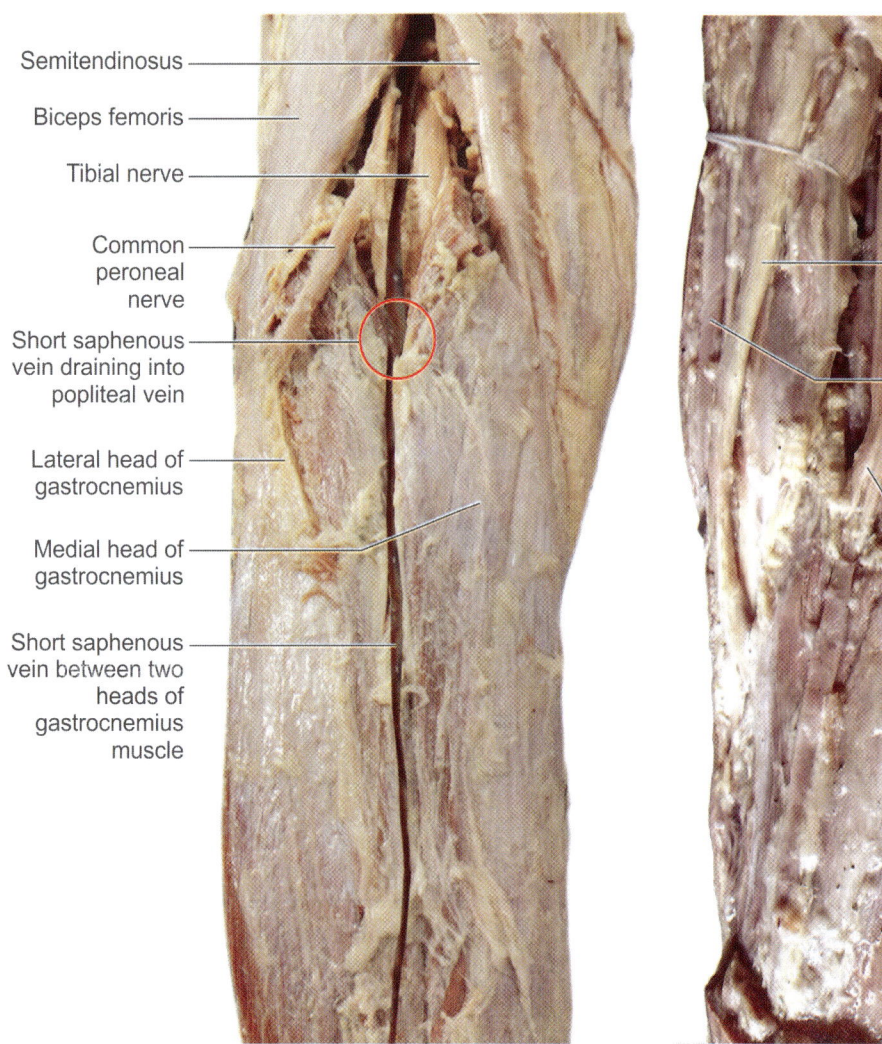

Semitendinosus

Biceps femoris

Tibial nerve

Common peroneal nerve

Short saphenous vein draining into popliteal vein

Lateral head of gastrocnemius

Medial head of gastrocnemius

Short saphenous vein between two heads of gastrocnemius muscle

Fig. 19.4: Muscles forming lower lateral and lower medial boundaries of popliteal fossa

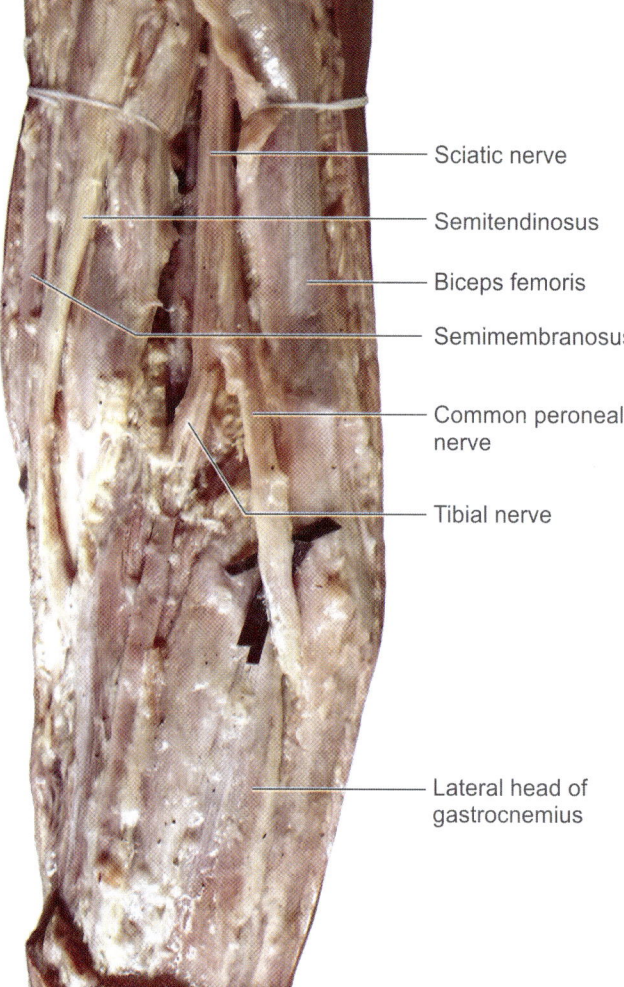

Sciatic nerve

Semitendinosus

Biceps femoris

Semimembranosus

Common peroneal nerve

Tibial nerve

Lateral head of gastrocnemius

Fig. 19.5: Popliteal fossa. Common peroneal lying along medial border of biceps femoris muscle

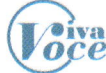

Viva Voce

- Name the boundaries of popliteal fossa. Which muscles form its upper medial boundary?
- Name the genicular branches of common peroneal nerve.

- What structures form the floor of fossa?
- What is direction of popliteal artery in the fossa from above downwards?
- What is the effect of injury to common peroneal nerve?

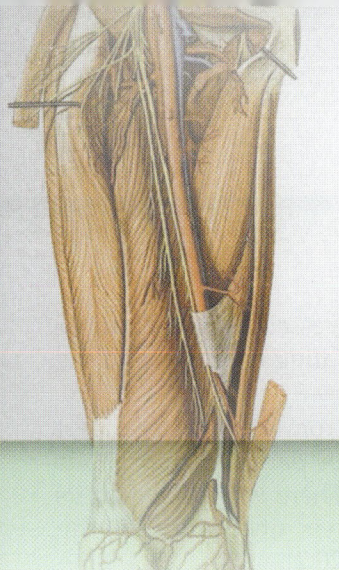

Back of Thigh

One should be able to
1. Identify all the hamstring muscles. Recapitulate their origin, insertion, nerve supply and actions.
2. Do these actions on yourself.
3. Identify the sciatic nerve and all its branches.
4. Identify the arteries taking part in the anastomoses on back of thigh.

OVERVIEW

Back of thigh is a small area between the gluteal region and the popliteal fossa.

The muscles here arise mainly from the ischial tuberosity and mostly get inserted into upper ends of tibia and fibula.

All are supplied by the thickest sciatic nerve from its medial side.

All these hamstrings are chief flexors of knee joint and weak extensors of hip joint.

Sciatic nerve—the terminal and thickest branch of lumbosacral plexus enters this region from the greater sciatic foramen, runs in gluteal region without giving any branches, enters the back of thigh, where it gives number of branches. Finally the nerve terminates close to the upper angle of popliteal fossa by dividing into larger tibial and smaller common peroneal nerves.

Competency achievement: The student should be able to:

AN 16.4 Describe and demonstrate the hamstrings group of muscles with their attachment, nerve supply and actions.

STEPS OF DISSECTION

- Give a vertical incision on the back of intact skin left after the dissections of gluteal region and the popliteal fossa (viii). Reflect the skin and fasciae on either side (Fig. 20.1).

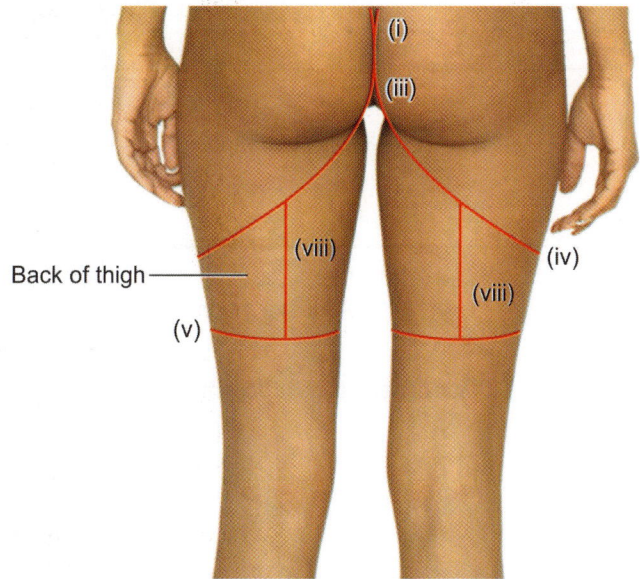

Back of thigh

Fig. 20.1: Lines of incision

149

- Sciatic nerve is seen in the gluteal region. Identify its branches in back of thigh to each of the hamstring muscles including occasionally for the short head of biceps femoris muscle. Trace the two terminal divisions of this nerve.
- Separate the hamstring muscles to expose the ischial part of the composite or hybrid adductor magnus muscle.
- Look for insertion of adductor longus, into the linea aspera of femur.

- Trace the profunda femoris vessels behind adductor longus including its perforating branches and the tributaries.

Semimembranosus arises from superolateral part of ischial tuberosity. Its upper part is membranous and lower part is muscular. There is a groove on its superficial surface which is occupied by the semitendinosus tendon (Fig. 20.2).

This muscle is inserted into a groove on the posterior surface of medial condyle if tibia. It gives a

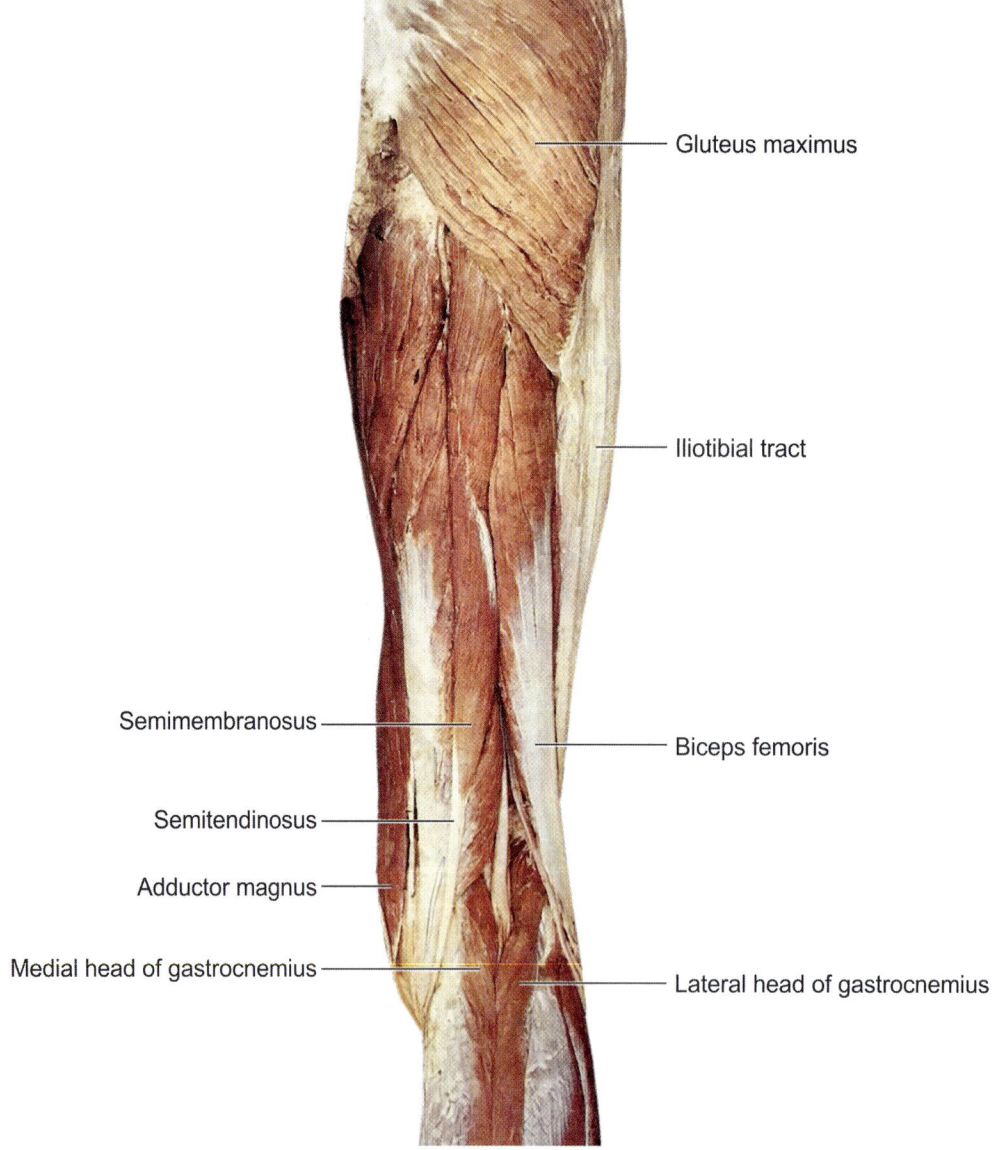

Fig. 20.2: Hamstring muscles arising from ischial tuberosity

number of expansions at its insertion, the important ones are oblique popliteal ligament of knee joint and the popliteal fascia.

Semitendinosus has its origin from inferomedial part of ischial tuberosity above the horizontal line along with long head of biceps femoris muscle. The muscle is muscular in upper part and tendinous in lower part (Fig. 20.2). It is inserted into upper medial surface of tibia just behind sartorius and gracilis muscles. This muscle with sartorius and gracilis stabilises the pelvis on the thigh.

Long head of biceps femoris arises in conjunction with semitendinosus. The two muscles soon diverge. Long head courses superficial to sciatic nerve to reach lateral side of femur, where it joins the short head of biceps femoris (Fig. 20.3). The two together get inserted into styloid process and head of fibula, being grooved by fibular collateral ligament.

Adductor magnus arises from lower lateral part of ischial tuberosity as the ischial head. Its other head, obturator head, arises from ischiopubic rami. The obturator head fans to be inserted into medial lip of

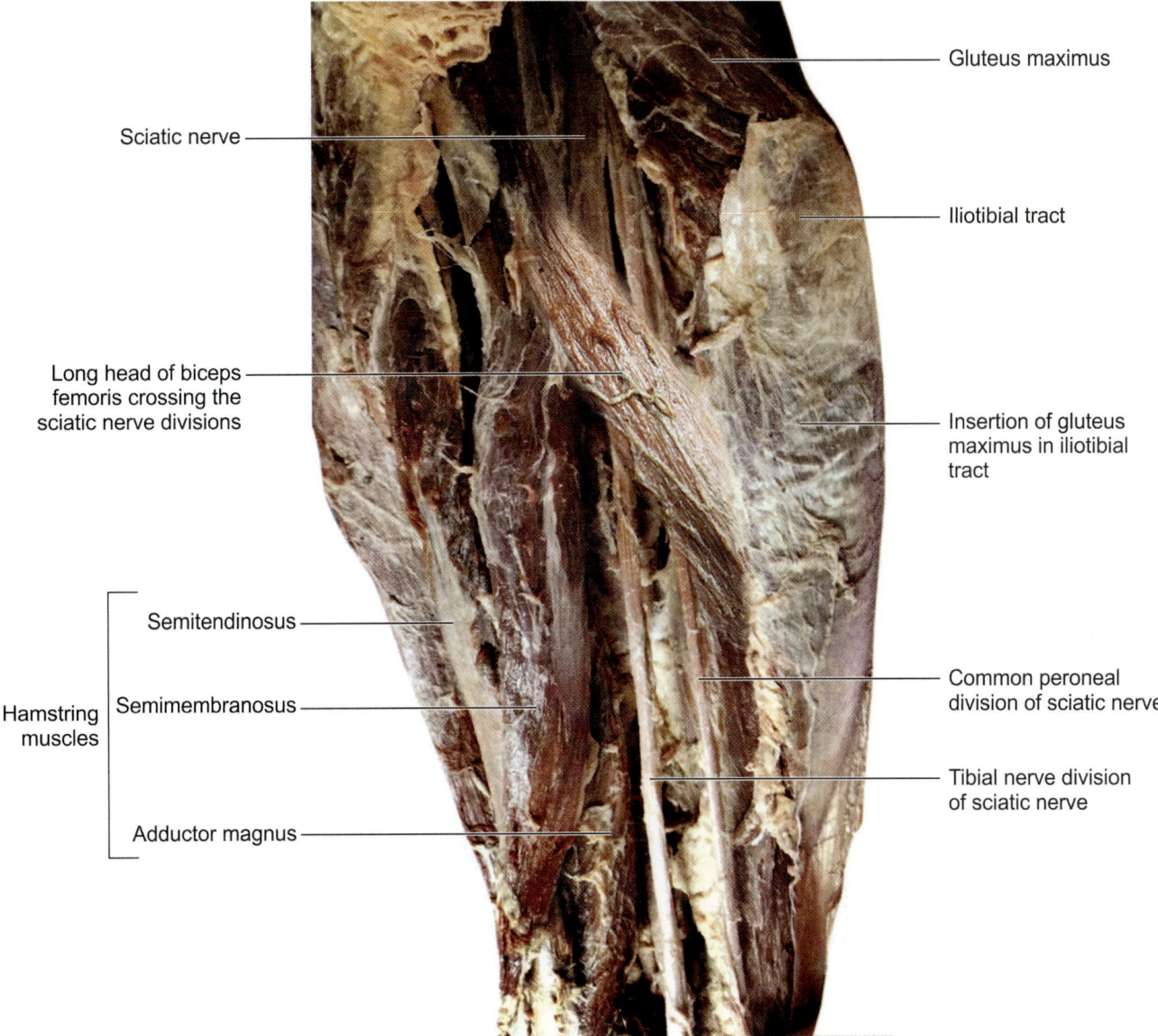

Fig. 20.3: Long head of biceps femoris crossing sciatic nerve to join its short head

linea aspera while the ischial head runs vertically to be inserted into adductor tubercle. Above and between the insertions of the two heads is an opening in the adductor magnus through which femoral vessels pass to reach popliteal fossa (*see* Fig. 19.2). These are renamed there as popliteal vessels.

Adductor magnus is a composite/hybrid muscle as its obturator head is innervated by obturator nerve while its ischial head is supplied by sciatic nerve. Thus this muscle has two origins, two insertions, two nerve supplies and two actions (flexor digitorum profundus of front of forearm is also a hybrid muscle). Adductor magnus continues distally as the medial collateral ligament which is attached to medial epicondyle of femur (which is 5 mm away from adductor tubercle) and upper medial surface of tibia.

> *Competency achievement:* The student should be able to:
>
> **AN 16.5** Describe and demonstrate the origin, course, relations, branches (or tributaries), termination of important nerves and vessels on the back of thigh.

ARTERIES ON BACK OF THIGH

Profunda (deep) femoris is the largest branch of femoral artery. It courses with the profunda vein through femoral triangle and reaches behind adductor longus muscle.

- At the apex of femoral triangle identify and appreciate the order of four vessels and muscle, viz. femoral artery, femoral vein, adductor longus, profunda vein, profunda artery. A sharp injury at this area can endanger all the four vessels.
- Look for the branches of profunda femoris artery. These are:
  – Lateral circumflex femoral artery giving three branches, i.e. ascending, transverse and descending.

– Medial circumflex femoral artery dividing into three branches, i.e. ascending, acetabular and transverse.
– 1st, 2nd and 3rd perforating arteries. The 1st and 2nd pierce adductor brevis and adductor magnus. 3rd and 4th (terminal part of profunda femoris) pierce only the adductor magnus as these arise below the level of adductor brevis. All these perforating arteries have to be traced towards vastus lateralis. All these arteries form an intercommunicating anastomoses.
- Look for the first perforating anastomosing with inferior gluteal and fourth one anastomosing with branch of popliteal artery.

Sciatic nerve is accompanied by a small artery which gets buried in its substance. It is called *arteria comitantes nervi ischidisi* and is a branch of inferior gluteal artery. Sciatic nerve resembles the median nerve of upper limb, which is also not accompanied by a big artery, but by a thin artery—the median artery; a branch of anterior interosseous artery.

Sciatic nerve is crossed by long head of biceps femoris muscle. The branches of this nerve innervate the hamstring muscles (Fig. 20.3).

Anastomoses on the Back of Thigh

- Many arteries are seen on back of thigh, anastomosing with each other. These are branches of:
  - i. Medial and lateral circumflex femoral arteries.
  - ii. 1st, 2nd, 3rd and 4th perforating arteries. 1st, 2nd and 3rd are branches of profunda femoris and 4th is terminal part of profunda femoris artery itself.
  - iii. Muscular branches of popliteal artery.
- All these form a rich network of anastomoses.

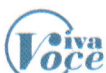

- Name the terminal branches of sciatic nerve.
- What artery runs in the substance of sciatic nerve? What is it a branch of?

- Which is the safe side of sciatic nerve?
- Enumerate the properties of hamstring muscles.

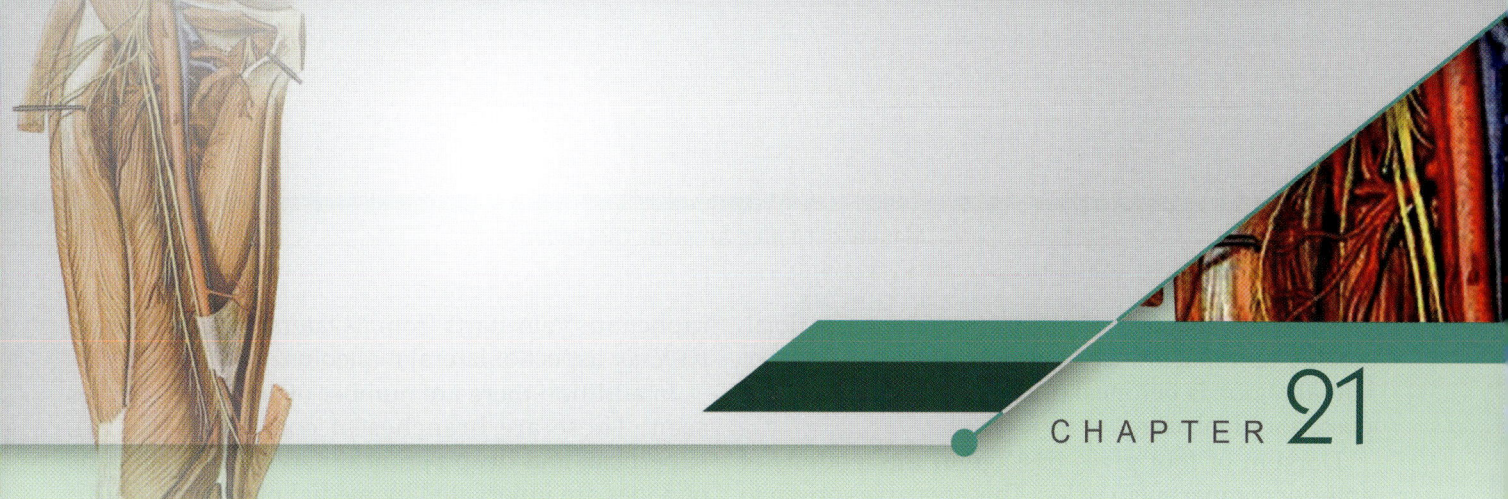

CHAPTER 21

Front of Leg with Dorsum of Foot and Lateral Compartment of Leg

Learning Objectives

One should be able to

1. Trace the full course of great/long saphenous vein from dorsal venous plexus into the leg. Trace the course of short saphenous vein from lateral side of dorsal venous plexus behind lateral malleolus into the region of calf.
2. Demarcate the areas innervated by various cutaneous nerves.
3. Identify muscles of anterior compartment of leg. Learn their attachments. Do the actions on yourself and your friends.
4. Trace the anterior tibial artery and its muscular branches in front of leg and branches of dorsalis pedis artery on dorsum of foot.
5. Show branches of deep peroneal nerve on front of leg and dorsum of foot.

Lateral compartment of leg
1. Recapitulate attachments, nerve supply and actions of peroneus longus and peroneus brevis.
2. Trace the course of superficial peroneal nerve.

Medial side of leg
1. One should be able to describe the course of great/long saphenous and small/short saphenous veins.
2. To trace the course of the three muscles belonging to medial side of leg.

OVERVIEW

Front of leg extends from front of knee joint to ankle joint. Dorsum of foot extends from ankle joint to the tips of toes. Bones in the region of leg are two long bones—tibia and fibula. Bones in the region of foot are seven tarsal bones, five metatarsal bones and fourteen very small phalanges.

Upper ends of the leg bones give insertion to the muscles of three compartments of thigh, viz. ligamentum patellae on the tibial tuberosity from anterior compartment of thigh; sartorius, gracilis and semitendinosus on upper medial surface of tibia. These are one each from the anterior, medial and posterior compartments of thigh respectively. Semimembranosus gets attached to back of medial condyle of tibia.

The muscles of leg are also disposed in three main compartments, these being anterior, lateral and posterior (in thigh the compartments are anterior, medial and posterior).

Muscles of anterior and lateral compartments of leg take origin from the two long bones. These course down in front of and on lateral sides of the leg to reach their destination—the foot. The tendons of these muscles are kept in proper position by two extensor retinacula and two peroneal retinacula.

The two branches of common peroneal nerve supply these two muscle groups.

Common peroneal nerve lies in intimate relation to the neck of fibula where it divides into deep peroneal for muscles of anterior compartment and superficial peroneal for muscles of lateral compartment. It is vulnerable to injury at neck of fibula.

The artery of anterior compartment is anterior tibial, smaller terminal branch of popliteal artery. Artery of lateral region is peroneal (fibular) artery, a branch of posterior tibial artery.

Dorsum of foot gives passage to the tendons of anterior compartment of leg. This area gives origin to one muscle only, the extensor digitorum brevis. Anterior tibial artery also travels down on dorsum of foot as dorsalis pedis artery and then slips down into the sole of foot.

The nerve accompanying the dorsalis pedis artery remains as deep peroneal nerve. On entering the foot, the nerve divides into a lateral branch for the only muscle of dorsum of foot, extensor digitorum brevis and medial cutaneous branch which gives digital branches to adjacent sides of 1st and 2nd toes.

Next to the skin in the superficial fascia on dorsum of foot lies the dorsal venous plexus. The long saphenous vein starts from its medial end and lies on *anterior* aspect of medial malleolus. The short saphenous vein starts from its lateral end and lies on *posterior* aspect of lateral malleolus.

In addition there are number of cutaneous nerves seen. These are branches of common peroneal, superficial and deep peroneal nerves. The nail beds of 5 toes are innervated by medial plantar nerve (3½ toes) and by lateral plantar nerve (1½ toes).

STEPS OF DISSECTION

Superficial Fascia

- Make a horizontal incision across the leg at its junction with foot, i.e. at ankle joint (Fig. 21.1).
- Provide a vertical incision up from the centre of incision to the middle of incision drawn just below the level of tibial tuberosity.
- Carry this vertical incision onto the dorsum of foot till the middle of the second toe.
- Reflect the skin on both the sides. Look for various veins and cutaneous nerves in the leg and foot according to the description given in the text.

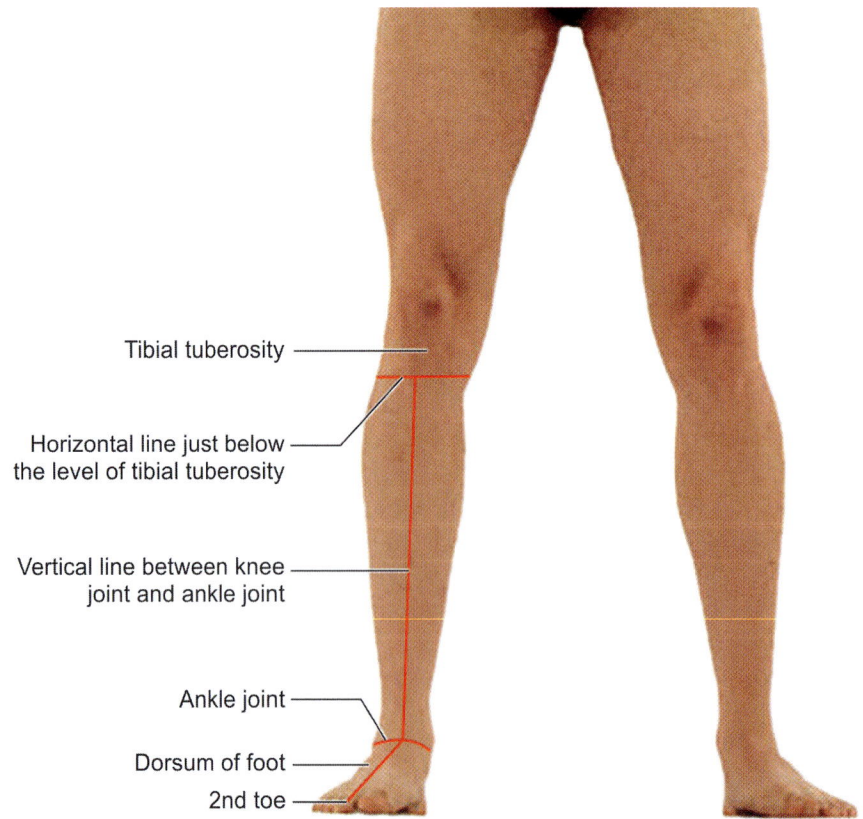

Fig. 21.1: Lines of incision

The nerves seen in this region are:

1. Infrapatellar branch of saphenous nerve.
2. Saphenous nerve itself
3. Lateral cutaneous nerve of the calf.
4. Superficial peroneal nerve
5. Sural nerve
6. Deep peroneal nerve
7. Digital branches of medial plantar nerve
8. Digital branches of lateral plantar nerve
- Vein seen in great saphenous vein lying anterior to the medial malleolus of tibia (Fig. 21.2).

Deep Fascia

- Underlying the superficial fascia is the dense deep fascia of leg. Divide this fascia longitudinally as it stretches between tibia and fibula.

- Expose the superior extensor retinaculum 5 cm above the ankle joint and the inferior extensor retinaculum in front of the ankle joint

- See the attachments of superior extensor retinaculum medially to lower part of anterior border of tibia and laterally to lower part of anterior border of

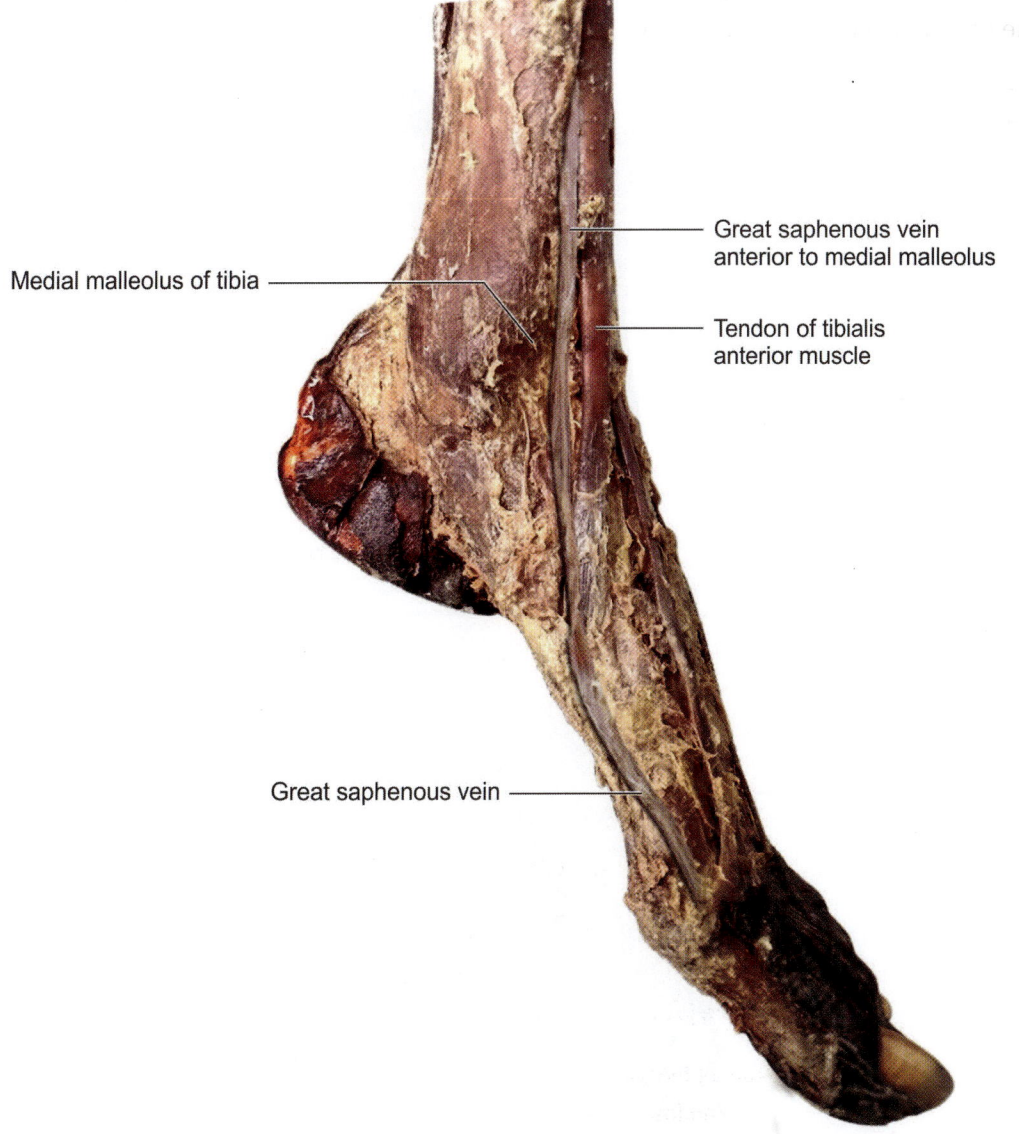

Medial malleolus of tibia

Great saphenous vein anterior to medial malleolus

Tendon of tibialis anterior muscle

Great saphenous vein

Fig. 21.2: Beginning of great saphenous vein

fibula forming anterior boundary of elongated triangular area just above lateral malleolus.

- Identify and clean the attachments of 'Y' shaped inferior extensor retinaculum, the stem of 'Y' is attached to superficial surface of calcaneus in front of sulcus calcanei (Fig. 21.3). The upper band gets attached to anterior border of medial malleolus. Lower band passes downwards and medially into the sole to be attached to the plantar aponeurosis.
- See the structures passing under both the retinacula from medial to lateral side. These are:
  1. Tendon of tibialis anterior
  2. Tendon of extensor hallucis longus
  3. Anterior tibial vessels
  4. Deep peroneal nerve
  5. Tendon of extensor digitorum longus
  6. Tendon of peroneus tertius

Competency achievement: The student should be able to:

AN 18.1 Describe and demonstrate major muscles of anterior compartment of leg with their attachment, nerve supply and actions.

Muscles of Front of Leg

- Identify the muscles of anterior compartment of leg as these are lying close together on the lateral surface of tibia, adjoining interosseous membrane and medial surface of fibula.

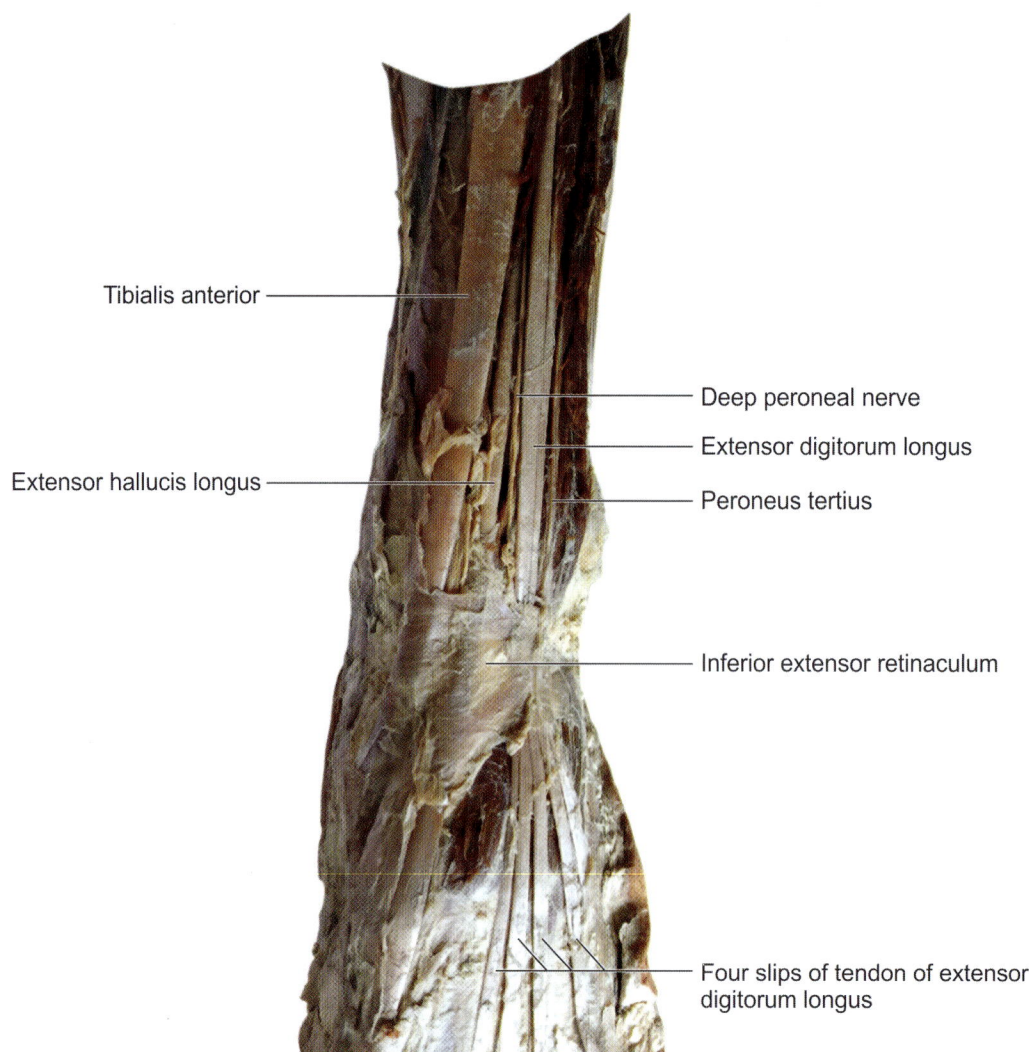

Fig. 21.3: Inferior extensor retinaculum and the tendons underlying it

- Trace these tendons deep to the two retinacula on the dorsum of foot till their insertion. Look for anterior tibial artery and accompanying deep peroneal nerve as these lie on the upper part of interosseous membrane of leg. Study their course, relations and branches.

The muscles of anterior compartment are crowded as these lie between lateral surface of tibia and medial surface of fibula.

Tibialis anterior is the most medial one. It passes downwards and medially on the leg and then under both superior and inferior retinacula to be inserted into medial cuneiform and base of 1st metatarsal.

Extensor hallucis longus arises from lower part of fibula, descends down deep to the two retinacula. It crosses anterior tibial vessels and deep peroneal nerve to become medial to these structures.

Extensor digitorum longus arises from most part of fibula. It courses downwards to lie on lateral side of neurovascular bundle, then deep to retinacula in dorsum of foot. Here, it divides into four tendons for 2nd to 5th digits (Fig. 21.4).

Peroneus tertius is seen to arise from medial surface of lower one-fourth of fibula and gets inserted into dorsal surface of base of 5th metatarsal.

Extensor digitorum brevis is the only muscle on dorsum of foot. It is seen to arise from anterior part of superior surface of calcaneum. The muscle is seen to divide into four tendons for 1st to 4th digits (excluding 5th one).

All these muscles are innervated by deep peroneal nerve, the larger branch of common peroneal nerve. Look for anterior tibial vessels and deep peroneal nerve.

Competency achievement: The student should be able to:

AN 18.2 Describe and demonstrate origin, course, relations, branches (or tributaries), termination of important nerves and vessels of anterior compartment of leg.

Anterior tibial artery is the smaller terminal branch of popliteal artery. It enters anterior compartment through an opening in the upper part of interosseous membrane. At first it runs between tibialis anterior and extensor digitorum longus. Then in the middle part it lies between tibialis anterior and extensor hallucis longus. In the lower part extensor hallucis longus crosses in front of the artery and lies on the

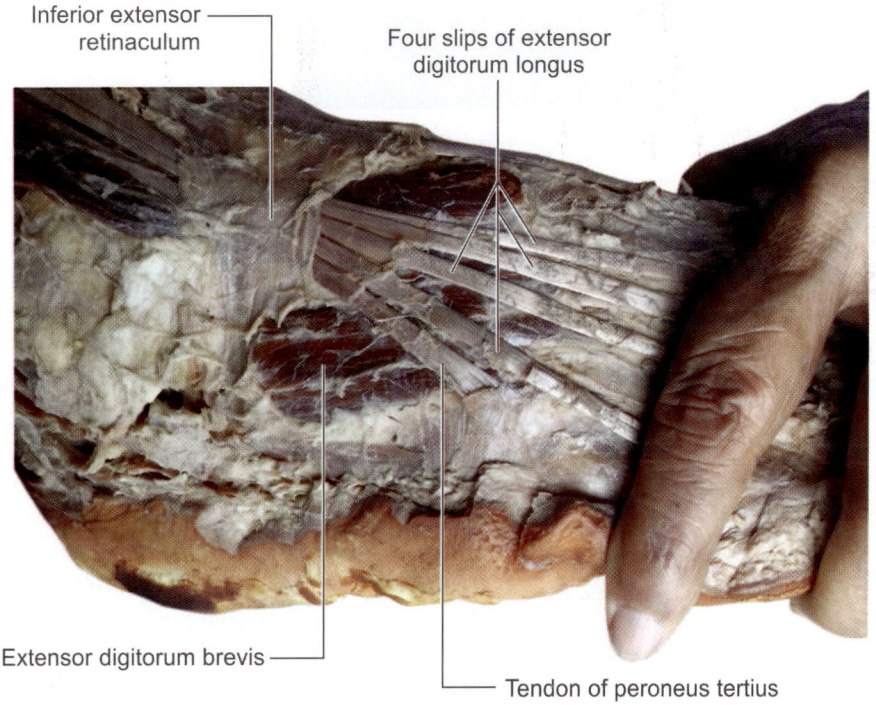

Fig. 21.4: 4 Slips of extensor digitorum longus

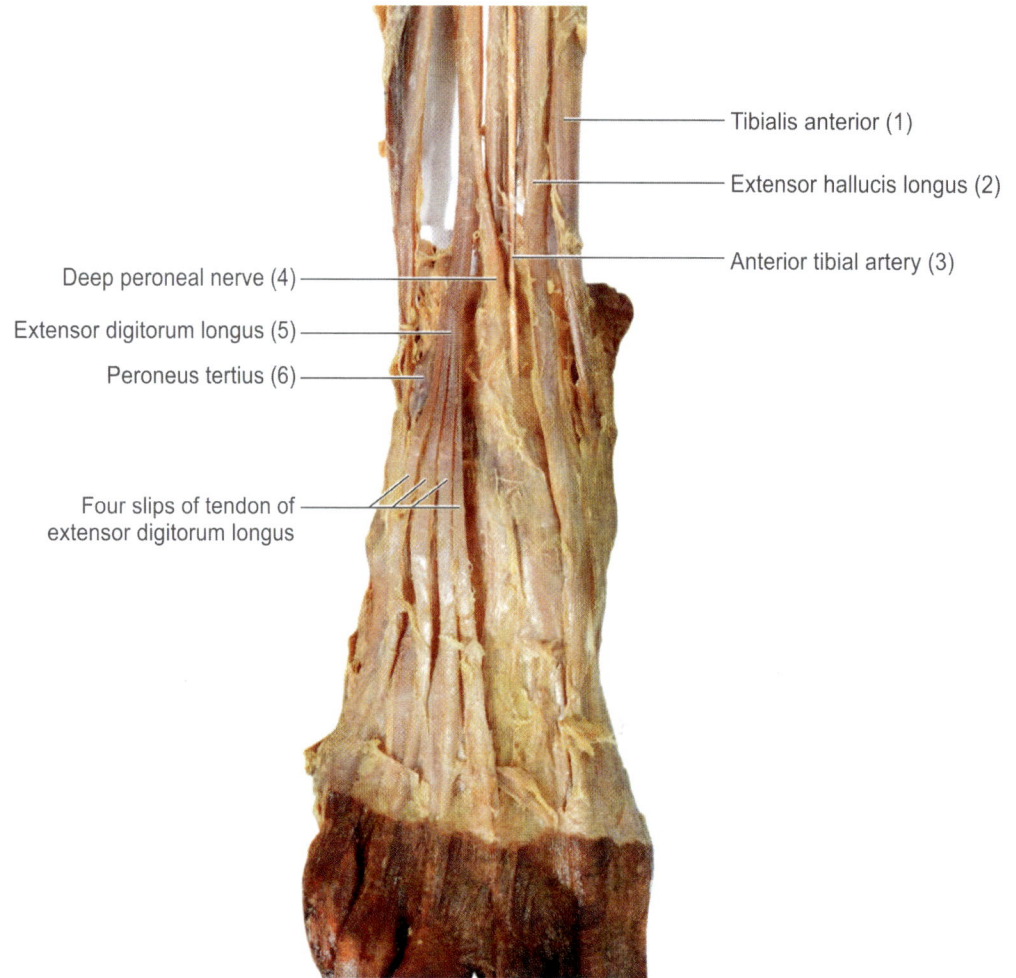

Tibialis anterior (1)

Extensor hallucis longus (2)

Anterior tibial artery (3)

Deep peroneal nerve (4)

Extensor digitorum longus (5)

Peroneus tertius (6)

Four slips of tendon of
extensor digitorum longus

Fig. 21.5: Structures under extensor retinacula in order 1 to 6

medial side of the artery. So the artery lies between extensor hallucis longus and extensor digitorum longus. The nerve almost follows the artery. Thus the order of structures under extensor retinacula is:

1. Tendon of tibialis anterior (Fig. 21.5)
2. Tendon of extensor hallucis longus
3. Anterior tibial vessels
4. Deep peroneal nerve
5. Tendon of extensor digitorum longus
6. Tendon of peroneus tertius

DORSUM OF FOOT

Steps of Dissection

- Identify the small muscle extensor digitorum brevis situated on the lateral side of dorsum of foot. Its

tendons are deep to the tendons of extensor digitorum longus. Its most medial tendon is called extensor hallucis brevis (Fig. 21.6).

- Dissect the dorsalis pedis artery and its branches on the dorsum of the foot.
- Identify the four tendons of extensor digitorum longus for 2nd–5th toes and four tendons of extensor digitorum brevis for 1st–4th toes (Fig. 21.6). Their insertions into toes will be studied later.
- Identify dorsalis pedis artery as the continuation of anterior tibial artery (Fig. 21.5). See that it is palpable on the dorsum of your foot between tendon of extensor hallucis longus and 1st tendon of extensor digitorum longus on the middle cuneiform bone. It reaches the proximal part of 1st intermetatarsal space. There it is seen to dip down

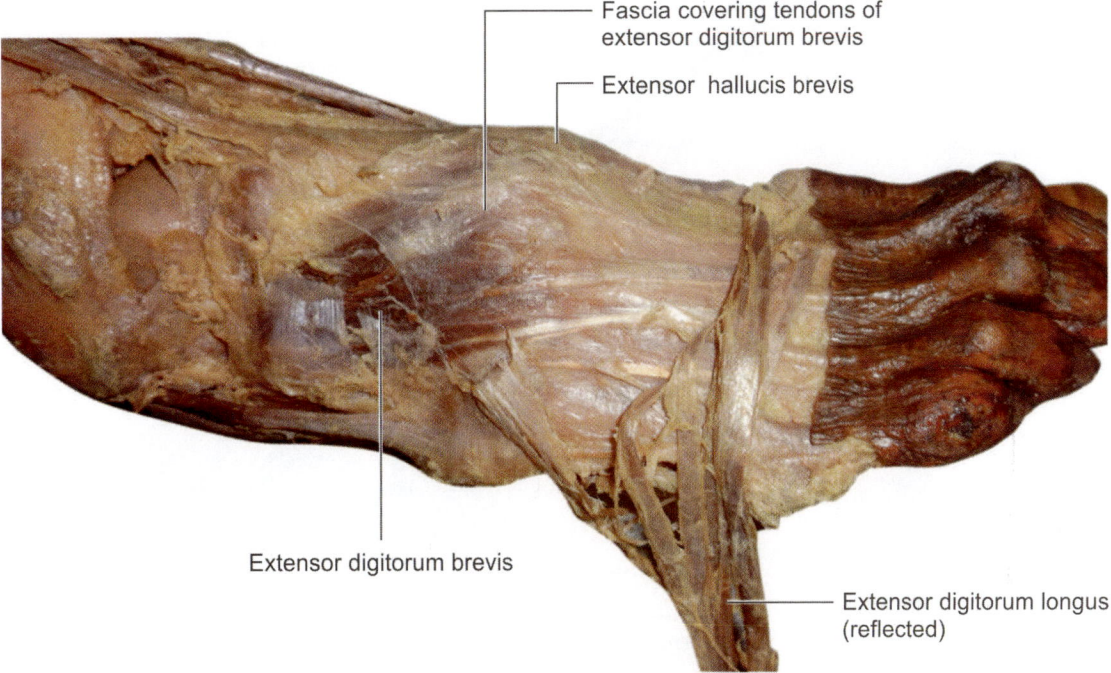

Fascia covering tendons of
extensor digitorum brevis

Extensor hallucis brevis

Extensor digitorum brevis

Extensor digitorum longus
(reflected)

Fig. 21.6: Muscles and tendons on the dorsum of foot

into the sole between the two heads of 1st dorsal interosseous muscle and ends by completing the plantar arch.

- Identify its branches as lateral tarsal and medial tarsal arteries.
- Arcuate artery may be seen.

LATERAL COMPARTMENT OF LEG

OVERVIEW

The lateral compartment is localised between anterior and posterior intermuscular septa of leg attached to the anterior and posterior borders of fibula.

Contents of this compartment are two muscles viz. the peroneus longus and peroneus brevis along with superficial peroneal nerve. Both these muscles arise from fibula, peroneus brevis from middle and lower parts while peroneus longus from most of fibula's shaft including its head. Peroneus longus and brevis are kept in position by superior and inferior peroneal retinacula. Peroneus brevis gets attached to tuberosity of 5th metatarsal, while peroneus longus lies in the groove in the cuboid bone, runs across the sole to be attached to medial cuneiform and base of 1st metatarsal (same as tibialis anterior muscle).

Peroneus longus and brevis evert the foot as while walking on uneven surfaces.

The lateral side/compartment of leg is small as it contains only two muscles, peroneus longus and peroneus brevis with their nerve, i.e. superficial peroneal nerve. Peroneal artery supplies blood to these muscles.

STEPS OF DISSECTION

- Reflect the lateral skin flap of leg further laterally till peroneal muscles are seen.
- Divide the deep fascia longitudinally over peroneal muscles.
- Identify and clean the superior and inferior peroneal retinacula situated just above and below the lateral malleolus. These are modifications of deep fascia and keep the peroneal tendons in place.
- Superior peroneal retinaculum is attached to posterior margin of lateral malleolus and to the posterior part of lateral surface of calcaneum.
- Inferior peroneal retinaculum is attached to anterior part of superior surface of calcaneum and to lateral surface of calcaneum. The space is divided into two parts by a septum attached to peroneal tubercle.

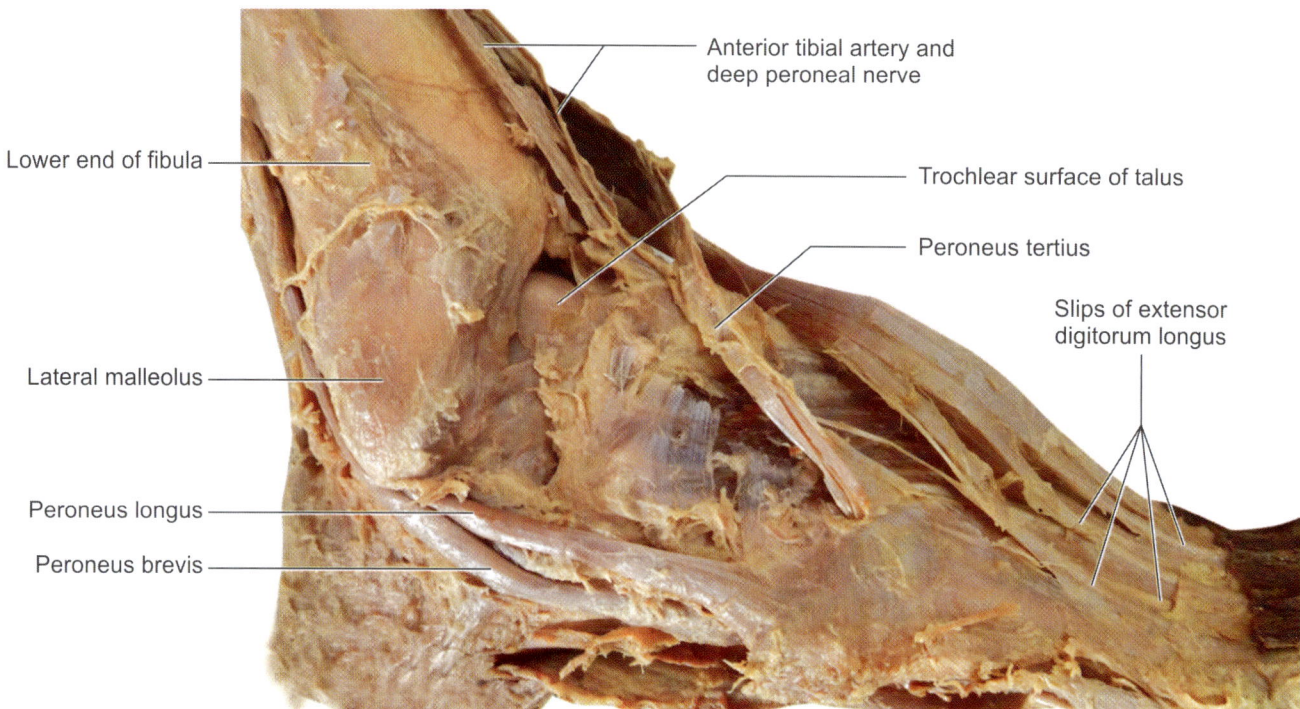

Fig. 21.7: Structures on the anterior and lateral aspects of ankle joint

- The tendons are surrounded by a common synovial sheath under superior peroneal reticulum while under the inferior peroneal retinaculum each tendon is enclosed in a separate synovial sheath.

Peroneal muscles are seen in the upper part of lateral side of leg. Both the muscles arise from parts of lateral surface of fibula. Peroneus brevis is shorter and is inserted into the tuberosity at base of 5th metatarsal bone (Fig. 21.7). Peroneus longus is longer. Its tendon travels through a groove on the lateral surface and plantar surface of cuboid bone in the sole (Fig. 21.8). In the sole the tendon lies across the sole to reach its medial side. Finally it gets attached to lateral side of distal surface of medial cuneiform and adjoining part of base of 1st metatarsal, the insertion of peroneus longus is similar to that of tibialis anterior muscle; except that insertion of peroneus longus into 1st metatarsal bone is more than into medial cuneiform bone.

SUPERFICIAL PERONEAL NERVE

- Identify and clean the superficial peroneal nerve lying in relation to neck of fibula. Trace it as it runs through the peroneal muscles to become cutaneous at the junction of upper 2/3rd and lower 1/3rd of leg.

It pierces the deep fascia, divides into two branches which lie in the distal 1/3rd of leg to run superficial to the extensor retinaculum. These two branches—medial and lateral enter the dorsum of foot and supply skin of most of the dorsum of foot.

The medial branch carries sensations from medial side of big toe and adjoining sides of 2nd and 3rd toes (adjoining sides of 1st and 2nd toes are supplied by deep peroneal nerve).

The lateral branch gives digital branches for the adjoining sides of 3rd and 4th and 4th and 5th toes.

MEDIAL SIDE OF LEG

OVERVIEW

This is a small area on upper medial surface of tibia where sartorius from anterior compartment, gracilis from medial compartment and the semitendinosus from posterior compartment of leg get attached. These three muscles support the pelvis from the leg.

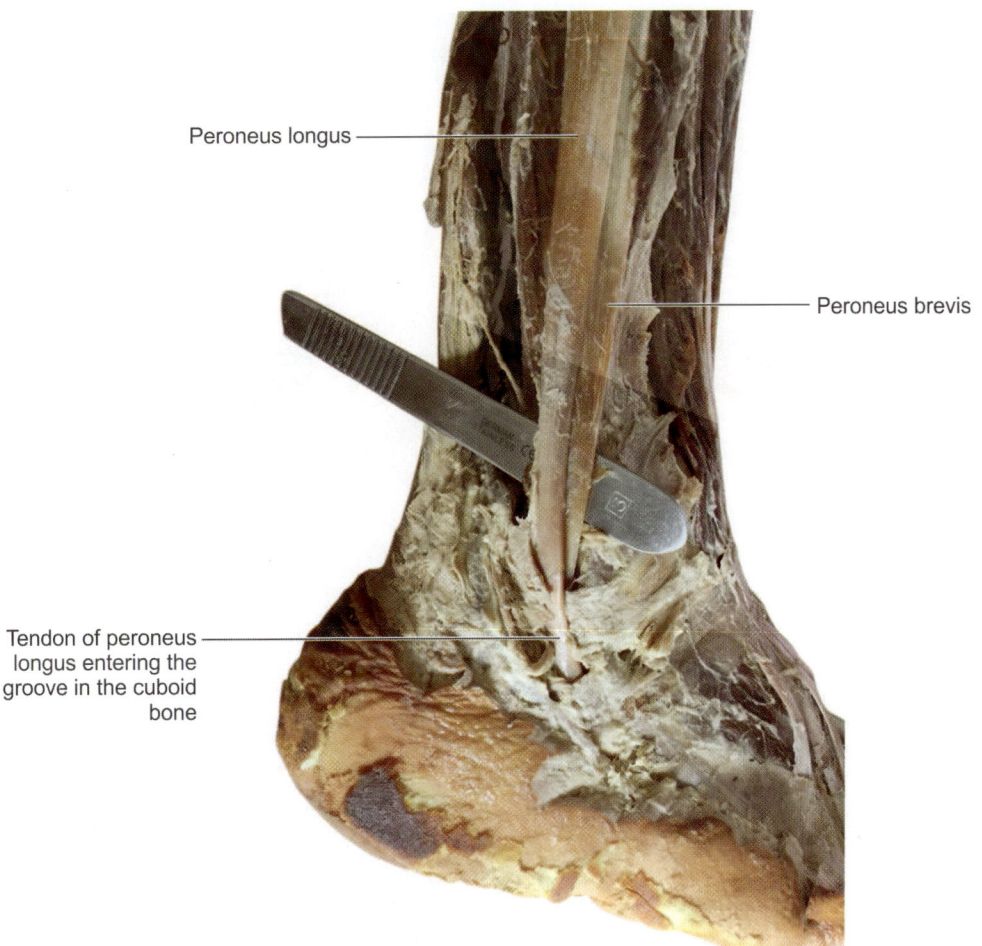

Peroneus longus

Peroneus brevis

Tendon of peroneus longus entering the groove in the cuboid bone

Fig. 21.8: Muscles in the lateral compartment of leg with their tendons on lateral side of ankle joint

STEPS OF DISSECTION

- Identify the 3 tendons of a tripod formed by sartorius, gracilis and semitendinosus at their insertion on the upper medial side of tibia (Fig. 21.9).
- Behind these tendons is present the tibial collateral ligament of knee joint.
- Great saphenous vein (GSV) is visualised on the lower 1/3rd of tibia. From there it ascends along the medial border of tibia to reach posteromedial aspect of knee joint. The GSV is accompanied by saphenous (easily seen) nerve. Both these lie anterior to medial malleolus of tibia. The saphenous nerve runs along the medial border of foot till the 1st metatarsophalangeal joint.
- Sartorius is the longest muscle of the body with parallel fibres. It belongs to front of thigh and is

supplied by femoral nerve, the nerve of the front of thigh/anterior compartment of thigh.
- Gracilis belongs to medial/adductor compartment of thigh and is supplied anterior division of obturator nerve, the nerve of this compartment.
- Semitendinosus lies in the posterior compartment of thigh to be innervated by sciatic nerve.
- As these muscles arising from three parts of hip bone, travel through three compartments of thigh, get inserted into upper medial surface tibia close to each other and support and stabilise the pelvis. These thus act as guy ropes.
- Try and identify a complicated bursa—bursa anserina with diverticula which separates the three tendons from each other. The diverticula also separate tendons from medial surface of tibia and from strong tibial collateral ligament.

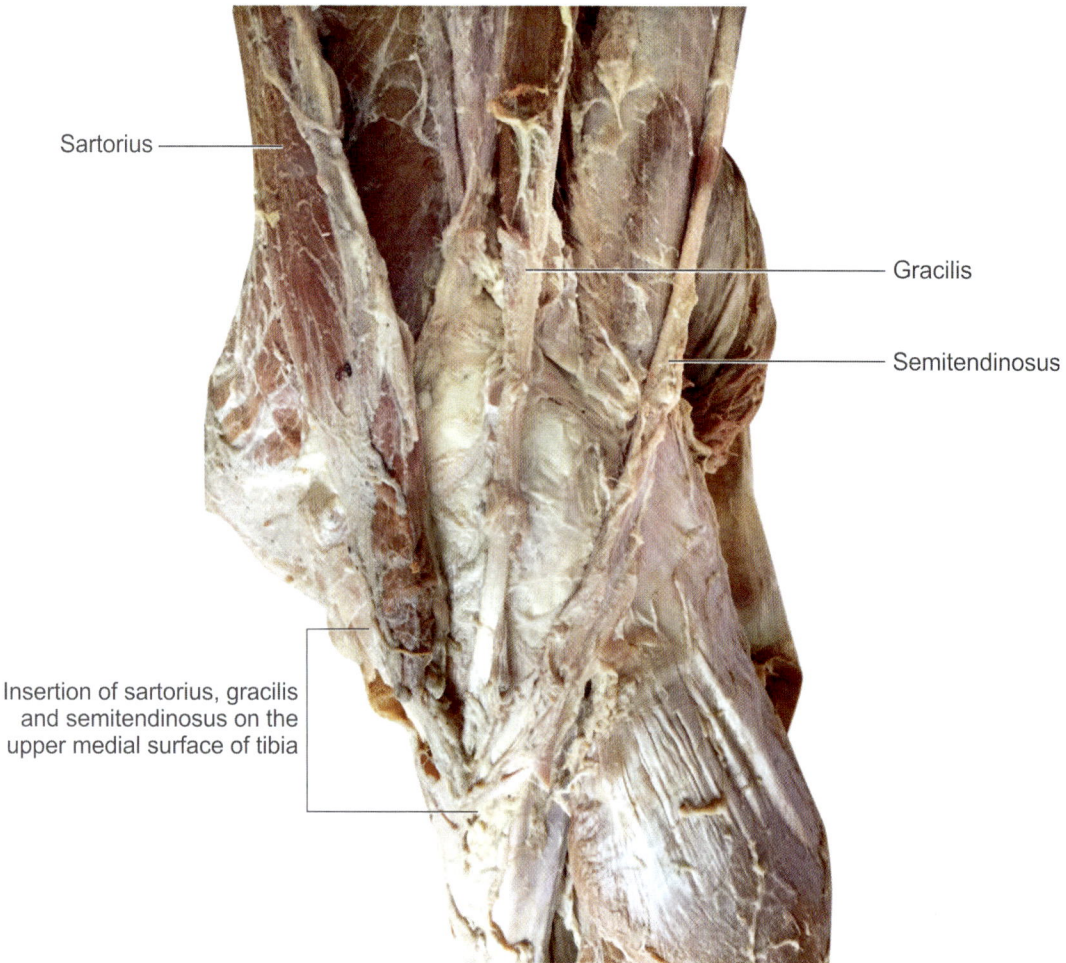

Sartorius

Gracilis

Semitendinosus

Insertion of sartorius, gracilis
and semitendinosus on the
upper medial surface of tibia

Fig. 21.9: Insertions of three muscles on upper medial surface of tibia

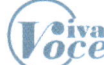

- How does anterior tibial artery enter the front of leg?
- How does common peroneal nerve enter the front of leg?
- Which tendon crosses the anterior tibial artery and deep peroneal nerve in the distal part of the leg?
- Name the attachments of inferior peroneal retinaculum.
- Enumerate the structures in order passing under extensor retinacula of ankle.
- Which muscle joins the slips of extensor digitorum longus?

- What nerve supplies the skin of adjacent sides of 1st and 2nd toes?
- Where is the insertion of peroneus brevis?
- Trace the insertion of peroneus longus.
- What is the difference in the insertions of tibialis anterior and peroneus longus?
- What is the cause of footdrop and what are its symptoms?
- Name the three muscles inserted on the upper medial surface of tibia. Name their nerve supply.
- What bursa separates the attachments of these muscles?

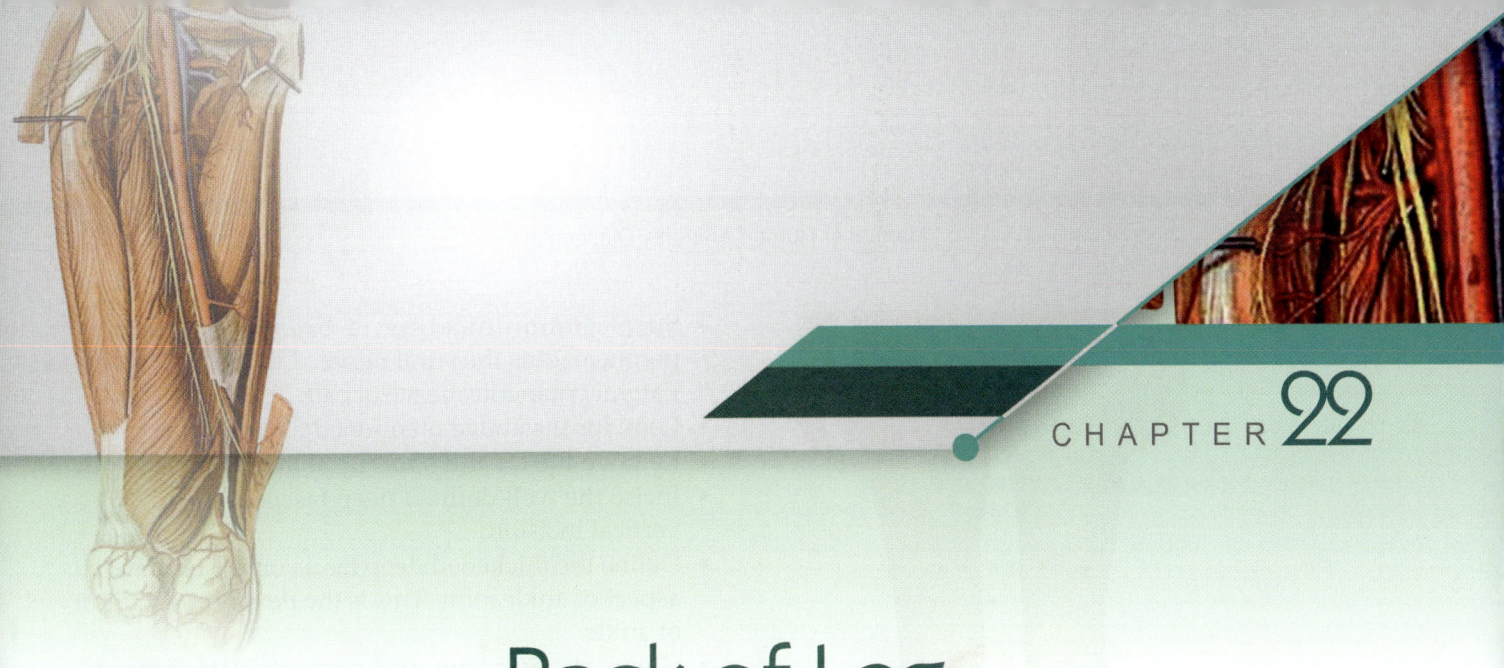

CHAPTER 22

Back of Leg

Learning Objectives

One should be able to

1. Learn the attachments of the soleus muscle. Why it is called "peripheral heart".

2. Do the action of tendo calcaneous
3. Recapitulate branches of tibial nerve and posterior tibial artery.

OVERVIEW

Back of leg (calf region) extends from the lower end of popliteal fossa till the flexor retinaculum. It is the bulkiest region of the leg, comprising of:

a. Eight muscles—four superficial and four deep muscles

b. One tibial nerve innervating all eight muscles

c. One posterior tibial artery providing blood to all these eight muscles

d. One peroneal artery—a branch of posterior tibial artery supplying the two peroneal muscles of the lateral compartment of the leg

e. Venae comitantes with these two arteries and the small/short saphenous vein, which starts from dorsum of foot to end in the popliteal vein.

Four superficial muscles form the longest and strongest tendon of the body, the tendo calcaneus, which gets attached to the posterior surface of the calcaneus.

Out of the four superficial muscles one is small triangular muscle which forms the floor of popliteal fossa. The other three long bipennate muscles course deep to the flexor retinaculum to enter the sole where these are inserted.

STEPS OF DISSECTION

- The horizontal incision (vi) in the skin is already given. Carry this incision along the lateral and medial borders of the leg (Fig. 22.1). Reflect whole skin of the back of leg distally till the heel (ix).
- Identify small and great saphenous veins and cutaneous nerves.
- See that small/short saphenous vein, the main vein of calf, starts by the union of lateral marginal vein of foot with lateral end of the dorsal venous arch. This vein lies *behind* lateral malleolus. It is accompanied by sural nerve in the calf region. Trace the vein ascending lateral to tendo calcaneus and then along midline of calf.
- See how it pierces the deep fascia of the popliteal region to drain into the popliteal vein.
- Only a part of great saphenous vein is seen as it lies on the posteromedial aspect of knee.

Cutaneous nerves seen in this region are:

1. Saphenous nerve gives few branches to posteromedial side of leg.
2. Posterior cutaneous nerve of thigh
3. Sural nerve from tibial nerve accompanies the short saphenous vein.

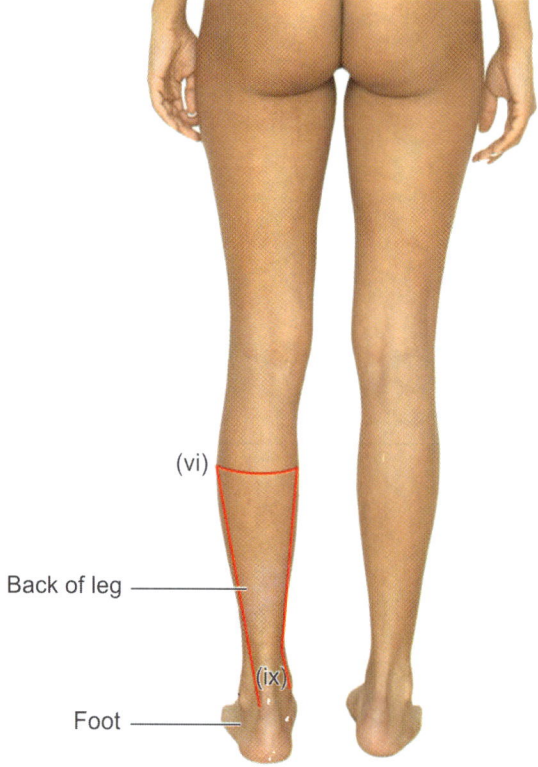

(vi)

Back of leg

(ix)

Foot

Fig. 22.1: Lines of dissection

4. Sural communicating, a branch of common peroneal joins the sural nerve.
5. Lateral cutaneous nerve of calf.
- Look for the above mentioned cutaneous nerves
- Remove the fat and superficial fascia
- Incise the well defined deep fascia of the calf by a vertical incision.
- Define the thickened deep fascia on posteromedial aspect of ankle joint. This is the flexor retinaculum of ankle.
- Clean its margins and note its attachments, anteriorly to posterior border of medial malleolus and posteriorly to medial tubercle of calcaneum.
- Identify the structures passing deep to this retinaculum. These are from medial to lateral side:
  1. Tendon of tibialis posterior enclosed in the synovial sheath (Fig. 22.2).
  2. Tendon of flexor digitorum longus enclosed in its synovial sheath
  3. Posterior tibial artery and vein
  4. Tibial nerve
  5. Tendon of flexor hallucis longus

The flexor retinaculum with the underlying bones form "tarsal tunnel" through which the above

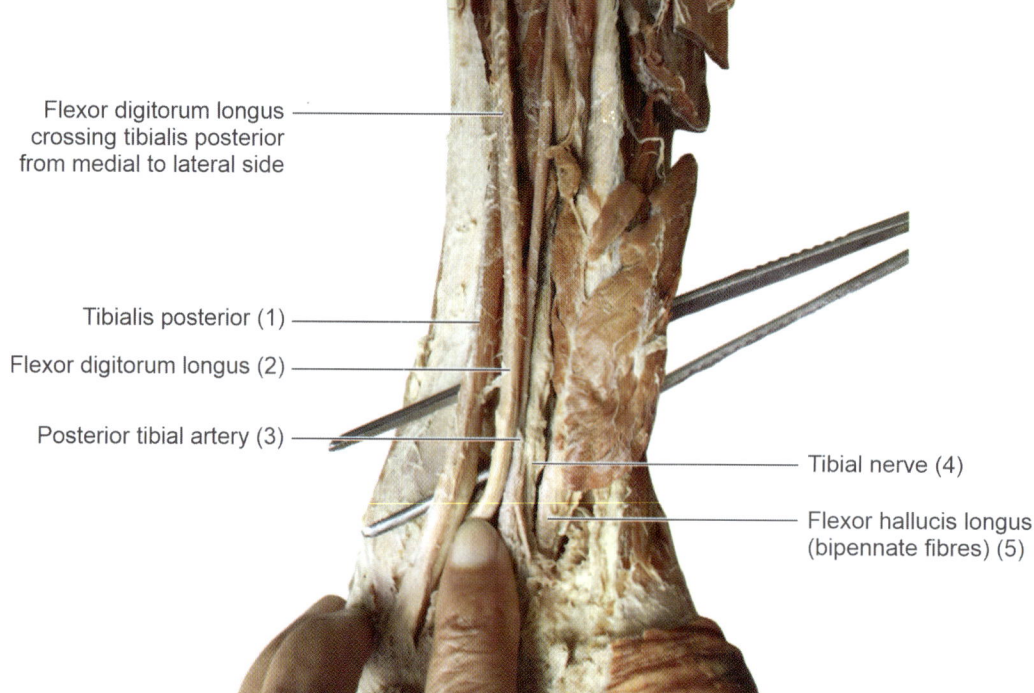

Flexor digitorum longus crossing tibialis posterior from medial to lateral side

Tibialis posterior (1)

Flexor digitorum longus (2)

Posterior tibial artery (3)

Tibial nerve (4)

Flexor hallucis longus (bipennate fibres) (5)

Fig. 22.2: Structures 1–5 passing under flexor retinaculum of ankle

mentioned structures are passing. In case of pressure on the nerve, the symptoms and signs are called "Tarsal tunnel syndrome".

> *Competency achievement:* The student should be able to:
> **AN 19.1** Describe and demonstrate the major muscles of back of leg with their attachment, nerve supply and actions.

- After the study of flexor retinaculum, look at the muscles of calf. The superficial layer is formed by medial and lateral heads of gastrocnemius muscles. Remember that the two heads arise from lower end of femur. Medial head arises from medial side of popliteal surface of femur and lateral head from an impression above the lateral condyle of femur (Fig. 22.3).
- Cut the medial belly 5 cm distal to its origin and reflect its proximal part laterally.

- Identify the popliteal vessels and tibial nerve in deep part of back of leg.
- On the lateral side, identify a small belly of the plantaris muscle, with the longest tendon, posteromedial to the lateral head of gastrocnemius. The tendon then lies between gastrocnemius and soleus muscles (Fig. 22.4).
- Incise the belly of lateral head of gastrocnemius 5 cm distal to its origin and reflect the proximal part laterally.
- Identify the distal parts of both bellies of gastrocnemius muscle. Reflect these distal parts towards the calcaneum.
- Identify and clean the strong soleus muscle deep to the gastrocnemius muscle.
- Once the soleus has been studied, separate it from its attachment on tibia and reflect it laterally

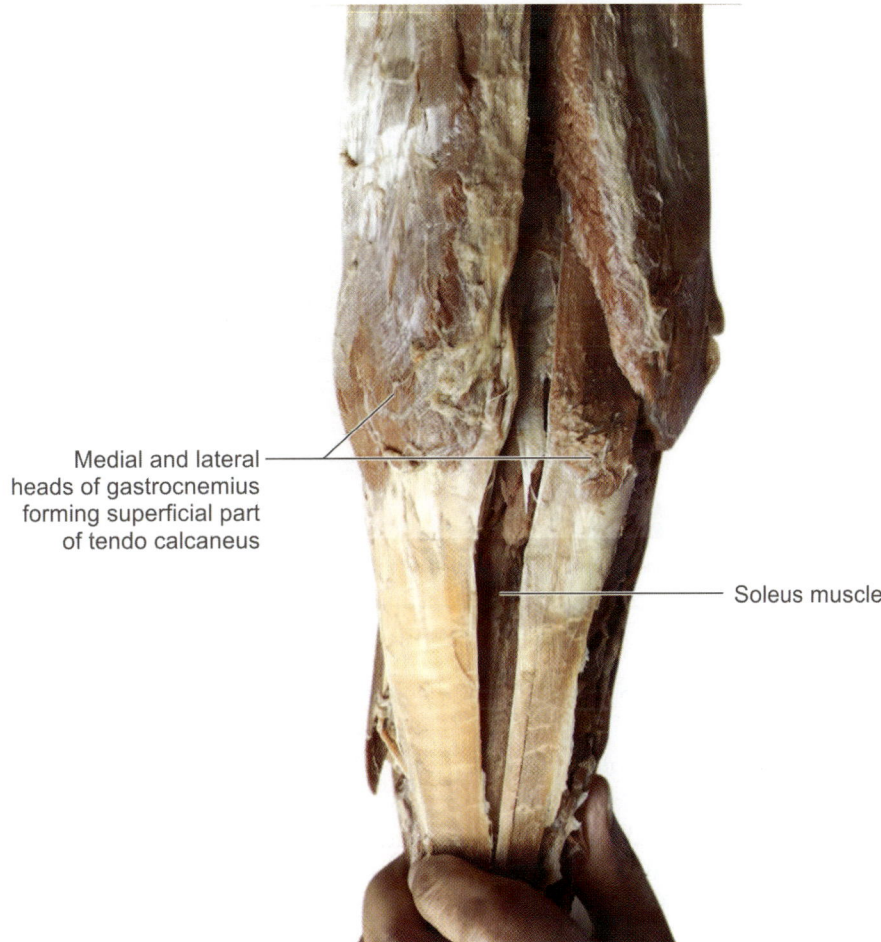

Medial and lateral heads of gastrocnemius forming superficial part of tendo calcaneus

Soleus muscle

Fig. 22.3: Formation of tendo calcaneus

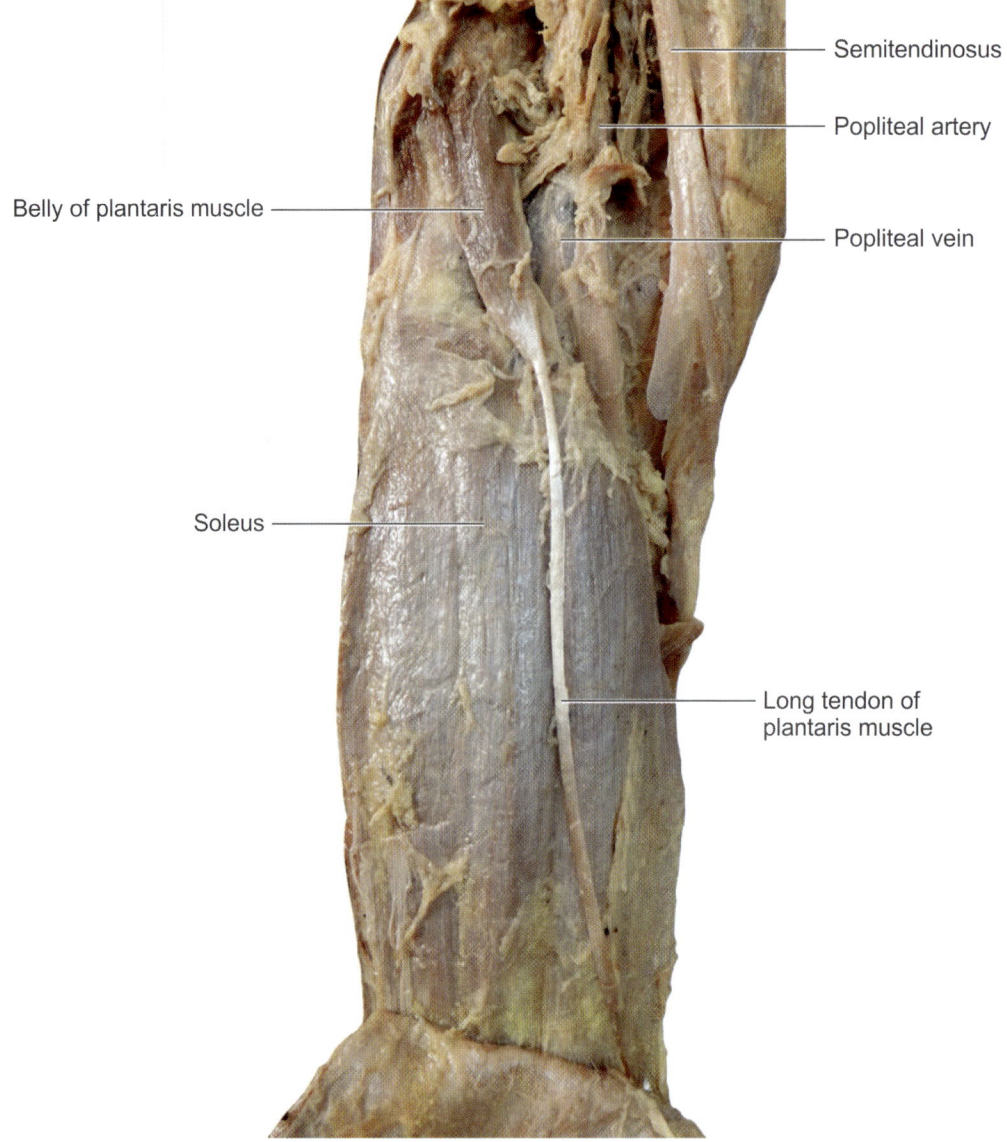

Semitendinosus

Popliteal artery

Belly of plantaris muscle

Popliteal vein

Soleus

Long tendon of
plantaris muscle

Fig. 22.4: Tendon of plantaris seen after removal of the both heads of gastrocnemius muscle

(Fig. 22.5). Look for a number of deep veins which emerge from this muscle.

- Identify popliteus, situated above the soleus muscle.
- Deep to soleus, identify the superficial transverse fascial septum attached to medial border of tibia and posterior intermuscular septa attached to fibula.
- Incise this septum vertically to reach the long flexors of the toes, e.g. flexor hallucis longus laterally and flexor digitorum longus medially.

Competency achievement: The student should be able to:

AN 19.2 Describe and demonstrate the origin, course, relations, branches (or tributaries), termination of important nerves and vessels of back of leg.

- Identify posterior tibial vessels and tibial nerve between these two long muscles (Fig. 22.5).
- Follow the tendons of flexor hallucis longus (Fig. 22.6) and flexor digitorum longus till the flexor retinaculum.

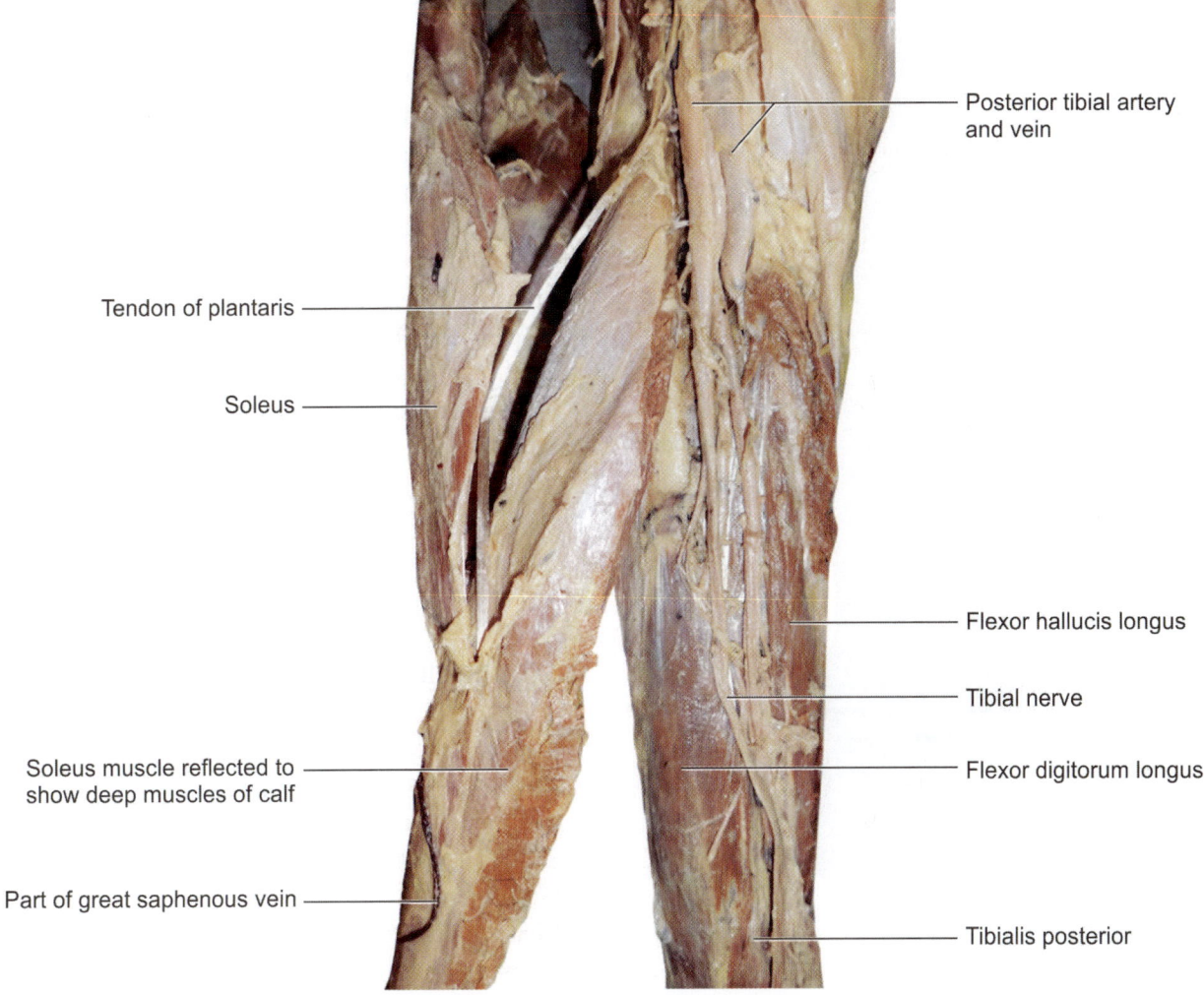

Posterior tibial artery and vein

Tendon of plantaris

Soleus

Flexor hallucis longus

Tibial nerve

Soleus muscle reflected to show deep muscles of calf

Flexor digitorum longus

Part of great saphenous vein

Tibialis posterior

Fig. 22.5: Superficial muscles of calf reflected to show the deep muscles

- Turn the flexor hallucis longus muscle laterally to expose the deep transverse fascial septum. See that this deep septum is attached to medial crest of fibula and vertical ridge on posterior surface of tibia. The deep septum contains peroneal vessels.
- Divide this deep septum to reveal the deepest muscle of calf, tibialis posterior.
- Study the attachment of these four muscles—popliteus, flexor hallucis longus, flexor digitorum longus and tibialis posterior on dried bones and articulated foot. For details see BD Chaurasia's *Human Anatomy.*

- Clean the lowest part of popliteal vessels to trace its two terminal branches—anterior tibial for the anterior compartment and posterior tibial for the posterior compartment of leg.
- Clean the posterior tibial vessels and tibial nerve in the fibrofatty tissue between the two long muscles, i.e. flexor hallucis longus and flexor digitorum longus (Fig. 22.5).
- See the beginning of posterior tibial artery at the lower border of popliteus. Trace it passing deep to tendinous arch of soleus (Fig. 22.5). Then it runs downwards and medially to reach the flexor

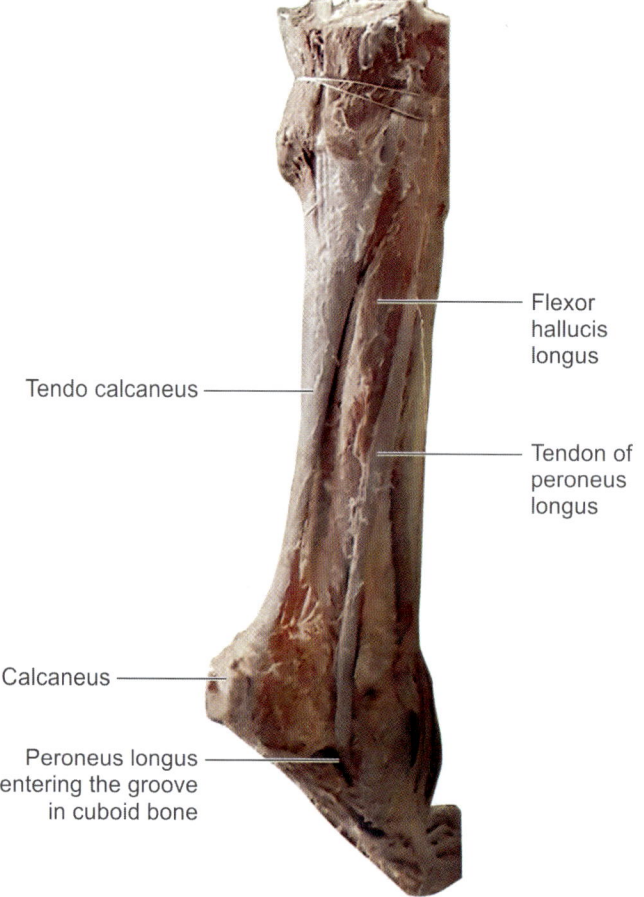

Flexor hallucis longus

Tendo calcaneus

Tendon of peroneus longus

Calcaneus

Peroneus longus entering the groove in cuboid bone

Fig. 22.6: Flexor hallucis longus and peroneus longus along with tendo calcaneous

retinaculum. Under the flexor retinaculum see the artery dividing into its two terminal branches, the medial plantar and lateral plantar arteries.

- Trace the branches of posterior tibial artery:
  1. The largest branch is the peroneal artery lying in the deep transverse fascial septum.

2. Muscular branches to the muscles seen in the region.

3. Nutrient artery to tibia

4. Medial malleolar branch and calcaneal branches

- See the large peroneal artery 2.5 cm below the lower border of popliteus.
- Trace it descending along medial crest of fibula, then behind ankle joint.
- Identify its terminal calcaneal branches.
- Identify the branches of peroneal artery. These are:
  - Muscular to the muscles of posterior and lateral compartments of leg.
  - Nutrient artery to fibula.
  - Lateral malleolar branch.
  - Perforating branch pierces the lower part of interosseous membrane to reach anterior compartment of leg.

POSTERIOR TIBIAL VEIN AND TIBIAL NERVE

- Trace posterior tibial vein formed by union of two plantar veins under flexor retinaculum. It accompanies posterior tibial artery. Identify its tributaries—muscular veins and peroneal vein.
- See posterior tibial vein uniting with anterior tibial vein to form popliteal vein.
- Identify tibial nerve accompanying posterior tibial vessels in whole of its course (Fig. 22.5).
- See it dividing into medial plantar and lateral plantar branches under the flexor retinaculum.
- Trace its branches to tibialis posterior, flexor digitorum longus, flexor hallucis longus, deep part of soleus and medial calcaneal for the skin on medial side of calcaneus.

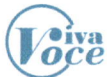

- Name the superficial vein in calf region. Where does it drain?
- Which muscle of calf is called 'peripheral heart' and why?

- Name 'in order' the structures passing under flexor retinaculum of the ankle.
- Name the bone where most of tibialis posterior is inserted. Show its actions.

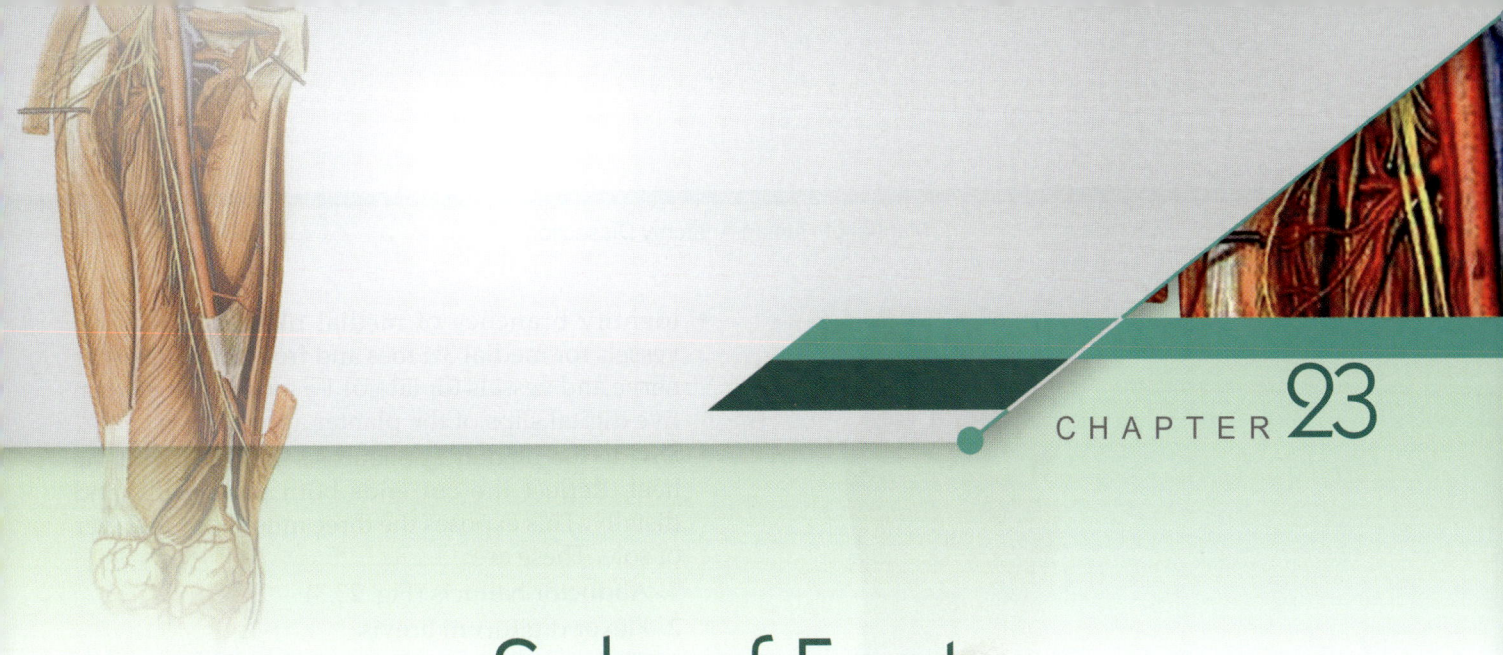

Sole of Foot

Learning Objectives

One should be able to
1. Name the branches of medial plantar nerve.

2. Name the branches of lateral plantar nerve.
3. Describe how plantar arch is formed?

OVERVIEW

Sole of the foot corresponds to the palm of hand. The skin of the sole is thicker than that of the palm. The superficial fascia contains cutaneous nerves and vessels. The deep fascia is modified to form the thick "plantar aponeurosis" in the centre of the sole. The muscle layers are well organised and are seen in four layers.

First layer has three muscles—one each on lateral and medial sides and one in the centre of the sole.

Second layer comprises two long muscles from the calf. Tendons of one of these—the flexor digitorum longus, gives origin to the four lumbrical muscles. This tendon also receives the insertion of flexor digitorum accessories. Thus the second layer in total has seven muscles.

The third layer has three small muscles; one is a flexor each of 1st and 5th toes, and third is adductor of 1st toe.

Fourth layer contains three plantar interossei, attached to 3rd, 4th and 5th metatarsals; four dorsal interossei in between the five metatarsal bones. In addition it also contains tendons of peroneus longus and tibialis posterior muscles.

The nerve supply and blood supply is derived from lateral plantar and medial plantar nerves and blood vessels. Medial plantar nerve innervates *four* intrinsic muscles while the lateral plantar nerve innervates *fourteen* muscles. Muscles of leg which reach the sole are innervated by nerves of respective compartments.

STEPS OF DISSECTION

Skin of the sole usually becomes very hard. To remove it, the incision is given from back of heel through the root to the tip of the middle toe. Reflect the skin and fatty superficial fascia to each side of the sole. Look for cutaneous nerves and vessels (Fig. 23.1).

The cutaneous nerves and vessels are:
1. Medial calcanean
2. Medial plantar
3. Lateral plantar
4. Saphenous along part of medial border
5. Sural along lateral border

- Identify the deep fascia. It is thickened in the central part to form plantar aponeurosis (Fig. 23.2). See that the aponeurosis divides into five slips for all five toes.
- See the fibrous flexor sheaths along the toes.
- Identify cutaneous branches from medial and lateral plantar arteries and nerves along the respective sides of plantar aponeurosis.

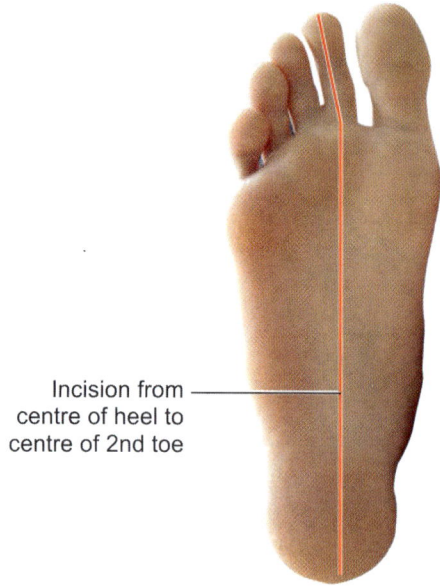

Incision from centre of heel to centre of 2nd toe

Fig. 23.1: Line of incision

- Identify branches of medial plantar nerve and vessels for medial 3½ toes and from lateral plantar nerve and vessels for lateral 1½ toes lying between five digital slips of the plantar aponeurosis.
- Divide the plantar aponeurosis 4 cm distal to the heel. Reflect the cut ends both proximally and distally. This exposes the three muscles of 1st layer of sole. These are:
  1. Abductor hallucis (Fig. 23.3)
  2. Flexor digitorum brevis
  3. Abductor digiti minimi
- See medial plantar nerve and vessels which are easily visualised close to the medial border of sole (Fig. 23.4). Also see stems of lateral plantar nerve and vessels and their superficial division.
- Trace the medial plantar artery from beneath the flexor retinaculum to run along the medial border of sole. See its branches:

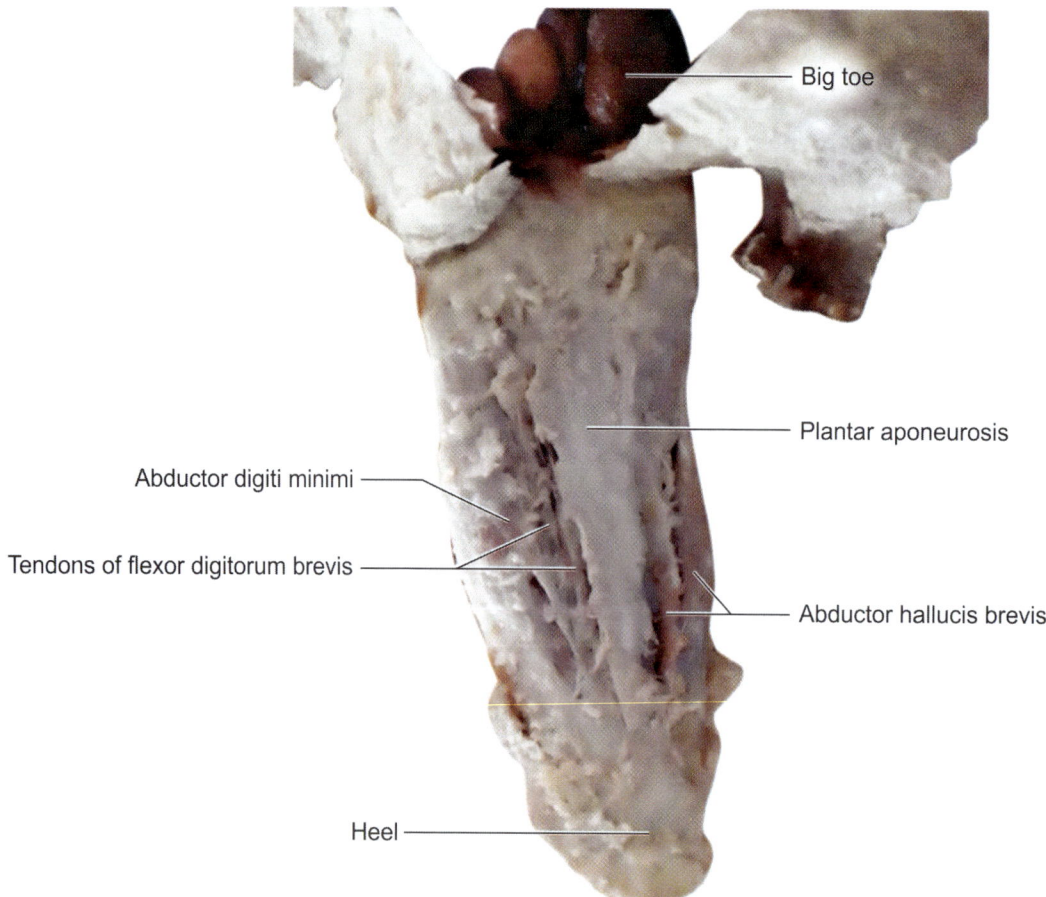

Big toe

Plantar aponeurosis

Abductor digiti minimi

Tendons of flexor digitorum brevis

Abductor hallucis brevis

Heel

Fig. 23.2: Plantar aponeurosis and muscles of 1st layer of sole

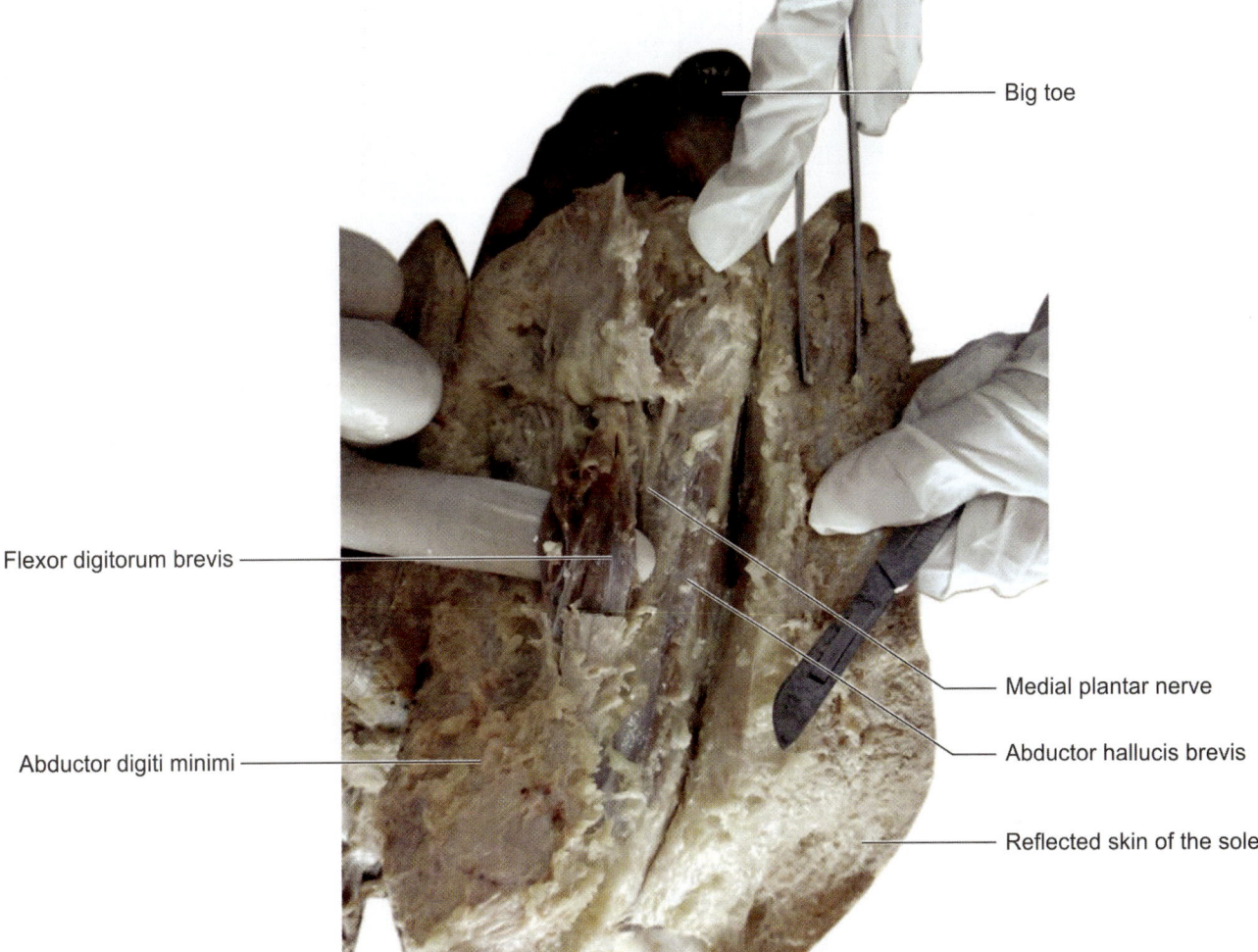

Big toe

Flexor digitorum brevis

Abductor digiti minimi

Medial plantar nerve

Abductor hallucis brevis

Reflected skin of the sole

Fig. 23.3: Muscles of 1st layer of sole

1. Muscular to muscles of 1st and 2nd layers of sole.
2. Cutaneous to skin of medial side of sole
3. Three superficial digital branches which end by joining 1st, 2nd and 3rd plantar metatarsal arteries which are branches of plantar arch.
- Trace medial plantar nerve as a larger branch of tibial nerve. See it running between abductor hallucis and flexor digitorum brevis which it supplies. Trace its branches which are:
  1. 1st lumbrical of second layer
  2. Muscular to two medial muscles of first layer
  3. Flexor hallucis brevis of third layer, i.e. total of four muscles
  4. Cutaneous branches to skin of medial side of sole
  5. Digital branches to medial 3½ toes
  6. Articular branches.

- Identify the lateral plantar artery as the larger branch of posterior tibial artery. See it entering the sole from medial side of sole (Fig. 23.4).
- Follow it between 1st and 2nd layers of sole till the base of 5th metatarsal bone where it gives a small superficial branch and then continues as plantar arch between 3rd and 4th muscular layers of sole.
- Trace its muscular and cutaneous branches. See the superficial branch running along lateral border of sole. It gives digital branches to lateral 1½ toes.
- See the lateral plantar nerve as the smaller terminal branch of tibial nerve. It enters the sole with the lateral plantar artery. See it travelling forwards and laterally till the base of 5th metatarsal, where it divides into superficial and deep branches.

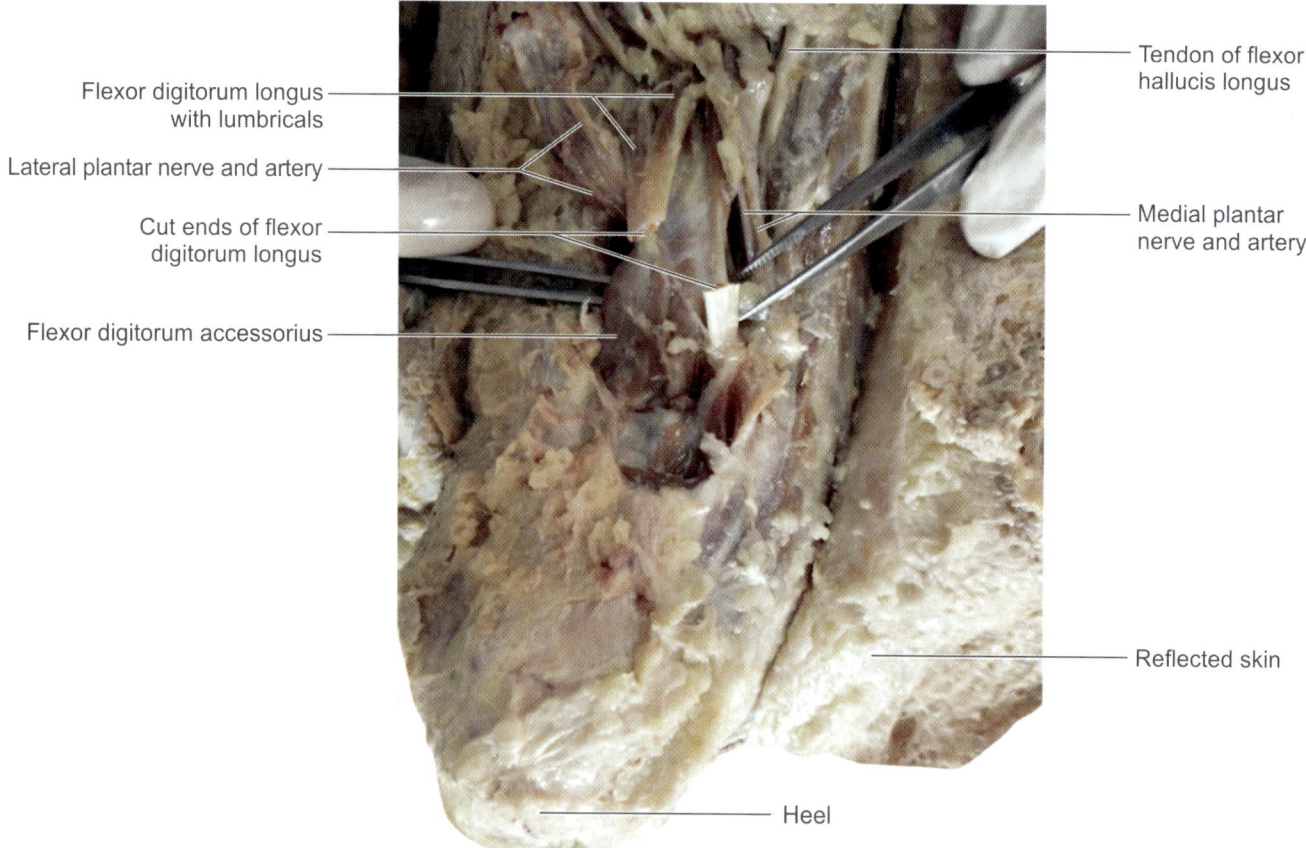

Flexor digitorum longus with lumbricals

Lateral plantar nerve and artery

Cut ends of flexor digitorum longus

Flexor digitorum accessorius

Tendon of flexor hallucis longus

Medial plantar nerve and artery

Reflected skin

Heel

Fig. 23.4: Tendons and muscles of 2nd layer of sole

- Trace the branches from main trunk to:
  - Abductor digiti minimi of 1st layer
  - Flexor digitorum accessorius of 2nd layer
- Trace two branches from superficial division. These are:
  1. Lateral muscular for:
     - Flexor digiti minimi brevis of 3rd layer
     - 3rd plantar and 4th dorsal interossei of 4th layer
     - Skin on lateral side of little toe
  2. Medial branch gives digital branches to adjoining sides of 4th and 5th toes.
     The deep branch will be traced later for muscles and tendons of 3rd and 4th layers
- Identify muscles of 2nd layer, e.g. flexor digitorum longus with four lumbricals and flexor digitorum accessorius inserted in the tendon of flexor digitorum longus (Fig. 23.5). Medially lies the tendon of flexor hallucis longus (Fig. 23.4).

- Identify muscles of 3rd layer. These are:
  1. Flexor hallucis brevis (Fig. 23.6)
  2. Adductor hallucis
  3. Flexor digiti minimi brevis
- Separate flexor hallucis brevis from oblique head of adductor hallucis from their origin and reflect them distally. Look for sesamoid bone at insertion of flexor hallucis brevis.
- Carefully preserve the plantar arch and deep branch of lateral plantar nerve. Reflect the transverse head of adductor hallucis medially. On cutting the deep transverse metatarsal ligament on both sides of 2nd toe, tendons of interossei muscles are recognised.
- Detach the flexor digiti minimi brevis from its origin and reflect it forwards. Now see the laterally situated interossei muscles.
- Identify and examine the main attachment of tendon of tibialis posterior into tuberosity of navicular bone.

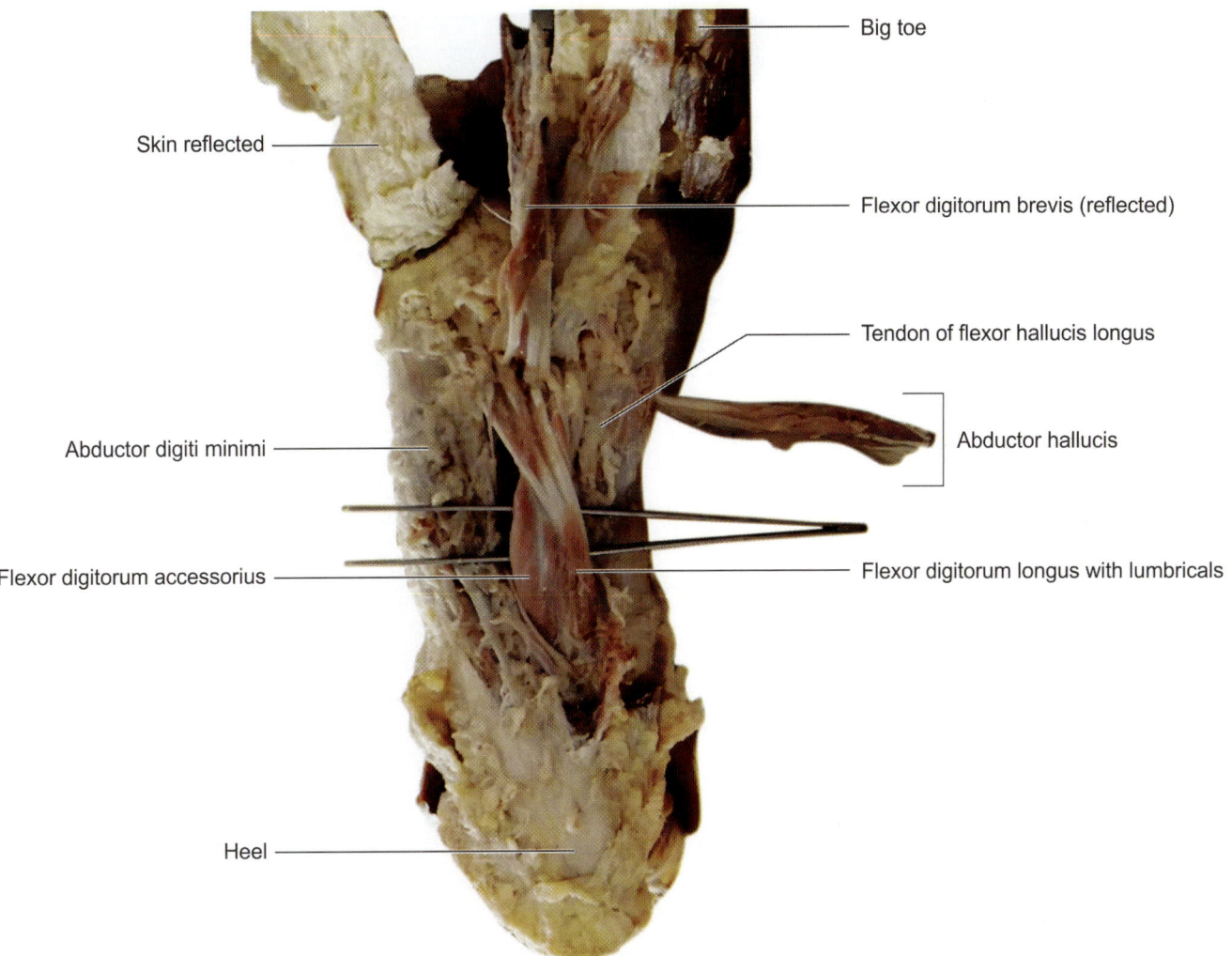

Big toe

Skin reflected

Flexor digitorum brevis (reflected)

Tendon of flexor hallucis longus

Abductor hallucis

Abductor digiti minimi

Flexor digitorum accessorius

Flexor digitorum longus with lumbricals

Heel

Fig. 23.5: Muscles of 2nd layer of sole

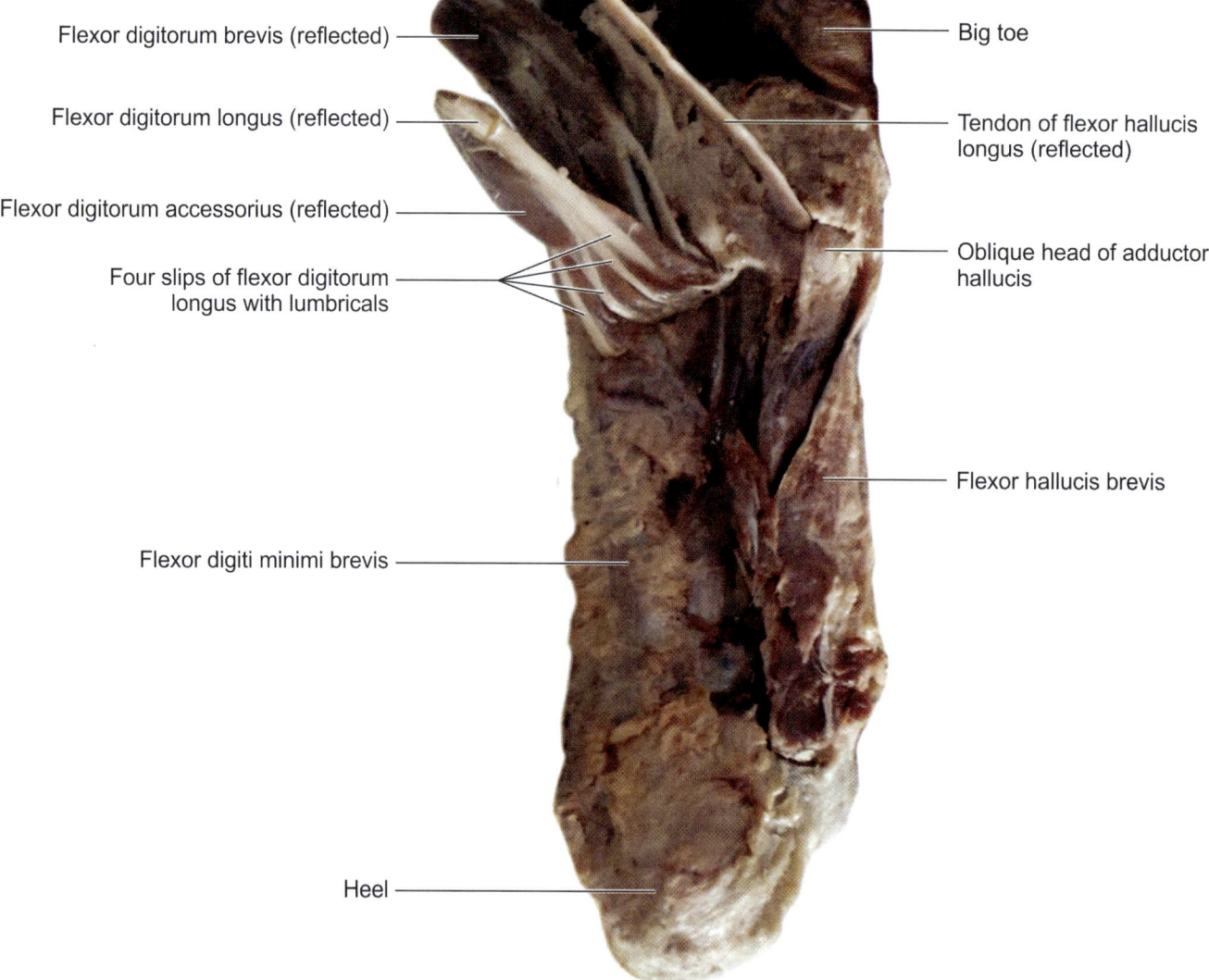

Flexor digitorum brevis (reflected)

Flexor digitorum longus (reflected)

Flexor digitorum accessorius (reflected)

Four slips of flexor digitorum longus with lumbricals

Flexor digiti minimi brevis

Heel

Big toe

Tendon of flexor hallucis longus (reflected)

Oblique head of adductor hallucis

Flexor hallucis brevis

Fig. 23.6: Muscles of 3rd layer of sole

- Trace the course of tendon of peroneus longus through the groove of the cuboid bone, across the sole to its insertions into lateral sides of base of 1st metatarsal and medial cuneiform bone.

- Now detach these muscles of 3rd layer from their origins and reflect towards their insertion. Muscles of the 4th layer will now be visible.

- Between the 3rd and 4th muscular layers is the plantar arch.

- Trace the plantar arch as a continuation of deep branch of lateral plantar artery. See the arch getting completed medially by dorsalis pedis artery which dips down into the sole (Fig. 23.7).

- Trace the four metatarsal arteries which are branches of the plantar arch. The 3 medial metatarsal arteries give two branches each to the adjacent sides of 2nd–5th toes. The fourth metatarsal artery runs along the lateral side of 5th toe.

- Trace the deep branch of lateral plantar nerve in the concavity of the plantar arch. It gives branches to nine muscles:
  - 2nd, 3rd and 4th lumbricals of 2nd layer
  - Adductor hallucis of 3rd layer
  - 1st, 2nd and 3rd dorsal interossei of 4th layer
  - 1st and 2nd plantar interossei of 4th layer.

MUSCLES OF FOURTH LAYER OF SOLE

- Identify three unipennate plantar interossei muscles. Deep to these, identify four bipennate dorsal interossei muscles. These seven muscles are intrinsic muscles of the sole, i.e. their origin and insertions are in the foot and sole only (Fig. 23.7).

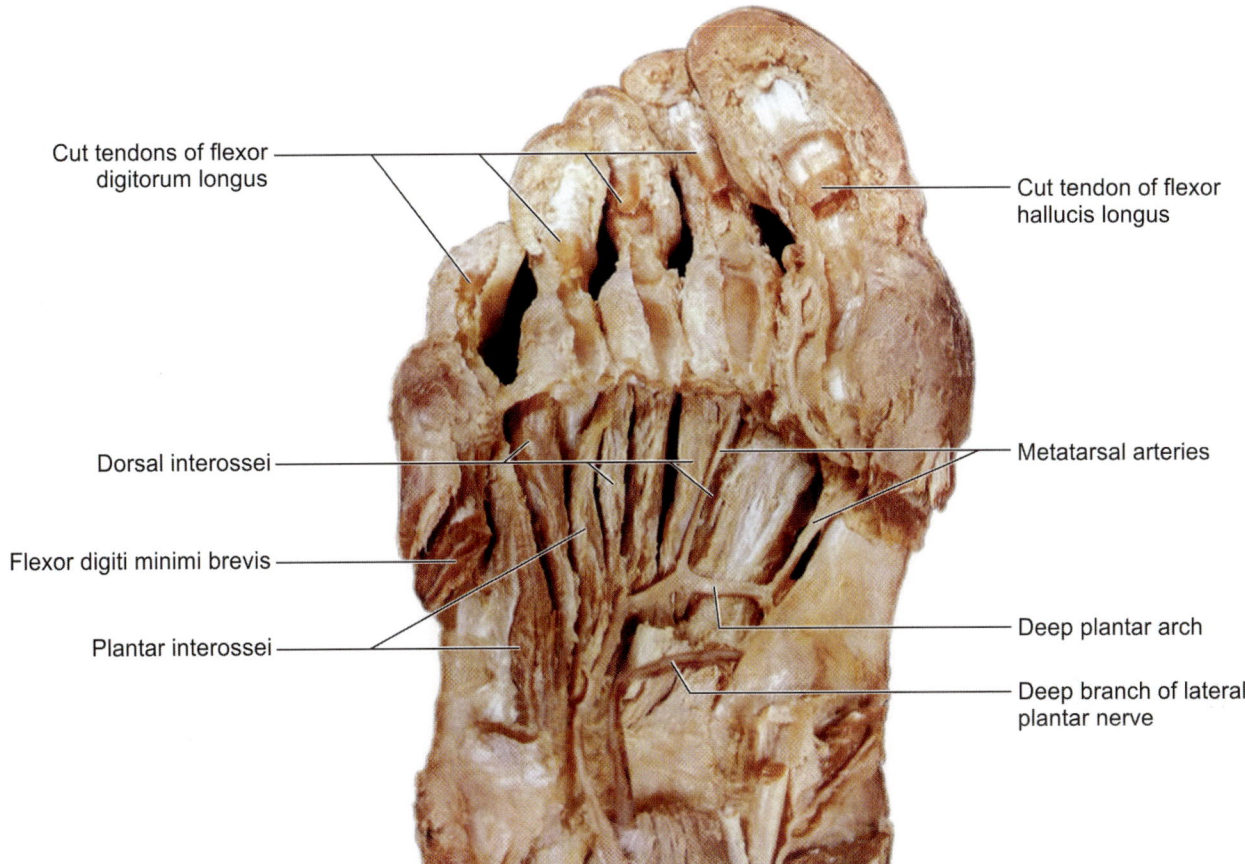

Fig. 23.7: Interossei muscles of 4th layer of sole with plantar arch and deep branch of lateral plantar nerve

- Trace the tendons of tibialis posterior on medial side of foot into tuberosity of navicular and many other bones.

- Follow the tendon of peroneus longus from lateral side across the sole to the medial side. These two muscles are the extrinsic muscles of sole, arriving in the sole from posterior and lateral compartments respectively.

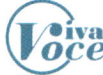

- Name the muscles supplied by medial plantar nerve.
- How many digital branches are given by medial plantar nerve and lateral plantar nerve?
- How is the plantar arch formed?

- Name the muscles and tendons of 2nd layer of sole. What is their nerve supply?
- What is the axis of abduction and adduction of the toes?
- Where is the main insertion of tibialis posterior muscle?

CHAPTER 24

Veins of Lower Limb

Learning Objectives

One should be able to
1. Mark the dorsal venous arch
2. Mark the course of great saphenous vein in relation to medial malleolus and medial surface of lower third of tibia
3. Trace the course of short saphenous vein in relation to lateral malleolus. Which nerve accompanies this vein?

Dorsal venous arch/plexus lies on the dorsum of foot. It is formed by 4 dorsal metatarsal veins, each of which is formed by the union of 2 dorsal digital veins.

GREAT/LONG SAPHENOUS VEIN

Great/long saphenous vein is formed by the union of medial end of dorsal venous arch and medial marginal vein from the medial side of the big toe (Fig. 24.1). It runs upwards *anterior* to medial malleolus, crosses obliquely the lower 1/3rd of medial surface of tibia to reach the medial border of tibia and back of knee joint. This vein is accompanied by saphenous nerve, branch of femoral nerve. From back of knee, it courses upwards and forwards in the front of thigh to reach the saphenous opening (below and lateral to pubic tubercle) where it pierces cribriform fascia to drain into the femoral vein. It receives tributaries from the front of leg and thigh.

Before its termination it receives three superficial veins, namely superficial external pudendal, superficial epigastric and superficial circumflex iliac (Fig. 24.2).

There are 10–15 valves which divide the long column of blood into short columns relieving the pressure on the distal part of the vein.

SMALL/SHORT SAPHENOUS VEIN

Small saphenous vein is formed on the lateral side of dorsum of foot by union of lateral end of dorsal venous plexus with the lateral marginal vein. The latter vein drains the lateral side of the little toe. The vein runs up by passing *behind* the lateral malleolus of fibula. Then it ascends lateral to tendocalcaneous to the midline of the calf and the lower part of popliteal fossa. In the popliteal fossa (Fig. 24.3), the vein pierces deep fascia to drain into the popliteal vein. This vein is accompanied by sural nerve.

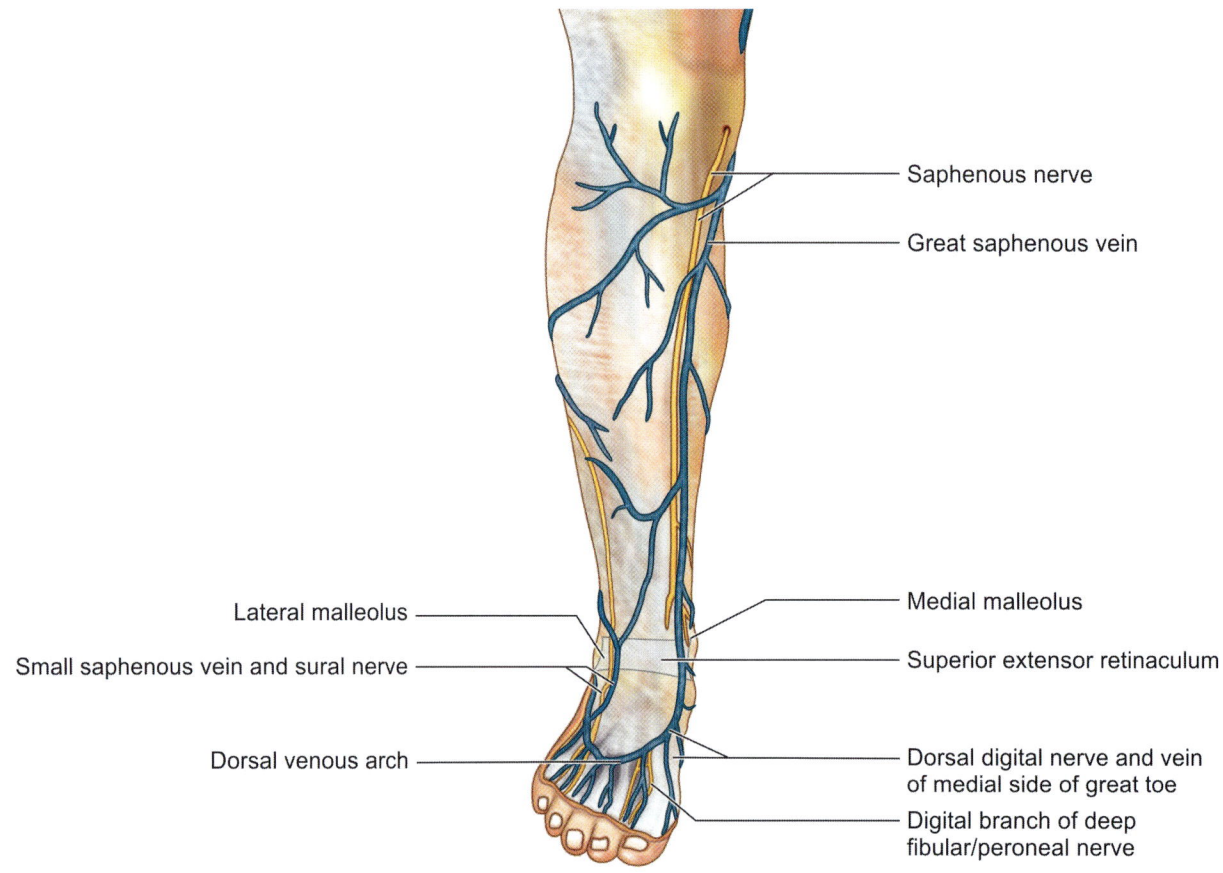

Fig. 24.1: Superficial veins with cutaneous nerves

Saphenous nerve

Great saphenous vein

Medial malleolus

Superior extensor retinaculum

Lateral malleolus

Small saphenous vein and sural nerve

Dorsal venous arch

Dorsal digital nerve and vein of medial side of great toe

Digital branch of deep fibular/peroneal nerve

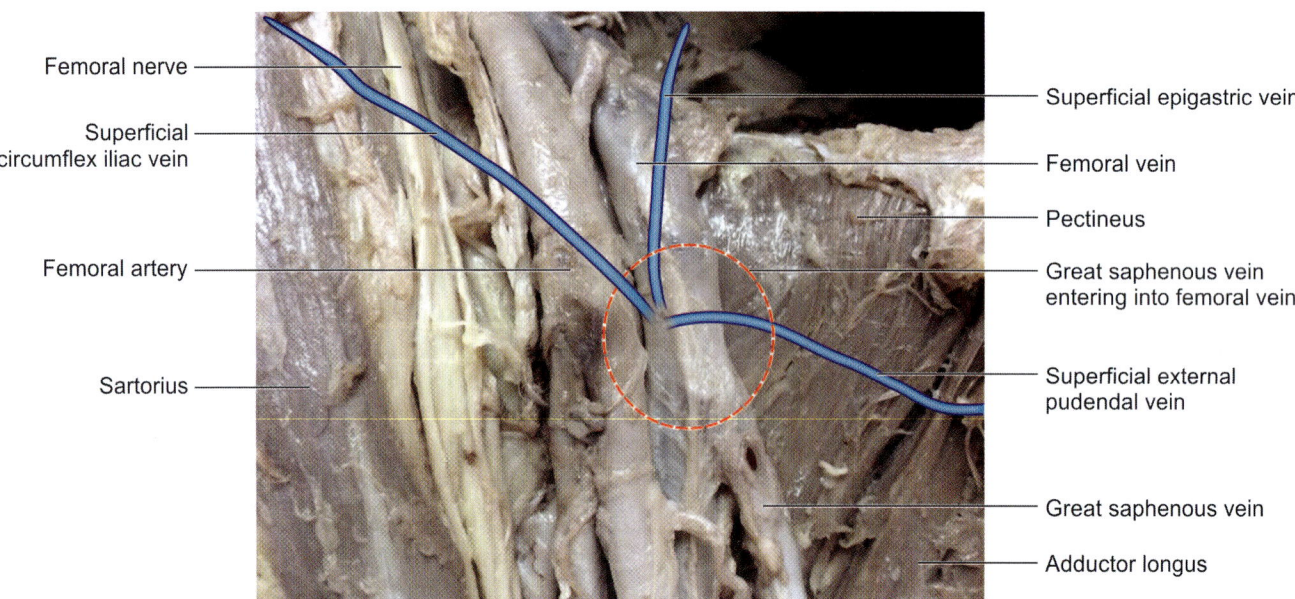

Fig. 24.2: Tributaries of great saphenous vein

Femoral nerve

Superficial circumflex iliac vein

Femoral artery

Sartorius

Superficial epigastric vein

Femoral vein

Pectineus

Great saphenous vein entering into femoral vein

Superficial external pudendal vein

Great saphenous vein

Adductor longus

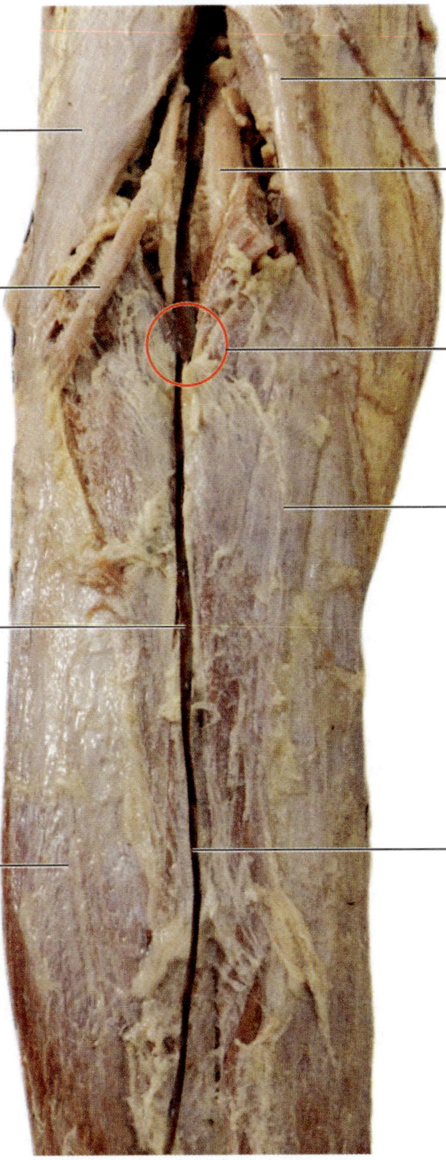

Biceps femoris

Common peroneal nerve

Short saphneous vein between
two heads of gastrocnemius muscle

Lateral head of gastrocnemius

Semitendinosus

Tibial nerve

Short saphenous vein
draining into popliteal
vein

Medial head of
gastrocnemius

Short saphenous vein

Fig. 24.3: Course of short saphenous vein

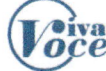

Viva Voce

- What is the relation of great saphenous vein (GSV) to medial malleolus?
- What nerve accompanies GSV? What is its clinical importance?

- Why are varicose veins common in lower limb?
- What are indirect perforators?
- What area drains into lower vertical group of superficial inguinal lymph nodes?
- What is lymph shed area of back of thigh?

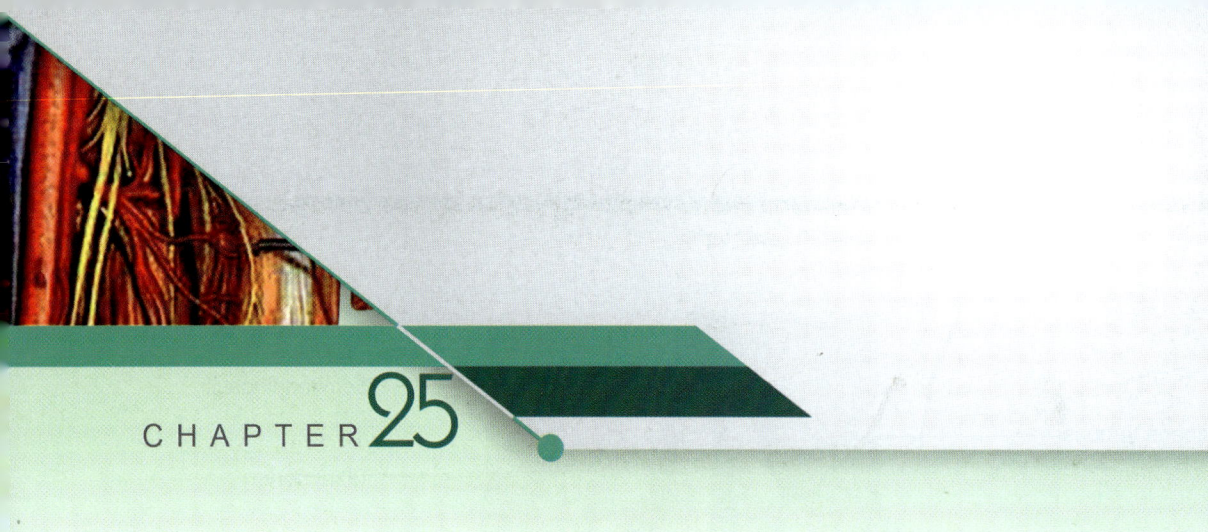
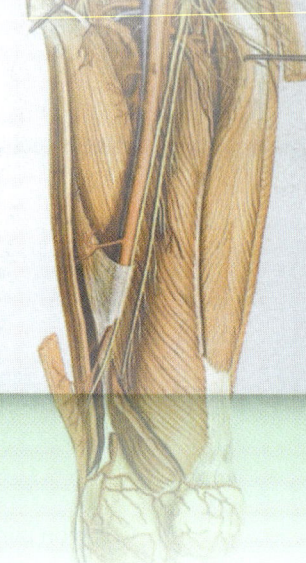

CHAPTER 25

Bones and Joints of Lower Limb

Learning Objectives

One should be able to

1. Show movements of hip joint. Name the muscles responsible for the movements with their nerve supply.

2. Name the bursae around knee joint.

3. Show the insertions of the muscles causing inversion and eversion of the foot.

Keep a set of bones of lower limb while dissecting the joints of lower limb.

OVERVIEW

Bones and joints of the lower limb are stronger as they are weight transmitting joints.

Stable hip joint corresponds to the highly mobile shoulder joint. The range of movements is limited as compared to shoulder joint.

The ligaments especially iliofemoral ligament is very strong. The joint is related anteriorly to femoral vessels and posteriorly to sciatic nerve and gluteus maximus.

The movements permitted are flexion and extension; abduction and adduction; medial and lateral rotation and circumduction.

Knee joint is the most complicated joint in the body. It has 12–13 bursae around it to provide smooth movements. The cavity of the joint is divided into upper and lower joint cavities by the medial and lateral menisci, permitting different movements in each of the two cavities. Besides lower end of femur and upper end of tibia, the patella also takes part in this joint. This joint gets locked during end stage of extension. Popliteus on the back of the joint unlocks the knee joint before hamstring muscles take up the job of flexing the knee joint.

Tibiofibular joints are three in number: Superior, middle and inferior.

Superior/upper end of fibula articulates with tibia, not with femur. So fibula does not take part in the formation of knee joint and thus it remains thin and delicate. This joint is plane variety of synovial joint.

Middle tibiofibular joint is formed by interosseous membrane keeping the bones together and increases the surface area for attachment of muscles.

Inferior tibiofibular joint is a strong joint of syndesmosis type, united by ligaments only.

Lower end of fibula takes part in the formation of ankle joint.

Ankle joint is formed by the lower ends of tibia and fibula articulating with the talus. It permits movements of dorsiflexion and plantar flexion only.

Joints of the foot: There are six joint cavities amongst the seven tarsal and bases of five metatarsal bones. These are:

1. Subtalar joint

2. Talocalcaneonavicular joint

3. Calcaneocuboid joint

4. Cuneometatarsal joint
5. Talonavicular with extensions
6. Cubometatarsal joint

The joints in the forepart of the foot are metatarsophalangeal, proximal and distal interphalangeal joints.

The lower limb comprises hip bone, femur, patella, tibia, fibula, seven tarsal bones, five metatarsals and fourteen phalanges.

HIP JOINT

See the bones taking part in the formation of hip joint on a skeleton. These are all three elements of the hip bone, i.e. ilium, ischium and pubis proximally (Fig. 25.1a and b) and upper end of femur distally (Fig. 25.2a and b).

Competency achievement: The student should be able to:

AN 17.1 Describe and demonstrate the type, articular surfaces, capsule, synovial membrane, ligaments, relations, movements and muscles involved, blood and nerve supply, bursae around the hip joint.

Steps of Dissection

- Identify head of femur with a pit for the round ligament of head of femur, narrow neck of femur, intertrochanteric line anteriorly and intertrochanteric crest posteriorly (Fig. 25.3).
- Identify muscles close to the hip joint. These are sartorius, rectus femoris and pectineus. Remove these muscles. Identify iliopsoas attached to lesser trochanter of femur. Incise the muscle close to lesser trochanter and reflect it upwards (Fig. 25.4).
- Now the ligaments of the hip joint are visible. Anteriorly a big ligament is seen. Identify the 'inverted Y" shaped iliofemoral ligament attached to anterior inferior iliac spine proximally and to intertrochanteric line distally. The upper oblique and lower vertical bands form strong bands, while middle fibres are weak.
- Cut the iliofemoral ligament. Open the capsule of the joint from the anterior aspect. See the articular cartilage on head of femur.
- Abduct the femur and rotate it laterally to identify the ligament of head of femur. Note the obturator

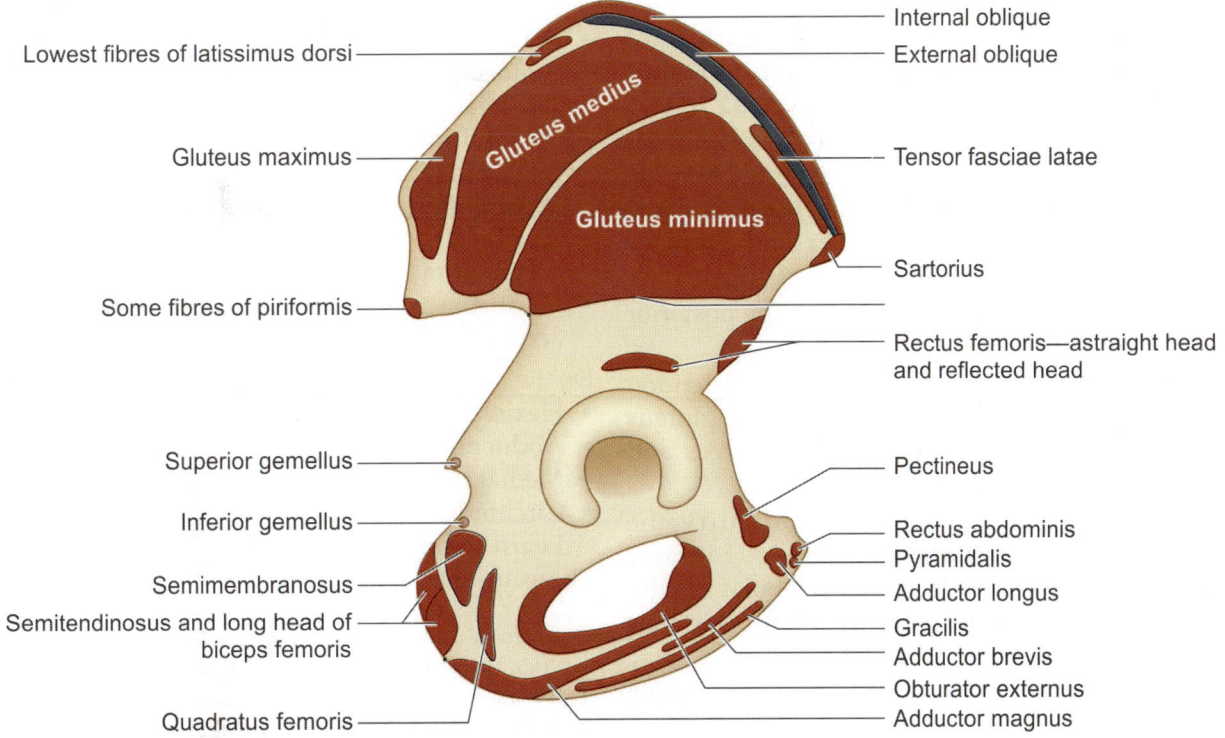

Fig. 25.1a: Attachments on the outer surface of the right hip bone

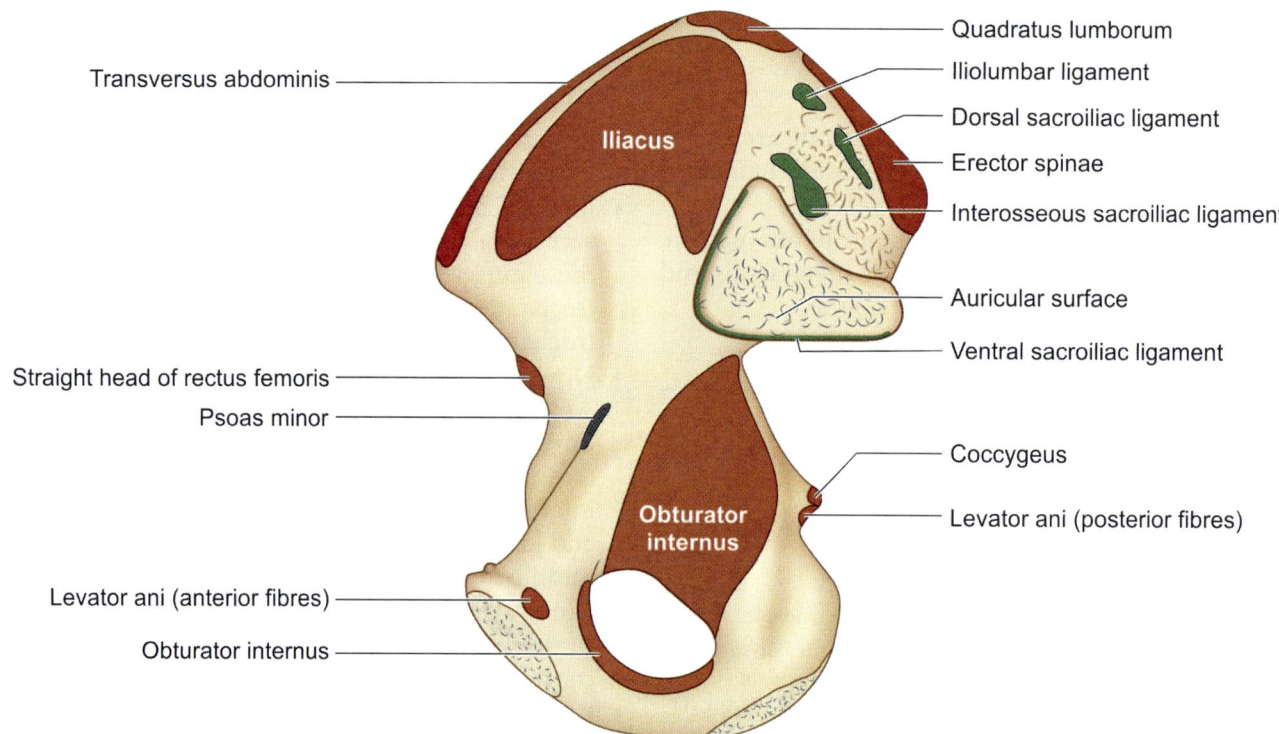

Fig. 25.1b: Attachments on the inner surface of the right hip bone

externus situated between external surface of obturator membrane and trochanteric fossa of greater trochanter of femur.

- Cut the muscle from both the ends and remove it (Fig. 25.4). Now identify the exposed pubofemoral ligament attached to iliopubic eminence proximally and fusing with the lower vertical band of iliofemoral ligament distally.
- Put the limb in prone position to see the posterior relations of hip joint.
- Posteriorly there is piriformis, two gemelli, tendon of obturator internus, quadratus femoris, gluteus minimus and medius muscles with nerves and blood vessels (*see* Fig. 18.5).
- Remove all these structures to identify the posterior part of the joint capsule. Identify ischiofemoral ligament from the acetabular margin to neck of femur. It does not reach intertrochanteric crest.
- Now incise the posterior part of the joint capsule of hip joint.
- Turn the limb in supine position.

- Put a probe under the round ligament of femur and cut the ligament. Rotate the femur laterally and take the head of femur out of from the socket of acetabulum. See the upper end of femur including its articular cartilage (Fig. 25.3). Identify the artery accompanying the ligament of head of femur. Appreciate the articular lunate surface of the acetabulum.
- Clean the transverse acetabular ligament lying across the acetabular notch.

Do the movements of hip joint on yourself. These are:
- Flexion, extension
- Abduction, adduction
- Medial rotation, lateral rotation
- Circumduction

Learn the muscles performing these movements. These are shown in Table 25.1.

Competency achievement: The student should be able to:

AN 18.4 Describe and demonstrate the type, articular surfaces, capsule, synovial membrane, ligaments, relations, movements and muscles involved, blood and nerve supply, bursae around the knee joint.

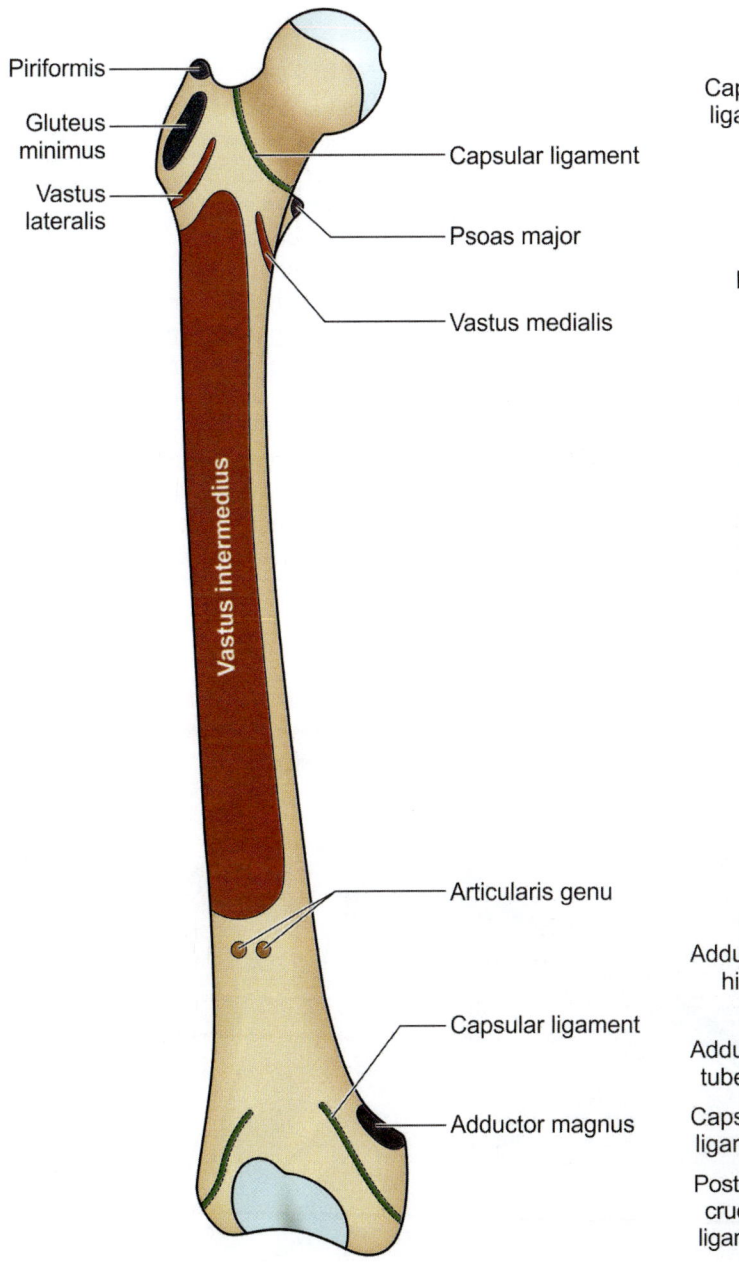

Fig. 25.2a: Attachments on the anterior aspect of the right femur

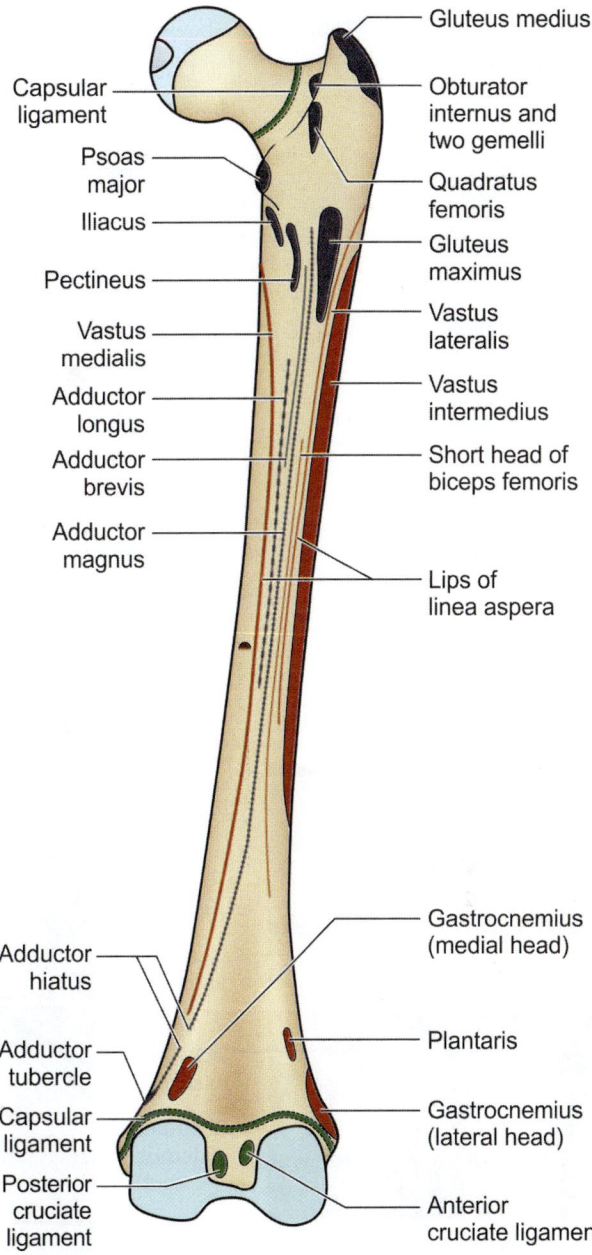

Fig. 25.2b: Attachments on the posterior aspect of the right femur

KNEE JOINT

- Study the bones taking part in knee joint. These are lower end of femur (Fig. 25.2a and b), upper end of tibia (Fig. 25.5a to c) and patella (Fig. 25.6a and b).
- Identify the medial and lateral condyles of femur (Fig. 25.7). On the medial surface of medial condyle feel the prominent medial epicondyle. See the adductor tubercle a little above this epicondyle.
- On the lateral surface of lateral condyle see the prominent lateral epicondyle.
- See the intercondylar notch with impressions for attachments of anterior and posterior cruciate ligaments (Fig. 25.7).

Table 25.1: Showing movements at hip joint with their muscles and nerves

Movement	Chief muscles	Nerve supply
Flexion	Psoas major	Ventral rami of L2 and L3
	Iliacus	Femoral nerve
Extension	Gluteus maximus	Inferior gluteal nerve
	Hamstrings	Sciatic nerve
Adduction	Adductor longus	Obturator nerve
	Adductor part of adductor magnus	Obturator nerve
Abduction	Gluteus medius and minimus	Superior gluteal nerve
Medial rotation	Tensor fascia latae	Superior gluteal nerve
	Anterior fibres of gluteus medius	Superior gluteal nerve
	and minimus	Superior gluteal nerve
Lateral rotation	Obturator externus	Obturator nerve
	Obturator internus	Nerve to obturator internus
	Superior gemellus	Nerve to obturator internus
	Inferior gemellus	Nerve to quadratus femoris
	Quadratus femoris	Nerve to quadratus femoris

Circumduction: A movement involving above movements in a sequence.

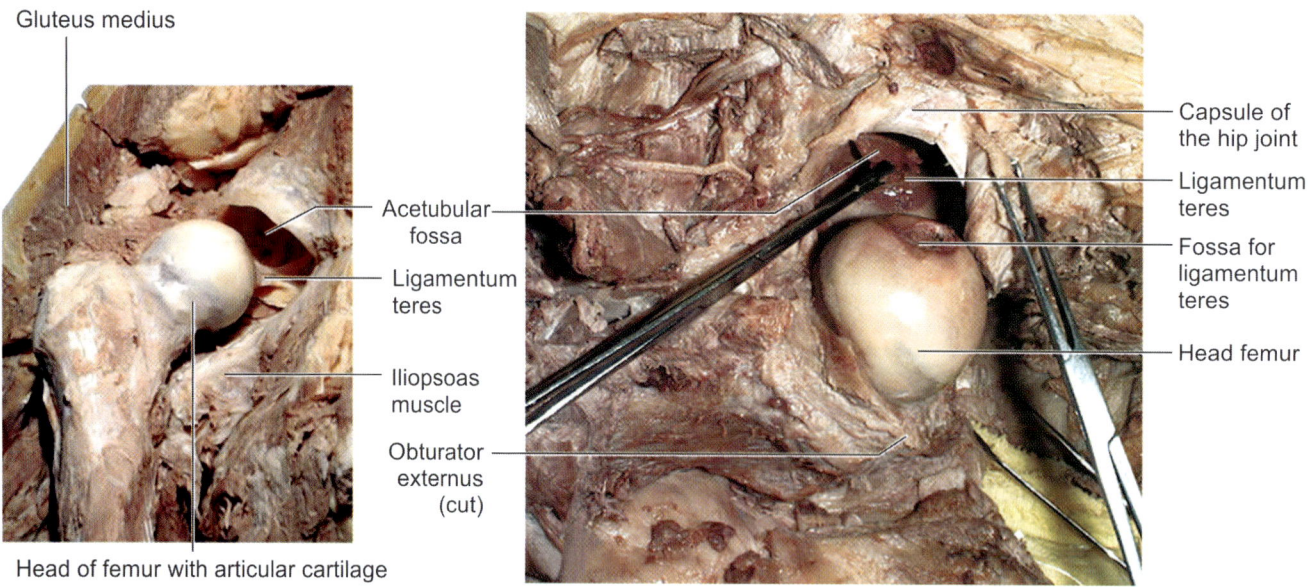

Fig. 25.3: Dissection of hip joint

Fig. 25.4: Dissection of hip joint

- Identify the upper surface of the medial and lateral condyles of tibia with intercondylar eminence (Fig. 25.5c).
- See the prominent tibial tuberosity on the anterior aspect close to upper end of tibia. It comprises an upper smooth part for the attachment of ligamentum patellae and a lower rough part for a bursa.

- Patella shows a rough anterior surface and a posterior articular surface (Figs 25.6 and 25.7).
- Recollect the structures attached to upper surface of tibia from before backwards (Fig. 25.5c). These are:
  - Anterior horn of medial meniscus
  - Anterior cruciate ligament
  - Anterior horn of lateral meniscus

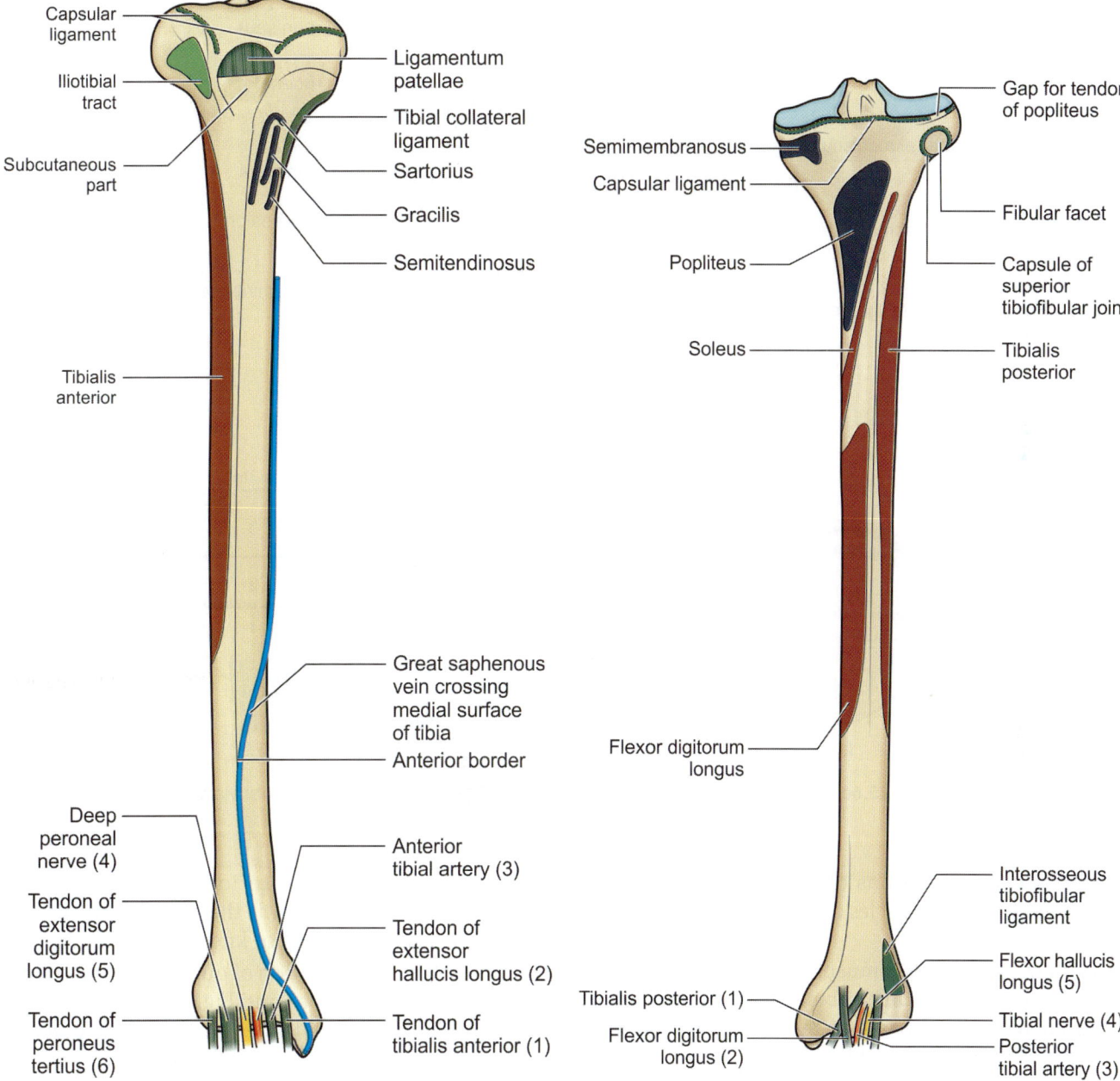

Fig. 25.5a: Attachments and relations on the anterior aspect of the right tibia

Fig. 25.5b: Attachments and relations on the posterior aspect of the right tibia

- Posterior horn of lateral meniscus
- Posterior horn of medial meniscus
- Posterior cruciate ligament
- Identify the tendon of biceps femoris on the lateral side of knee joint.
- Incise the tendon of biceps femoris close to its insertion on fibula. Reflect the tendon upwards

and identify fibular collateral ligament which is not attached to lateral meniscus (Fig. 25.7b). Trace the tendon of popliteus muscle deep to the ligament.

- Deep to the tendon of popliteus lies the fibrous joint capsule. Thus popliteus lies between the capsule and fibular collateral ligament.

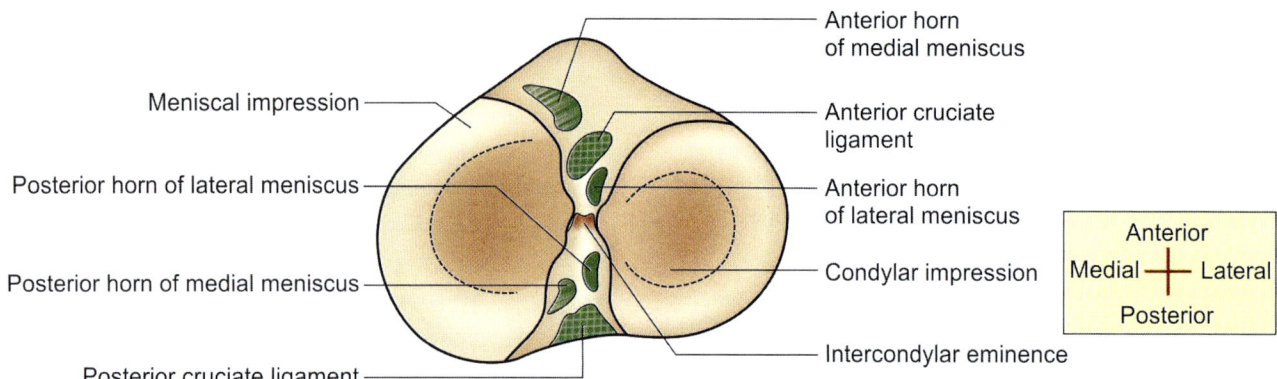

Fig. 25.5c: Superior veiw of the upper end of the right tibia

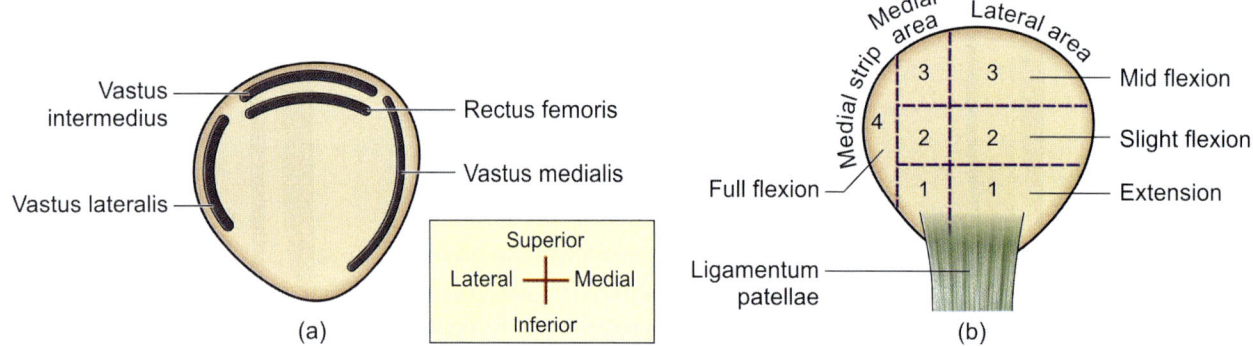

Fig. 25.6a and b: Features of the right patella: (a) Anterior view; (b) Posterior view

- Identify the insertions of sartorius, gracilis and semitendinosus muscles on the medial side of knee joint (*see* Fig. 21.9).
- Reflect these three muscles and identify tibial collateral ligament. The tibial collateral ligament is fused with the capsule of the joint and also with the medial meniscus of knee joint.
- Now put the limb in prone position. Remove the popliteal vessels, tibial and common peroneal nerves.
- Detach semimembranosus muscle
- See the oblique popliteal ligament supplementing the posterior surface of capsule of knee joint.
- Incise and reflect the attachment of plantaris, medial and lateral heads of gastrocnemius muscles.
- Now remove the popliteus muscle from both its attachments. Identify the posterior cruciate

ligament as well as anterior cruciate ligament (Fig. 25.7a). These lie inside the capsule but outside the synovial membrane of knee joint.
- Identify the strong tendon of quadriceps muscle on anterior aspect of knee joint (Fig. 25.8). On each side of the tendon notice the medial and lateral patellar retinacula.
- Give the transverse incision through the quadriceps femoris muscle above the patella. Extend it both on lateral and medial sides till the medial and lateral collateral ligaments of knee joint.
- Reflect the patella with the ligamentum patellae upwards. As the patella is reflected upwards note the huge infrapatellar synovial fold and pad of fat in it (Fig. 25.8).
- Remove the fat and posterior part of fibrous capsule to see the cruciate ligaments and the menisci.

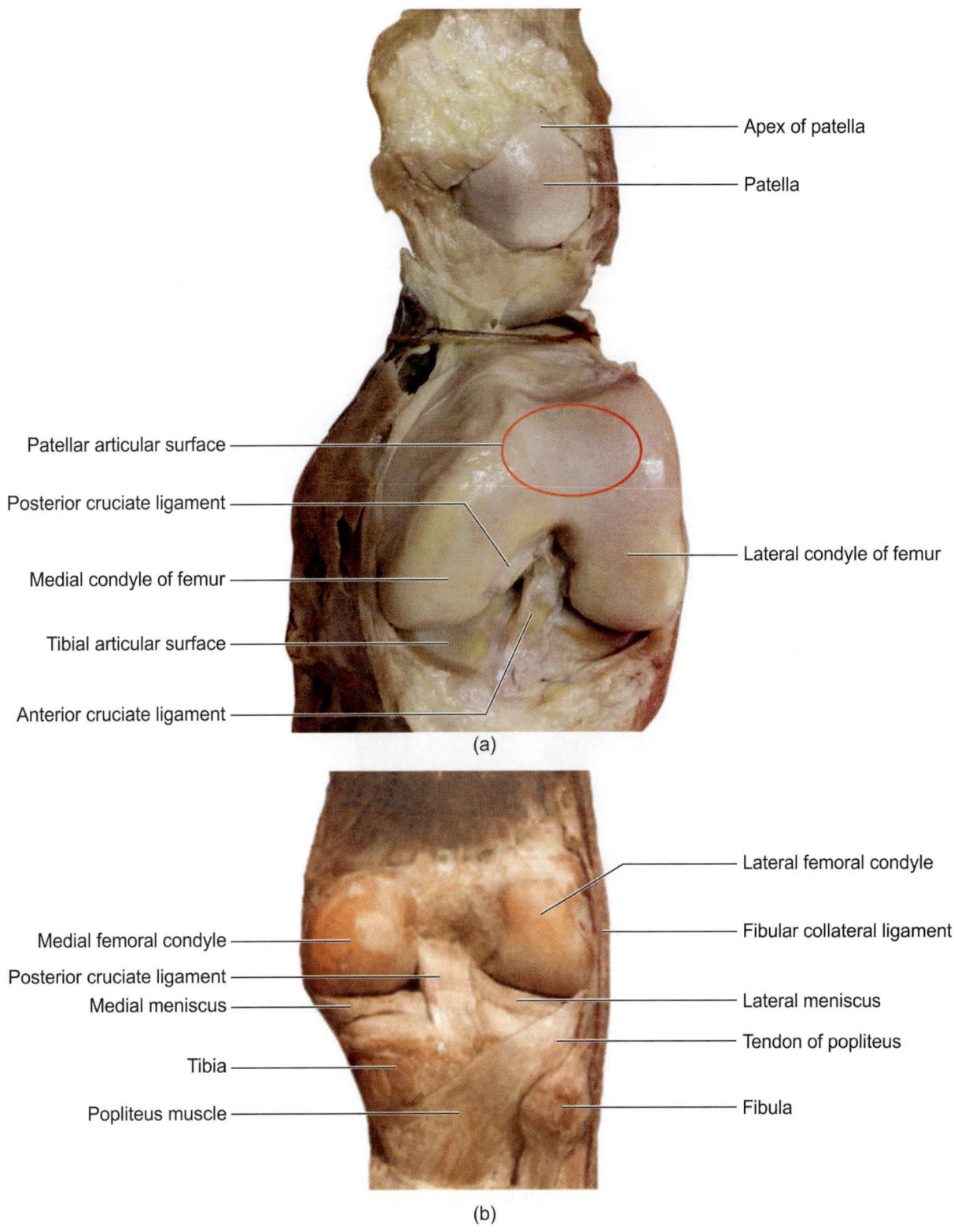

Apex of patella

Patella

Patellar articular surface

Posterior cruciate ligament

Medial condyle of femur

Tibial articular surface

Anterior cruciate ligament

Lateral condyle of femur

(a)

Lateral femoral condyle

Medial femoral condyle

Fibular collateral ligament

Posterior cruciate ligament

Medial meniscus

Lateral meniscus

Tibia

Tendon of popliteus

Popliteus muscle

Fibula

(b)

Fig. 25.7: Knee joint: (a) Anterior aspect; (b) Posterior aspect

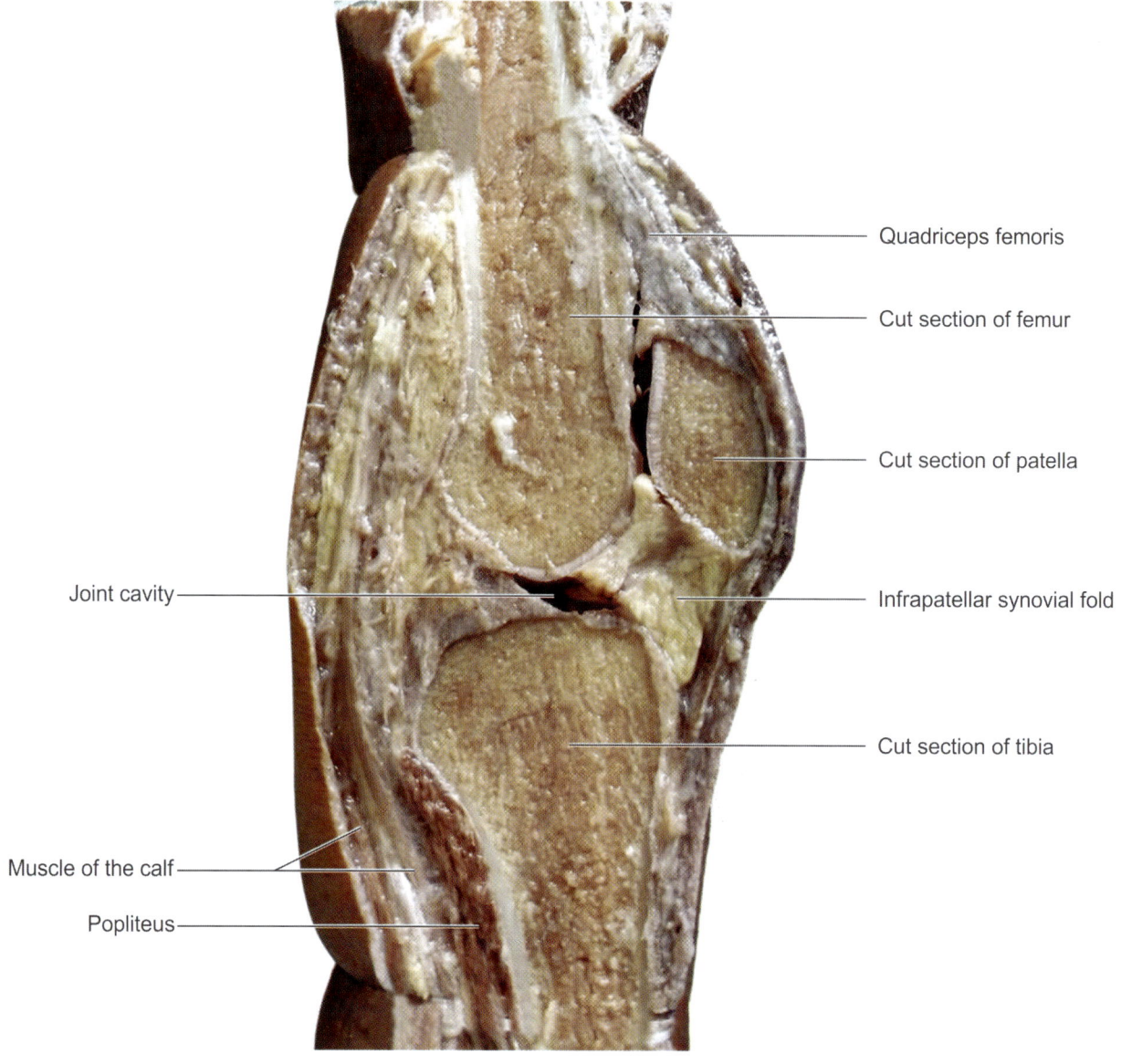

Quadriceps femoris

Cut section of femur

Cut section of patella

Joint cavity

Infrapatellar synovial fold

Cut section of tibia

Muscle of the calf

Popliteus

Fig. 25.8: Sagittal section through knee joint

- Identify the anterior and posterior cruciate ligaments (Fig. 25.7a and b). See that these form an important bond of union between femur and tibia.
- See that the menisci are medial and lateral. The medial meniscus is "C shaped" and the lateral is "O" shaped. Notice the attachment of medial meniscus to tibial collateral ligament.

Analyse the movements of knee joint on the femur, tibia and patella. Try all these movements on your body. These are shown in Table 25.2.

TIBIOFIBULAR JOINTS

These joints are seen between tibia and fibula (Fig. 25.9a and b).

Competency achievement: The student should be able to:

AN 20.1 Describe and demonstrate the type, articular surfaces, capsule, synovial membrane, ligaments, relations, movements and muscles involved, blood and nerve supply of tibiofibular and ankle joint.

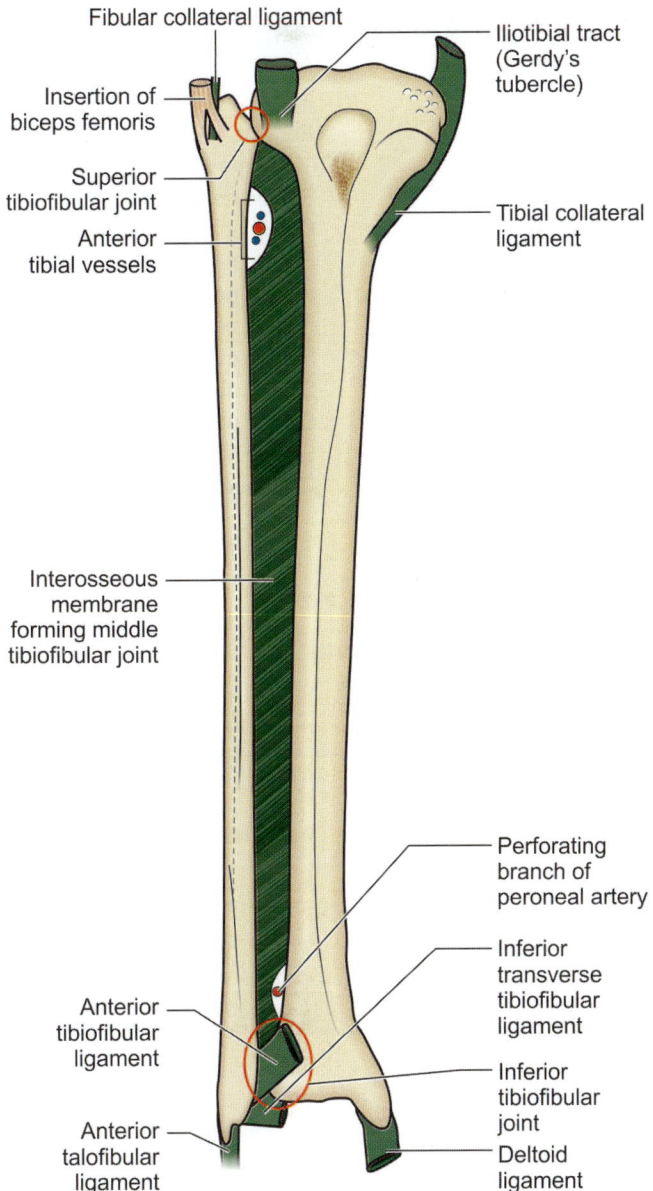

Fig. 25.9a: Anterior view of right tibia and fibula including the ligaments to form inferior tibiofibular joint

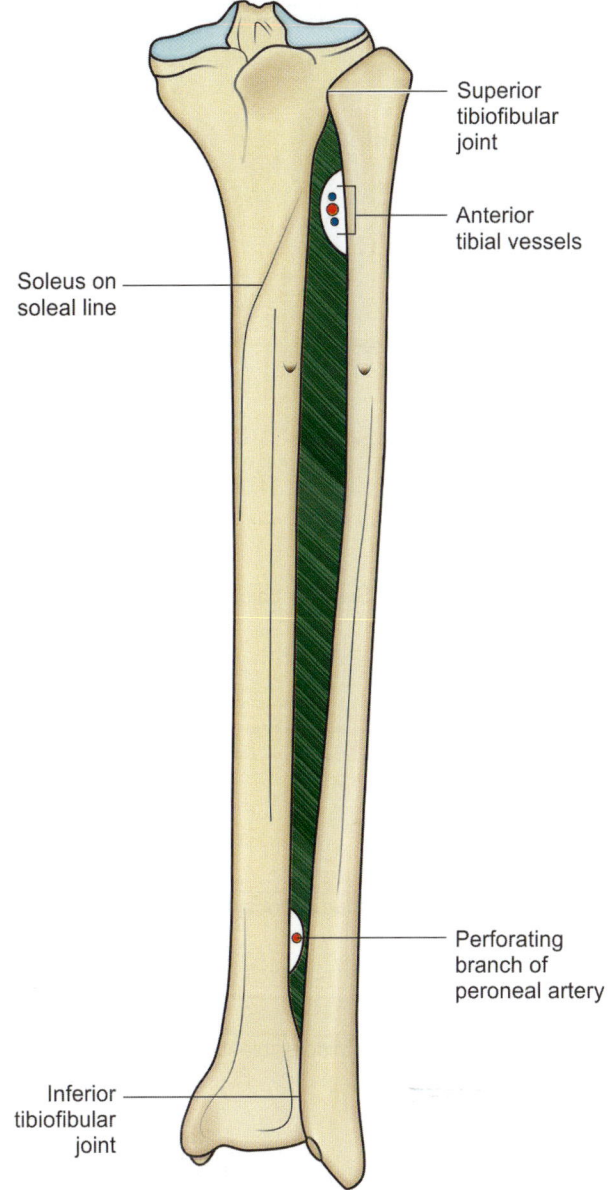

Fig. 25.9b: Posterior view of right tibia and fibula

Superior Tibiofibular Joint

- Remove the muscles around the superior tibio-fibular joint (Fig. 25.10). Define the tendon of popliteus muscle on its posterior surface.
- Open the joint.

Middle Tibiofibular Joint

- Remove the muscles from anterior and posterior surfaces of the interosseous membrane. This membrane forms the middle tibiofibular joint (Fig. 25.10).

- Identify the opening in upper part of membrane for anterior tibial vessels and in lower part for perforating branch of peroneal artery.

Inferior Tibiofibular Joint

- Define the attachments of anterior tibiofibular, posterior tibiofibular and inferior transverse tibiofibular ligaments.

Table 25.2: Showing movements at knee joint with their muscles and nerves

Movement	Principal muscles	Nerve supply
Extension	Quadriceps femoris	Femoral nerve
Locking	Vastus medialis	Femoral nerve
Unlocking	Popliteus	Tibial nerve
Flexion	Long head of biceps femoris	Sciatic nerve
	Short head of biceps femoris	Common peroneal nerve
	Semitendinosus	Sciatic nerve
	Semimembranosus	Sciatic nerve
	Ischial part of adductor magnus	Sciatic nerve
Medial rotation of flexed knee	Popliteus	Tibial nerve
	Semimembranosus	Sciatic nerve
	Semitendinosus	Sciatic nerve
Lateral rotation of flexed knee	Long head of biceps femoris	Sciatic nerve
	Short head of biceps femoris	Common peroneal nerve

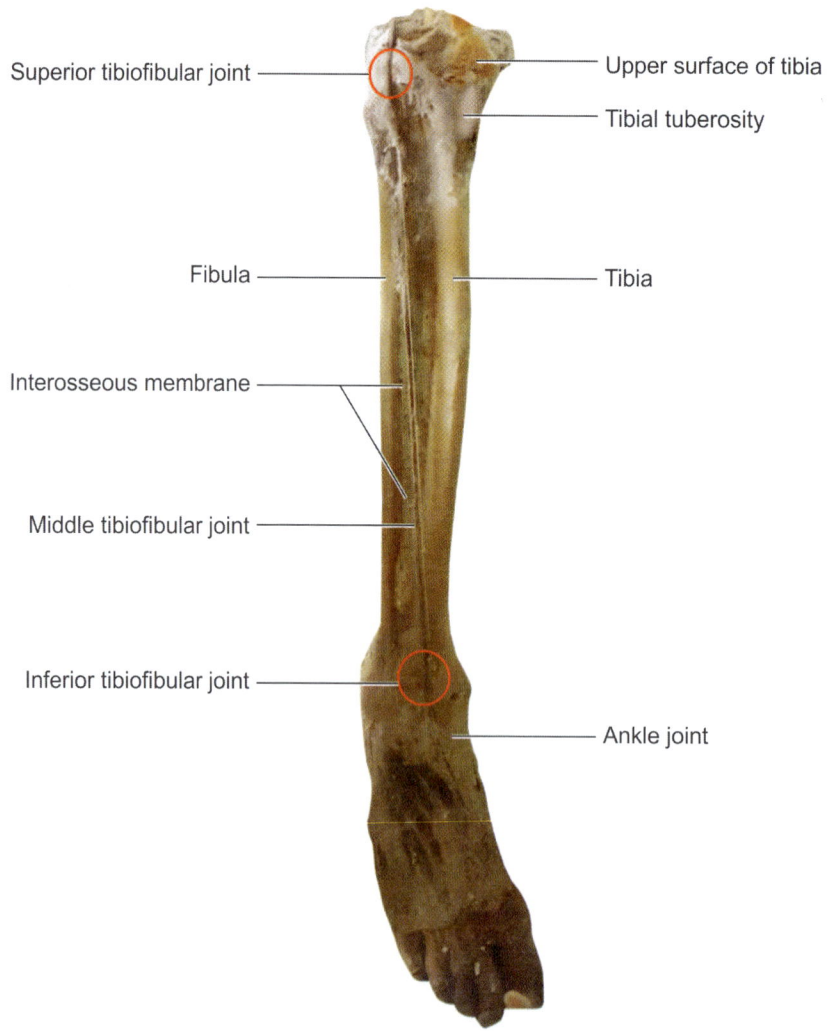

Fig. 25.10: Tibiofibular joints

- Divide these ligaments to expose the strong interosseous tibiofibular ligament.
- Use dry bones and articulated foot to understand the attachments of the ligaments.

ANKLE JOINT

- Study the lower ends of tibia, fibula and the superior surface of talus (Figs 25.5a,b, 25.9a,b and 25.11).
- Define the margins of superior and inferior extensor retinacula from anterior aspect of leg (*see* Fig. 21.3).
- Clean the flexor retinaculum from medial side of ankle.
- Define margins of superior and inferior peroneal retinacula on lateral side of ankle joint.
- Incise all these retinacula from the middle and reflect them on either side.
- Cut the tendons, nerves and vessels in the middle and reflect them on either side. Do this procedure in relation to the retinacula on all three sides of ankle.
- Now the ankle joint can be viewed. See the articular ends covered by articular cartilage.
- On the medial side of ankle joint, identify the strong deltoid ligament with its parts. These are:
  - Anterior tibiotalar

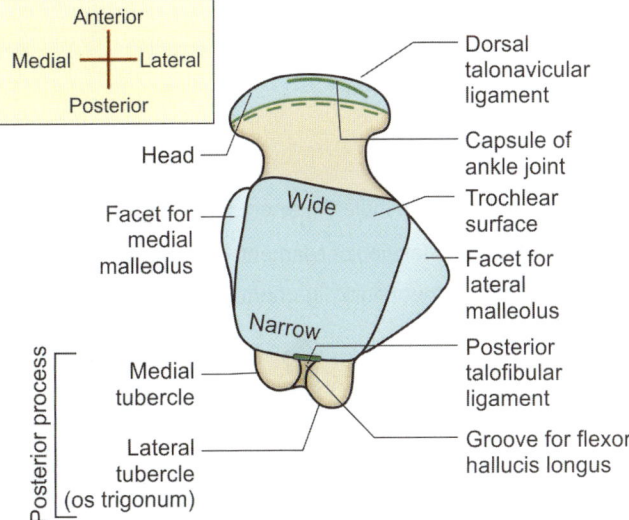

Fig. 25.11: Right talus superior view

  - Posterior tibiotalar
  - Tibiocalcanean
  - Tibionavicular (Fig. 25.12)
- Identify the lateral ligament of ankle joint. Its parts are:
  - Anterior talofibular
  - Posterior talofibular
  - Calcaneofibular (Fig. 25.13)

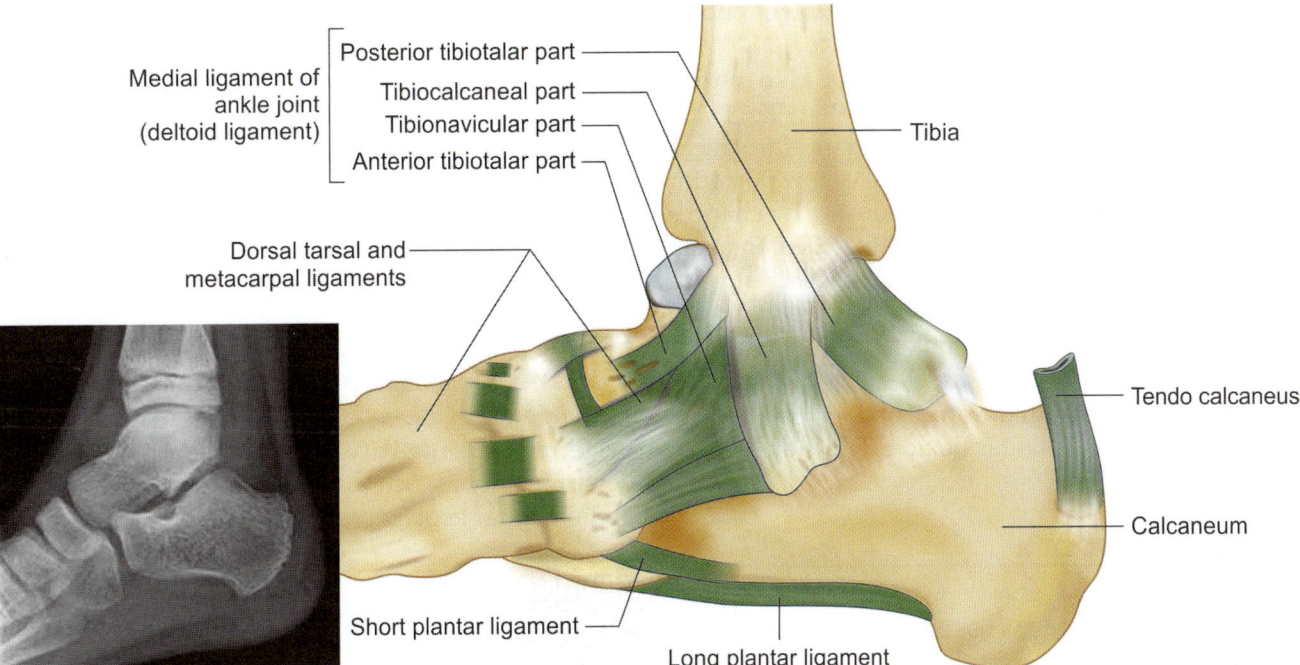

Fig. 25.12: Medial aspect of ankle joint

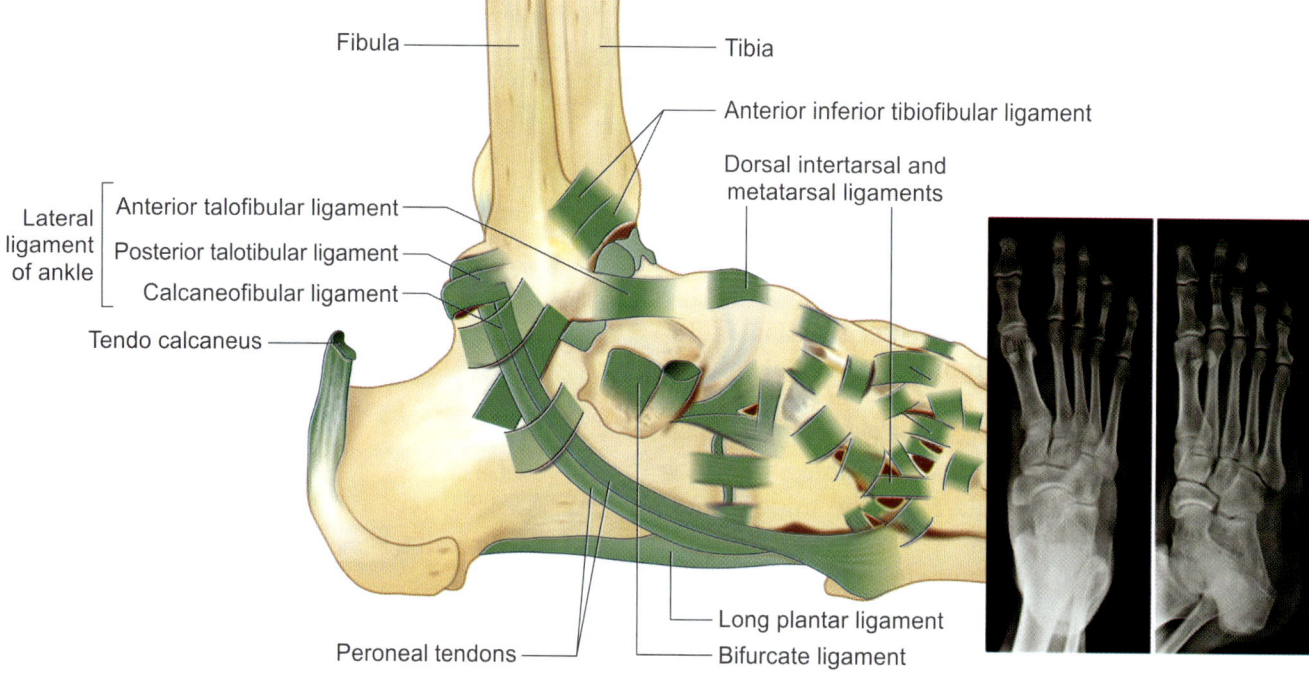

Fig. 25.13: Lateral aspect of ankle joint

- See tendons of peroneus brevis and peroneus longus on the lateral side of ankle joint (Fig. 25.13, *see* Fig. 21.7).
- Observe that the anterior surface of lower end of tibia is wider than its posterior surface.

  The trochlear surface of talus is also wider anteriorly and narrow posteriorly (Fig. 25.11). So in dorsiflexion the wider anterior part of trochlear surface of talus fits tightly into the narrow posterior surface of lower end of tibia. There are no chances of dislocation of the joint. In plantar flexion, as in wearing high heels, the narrow posterior surface of talus fits loosely into the wider anterior surface of lower end of tibia. This increases the chances of dislocation.

- Movements permitted at the ankle joint are only dorsiflexion and plantar flexion. These are shown in Table 25.3.

JOINTS OF THE FOOT

Competency achievement: The student should be able to:

AN 20.2 Describe the subtalar and transverse tarsal joints.

Table 25.3: Showing movements at ankle joint with their muscles and nerves

Movement	Main muscle	Nerve supply
Dorsiflexion	Tibialis anterior	Deep peroneal nerve
	Extensor hallucis longus	Deep peroneal nerve
Plantar flexion	Gastrocnemius, soleus	Tibial nerve

The proximal part of foot comprises 7 tarsal bones, 5 metatarsals and 14 phalanges. The tarsal bones are talus, calcaneum, navicular, 3 cuneiforms and cuboid (Fig. 25.14a and b)

- Remove all the tendons and muscles from both dorsal and plantar aspects of tarsal, metatarsals and phalanges.
- Define and identify the ligaments joining the various bones. See that ligaments are stronger on the plantar aspect than dorsal aspect.

SUBTALAR JOINTS

- See that the two big tarsal bones, i.e. talus and calcaneum are united at talocalcanean and talocalcaneonavicular joints (Fig. 25.10).

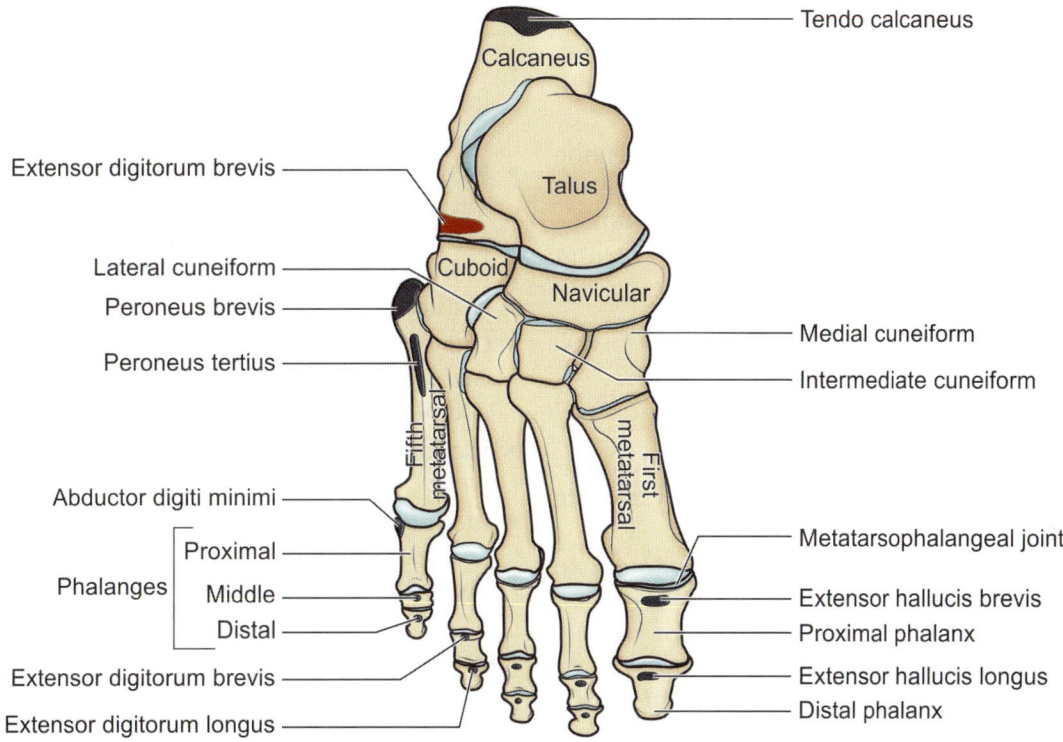

Tendo calcaneus

Calcaneus

Talus

Extensor digitorum brevis

Lateral cuneiform
Cuboid
Navicular

Peroneus brevis

Peroneus tertius

Medial cuneiform

Intermediate cuneiform

Fifth metatarsal

First metatarsal

Abductor digiti minimi

Metatarsophalangeal joint

Phalanges
Proximal
Middle
Distal

Extensor hallucis brevis

Proximal phalanx

Extensor digitorum brevis

Extensor hallucis longus

Extensor digitorum longus

Distal phalanx

Fig. 25.14a: Attachment of muscles to skeleton of the foot (dorsal aspect) except interossei

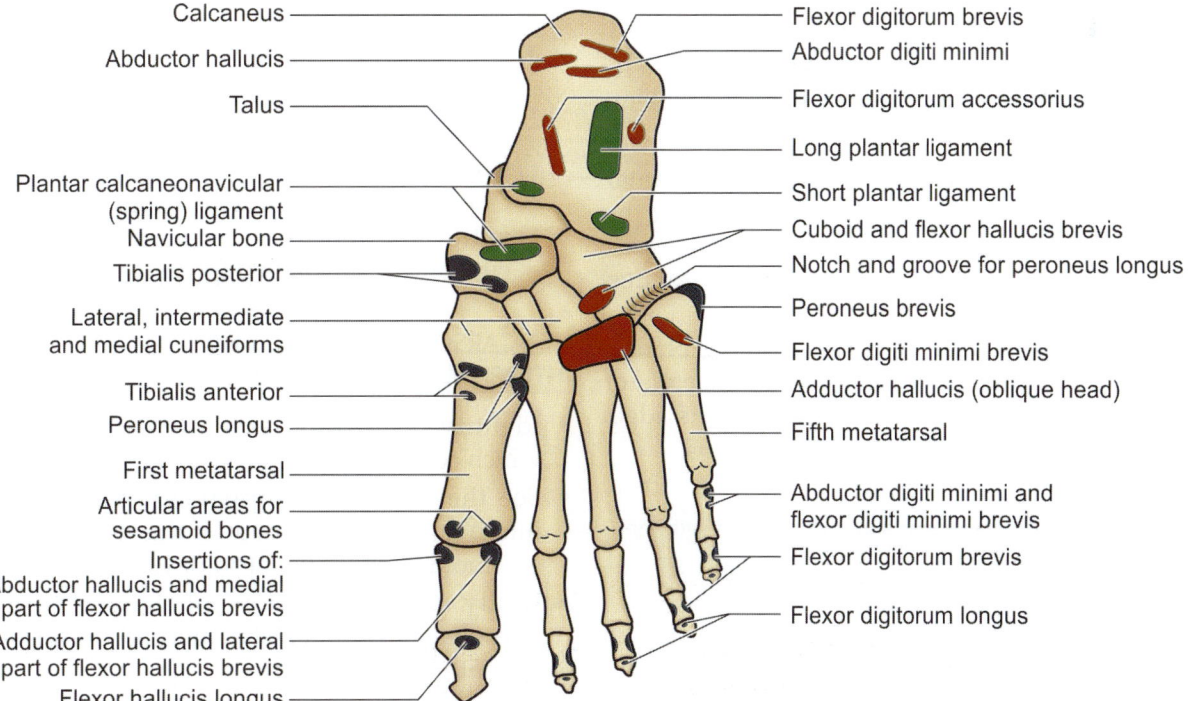

Calcaneus

Flexor digitorum brevis

Abductor hallucis

Abductor digiti minimi

Talus

Flexor digitorum accessorius

Plantar calcaneonavicular (spring) ligament

Long plantar ligament

Navicular bone

Short plantar ligament

Tibialis posterior

Cuboid and flexor hallucis brevis

Notch and groove for peroneus longus

Lateral, intermediate and medial cuneiforms

Peroneus brevis

Tibialis anterior

Flexor digiti minimi brevis

Peroneus longus

Adductor hallucis (oblique head)

First metatarsal

Fifth metatarsal

Articular areas for sesamoid bones

Abductor digiti minimi and flexor digiti minimi brevis

Insertions of:
Abductor hallucis and medial part of flexor hallucis brevis

Flexor digitorum brevis

Adductor hallucis and lateral part of flexor hallucis brevis

Flexor digitorum longus

Flexor hallucis longus

Fig. 25.14b: Attachment of skeleton of the foot (plantar aspect) except interossei

Movements of inversion and eversion occur at talocalcanean and talocalcaneonavicular joints. These also occur at talonavicular and calcaneo-cuboid joints (transverse tarsal joints).

See talocalcanean joint on dried bones between the undersurface of body of talus and convex facet on middle 1/3rd of superior surface of calcaneum.

- Identify the fibrous capsule and very strong interosseous talocalcanean ligament.
- Movements occurring at this joint are inversion and eversion.
- Identify talocalcaneonavicular ligament looking like a ball and socket joint.
- See the spring ligament or plantar calcaneo-navicular ligament and medial limb of bifurcate ligament.
- Identify the attachments of spring ligament to anterior margin of sustentaculum tali and to plantar surface of navicular bone. Tendons of tibialis posterior, flexor hallucis longus and flexor digitorum longus support the ligament inferiorly. This ligament also supports medial longitudinal arch of the foot.
- Identify calcaneocuboid joint—a saddle shaped joint between calcaneum and cuboid bones. See the following ligaments in addition to its capsule:

Bifurcate ligament—see its stem attached to sulcus calcanei; medial limb to navicular bone and lateral limb to cuboid bone.

Long plantar ligament—identify this ligament to plantar surface of calcaneum and to lips of groove on the cuboid bone and to bases of middle three metatarsals. See the groove is converted into a tunnel for tendon of peroneus longus.

Short plantar ligament is seen deep to long plantar ligament. See it extending from anterior tubercle of calcaneum to plantar surface of cuboid behind its ridge.

Table 25.4 shows movements at these joints.

Table 25.4: Showing movements at subtalar joint with their muscles and nerve supply

Movement	Main muscle	Nerve supply
Inversion	Tibialis anterior	Deep peroneal nerve
	Tibialis posterior	Tibial nerve
Eversion	Peroneus longus	Superficial peroneal nerve
	Peroneus brevis	Superficial peroneal nerve

SMALLER JOINTS OF FOREFOOT

- Cut across the cuneocuboid, cuneonavicular and intercuneiform joints to expose the articulating surfaces.
- With a strong knife cut through tarsometatarsal and intermetatarsal joints. Try to separate the bones to see interosseous ligaments. Detach abductor hallucis, flexor hallucis brevis, and adductor hallucis from the sesamoid bones of the big toe.
- Cut the deep transverse metatarsal ligaments on each side of third toe. Now the tendons of dorsal and plantar interossei can be seen till their insertion.
- Identify distal attachments of lumbrical muscles as well.
- Identify extensor expansion on the dorsum of digits and see its continuity with the collateral ligaments. Study these joints on an articulated foot.

JOINT CAVITIES OF FOOT

- There are only six joint cavities on proximal part of foot. These are intertarsal, tarsometatarsal, and intermetatarsal joints (Fig. 25.13).
- See the cavities as mentioned:
  - Talocalcanean
  - Talocalcaneonavicular
  - Calcaneocuboid
  - 1st cuneometatarsal
  - Cubometatarsal
  - Cuneonavicular with extensions, i.e. navicular with three cuneiforms including 2nd and 3rd cuneometarsal joints (Fig. 25.15).

METATARSOPHALANGEAL AND INTERPHALANGEAL JOINTS

- Identify deep transverse metatarsal ligaments which connect all five toes.
- See the 1st metatarsophalangeal joint and 1st interphalangeal joint both of the big toe. Look for sesamoid bones at the head of 1st metatarsal bone.
- Lastly identify metatarsophalangeal, proximal interphalangeal and distal interphalangeal joints of 2nd–5th toes (Fig. 25.16).

The toes are adducted and abducted with reference to the 2nd toe and not the 3rd digit as in the hand.

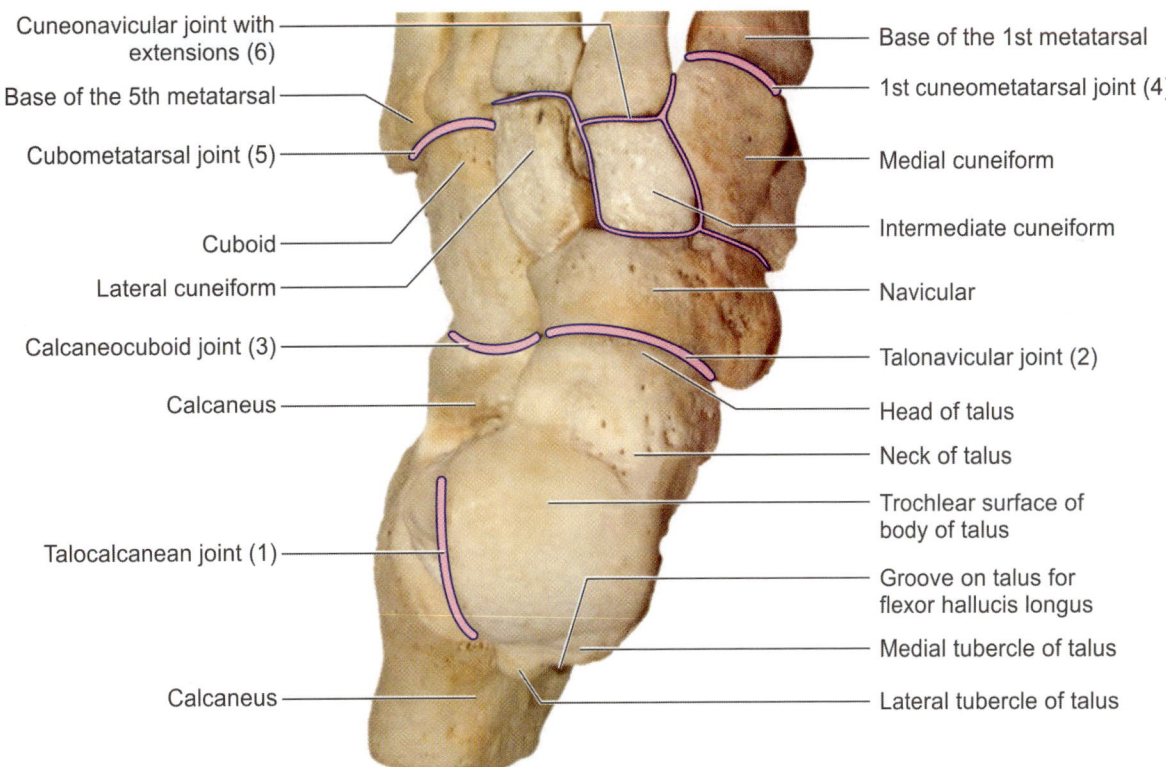

Cuneonavicular joint with extensions (6)

Base of the 5th metatarsal

Cubometatarsal joint (5)

Cuboid

Lateral cuneiform

Calcaneocuboid joint (3)

Calcaneus

Talocalcanean joint (1)

Calcaneus

Base of the 1st metatarsal

1st cuneometatarsal joint (4)

Medial cuneiform

Intermediate cuneiform

Navicular

Talonavicular joint (2)

Head of talus

Neck of talus

Trochlear surface of body of talus

Groove on talus for flexor hallucis longus

Medial tubercle of talus

Lateral tubercle of talus

Fig. 25.15: Joint cavities of foot

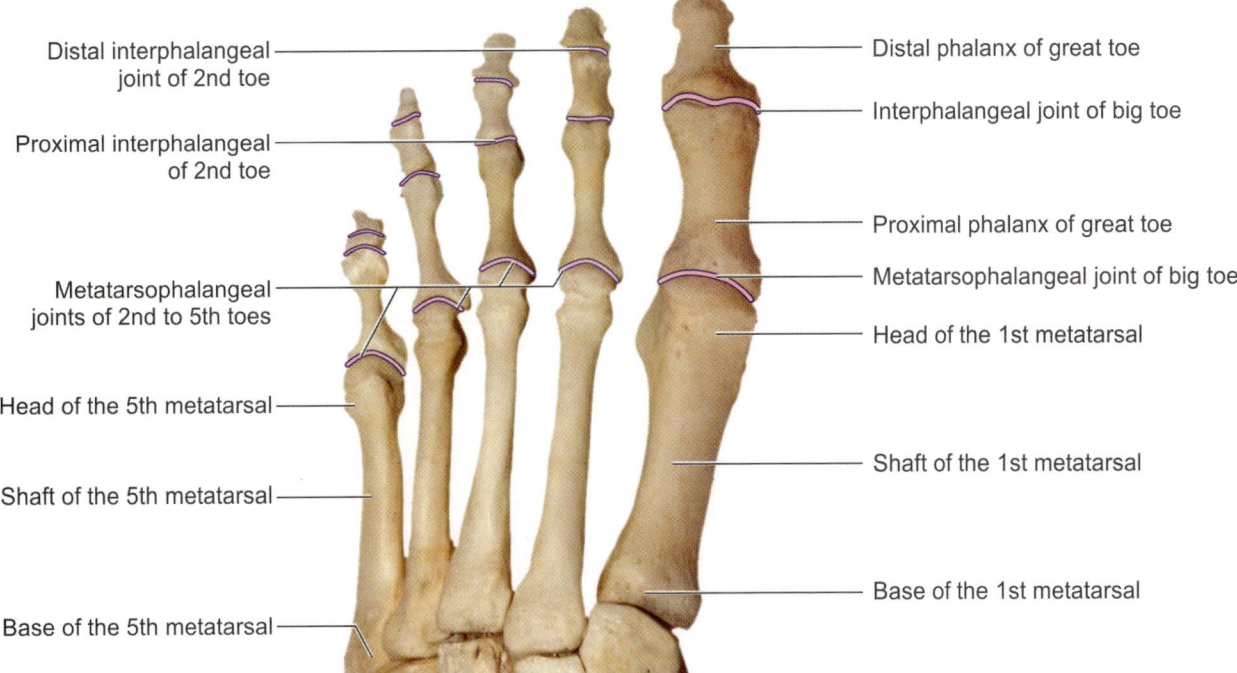

Distal interphalangeal joint of 2nd toe

Proximal interphalangeal of 2nd toe

Metatarsophalangeal joints of 2nd to 5th toes

Head of the 5th metatarsal

Shaft of the 5th metatarsal

Base of the 5th metatarsal

Distal phalanx of great toe

Interphalangeal joint of big toe

Proximal phalanx of great toe

Metatarsophalangeal joint of big toe

Head of the 1st metatarsal

Shaft of the 1st metatarsal

Base of the 1st metatarsal

Fig. 25.16: Metatarsophalangeal and interphalangeal joints of foot

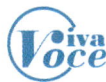

Viva Voce

- Which is the strongest ligament of hip joint?
- Name the muscles forming posterior relations of hip joint.
- What is coxa vara and coxa valga?
- Which important ligaments unite tibia and femur?
- Why is medial meniscus more prone to injury?
- What is the action of popliteus muscle?
- Which muscle causes locking of knee joint?
- Which muscle causes unlocking of knee joint?
- Name the attachments of deltoid ligament of ankle joint.
- What are the functions of interosseous membrane?
- What movements occur at tatocalcaneonavicular and transverse tarsal joints?
- Name the six joint cavities in the proximal part of the foot.

SPOTS ON LOWER LIMB

1. a. Identify the part of the marked muscle.
    b. Which nerves innervate this muscle?
    c. What is such a muscle called?

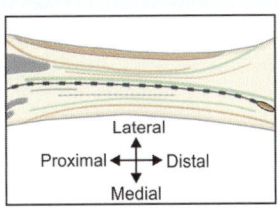

2. a. Name the fascial sheath around the structure shown.
    b. Which layers form the sheath?

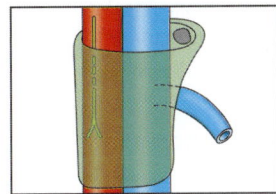

3. a. Identify the highlighted structure.
    b. What is the difference in root values of femoral nerve and this highlighted structure?

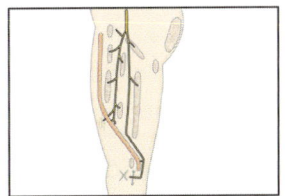

4. a. Name the marked structure.
    b. What is position of lower limb if it gets injured?

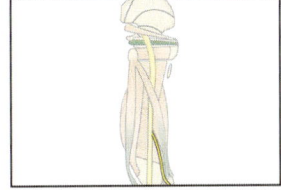

5. a. Name the three tendons
    b. Which nerves innervate the muscles of these tendons?

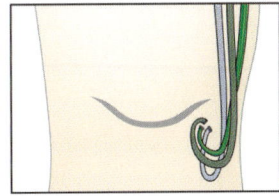

6. a. Identify the marked structure.
    b. Enumerate structures lying deep to it.

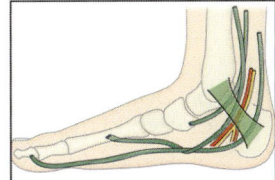

7. a. Identify the muscles arising from the tendons of flexor digitorum longus muscle.
    b. Name their nerve supply.

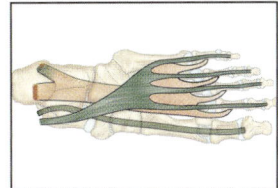

8. a. Identify the structure.
    b. What is its relation to medial malleolus?
    c. What is its clinical importance?

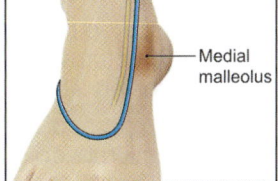

9. a. Identify the highlighted structure.
    b. Why is it commonly ruptured?

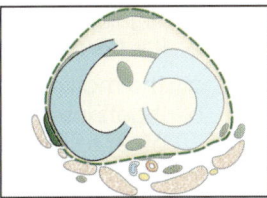

10. a. Name the marked tendon.
    b. Where all is it inserted?

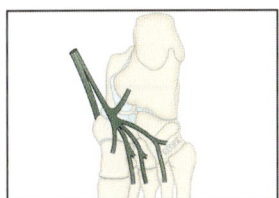

ANSWERS: SPOTS ON LOWER LIMB

1. a. Adductor magnus.
   b. Obturator nerve and sciatic nerve.
   c. Hybrid muscle.

2. a. Femoral sheath.
   b. Fascia transversalis anteriorly and psoas fascia posteriorly.

3. a. Obturator nerve.
   b. Femoral nerve arises from dorsal divisions of ventral primary rami of L2, L3, L4 spinal segments. Obturator nerve arises from ventral divisions of ventral primary of L2, L3, L4 spinal segments.

4. a. The marked structure is common peroneal nerve.
   b. In case of injury, the position of foot is "foot drop".

5. a. The three tendons are of sartorius, gracilis and semitendinosus.
   b. Nerve supply
      Sartorius—femoral nerve.
      Gracilis—obturator nerve.
      Semitendinosus—sciatic nerve.

6. a. Marked structure is flexor retinaculum of ankle.
   b. Structures underlying are: Tendon of tibialis posterior, tendon of flexor digitorum longus, posterior tibial vessels, tibial nerve and tendon of flexor hallucis longus.

7. a. 4 lumbrical muscles.
   b. 1st lumbrical supplied by medial plantar nerve 2nd–4th lumbricals by lateral plantar nerve.

8. a. The structure is great saphenous vein.
   b. It lies anterior to medial malleolus of tibia.
   c. "Cut open" procedure can be done to transfuse fluids, etc., if required.

9. a. Highlighted structure is medial meniscus of tibia.
   b. It is fixed to the tibial collateral ligament and so is more vulnerable to rupture.

10. a. The marked tendon is of tibialis posterior muscle.
    b. It gets inserted chiefly into tuberosity of navicular bone. The remaining part is attached by slips to all the other tarsal bones except talus. It also sends extensions to bases of 2nd and 3rd metatarsal bones.

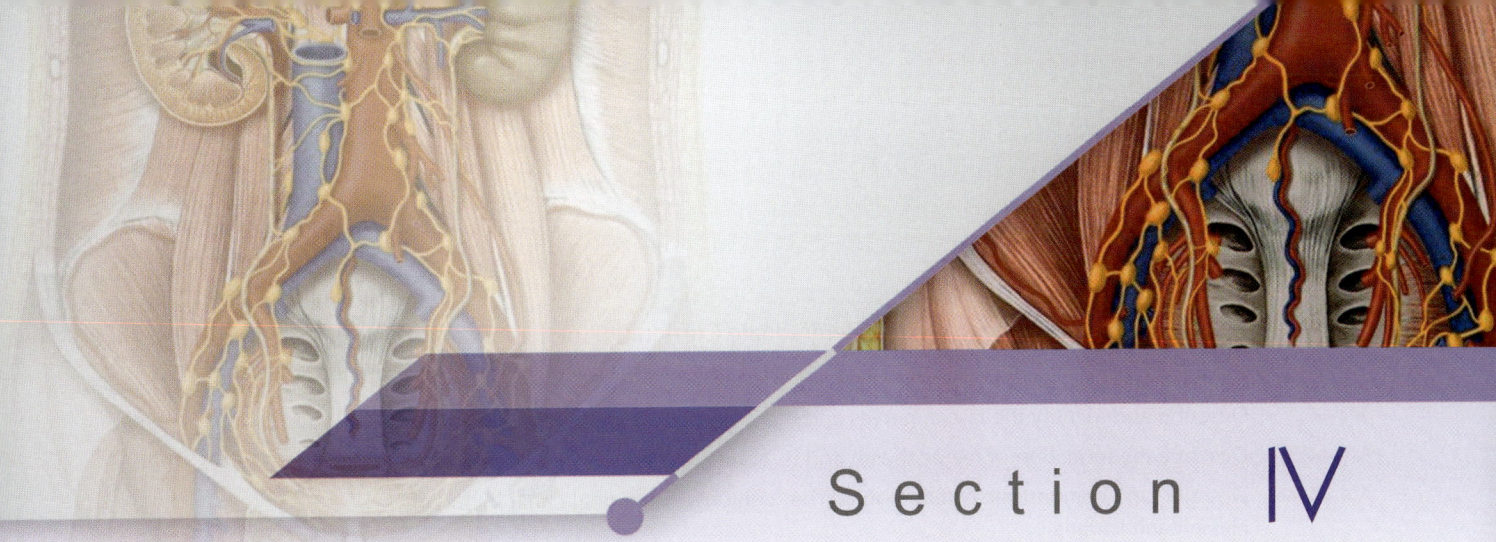

Section IV

Abdomen and Pelvis

CHAPTER 26

Anterior Abdominal Wall

Learning Objectives

One should be able to

1. Name the cutaneous nerve which supplies the region of umbilicus.
2. Name the coverings around the spermatic cord.
3. Mention the importance of arcuate line.
4. Discuss the actions of muscles of anterior abdominal wall.

OVERVIEW

Anterior abdominal wall also includes the lateral abdominal wall. It covers the abdominal cavity, giving it its deserved protection. Abdominal cavity is bounded by lower six ribs with their costal cartilages in the upper part. In the middle part it is only muscular and in the lower part, the hip bone forms the bony wall.

The skin of the anterior abdominal wall contains a depressed area—the umbilicus at the level between L3 and L4 vertebrae. There is a whitish vertical groove in the midline, which marks the position of the linea alba. Next to the skin are two layers of superficial fascia—a fatty superficial and deeper membranous. There is no deep fascia in the abdominal wall permitting the full stomach, distended intestines and the pregnant uterus to distend.

In the superficial fascia few cutaneous nerves and blood vessels can be cleaned and their courses can be read from BD Chaurasia's *Human Anatomy*.

Next to the superficial fascia are the three layers of muscles. These are external oblique, internal oblique and transversus abdominis. The direction of external oblique is downwards, forwards and medially; of internal oblique is upwards, forwards

and medially; of transversus abdominis in a transverse direction.

The straight muscle next to the anterior median line is the rectus abdominis. The attachments of these muscles have to be studied from **BD Chaurasia's** *Human Anatomy*.

The plane containing the main nerves and vessels is between internal oblique muscle and transversus abdominis muscle.

The nerves are the T7–T12 and branches of L1 nerve, e.g. iliohypogastric and ilioinguinal nerves. These nerves supply the muscles and overlying skin.

The arteries from above are terminal branches of anterior thoracic artery—musculophrenic laterally and superior epigastric medially. Arteries from below are inferior epigastric and deep circumflex iliac arteries.

Rectus Sheath

As the rectus abdominis extends from the pubic bone below to the 7th, 6th and 5th costal cartilages on each side of the anterior median line, it is enveloped by an aponeurotic sheath—the rectus sheath. This comprises an anterior wall, a posterior wall, lateral and medial walls. There is an arcuate line in relation to this sheath. This line is marked where the internal oblique and transversus abdominis lie anterior to the rectus muscle. It lies midway between umbilicus and pubic symphysis.

Contents of the sheath are rectus abdominis and pyramidalis muscle, if present, including the lower six thoracic nerves with superior and inferior epigastric vessels.

Deep to these four muscles is the transversalis fascia which lines the inner aspect of transversus abdominis muscle.
1. This fascia gives a tubular extension—the internal spermatic fascia to the spermatic cord.
2. It also forms anterior wall of femoral sheath.

Inguinal Canal

Since the testes have descended down, outside the abdominal cavity, an intermuscular canal is formed in lower part of anterior abdominal wall above the medial half of inguinal ligament. It lies between deep inguinal and superficial inguinal rings. Internal oblique muscle forms part of anterior wall, roof and part of posterior wall of this canal providing a shutter mechanism to the inguinal canal. Floor is formed by medial part of inguinal ligament and lacunar ligament. Internal oblique also takes part in the formation of conjoint tendon. This tendon forms part of posterior

wall of inguinal canal. Fascia transversalis also forms the posterior wall. Internal oblique also gives rise to fibres of cremasteric muscle.

Spermatic cord containing ductus deferens and associated nerves, blood vessels exit via superficial ring.

Hernia

Protrusion of abdominal organs/structures through any weakness in any of the abdominal walls is known as hernia. Inguinal hernia occurs more in males through its two openings or through the posterior wall of the inguinal canal. It may be congenital or acquired. Femoral hernia is never congenital and is more common in females.

Competency achievement: The student should be able to:

AN 44.2 Describe and identify the fascia, nerves and blood vessels of anterior abdominal wall.

STEPS OF DISSECTION

• Give an incision from xiphoid process till the umbilicus. Make a small circular incision around the umbilicus and extend it till the pubic symphysis. Carry the incision laterally from the umbilicus till the lateral abdominal wall on both sides. Give curved incisions 3 cm below from anterior superior

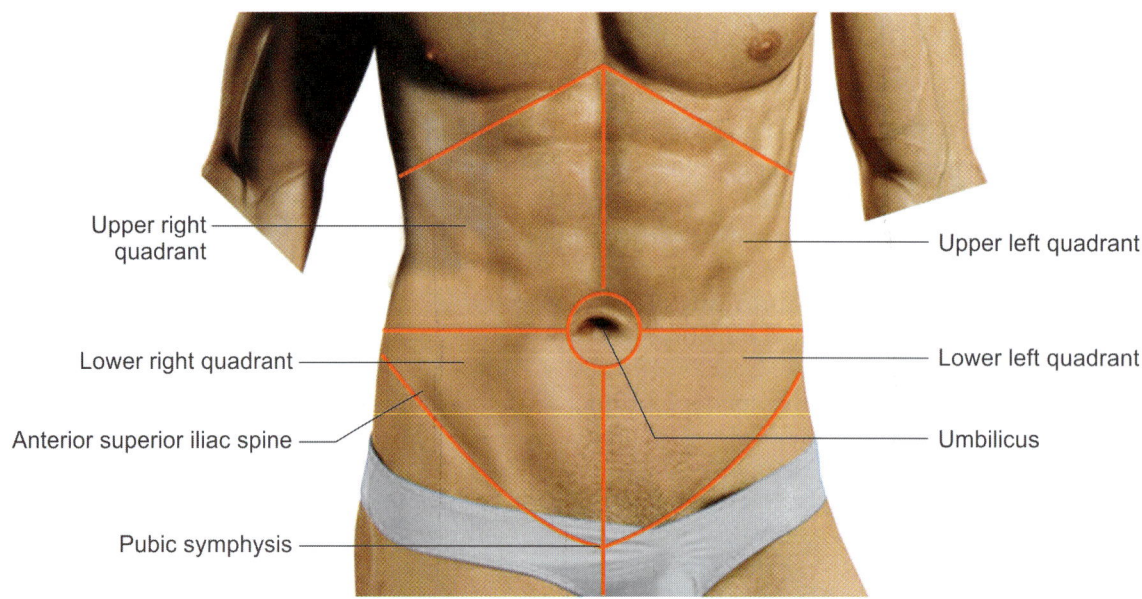

Fig. 26.1: Lines of incision

iliac spine to pubic symphysis on either side (Fig. 26.1).

- Finally, give an oblique incision from the xiphoid process along the costal margin till the lateral abdominal wall on either side.
- Carefully reflect the skin in four flaps leaving both the layers of superficial fascia on the anterior abdominal wall. Make a transverse incision through the entire thickness of the superficial fascia from the anterior superior iliac spine to the median plane. Raise the lower margin of the cut fascia and identify its fatty and membranous layers. Note that the fatty layer is continuous with the fascia of adjoining parts of the body. The membranous layer of anterior abdominal wall is continuous with the similar fascia (Colles' fascia) of the perineum. Note its attachment to pubic arch and posterior margin of perineal membrane (inferior fascia of urogenital diaphragm).
- Locate the superficial inguinal ring immediately superolateral to the pubic tubercle. Note the anterior cutaneous branch of the iliohypogastric

nerve piercing the aponeurosis of the external oblique muscle a short distance superior to the ring (Fig. 26.2).

- The spermatic cord/round ligament of uterus along with ilioinguinal nerve leave the abdomen through the superficial inguinal ring. Identify the external spermatic fascia attaching the spermatic cord to the margins of the ring. Divide the superficial fascia vertically in the median plane and in the line of the posterior axillary fold as far as the iliac crest.
- Reflect the fascia by blunt dissection from these two cuts and find the anterior and lateral cutaneous branches of the lower intercostal nerves along with respective blood vessels coming out from the anterior and lateral regions of the abdominal wall.

Cutaneous Nerves

- Observe that the anterior cutaneous branch of the T 7 nerve innervates the skin of epigastrium.

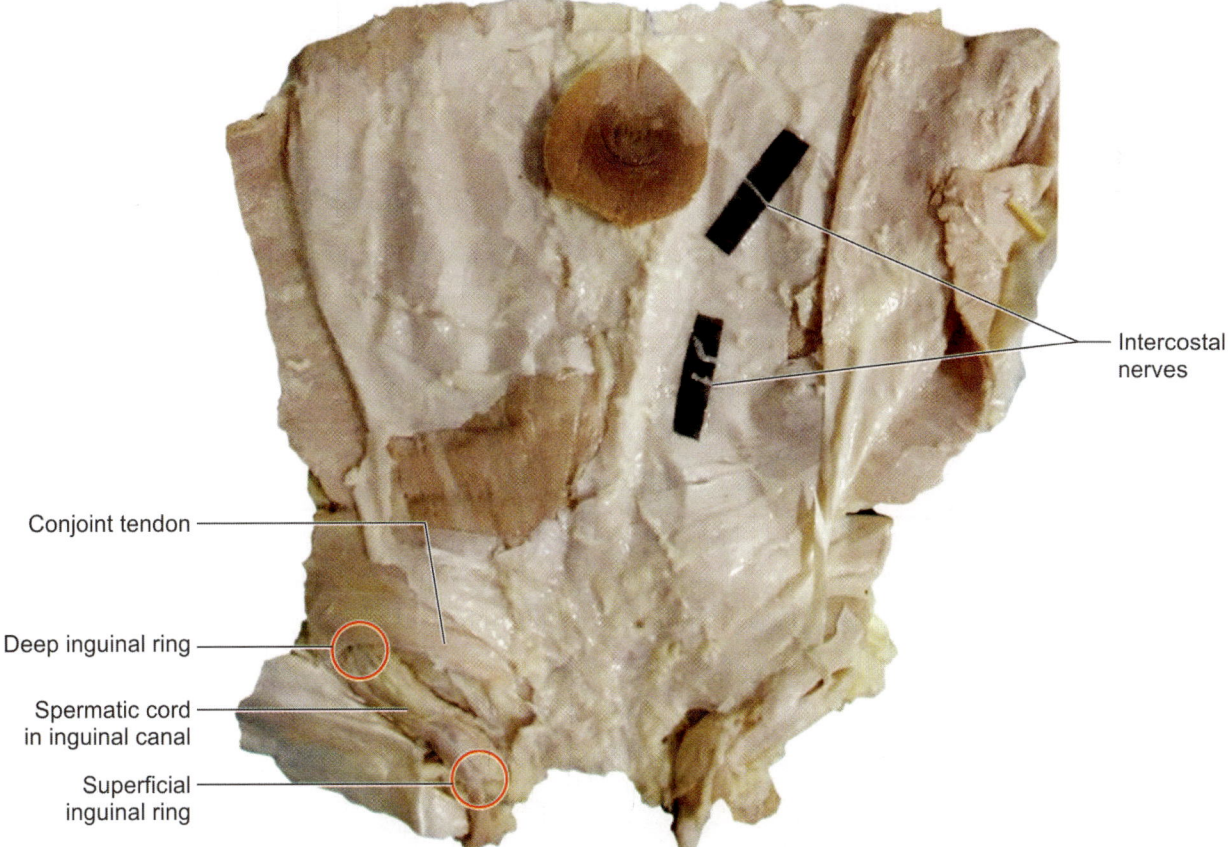

Fig. 26.2: Superficial region of anterior abdominal wall including inguinal canal

- Anterior cutaneous branch of T10 innervates the skin around the umbilicus.
- Anterior cutaneous branch of T12 innervates the skin of suprapubic region.
- Anterior cutaneous branch of iliohypogastric nerve (L1) pierces the aponeurosis of external oblique muscle a short distance superior to superficial inguinal ring.
- Identify and trace few lateral cutaneous branches of intercostal nerves near the midaxillary line.

Cutaneous Veins

- *Identify the following veins:*
  - Superficial epigastric vein running from the epigastric region towards inguinal region.
  - Superficial external pudendal vein from external genitalia to inguinal region.
  - Superficial circumflex iliac from iliac crest region to inguinal region.

All these three veins drain into the great saphenous vein before it pierces cribriform fascia to end in the femoral vein.

Note a vein—*thoracoepigastric vein* which joins the superficial epigastric vein with lateral thoracic vein of upper extremity. This forms a communicating channel between veins of the upper limb and lower limb and can open up in case of blockage. These veins are accompanied by cutaneous arteries.

Competency achievement: The student should be able to:

AN 44.6 Describe and demonstrate attachments of muscles of anterior abdominal wall.

Muscles of Anterolateral Abdominal Wall

The two layers of superficial fascia have been seen. There is no deep fascia in the abdominal wall. Its absence allows the abdomen to distend forwards when required. The distension is required in deep inspiration, after a heavy meal and during pregnancy. To allow for these activities the deep fascia is characteristically absent.

Next to superficial fascia are the three flat muscles of the abdominal wall. These are external oblique, internal oblique and transversus abdominis (Fig. 26.3).

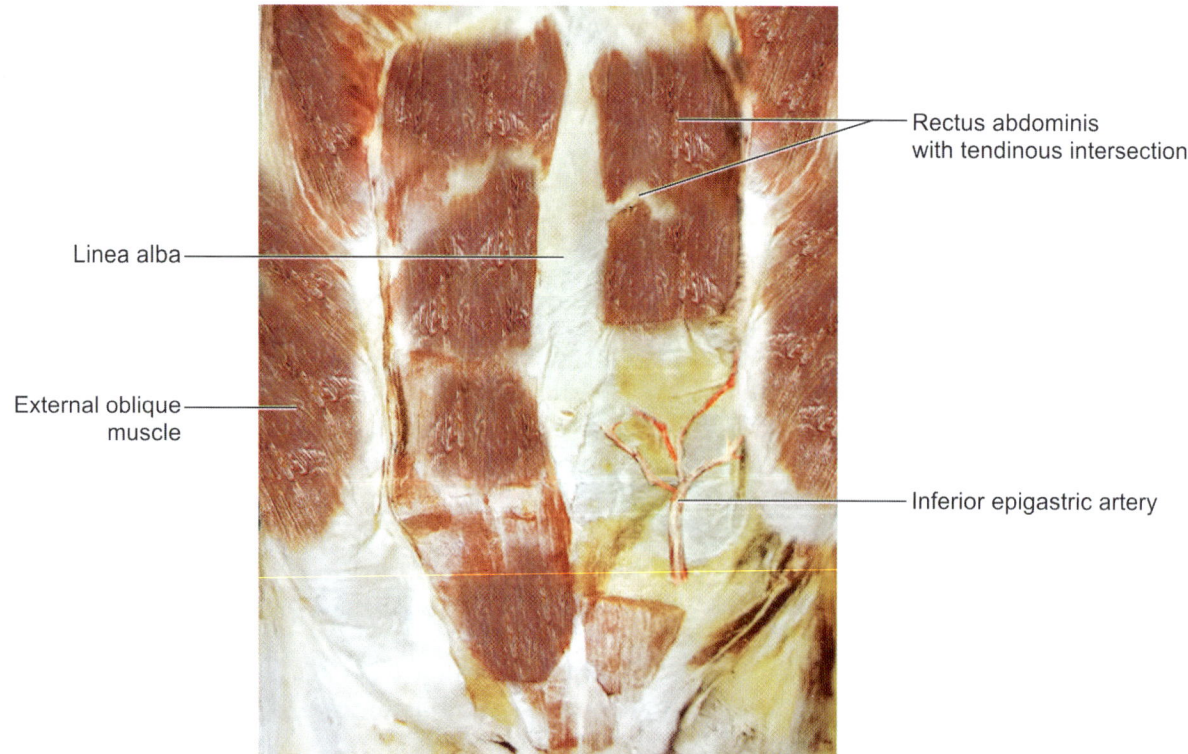

Linea alba

External oblique muscle

Rectus abdominis with tendinous intersections

Inferior epigastric artery

Fig. 26.3: Linea alba with rectus abdominis muscle

These reach the linea alba in the midline. But to strengthen the region of linea alba are rectus abdominis on each side of median plane (Fig. 26.3). The lowest part of anterior abdominal wall contains an intermuscular canal called the inguinal canal. It is located above the medial half of the inguinal ligament. The canal has two openings, superficial and deep inguinal rings (Fig. 26.2).

External Oblique Muscle

- Identify the origin of external oblique from the external surfaces of the lower eight ribs.
- See its interdigitations with serratus anterior in the upper part and with latissimus dorsi in the lower part of its origin. Direction of fibres is downwards, forwards and medially (Fig. 26.4).
- See the insertion of the muscle by a broad aponeurosis (flattened tendon) into xiphoid process, linea alba, pubic tubercle and outer lip of ventral 2/3rd segment of the iliac crest (Fig. 26.4).
- Clean the aponeurosis of external oblique by blunt dissection.
- The superficial inguinal ring (SIR) has been identified near the pubic tubercle. See the lateral and medial crus of this ring (Fig. 26.2).

Lateral crus is attached to pubic tubercle. It forms the lateral margin of the SIR. Medial crus is flat and is attached to medial half of pubic crest. It forms medial margin of SIR.

Inguinal ligament is the lower part of aponeurosis of external oblique muscle. It is attached to anterior superior iliac spine (laterally) and to pubic tubercle medially.

- Identify the gap between the inguinal ligament and the hip bone (parts of pubis and ilium). Through this gap structures course the abdominal cavity and the lower limb.

Pectineal part of inguinal ligament is a triangular fold of aponeurosis. Its apex is attached to pubic tubercle, one margin is continuous with inguinal ligament and the other is attached to pecten pubis. Its lateral margin is free and abuts against the femoral canal.

Pectineal ligament is the continuation of lower slip of pectineal part of inguinal ligament to pectineal line of pubis.

Intercrural fibres are the fibres that start from lower part of inguinal ligament, pass across both the lateral

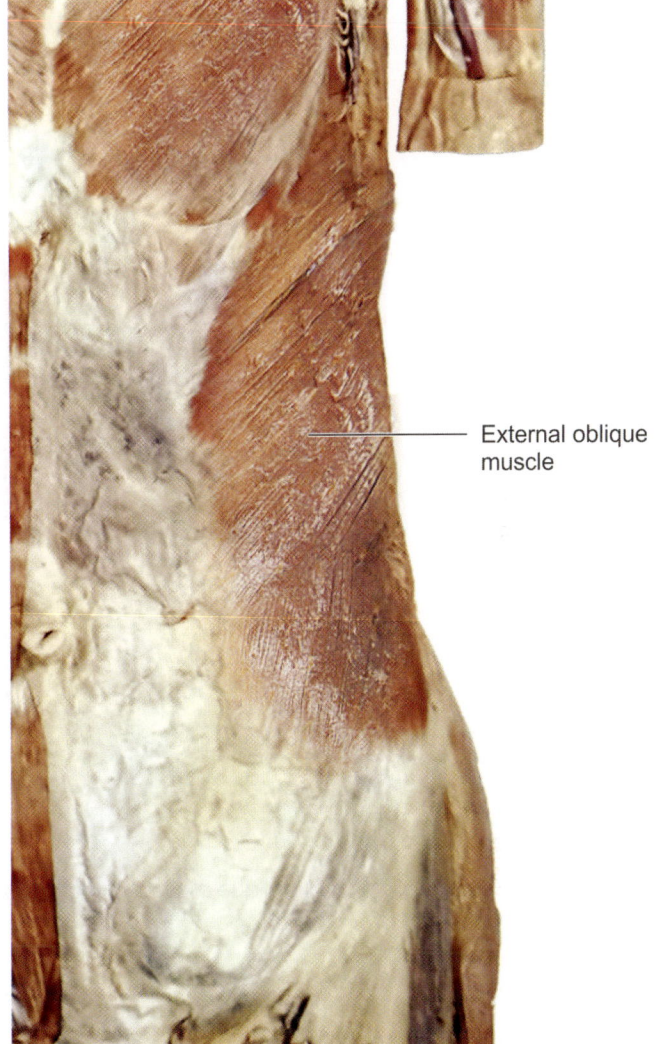

External oblique muscle

Fig. 26.4: External oblique muscle

and medial crus of SIR. These fibres maintain the integrity of SIR and prevent these from spreading.

The fibres of reflected ligament start from lateral crus, passing deep to SIR to fuse with linea alba. These strengthen the weakness caused by SIR.

- See a layer of fascia—external spermatic fascia arising from the aponeurosis of external oblique muscle to cover the spermatic cord.

STEPS OF DISSECTION

- Separate 1–6 digitations from the ribs.
- Cut vertically, through the muscle to the iliac crest posterior to the sixth digitation. Separate the

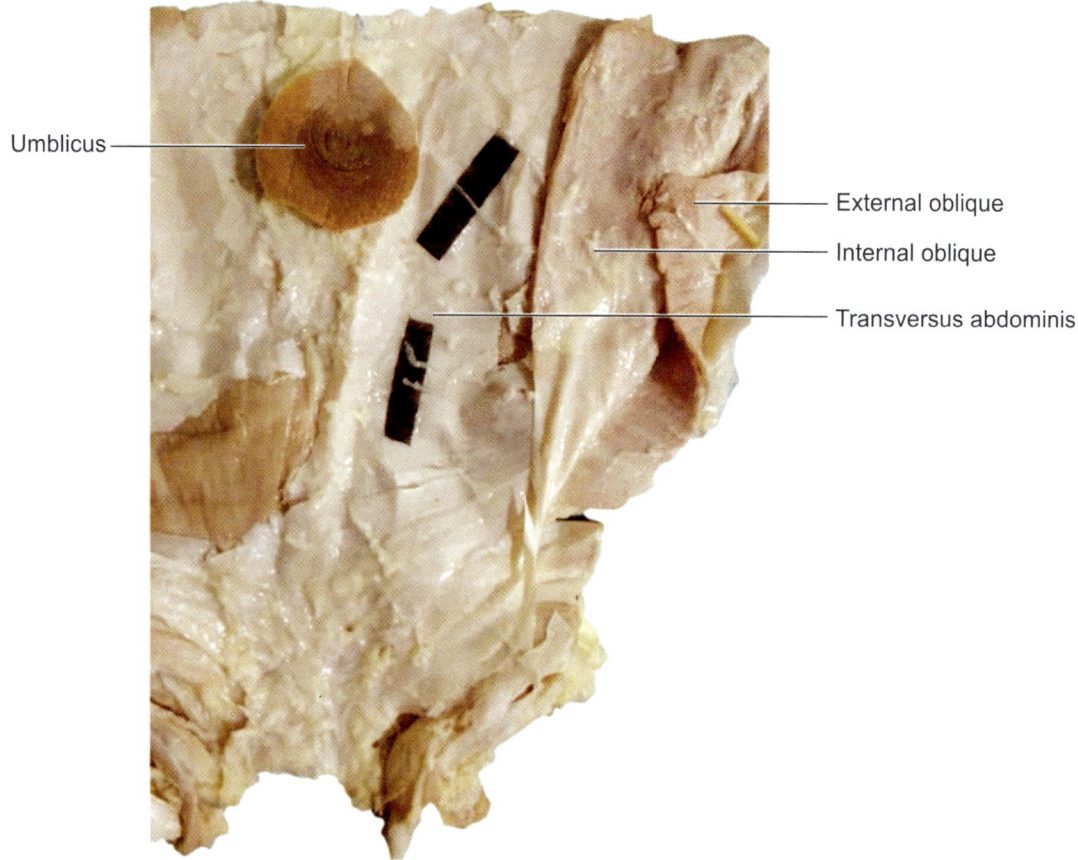

Umblicus

External oblique

Internal oblique

Transversus abdominis

Fig. 26.5: Internal oblique muscle reflected to show intercostal nerves in neurovascular plane

external oblique from the iliac crest in front of this. Try to avoid injury to the lateral cutaneous branches of the subcostal and iliohypogastric nerves which pierce it close to the iliac crest. Reflect the upper part of the external oblique forwards and expose the deeper internal oblique and its aponeurosis to the line of its fusion with the aponeurosis of the external oblique anterior to rectus abdominis. Just lateral to this line of fusion, divide the external oblique aponeurosis vertically till the pubic symphysis. Turn the muscle and aponeurosis inferiorly. This exposes the inferior part of the internal oblique and the lowest portion of aponeurosis of external oblique, i.e. the inguinal ligament. Identify the deep fibres of the inguinal ligament passing posteriorly to the pecten pubis. This is the lacunar ligament or pectineal part of the inguinal ligament.

Internal Oblique

Deep to external oblique is another flat muscle, the internal oblique (Fig. 26.5). It is visible as the external oblique has been reflected medially and downwards. It arises from lower part of abdomen, from lateral 2/3rd of inguinal ligament, anterior 2/3rd of ventral segment of iliac crest (intermediate area) and lumbar fascia (Fig. 26.6). The fibres are directed upwards forwards and medially at right angles to those of external oblique muscle.

This muscle is also inserted by a broad aponeurosis but it does not extend beyond the costal margin. Its insertion is into costal cartilages of 12th, 11th, 10th, 9th, 8th and 7th ribs.

As aponeurosis nears medially towards linea semilunaris (lateral border of rectus abdominis) it splits into two layers, one forming anterior wall and the other forming posterior wall of rectus sheath. This

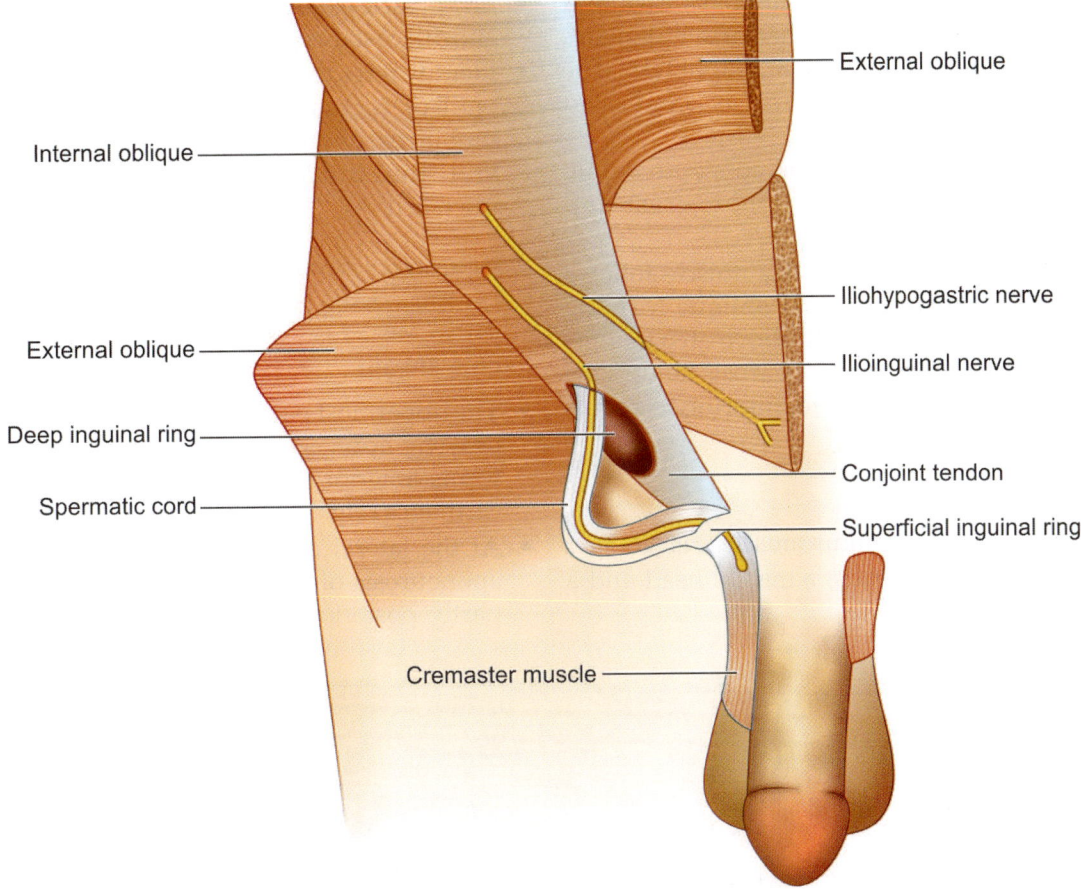

External oblique

Internal oblique

External oblique

Deep inguinal ring

Spermatic cord

Iliohypogastric nerve

Ilioinguinal nerve

Conjoint tendon

Superficial inguinal ring

Cremaster muscle

Fig. 26.6: Internal oblique muscle with conjoint tendon and cremaster muscle

arrangement persists till the midpoint of line joining umbilicus to pubic symphysis i.e. arcuate line/linea semilunaris in upper 3/4th of abdominal wall.

Identify arrangement of its aponeurosis below this line. It does not split and whole aponeurosis passes anterior to the rectus abdominis. Appreciate that lowest part of this muscle forms lateral part of anterior wall of inguinal canal, its roof and medial part of posterior wall of the canal in the form of conjoint tendon (Fig. 26.6).

- Lift the internal oblique and cut carefully through its attachments to the inguinal ligament, iliac crest and costal margin.
- Carefully preserve the nerves of the anterior abdominal wall which lie between internal oblique and transversus abdominis (Fig. 26.5). This is the neurovascular plane carried forwards from the ribs.
- Cut vertically through the internal oblique from the twelfth costal cartilage to the iliac crest and reflect

the muscle forwards from the transversus and the nerves.

Cremaster and Conjoint Tendon

- Remove the fascia from the surface of the internal oblique and its aponeurosis.
- Identify the part of the internal oblique which passes around the spermatic cord. This is the cremasteric muscle (Fig. 26.6).
- Trace the fibres of internal oblique into the conjoint tendon.
- Dissect the triple relation of internal oblique to the inguinal canal.

Transversus Abdominis

Transversus abdominis is the deepest muscle of the anterolateral region.

- Identify its origin from lateral half of inguinal ligament, anterior 2/3rd of inner lip of ventral segment of iliac crest, thoracolumbar fascia and inner aspects of 7th–12th ribs, where it interdigitates with fibres of thoracoabdominal diaphragm. The direction of its fibres is transverse as is indicated by its name (Fig. 26.7).

- Look for the insertion as a broad aponeurosis into xiphoid process, linea alba, pubic crest and pectineal line.
- Medially, the aponeurosis of this muscle follows the posterior layer of internal oblique forming posterior wall of rectus sheath above arcuate line. Below the arcuate line, the aponeurosis follows the whole internal oblique to lie anterior to rectus sheath.

Rectus Abdominis

- Identify the rectus abdominis muscle (Fig. 26.3).
- See its origin by two heads, a medial head and a lateral head.

- The muscle extends up and is inserted into 7th, 6th and 5th costal cartilages from medial to lateral side.
- Identify three tendinous intersections in the anterior wall of rectus abdominis, one at the level of umbilicus, another at the level of xiphoid process and the third one in between these two intersections.

Competency achievement: The student should be able to:

AN 44.3 Describe the formation of rectus sheath and its contents.

Rectus Sheath

- The uppermost part of rectus abdominis is covered only by aponeurosis of external oblique, which forms anterior sheath. Posterior wall is by costal cartilages (Fig. 26.8).
- At the lateral edge of the rectus abdominis, the aponeurosis of the internal oblique splits to pass partly posterior and partly anterior to the rectus

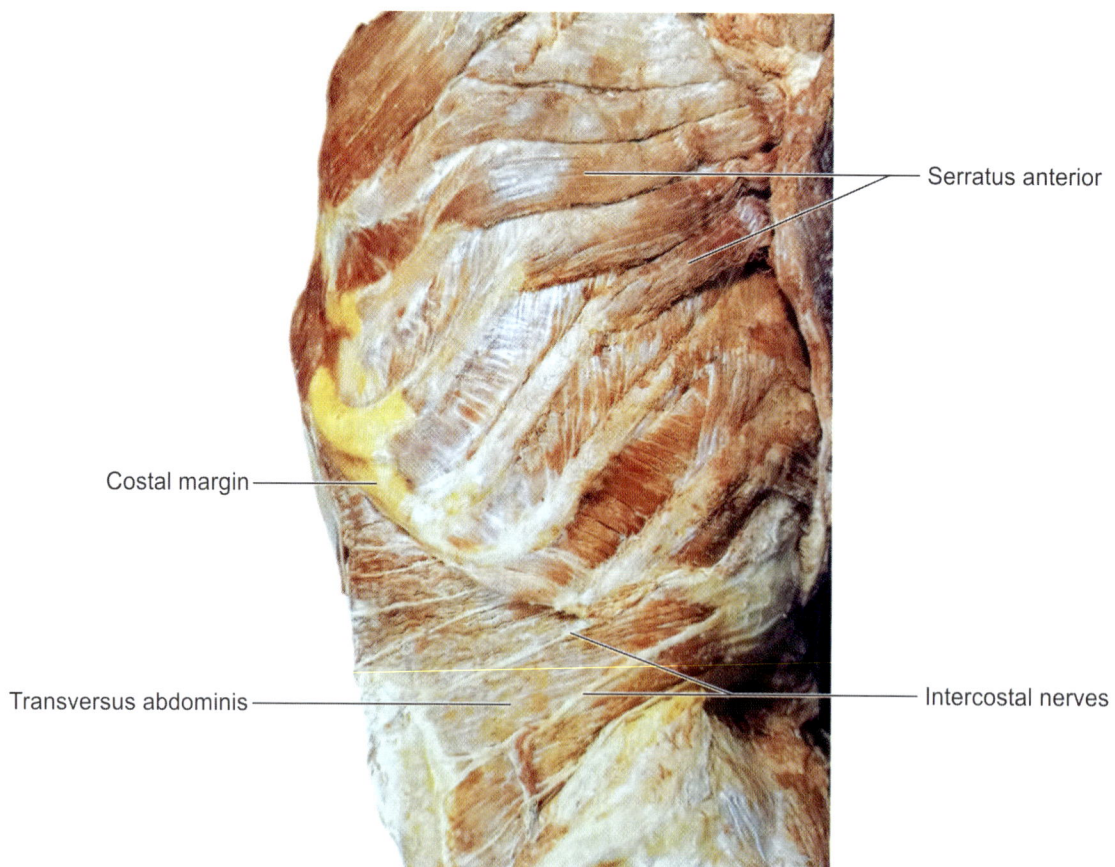

Serratus anterior

Costal margin

Transversus abdominis

Intercostal nerves

Fig. 26.7: Transversus abdominis muscle with intercostal nerves. Serratus anterior also seen

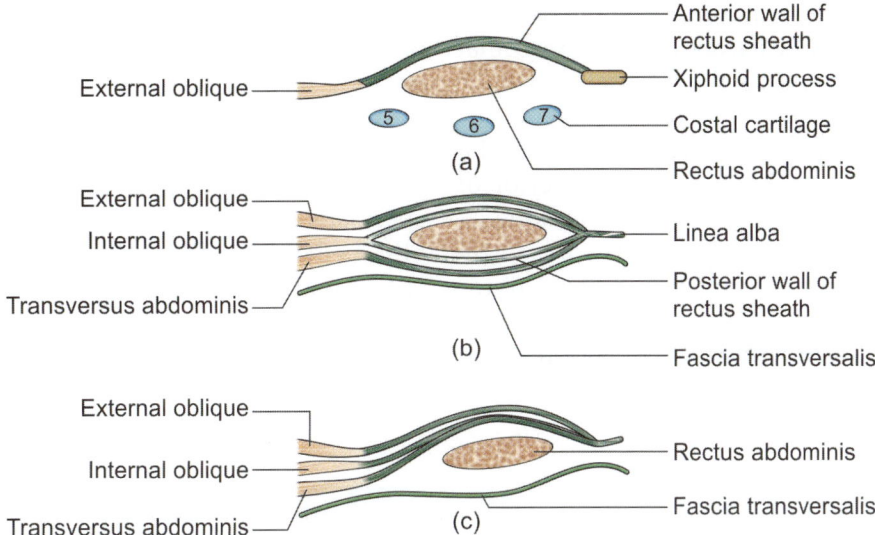

Fig. 26.8: Rectus sheath at different levels: (a) Above costal margin; (b) Between costal margin and arcuate line; (c) Below arcuate line

abdominis; the anterior layer fusing with the aponeurosis of external oblique and the posterior layer with that of the transversus abdominis. This is how most of the rectus sheath, i.e. upper 3/4th of the sheath is formed. Identify the arcuate line midway between umbilicus and pubic symphysis.
- Define the origins of the transversus abdominis and follow its aponeurosis to fuse with that of the internal oblique, posterior to the rectus abdominis above the arcuate line and anteriorly to the unsplit aponeurosis of internal oblique below the arcuate line. See that the aponeurosis of all three muscles pass anterior to rectus abdominis below the arcuate line. Inferior epigastric artery enters rectus sheath by passing up in front of arcuate line.
- Open the rectus sheath by a vertical incision along the middle of the muscle. Reflect the anterior layer of the sheath sideways, cutting its attachments to the tendinous intersections in the anterior part of the rectus muscle.
- Lift the rectus muscle and identify the 7–11 intercostal and subcostal nerves entering the sheath through its posterior lamina, piercing the muscle and leaving through its anterior wall (Fig. 26.5).
- Divide the rectus abdominis transversely at its middle. Identify its attachments and expose the posterior wall of the rectus sheath by reflecting its parts superiorly and inferiorly. Identify and trace

the superior and inferior epigastric arteries (Fig. 26.3).
- Define the arcuate line on the posterior wall of rectus sheath.
- Spermatic cord/round ligament of uterus with ilioinguinal nerve exit from superficial inguinal ring (Fig. 26.6).
- Palpate the firm tube-like ductus deferens in spermatic cord. Other structures are venous plexus, testicular artery, etc. Coverings are external spermatic fascia, cremasteric muscle and fascia and internal spermatic fascia.

Competency achievement: The student should be able to:

AN 44.4 Describe and demonstrate extent, boundaries, contents of inguinal canal including Hesselbach's triangle.

Inguinal Canal

- Identify again the superficial inguinal ring above the pubic tubercle. It lies in the aponeurosis of external oblique muscle and provides the external spermatic fascia to spermatic cord/round ligament of uterus (Fig. 26.2).
- Identify internal oblique muscle deep to external oblique. Note that its fibres lie anterior to deep inguinal ring, then arch over the inguinal canal and finally fuse with the transversus abdominis to form the conjoint tendon attached to pubic crest and pecten pubis (Fig. 26.6).

- Lastly identify the deep inguinal ring in the fascia transversalis situated 1.2 cm above the midinguinal point. This fascia provides the internal spermatic fascia to spermatic cord/round ligament of uterus.

Thus, see that external oblique forms whole of the anterior wall. Only lateral one-third of anterior of anterior wall is supplemented by internal oblique.

The entire floor of inguinal canal is formed by inguinal ligament. Roof is formed by arching fibres of internal oblique and transversus muscles. As these fibres fuse together to form the conjoint tendon which forms its posterior wall in medial half.

Fascia transversalis forms posterior wall in whole of its extent. 1.2 cm above the midinguinal point is an opening in the fascia transversalis. This opening is deep inguinal ring (DIR) situated lateral to inferior epigastric artery (Fig. 26.3). Internal spermatic fascia, a part of fascia transversalis, continues along spermatic cord. Above and lateral to pubic tubercle is SIR. As the spermatic cord exits through SIR, a fascial sheath is given off from external oblique aponeurosis. This fascial sheath is external spermatic fascia. Internal oblique also gives a muscular covering-the cremasteric muscle and fascia to the spermatic cord.

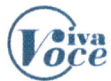

- What is caput medusae?
- What is the importance of umbilicus?
- Name the cutaneous nerve supplying the umbilical area.
- Name the main actions of muscles of anterior abdominal wall.
- What forms posterior wall of rectus sheath above the costal margin?
- Name the triple relation of internal oblique muscle to the inguinal canal.
- What are the contents of spermatic cord?
- Name two differences between direct and indirect inguinal hernia.

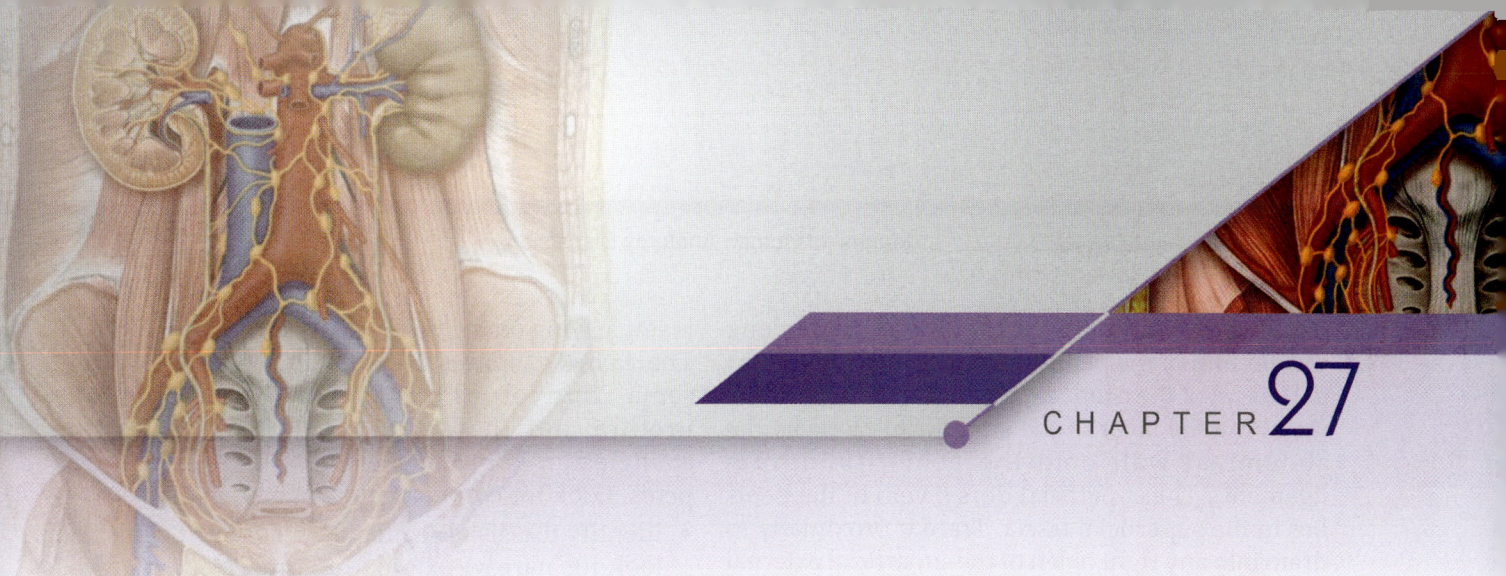

CHAPTER 27

Male External Genital Organs

Learning Objectives

One should be able to

1. To hold the testis in its anatomical position.
2. To identify the parts of epididymis.

3. To trace the course of testicular artery and veins of each side.
4. To learn descent of testis.

OVERVIEW

Male genital organs are both suspended outside the body and within the pelvis. Testis with its coverings and ducts are suspended outside the body in scrotal sac, as spermatogenesis needs 2–3 °C lower temperature than the inside temperature of the body.

Male external genital organs are:

Penis, scrotum enveloping the testes and epididymes and proximal parts of the vas/ductus deferens.

Penis is male copulatory organ conveying both the urine and semen at different time. It comprises one corpus spongiosum containing urethra and a pair of corpora cavernosa. The fascia enclosing these three bodies contains superficial and deep veins, a pair each of arteries and nerves.

Scrotum, a bag lies below the penis. It is partially divided into two compartments. Each compartment contains testis, epididymis and proximal part of ductus deferens. These are covered by two layers of peritoneum and spermatic fasciae.

Testis is divided into many compartments. Each compartment contains 2–3 seminiferous tubules.

STEPS OF DISSECTION

- From the superficial inguinal ring, make a longitudinal incision downwards through the skin of the anterolateral aspects of the scrotum till its lower part. Reflect the skin alone, if possible, otherwise reflect skin, dartos and the other layers together till the testis enveloped in its tunica vaginalis is visualised.

- Lift the testis and spermatic cord from the scrotum. Cut through the spermatic cord at the superficial inguinal ring and remove it together with the testis and put it in a tray of water.

- Incise and reflect the coverings, if any, e.g. remains of external spermatic fascia, cremasteric muscle, cremasteric fascia and internal spermatic fascia. Separate the various structures of spermatic cord. Feel ductus deferens as the important constituent of spermatic cord. Make a transverse section through the testis to visualise its interior.

- Identify the epididymis capping the superior pole and lateral surface of the testis. The slit-like sinus of epididymis formed by tucking-in of the visceral layer of peritoneum between the testis and the epididymis is seen on the posterolateral aspect of the testis. Cut through and reflect the skin along the dorsum of the penis from the symphysis pubis to the end of the prepuce. Find the extension of the membranous layer of the superficial fascia of the abdominal wall onto the penis (fundiform ligament). The superficial dorsal vein of the penis lies in the superficial fascia. Trace it proximally to drain into any right or left of the superficial external pudendal veins of thigh. Deep to this vein is the deep fascia and suspensory ligament of the penis. Divide the deep fascia in the same line as the skin incision. Reflect it to see the deep dorsal vein with the dorsal arteries and nerves on each side. Make a transverse section through the body of the penis, but leave the two parts connected by the skin of urethral surface or ventral surface. Identify two corpora cavernosa and single corpus spongiosum traversed by the urethra.

Competency achievement: The student should be able to:

AN 46.3 Describe penis under following headings: Parts, components, blood supply and lymphatic drainage.

STRUCTURE OF PENIS

Each corpus cavernosum, present on the dorsal aspect, contains the deep helicine artery of penis. The caverns are spaces bounded by septa. The corpus spongiosum is single lying on the ventral aspect of penis (Fig. 27.2). The caverns/spaces are smaller, bounded by fine septa. This corpus contains the important penile urethra and the arteries of the bulb. Corpus spongiosum is prolonged forwards to form glans penis. Look for corona glandis at base of glans.

- Identify the distal segment of transacted penis and look for narrow external urethral meatus, traced backwards urethra is dilated into a navicular fossa.
- Identify the prepuce (foreskin) covering the glans on under aspect of penis (Fig. 27.1). Look for a fold-the frenulum. The thin space between glans and prepuce is prepuitial sac.

SCROTUM

The scrotum is a cutaneous bag containing the right and left testes, the epididymes and the lower parts of the spermatic cords.

Externally the scrotum is divided into right and left parts by a ridge or raphe which is continued forwards onto the undersurface of the penis and backwards along the middle of the perineum to the anus (Fig. 27.1).

The left half of the scrotum hangs a little lower than the right, in correspondence with the greater length of the left spermatic cord.

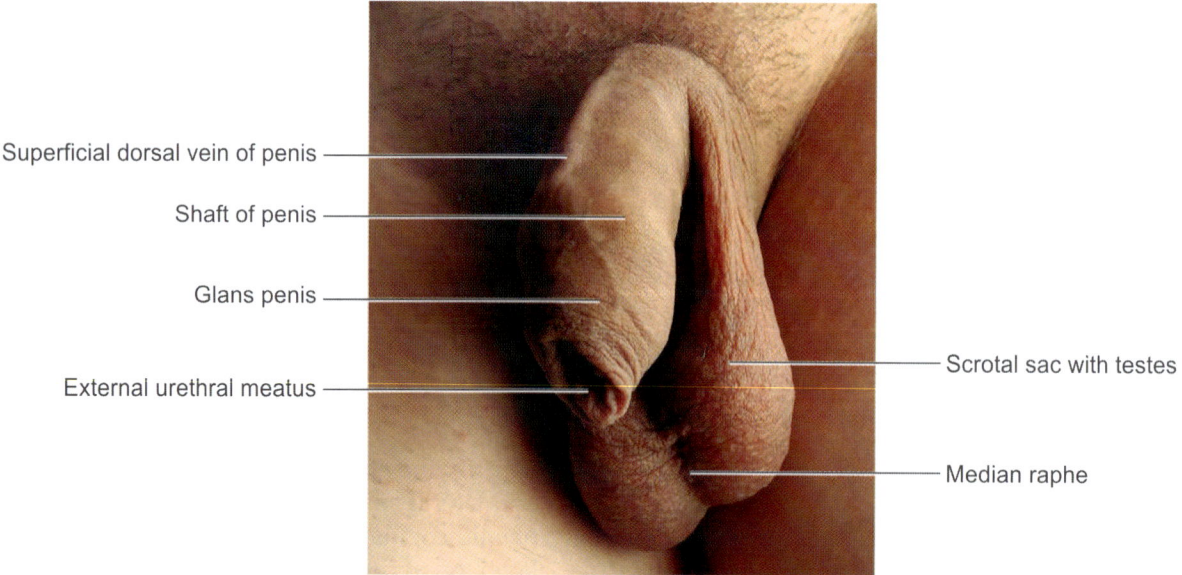

Superficial dorsal vein of penis

Shaft of penis

Glans penis

External urethral meatus

Scrotal sac with testes

Median raphe

Fig. 27.1: Male external genital organs

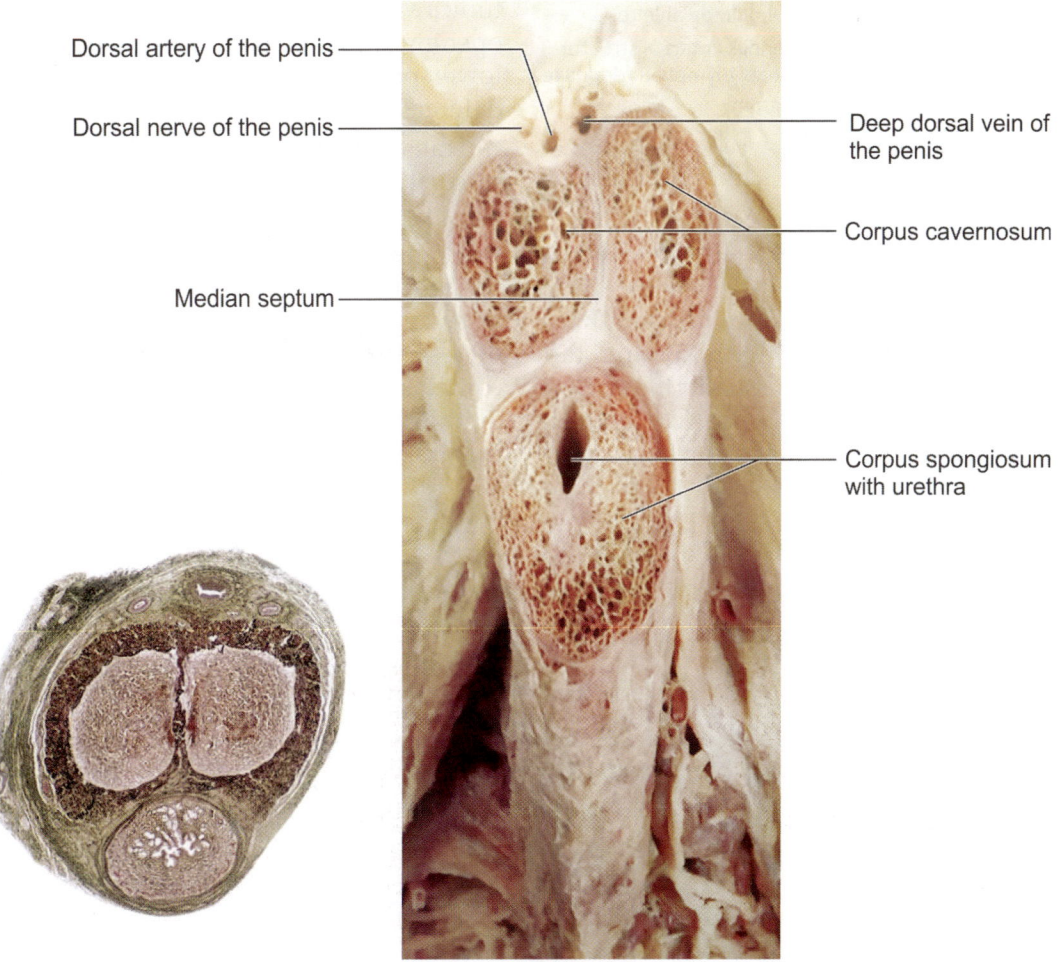

Dorsal artery of the penis

Dorsal nerve of the penis

Median septum

Deep dorsal vein of the penis

Corpus cavernosum

Corpus spongiosum with urethra

Fig. 27.2: Transverse section through the body of penis

Under the influence of cold, and in the young robust persons, the scrotum is short, corrugated and closely applied to the testis. This is due to contraction of the subcutaneous muscle of scrotum, called the dartos.

Layers of the Scrotum

The scrotum is made up of the following layers from outside inwards:

1. Skin
2. Dartos muscle which replaces the superficial fascia
3. The external spermatic fascia
4. The cremasteric muscle (*see* Fig. 26.6) and fascia.
5. The internal spermatic fascia. The dartos muscle is prolonged into a median vertical septum between the two halves of the scrotum.

Competency achievement: The student should be able to:

AN 46.1 Describe and demonstrate coverings, internal structure, side determination, blood supply, nerve supply, lymphatic drainage and descent of testis with its applied anatomy.

TESTIS

Testis comprises: 2 rounded poles—upper and lower; 2 borders—anterior and posterior; 2 surfaces—medial and lateral.

On the upper pole is the head of epididymis, like a helmet. It is continuous with its body and tail. Epididymis is fixed by areolar tissue to the back of testis along its posterolateral surface. The body of epididymis is separated from testis by an infolding of

tunica vaginalis, known as sinus of epididymis. The opening of the sinus faces postero-laterally. At the lower pole, tail of epididymis continues as ductus deferens.

Transverse section through the testis shows the thin visceral layer of tunica vaginalis.

Tough fibrous coat: The tunica albuginea, which gets thickened at the back of testis and is known as mediastinum testis. Radiating from mediastinum testis are fibrous septa which divide the parenchyma of testis into compartments. Each compartment contains 2–3 convoluted seminiferous tibules. Ends of these tubules open into rete testis inside the mediastinum testis. From the rete testis 15–20 vasa

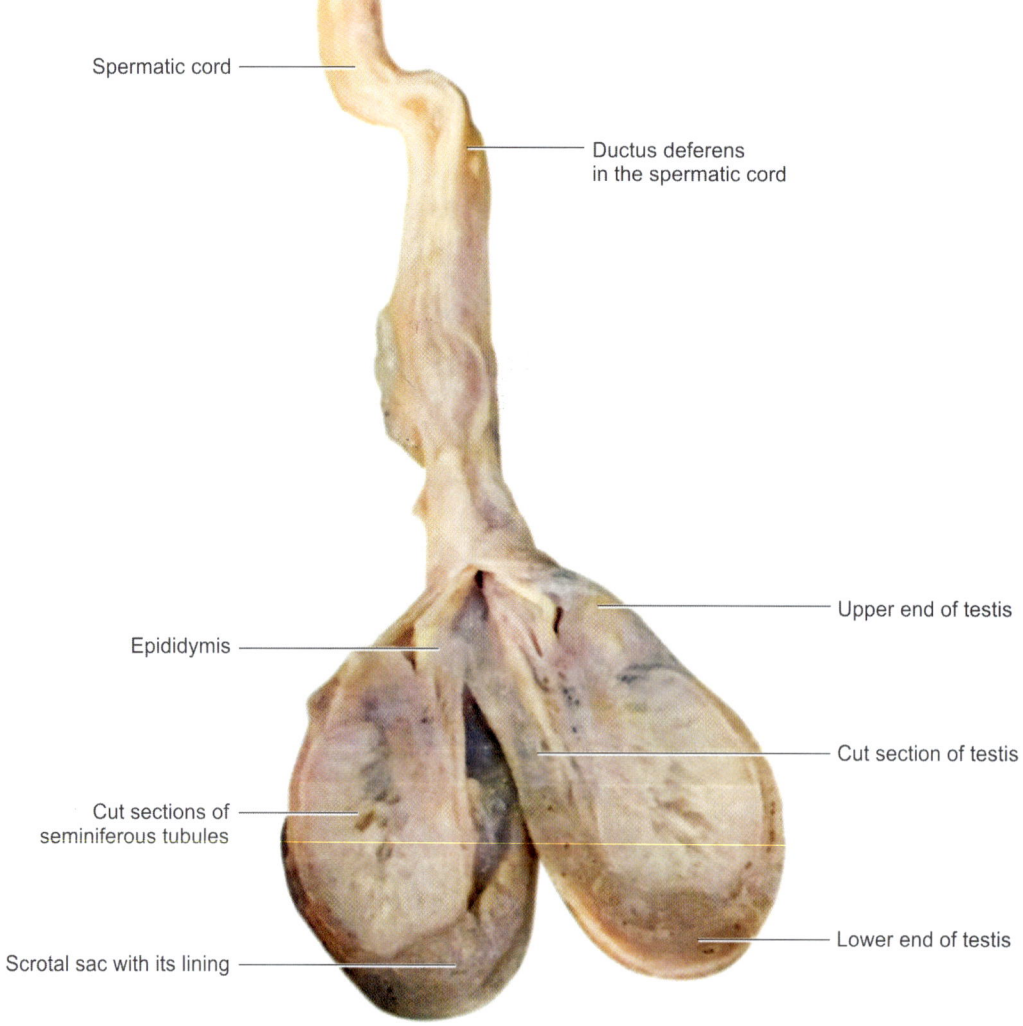

Spermatic cord

Ductus deferens
in the spermatic cord

Upper end of testis

Epididymis

Cut section of testis

Cut sections of
seminiferous tubules

Lower end of testis

Scrotal sac with its lining

Fig. 27.3: Opened up scrotal sac to show testis, epididymis, ductus deference in the spermatic cord

efferentia emerge and form a single duct in the head of epididymis.

Coverings of Testis

The testis is covered by three coats. From outside inwards, these are external spermatic fascia, cremasteric muscle and fascia and internal spermatic fascia (Fig. 27.4).

Competency achievement: The student should be able to:

AN 46.2 Describe parts of epididymis.

Epididymis

It is a highly coiled tube acting as a reservoir of spermatozoa. Its upper end is called head. It is connected to upper pole of testis by efferent ductules (Fig. 27.5). The middle part is body and the lower part is tail. This continues as ductus deferens.

Spermatic Cord

The cord starts at deep inguinal ring, courses through inguinal canal and exits at superficial inguinal ring. Then it reaches the upper pole and posterior border

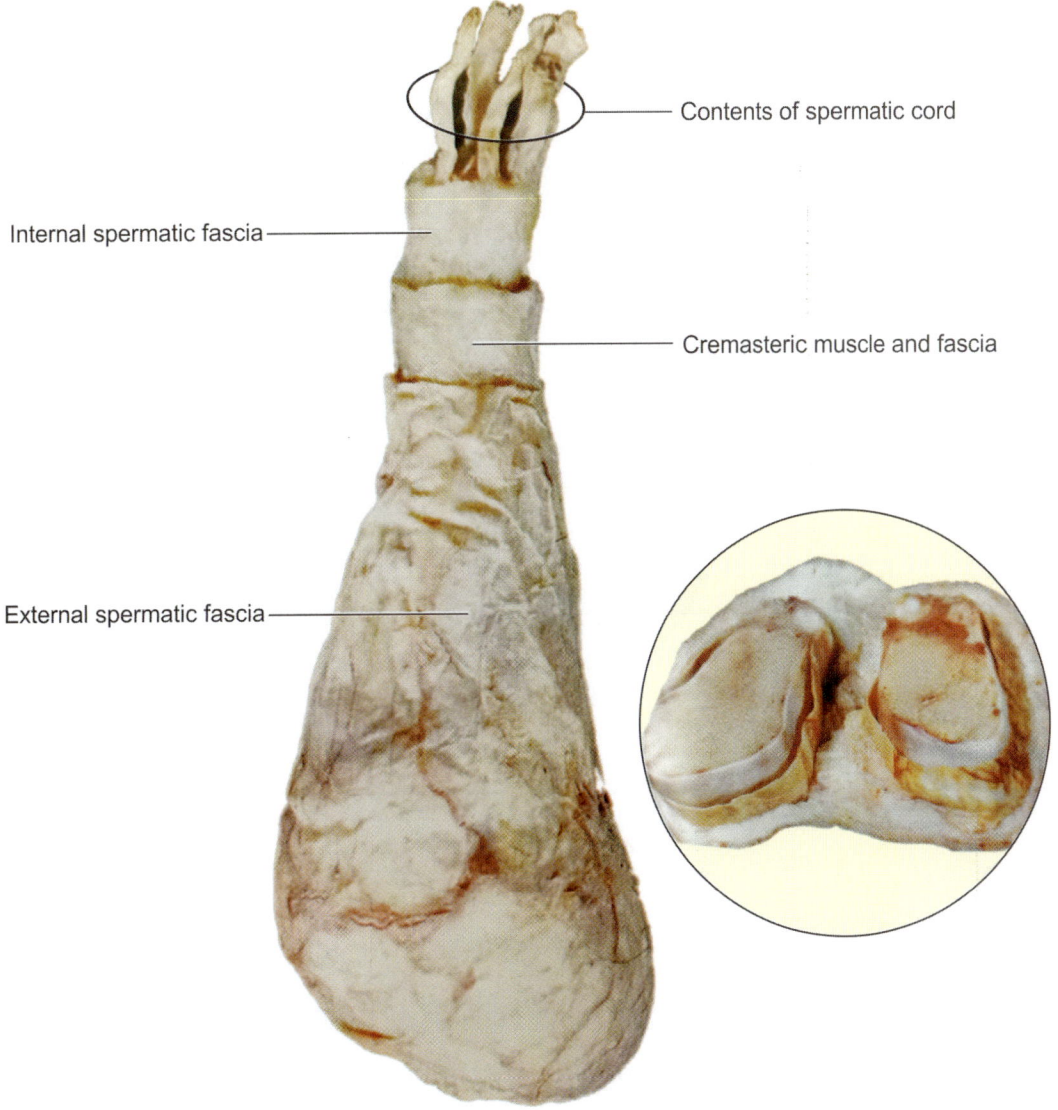

Contents of spermatic cord

Internal spermatic fascia

Cremasteric muscle and fascia

External spermatic fascia

Fig. 27.4: Testis with its coverings

of testis where its contents separate to enter/leave testis.

The contents of spermatic cord are:

i. Ductus deferens, remains of processes vaginalis.

ii. Testicular and cremasteric arteries and artery to ductus deferens.

iii. Pampiniform plexus of veins and lymph vessels.

iv. Genital branch of genitofemoral nerve with autonomic fibres.

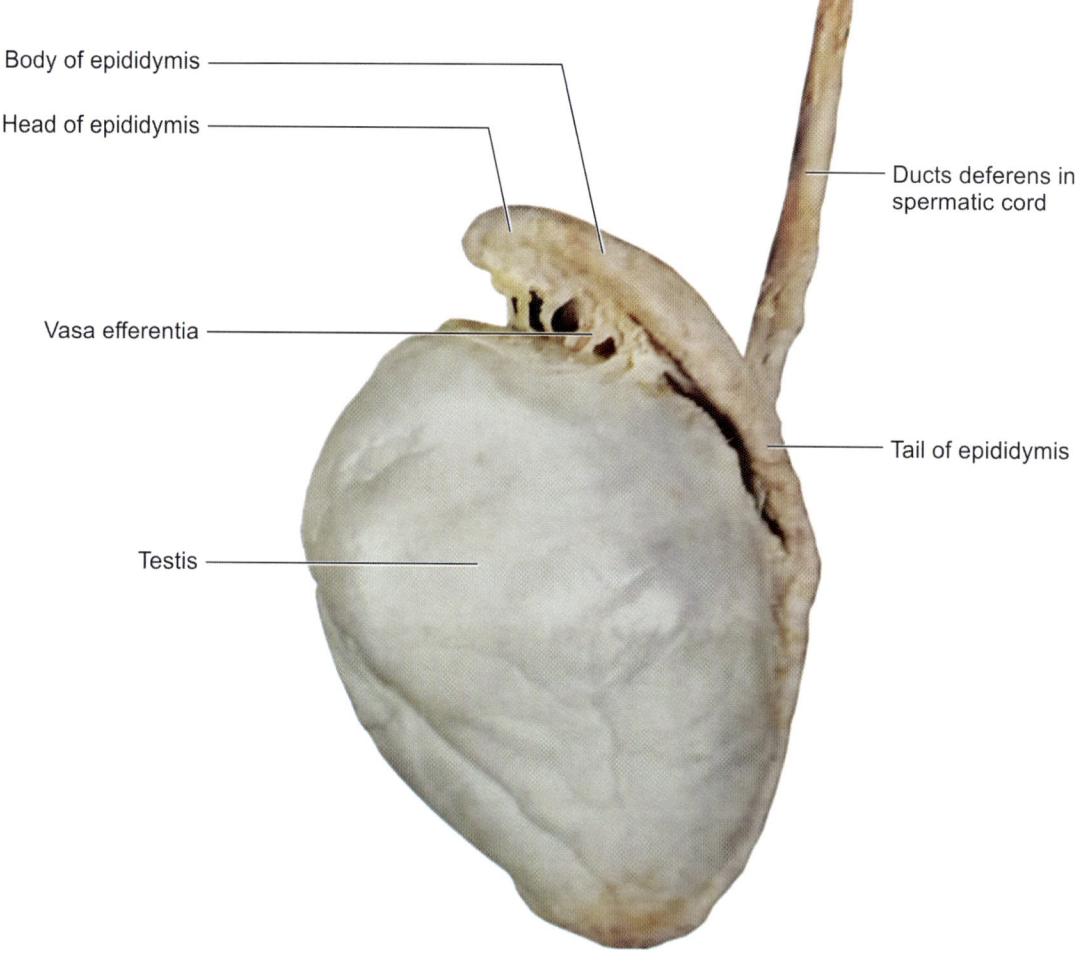

Body of epididymis

Head of epididymis

Vasa efferentia

Testis

Ducts deferens in spermatic cord

Tail of epididymis

Fig. 27.5: Parts of epididymis

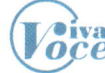

- What is the difference in cavernous tissues of corpus cavernous and corpus spongiosum?
- Why is varicocoele common on the left side?
- Name the parts of epididymis.

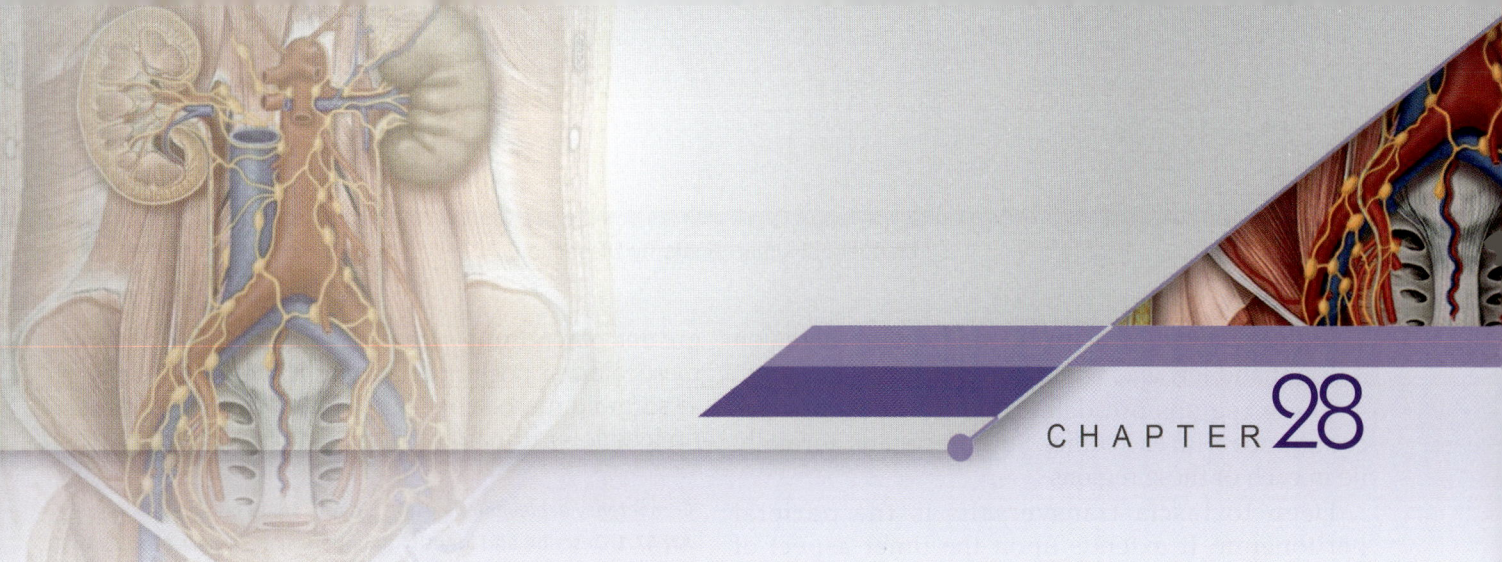

CHAPTER 28

Abdominal Cavity and Peritoneum

Learning Objectives

One should be able to

1. Trace the vertical disposition of peritoneum in female and male.
2. Clinical importance of Morrison's pouch and pouch of Douglas.

OVERVIEW

Abdominal cavity is divided into nine regions by two vertical lines (right and left midclavicular) and two horizontal lines (Fig. 28.1). The horizontal lines, one at the level of 9th costal cartilages and the other at the level of tubercles of iliac crest.

The nine regions are:

1. Right and left hypochondrium with epigastrium

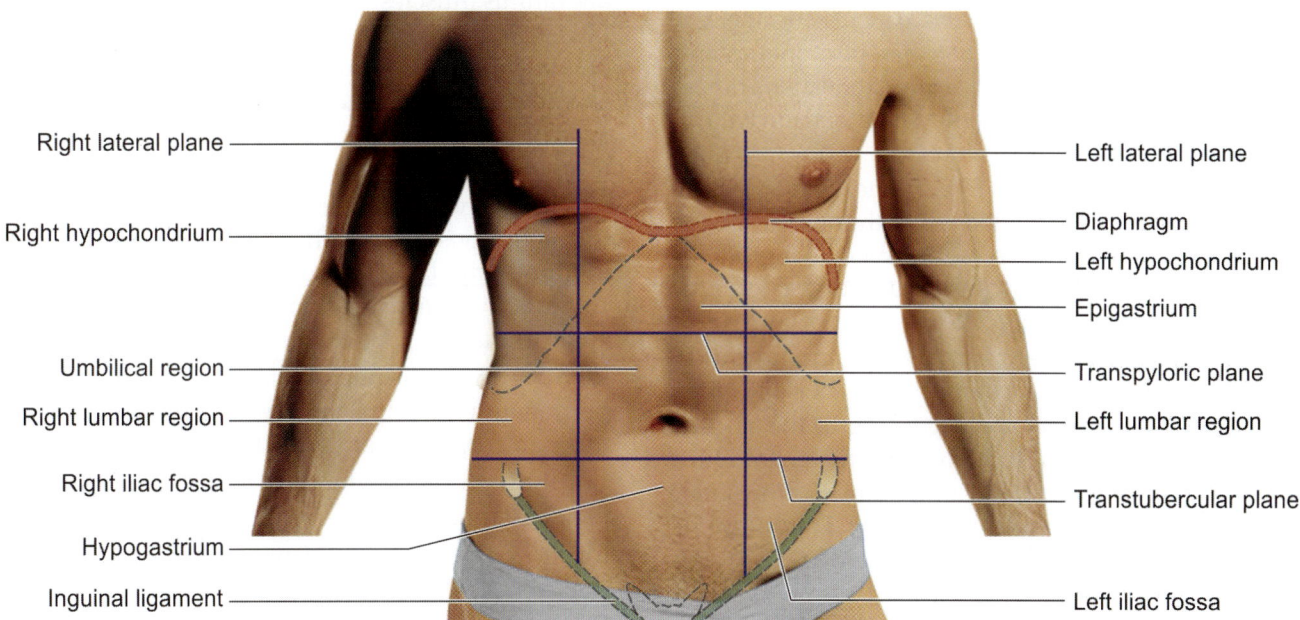

Right lateral plane	Left lateral plane
Right hypochondrium	Diaphragm
	Left hypochondrium
	Epigastrium
Umbilical region	Transpyloric plane
Right lumbar region	Left lumbar region
Right iliac fossa	Transtubercular plane
Hypogastrium	
Inguinal ligament	Left iliac fossa

Fig. 28.1: Four planes dividing the abdominal cavity into nine quadrants

2. Right and left lumbar regions with umbilical region
3. Right and left iliac with hypogastrium

These regions are delineated by lines, but are continuous with each other. Specific organs normally lie in each of these regions.

Deep to fascia transversalis is the parietal peritoneum. It extends upon the inner aspect of diaphragm; on the posterior abdominal wall as the posterior layer of peritoneum. Inferiorly it descends into the true pelvis to enclose the pelvic viscera.

A connecting fold of peritoneum starts from parietal peritoneum and extends into the abdominal cavity to cover the viscera, e.g. stomach, intestines, etc. This is the visceral peritoneum. The peritoneal fluid lies between parietal and visceral layers. Many viscera invaginate from above, behind and below to convert the simple peritoneal cavity into a complicated cavity.

Thus peritoneal cavity is divided into:
a. Greater sac
b. Lesser sac

Greater sac extends in most of the abdominal cavity (Fig. 28.2).

Lesser sac extends only behind stomach and liver in relation to upper part of posterior abdominal wall.

The two sacs are in communication with each other at the opening into the lesser sac.

Some organs, e.g. stomach, jejunum, ileum are intraperitoneal; others like kidneys, pancreas, duodenum are behind the peritoneum, between peritoneum and posterior abdominal wall, i.e. retroperitoneal; still others are covered on three sides: anterior, lateral and medial, e.g. ascending and descending colon.

There are some recesses in peritoneal cavity. Some part of intestine may get locked in them resulting in internal hernia. There are some special regions of peritoneum, e.g. Morrison's pouch and pouch of Douglas. These carry lots of clinical importance.

In females peritoneal cavity is in communication with exterior, so there are more chances of peritonitis.

Various folds are named according to the viscera to which these are attached. To the stomach, folds are lesser omentum and greater omentum. To the small intestine-fold is known as mesentery. To the colon-fold is the transverse and sigmoid mesocolon. To the liver and spleen, folds are known as ligaments.

Peritoneum can be traced from umbilicus → anterior abdominal wall → diaphragm → liver → stomach →

greater omentum → transverse colon → transverse mesocolon → posterior abdominal wall → mesentery → sigmoid mesocolon → in front of rectum → uterus (in female)→ urinary bladder and back to umbilicus.

Competency achievement: The student should be able to:

AN 47.1 Describe and identify boundaries and recesses of lesser and greater sac.

STEPS OF DISSECTION

- After the dissection of rectus sheath and the inguinal canal, reflect the muscles laterally to expose the parietal peritoneum and abdominal cavity. For reflection of muscles give an incision 1 cm left of linea alba (formed by fusion of three muscles of each side in the median plane) from the umbilical region above close to the xiphoid process.

- Extend this incision from umbilical region below to left of pubic symphysis.

- Give one transverse incision from umbilical region to right and left sides of the abdominal wall.

- Thus the abdominal muscles are reflected in quadrants, upper right, upper left, lower right and lower left quadrants.

- See the fascia transversalis lining the deeper aspect of the muscles, their aponeuroses and the rectus abdominis muscles. In relation to recti muscles this fascia alone forms the posterior wall of rectus sheath below the arcuate line. There is no aponeurotic sheath below the arcuate line. Observe the inferior epigastric artery entering the rectus sheath at the level of arcuate line.

- Fascia transversalis in the lowest part of abdomen forms the posterior wall of inguinal canal. Deep inguinal ring (DIR) is also an opening in this fascia 1.2 cm above the midinguinal point. See that inferior epigastric artery runs close to medial border of DIR.

- Identify the extraperitoneal tissue and parietal peritoneum covering the contents like a thin veil, through which viscera seem to be peeping out.

- Cut through the peritoneum in the same plane as the abdominal wall.

- Identify the viscera lying in these quadrants (Fig. 28.2).

The upper right quadrant is occupied by liver, falciform ligament, gallbladder, hepatic flexure of

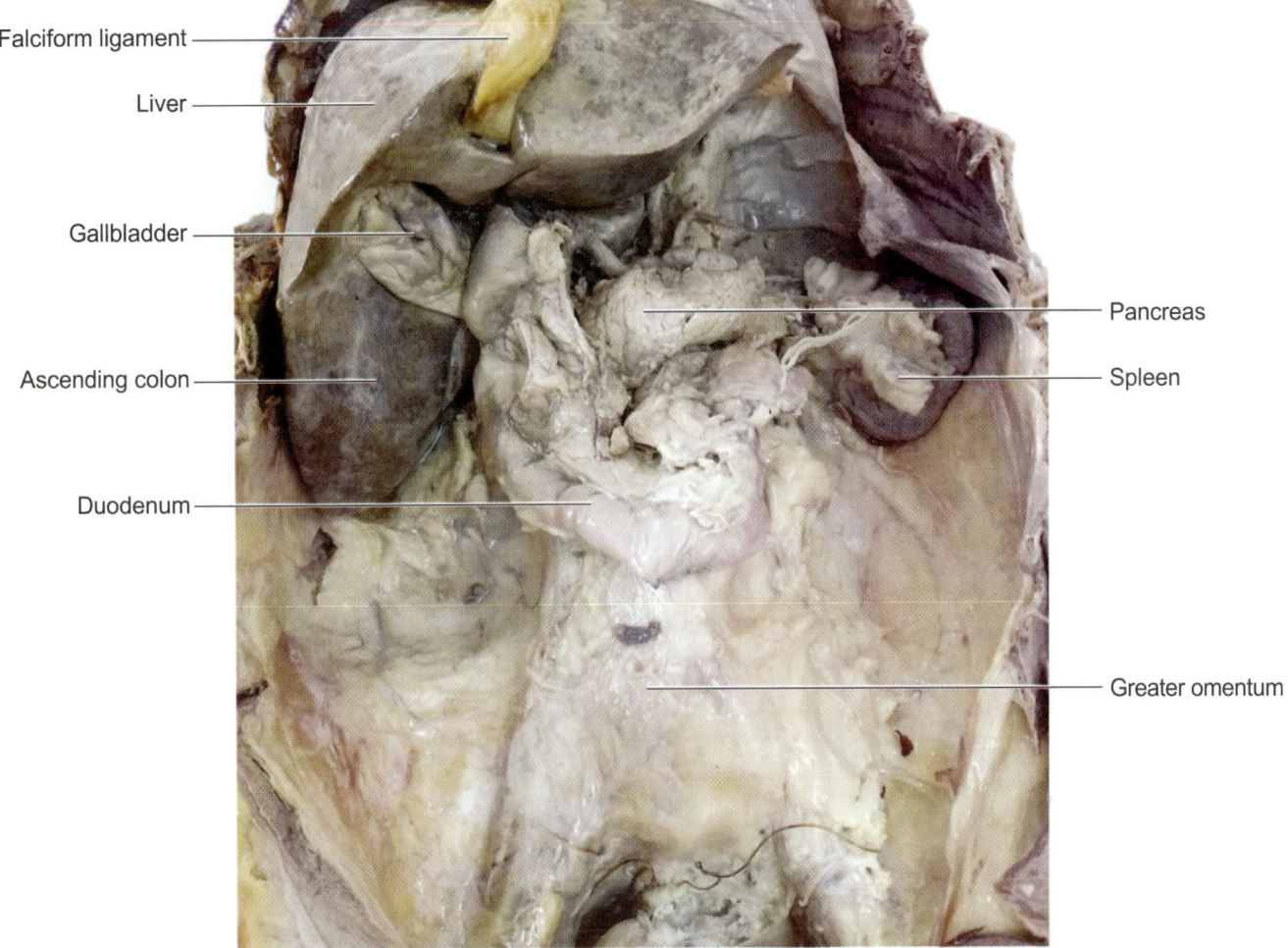

Falciform ligament

Liver

Gallbladder

Ascending colon

Duodenum

Pancreas

Spleen

Greater omentum

Fig. 28.2: Greater sac with organs in upper abdominal cavity

colon, pyloric part of stomach, part of duodenum and pancreas.

The upper left quadrant contains the left lobe of liver, stomach, greater omentum, spleen behind the stomach, splenic flexure of colon and proximal part of descending colon (Fig. 28.3).

The lower right quadrant is occupied by coils of ileum, mesentery, ileo-caecal junction, vermiform appendix and ascending colon (Fig. 28.4).

The lower left quadrant contains left part of transverse colon, descending colon till the left iliac fossa. The descending colon then continues as sigmoid colon in the pelvis.

The kidney and ureters of the urinary system lie on the posterior abdominal wall and are not visible from the anterior aspect.

Competency achievement: The student should be able to:

AN 47.2 Name and identify various peritoneal folds and pouches with its explanation.

• Observe a fold of peritoneum stretching from the umbilicus to the anterior abdominal wall; dome of diaphragm and anterior surface of liver. This fold is the falciform ligament. In its free posterior margin lies the round ligament of liver-ligamentum teres (remnant of left umbilical vein) which passes towards porta hepatis of liver to end in the left branch of portal vein. Other folds of peritoneum will be dealt while studying the liver. Examine the posterior surfaces of the reflected lowest parts of anterior abdominal wall. Identify five ill defined peritoneal folds which pass upwards towards the umbilicus.

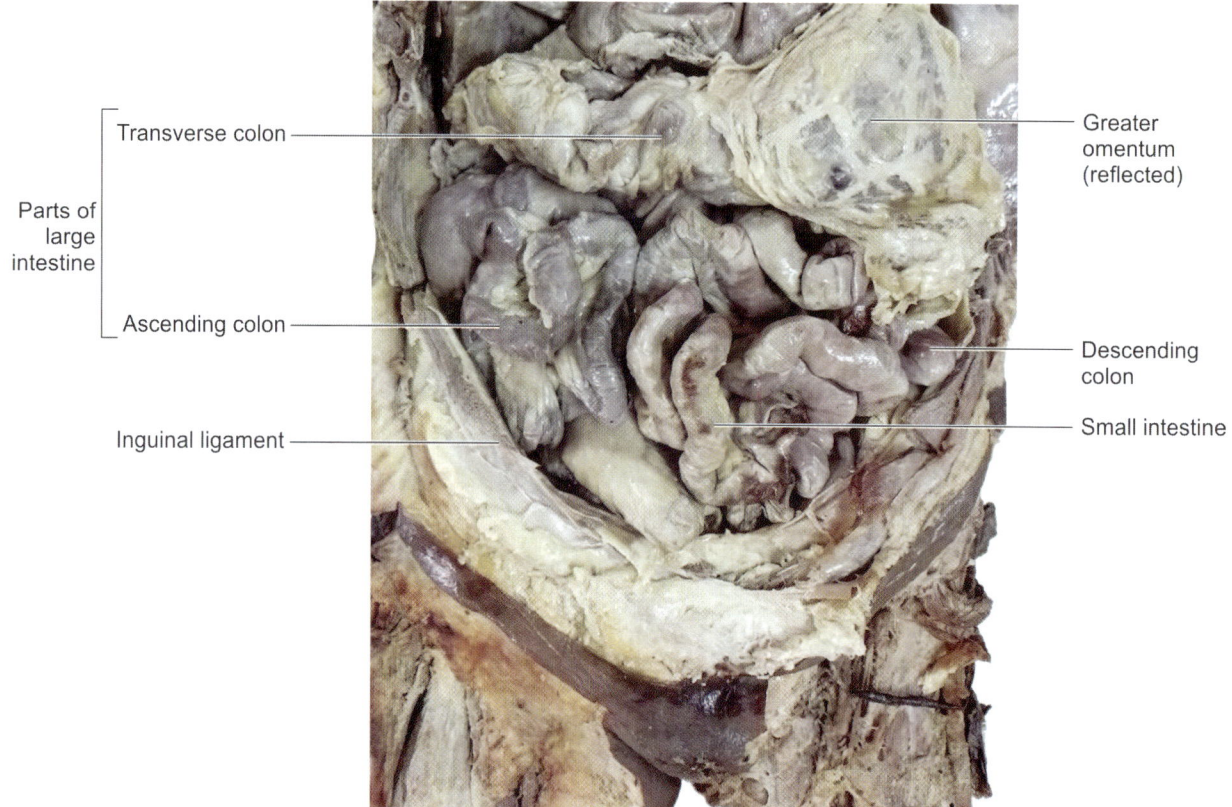

Transverse colon

Parts of large intestine

Ascending colon

Inguinal ligament

Greater omentum (reflected)

Descending colon

Small intestine

Fig. 28.3: Small and large intestine

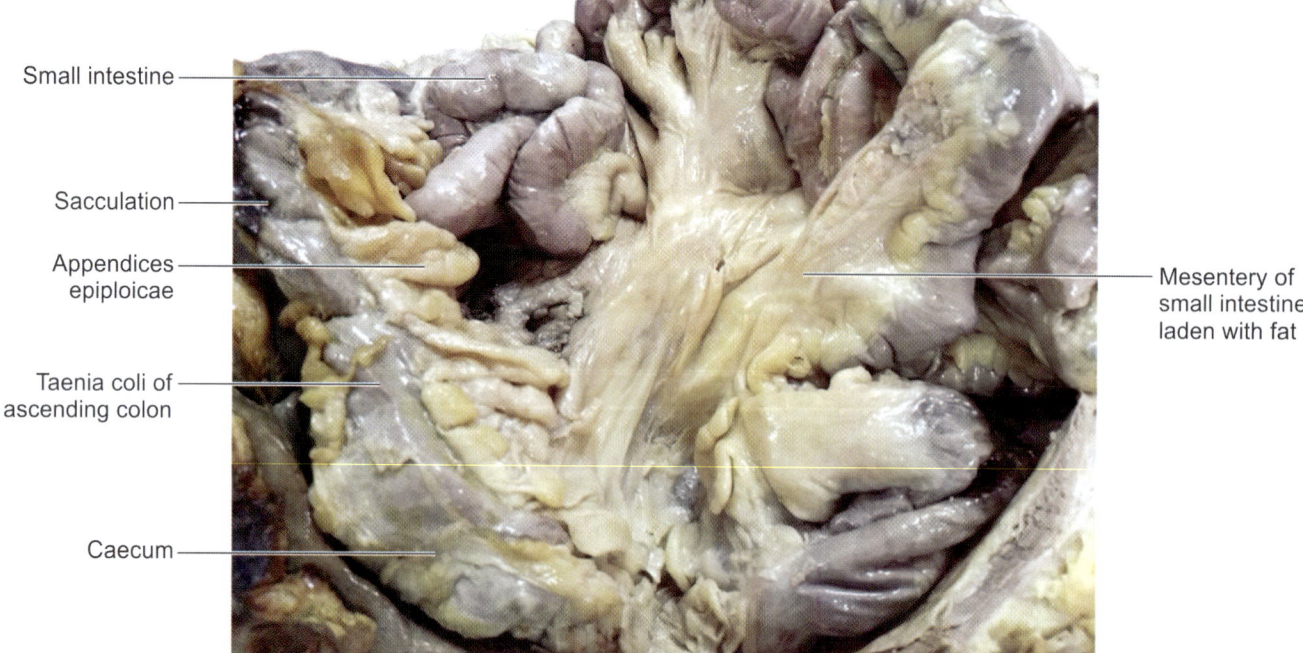

Small intestine

Sacculation

Appendices epiploicae

Taenia coli of ascending colon

Caecum

Mesentery of small intestine laden with fat

Fig. 28.4: Mesentery, caecum and ascending colon

The median fold is formed due to median umbilical ligament (remnant of urachus). The two medial umbilical folds are formed due to presence of medial umbilical ligaments (remnant of obliterated umbilical arteries).

The two lateral umbilical folds are formed due to presence of inferior epigastric arteries. These pass upwards and medially, cross the arcuate line to enter the rectus sheath.

- The parietal peritoneum has been identified. It is adherent to the parieties or wall of the abdominal cavity. Trace it from the walls to form various double layered folds which spread out to enclose the viscera as visceral peritoneum. Identify the prominent greater omentum (Fig. 28.5). Gently spread it out. It hangs down like a curtain covering the intestines.

- See the two layers of greater omentum hanging down almost till midway between umbilicus and pubic symphysis. Then it folds upon itself and as it passes upwards it encloses the transverse colon (Fig. 28.5). So the transverse colon seems to be

hanging from back of stomach. Thus, greater omentum comprises 4 layers—2 anterior (1, 2) and 2 posterior (3, 4 in Fig 28.8a).

- Cut through the 1 and 2 layers of the greater omentum, 2–3 cm inferior to the gastroepiploic arteries, to open the lower part of the omental bursa (inferior recess of lesser sac) sufficiently to admit a hand. Explore the bursa.

Greater omentum is attached along the greater curvature of stomach. On the left side there are 2 more folds, one passing from stomach to spleen-gastrosplenic ligament and the other stretching from fundus of stomach to the diaphragm-gastrophrenic ligament.

- Pull the liver superiorly and lift its inferior margin anteriorly to expose the lesser omentum. Examine the right free margin of lesser omentum, containing the bile duct, proper hepatic artery and portal vein.

- This free margin forms the anterior boundary of the opening into the lesser sac, i.e. epiploic foramen. The posterior boundary is the inferior vena cava. Superior to opening into the lesser sac is the caudate

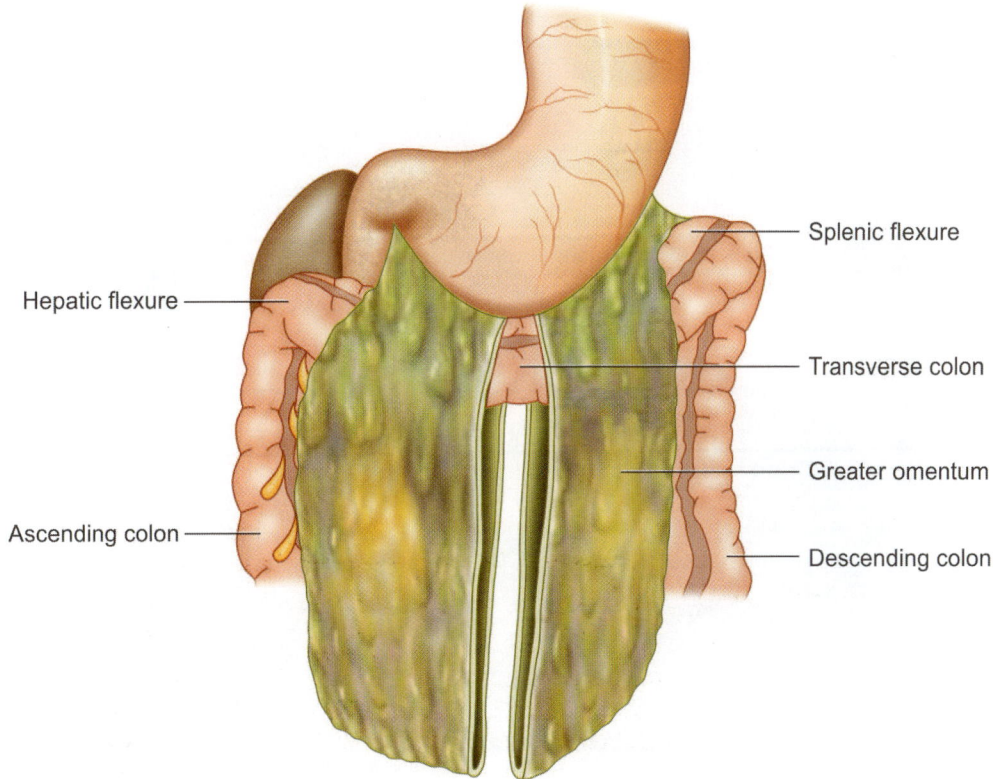

Hepatic flexure

Ascending colon

Splenic flexure

Transverse colon

Greater omentum

Descending colon

Fig. 28.5: Greater omentum like a curtain

process of liver and inferiorly is the first part of duodenum.

- Remove the anterior layer of peritoneum from the lesser omentum along the lesser curvature of the stomach.
- Find and trace the left gastric vessels along the lesser curvature of stomach. Trace the oesophageal branches to the oesophagus. Trace the right gastric artery to the proper hepatic artery and the vein to the portal vein.
- Expose the proper hepatic artery and trace its branches to the porta hepatis of liver.
- Identify the gallbladder with its fundus, body, neck and cystic duct. Trace the cystic duct from the gall bladder. Follow the common hepatic duct from the porta hepatis till it is joined by cystic duct to form the bile duct. Trace the bile duct till it passes behind the duodenum.

Lesser Omentum, Mesentery and Mesoappendix

- Remove the remains of the lesser omentum leaving the vessels and duct intact and examine the abdominal wall posterior to the omentum and the omental bursa.
- Turn the small intestine to the left. Cut through the right layer of peritoneum of the mesentery along the line of its attachment to the posterior abdominal wall and strip it from the mesentery. Remove the fat from the mesentery to expose the superior mesenteric vessels in its root and their branches and tributaries in the mesentery.
- Trace the superior mesenteric vessels proximally and distally. Dissect the branches to the jejunum, ileum, caecum, appendix, ascending colon, right two-thirds of transverse colon, the distal part of duodenum and pancreas.
- Turn the small intestine and its mesentery to the right. Remove the peritoneum and fat on the posterior abdominal wall between the mesentery and descending colon to expose the inferior mesenteric vessels and autonomic nerves and lymph nodes associated with them.
- Turn the caecum upwards and uncover the structures posterior to it. Trace the three taeniae on

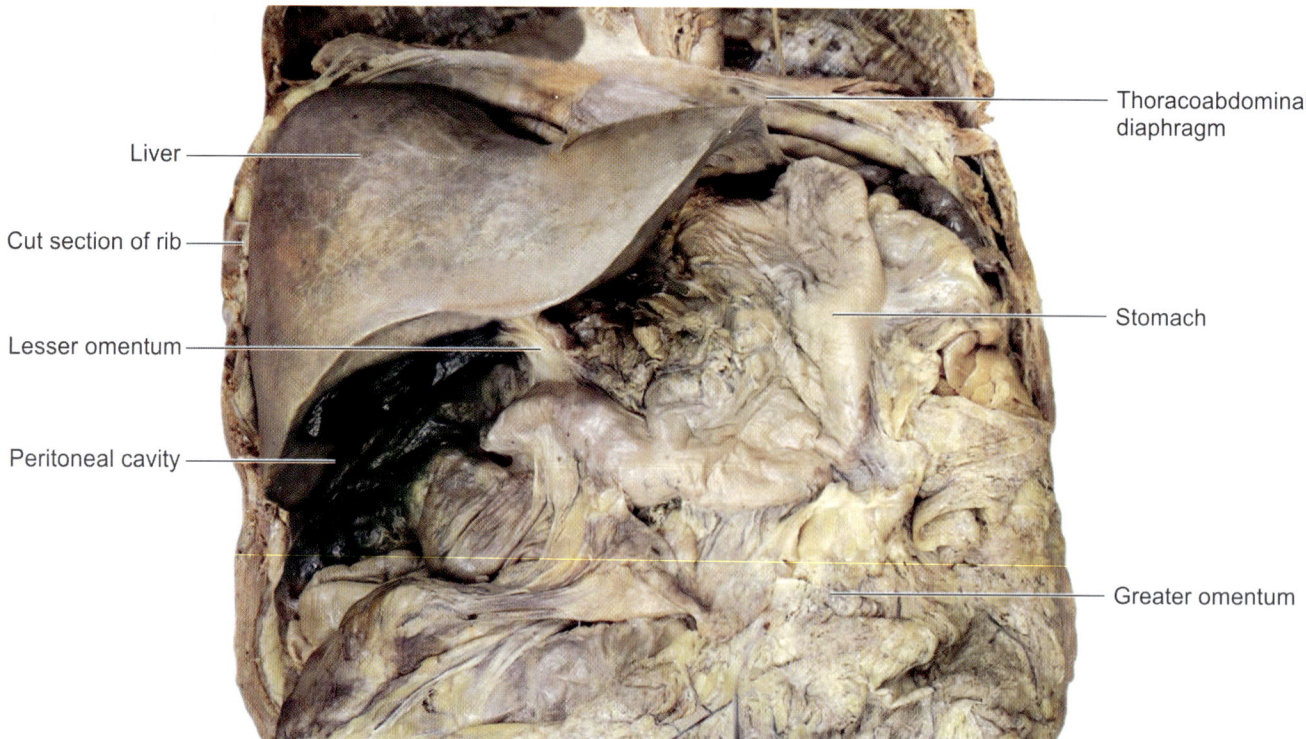

Fig. 28.6: Viscera in upper abdominal cavity including the lesser omentum (gateway to omental bursa)

the external surface of the colon and cranial to the root of the vermiform appendix (Fig. 28.7). The three taeniae are anterior or taenia libera, posterolateral or taenia omentalis and posteromedial or taenia mesocolica.

- At the hepatic flexure the ascending colon continues as transverse colon by bending at right angle (Fig. 28.7). There is some amount of twisting of the colon and the taeniae are repositioned.
  1. Taenia anterior/taenia libera is placed inferiorly in transverse colon.
  2. Posteromedial taenia is placed on posterior surface of transverse colon.
  3. Posterolateral taenia is placed on anterosuperior surface of transverse colon.

Peritoneal cavity is a closed cavity in males. The cavity is open to outside through vagina, uterus and fallopian tubes in females. So peritonitis is common even in young girls.

Various organs invaginate into the peritoneal cavity. Some are completely enveloped by peritoneum. These are intraperitoneal organs, e.g. stomach, jejunum, ileum, transverse colon and sigmoid colon.

Some organs are covered only on their anterior aspects. These organs are called retroperitoneal organs, e.g. most of duodenum, pancreas, kidneys and ureters.

Few organs are covered by peritoneum on three sides. These are called partially covered organs, e.g. ascending colon and descending colon.

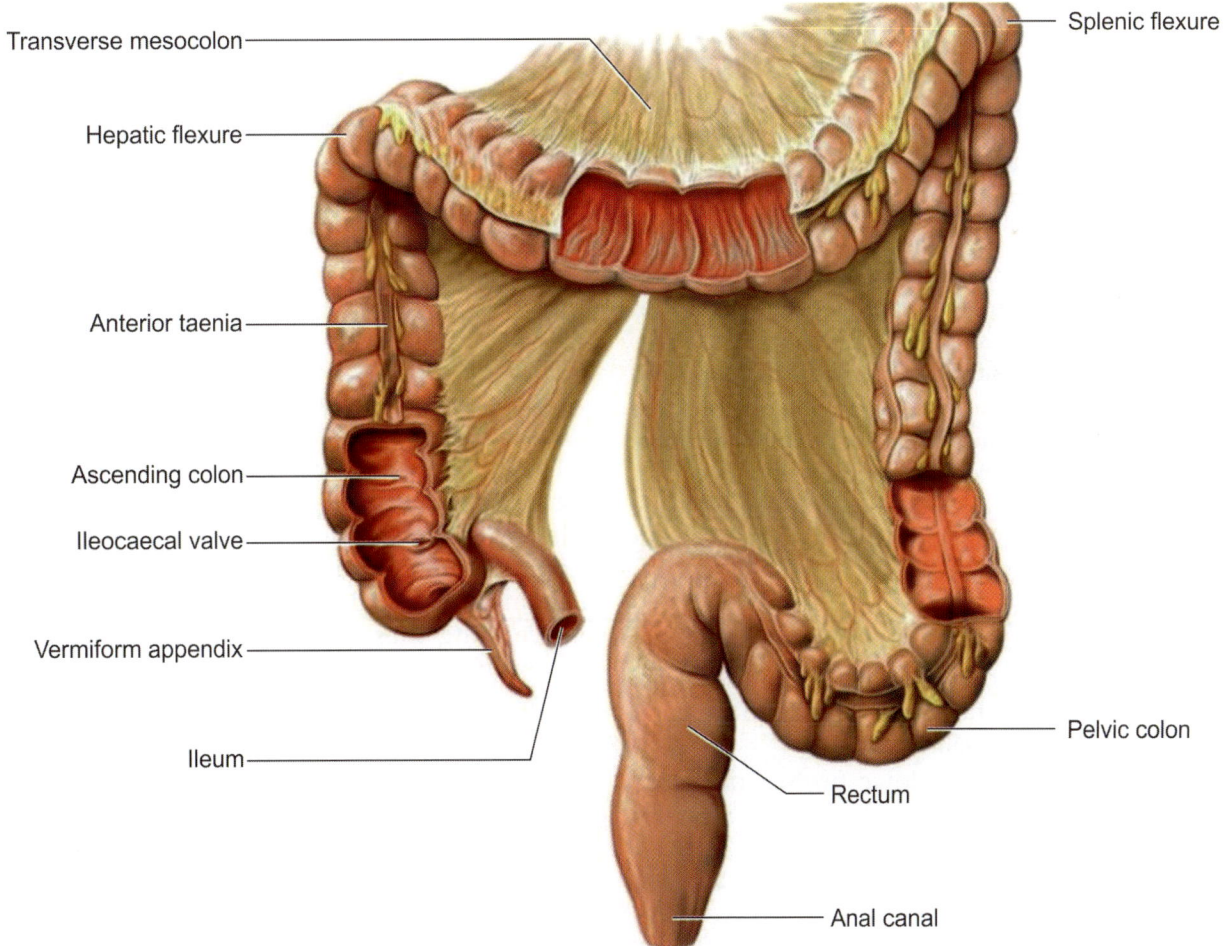

Fig. 28.7: Parts of large intestine including vermiform appendix

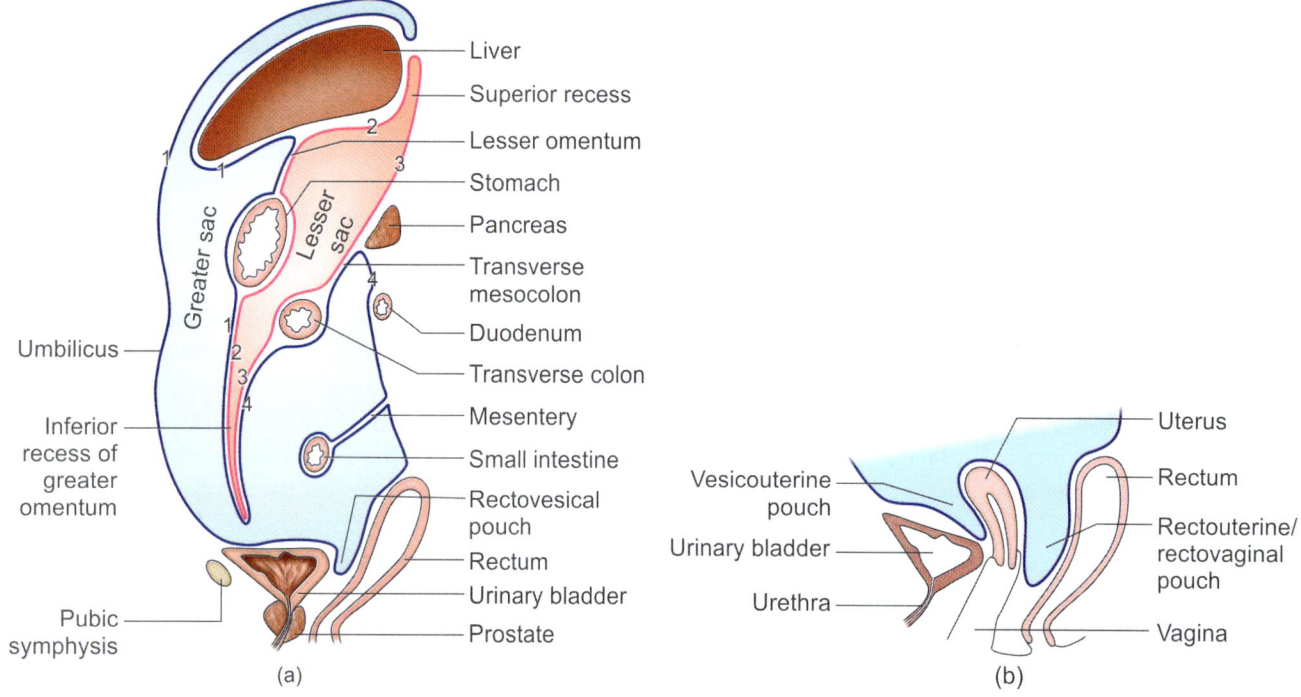

Fig. 28.8: Sagittal tracing of peritoneum: (a) Male pelvis; (b) Female pelvis

Transverse Mesocolon

It is already seen that 1st and 2nd layers of greater omentum are pleated and descend in abdominal cavity to varying degree. Then these layers fold on themselves, 1st layer becomes 4th layer and 2nd layer continues as 3rd layer. The 3rd and 4th layers on ascending, enclose the transverse colon and continue as transverse mesocolon (Figs 28.7 and 28.8), which is attached to anterior border of pancreas.

The third layer passes up covering the structures in upper part of posterior abdominal wall. From there it is reflected on posterior surface of liver and forms superior recess of lesser sac.

The fourth layer descends down covering the structures in lower part of posterior abdominal wall. At the level of L2 vertebra, it starts to enclose the small intestine forming its mesentery.

Then 4th layer descends down further to enclose sigmoid colon only on the left side. Finally it reaches the pelvic cavity.

Sagittal Tracing of Peritoneum

- Start from umbilicus. See double fold of peritoneum, the falciform ligament. Its two layers line the deep aspect of anterior abdominal wall, domes of diaphragm, superior surface, anterior surface and inferior surface of liver till porta hepatis (Fig. 28.8a).

- At porta hepatis it is joined by 3rd layer of greater omentum. Now these 2 layers of peritoneum form lesser omentum which descends down to lesser curvature of stomach. The 2 layers split to enclose stomach and at its greater curvature again come together. These 2 layers descend down as 1st and 2nd layers of greater omentum. These two layers fold upon themselves to form 3rd and 4th layers. While ascending these enclose transverse colon and then fuse to form transverse mesocolon.

- Third layer ascends up to form upper part of lesser sac.

- Fourth layer forms mesentery of small intestine and sigmoid mesocolon and then reaches pelvic cavity.

- In the pelvis in male, this layer forms rectovesical pouch between rectum and urinary bladder.

- Lastly it covers superior surface of urinary bladder, lines the deep aspect of muscles of anterolateral abdominal wall and reaches the umbilicus.

- In the pelvic cavity in female, this layer forms deep rectouterine pouch, covers whole posterior, superior and part of anterior surface of uterus (Fig. 28.8b). Then it forms shallow vesicouterine pouch, covers superior surface of urinary bladder and lines the deep aspect of muscles of anterolateral abdominal wall and reaches the umbilicus.

Epiploic Foramen/Foramen of Winslow/Opening to the Lesser Sac

- Identify the vertical slit like opening through which the lesser sac communicates with greater sac. This foramen is situated behind the right free margin of the lesser omentum at the level of 12th thoracic vertebra (Fig. 28.6).
- Above the foramen look for caudate process of liver. Identify first part of duodenum lying inferior to the epiploic foramen.

Peritoneal Recesses/Fossae

At the junction of intraperitoneal and retroperitoneal viscera there are small pockets of peritoneal cavity enclosed by small folds of peritoneum. These have clinical significance as being sites for internal hernia and strangulation. These are:

Duodenal Recesses

- Identify superior duodenal recess, if present. Put the finger in its orifice which looks downwards.
- Look for inferior duodenal recess, if present. Put your finger in it. Its orifice looks upwards.
- Orifice of paraduodenal recess looks to right. Identify inferior mesenteric vein in its free edge.
- See retroduodenal recess (if present) is about 3 cm deep. Its orifice looks downwards and to the left.

Ileocaecal Recesses

- Superior ileocaecal recess is mostly present. It contains a branch from ileocolic artery. Its orifice looks downwards and to the left.
- Inferior ileocaecal recess is covered by bloodless fold of Treves. Its orifice looks downwards and to the left.
- Retrocaecal recess lies behind the caecum, containing vermiform appendix.

Intersigmoid Recess

Intersigmoid recess lies behind apex of sigmoid mesocolon. See that its orifice looks downwards.

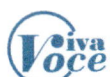

- Name the nine regions of the abdominal cavity proper.
- Which viscera lies in right iliac fossa?
- Why is greater omentum called 'abdominal policeman'?
- Name the viscera which are retroperitoneal.
- Name the boundaries of hepatorenal pouch.
- Name the boundaries of rectouterine pouch.
- Why is peritonitis common in females?

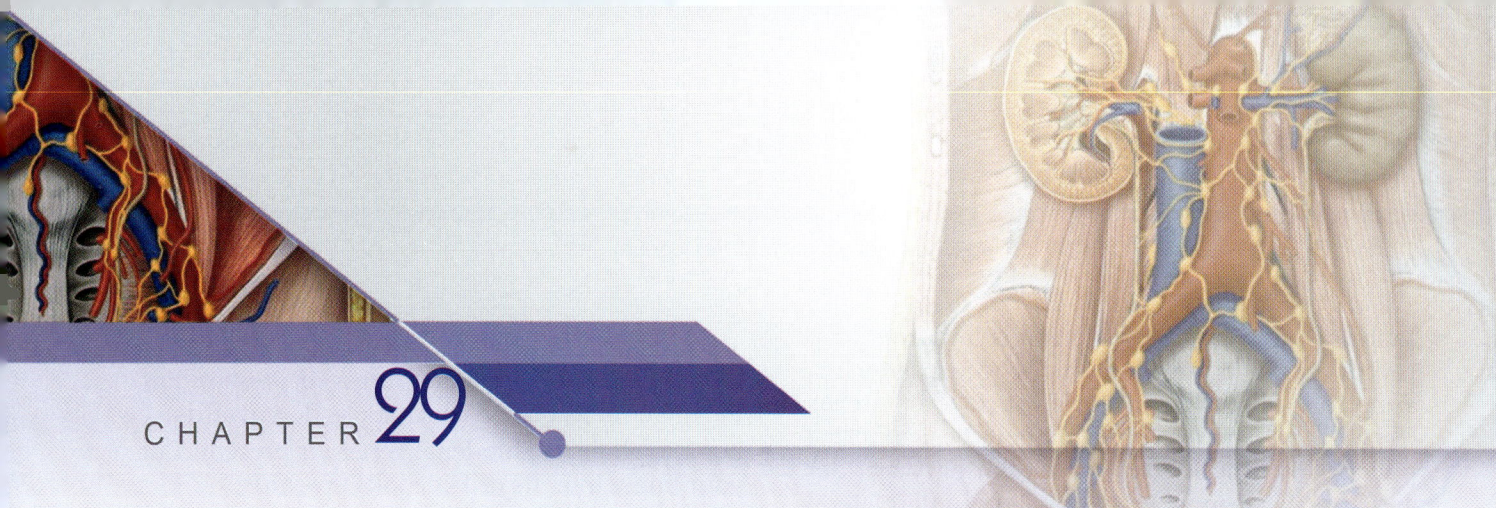

CHAPTER 29

Abdominal Part of Oesophagus and Stomach

Learning Objectives

One should be able to

1. Name the veins which form portosystemic anastomosis at the lower end of oesophagus.

2. What is the importance of gastric canal

3. Effects of parasympathetic nerves on the stomach.

OVERVIEW

Oesophagus is a long tube starting in the neck, coursing through the thorax, piercing the diaphragm and terminating in the abdomen. The abdominal part of oesophagus is only 1.25 cm. The artery to this part of oesophagus is by branches of left gastric artery. The venous drainage is partly into accessory hemiazygos → vena azygos and into superior vena cava; and partly into portal vein via left gastric vein. Thus, this is an important site of portocaval anastomosis. In liver cirrhosis, these veins may get dilated, tortuous and even rupture resulting in haematemesis.

Stomach is the most distensible part of gastro-intestinal tract, occupying epigastrium, left hypochondriac and umbilical regions. It comprises cardiac, fundus, body and pyloric regions. The stomach is resting on its bed, comprising of transverse colon, mesocolon, pancreas, splenic artery, left kidney, left suprarenal gland and diaphragm. All these organs do not get compressed by full stomach due to the presence of fluid in lesser sac of peritoneum.

Stomach is supplied by branches of coeliac axis artery; the first ventral branch of the abdominal aorta.

Active or parasympathetic nerve supply is by vagus. It increases the secretion of gastric juice,

stimulates peristalsis and inhibits the pyloric sphincter. Sympathetic supply is from T2 to T5 sympathetic ganglia and has opposite effects.

The inside of stomach shows longitudinal folds of mucous membrane. The muscular coat comprises outer longitudinal, middle circular and innermost oblique layer of muscle fibres.

Competency achievement: The student should be able to:

AN 47.5 Describe and demonstrate major viscera of abdomen under following headings (anatomical position, external and internal features, important peritoneal and other relations, blood supply, nerve supply, lymphatic drainage and applied aspects).

STEPS OF DISSECTION

- Cut and remove 6th and 7th costal cartilages. Identify the stomach and trace it towards the abdominal part of oesophagus. Clean this part of oesophagus.

- See the arterial supply of this part of oesophagus from branches of left gastric artery and from aorta.

- Venous drainage is partly into left gastric vein (tributary of portal vein) and partly into accessory hemiazygos vein which ends in vena azygos. The vena azygos drains into superior vena cava (systemic circulation).

There is some amount of venous anastomoses between portal venous system and caval venous system.

- Identify the biggest component of gastrointestinal tract—the stomach.
- Note various parts of stomach, e.g. cardiac end, fundus, body and pyloric parts (Fig. 29.1).
- Fundus is the part of stomach above the oesophageal opening.
- Trace the right and left gastric arteries along the lesser curvature of stomach.
- Similarly identify the right and left gastroepiploic arteries along the greater curvature.

- Tie two ligatures close to each other at the lowest part of oesophagus and another two ligatures at the pylorus. Pylorus can easily be identified by thickened musculature.
- Now incise oesophagus, left gastric artery, gastro-phrenic ligament between upper two ligatures.
- Similarly incise pyloric part between lower two ligatures. Free the stomach from the adjacent peritoneum, if any and put it in a tray for further dissection. Identify the cardiac end and thick pyloric end.
- Identify the concave lesser curvature and a big convex greater curvature of stomach.

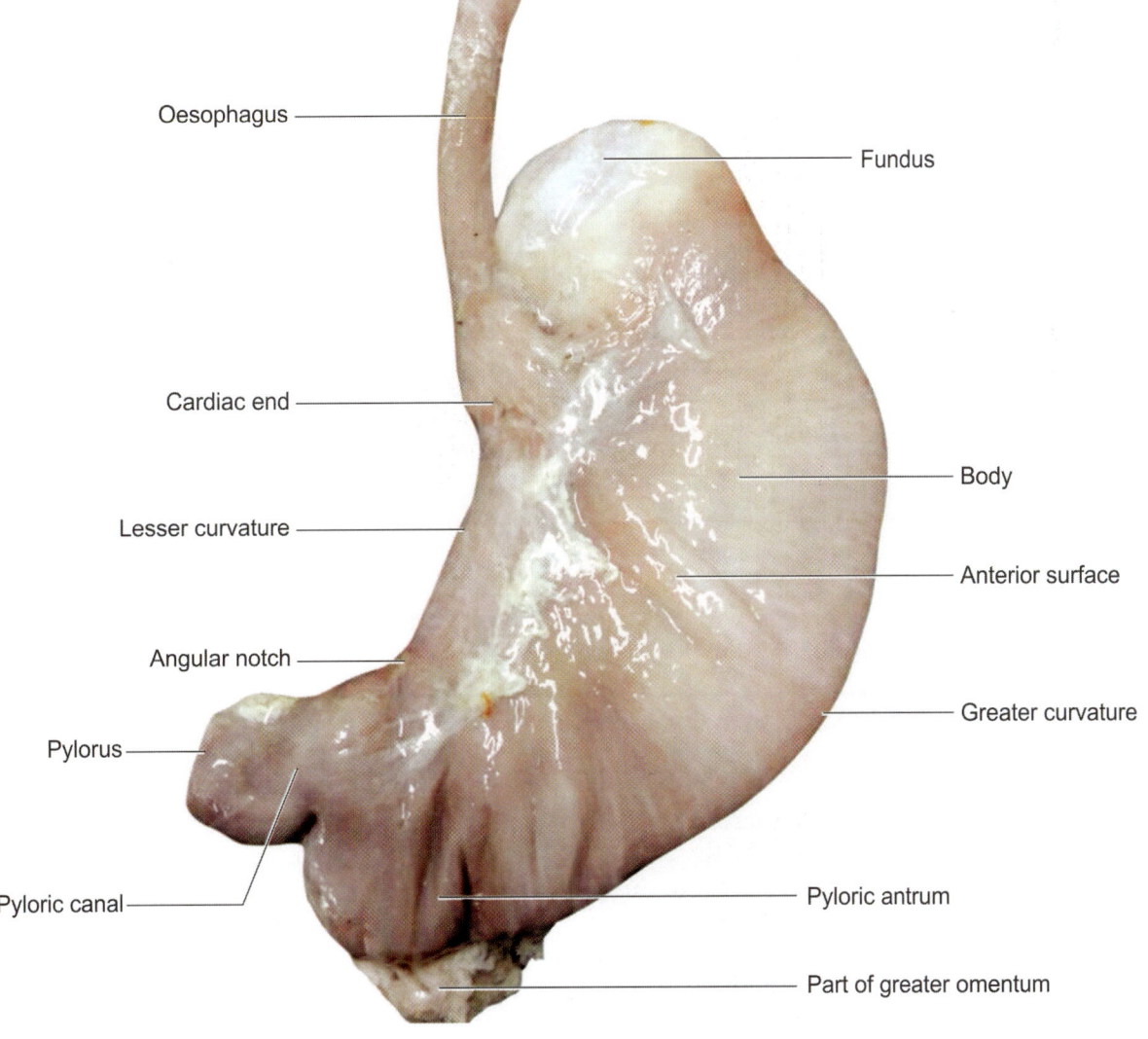

Fig. 29.1: Parts of stomach

- Identify the angular notch at the lowest part of lesser curvature.
- The larger cardiac part is subdivided into fundus and body.
- The smaller pyloric part is subdivided into pyloric antrum, pyloric canal and the thickened pylorus.

Peritoneal Relations

Lesser omentum from porta hepatis and fissure for ligamentum venosum extends to lesser curvature of stomach and first 5 cm of duodenum. It splits at lesser curvature of stomach to enclose the stomach. So it forms visceral peritoneum of the stomach.

The greater omentum is formed at the greater curvature of stomach by fusion of two layers which have enclosed the stomach (Fig. 29.2).

- From the back of fundus identify a fold of peritoneum which goes towards diaphragm. This is the gastrophrenic ligament.

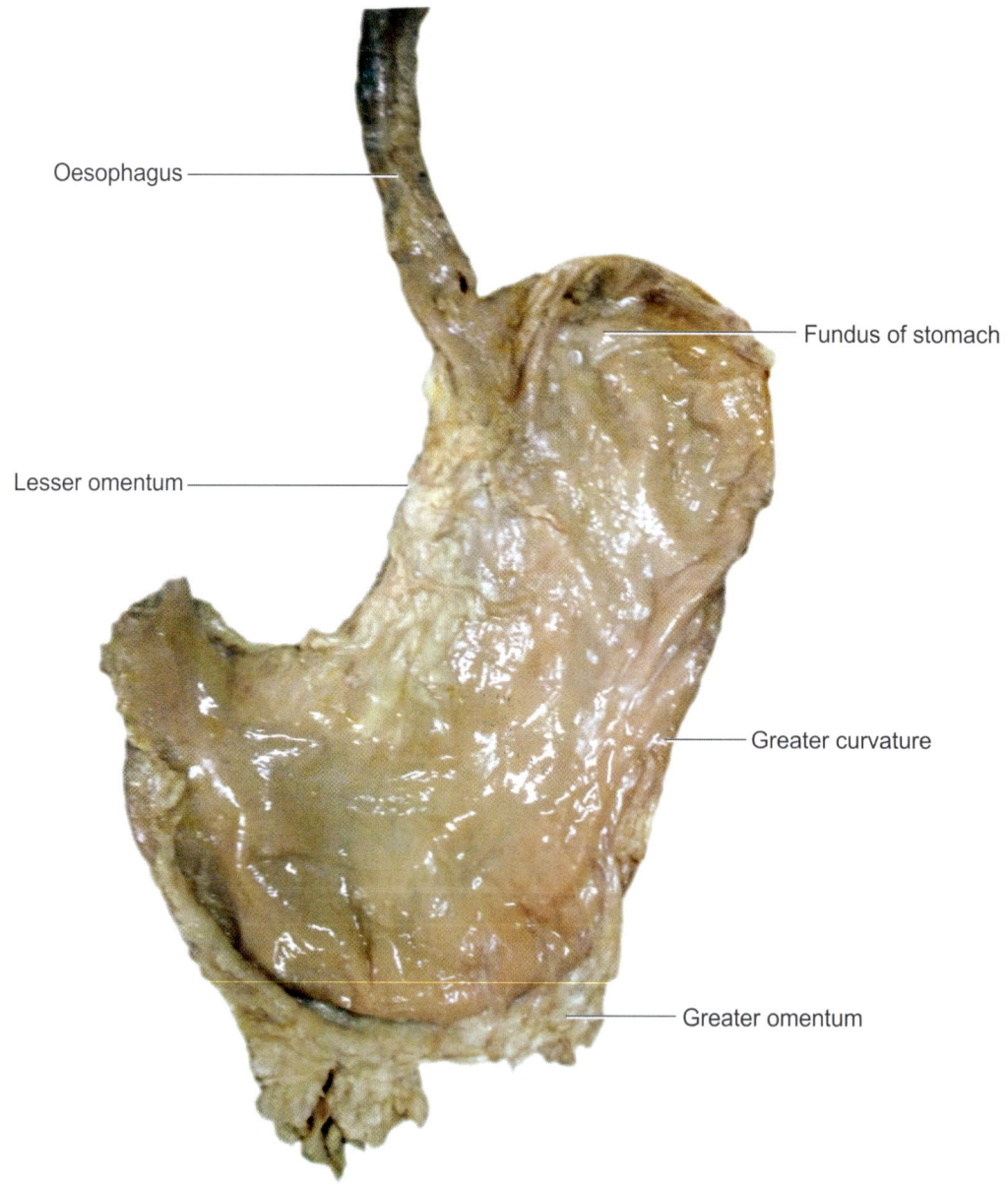

Oesophagus

Lesser omentum

Fundus of stomach

Greater curvature

Greater omentum

Fig. 29.2: Lesser and greater omenta

The stomach is related posteriorly to left dome of diaphragm, left kidney, left suprarenal, pancreas, splenic artery and transverse mesocolon. Identify all these structures as these form the stomach bed.

Blood Supply

- See the arteries supplying the stomach.
    1. Left and right gastric arteries along the lesser curvature of stomach.
    2. Left and right gastroepiploic arteries along the greater curvature.
    3. Five to seven short gastric branches to the fundus of stomach.

- Venous drainage
    1. Left and right gastric veins drain into the portal vein.
    2. Left gastroepiploic and short gastric veins drain into the splenic vein.
    3. Right gastroepiploic vein ends in the superior mesenteric vein.

Interior of Stomach

- Cut open the stomach by an incision on the anterior surface 2 cm away from the lesser curvature. Extend the incision from its upper end till the greater curvature of stomach and examine the mucous membrane (Fig. 29.3). Identify the longitudinal

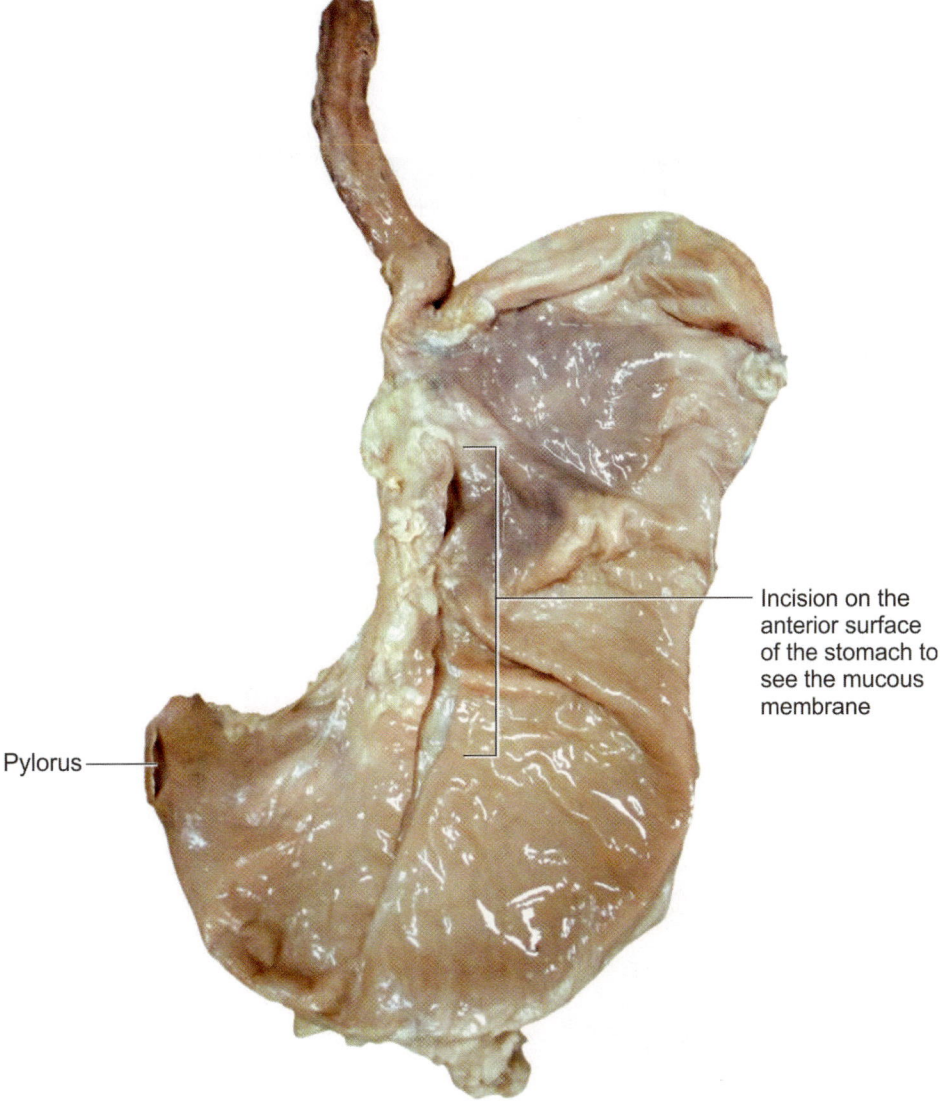

Pylorus

Incision on the anterior surface of the stomach to see the mucous membrane

Fig. 29.3: Incision on the anterior surface of stomach

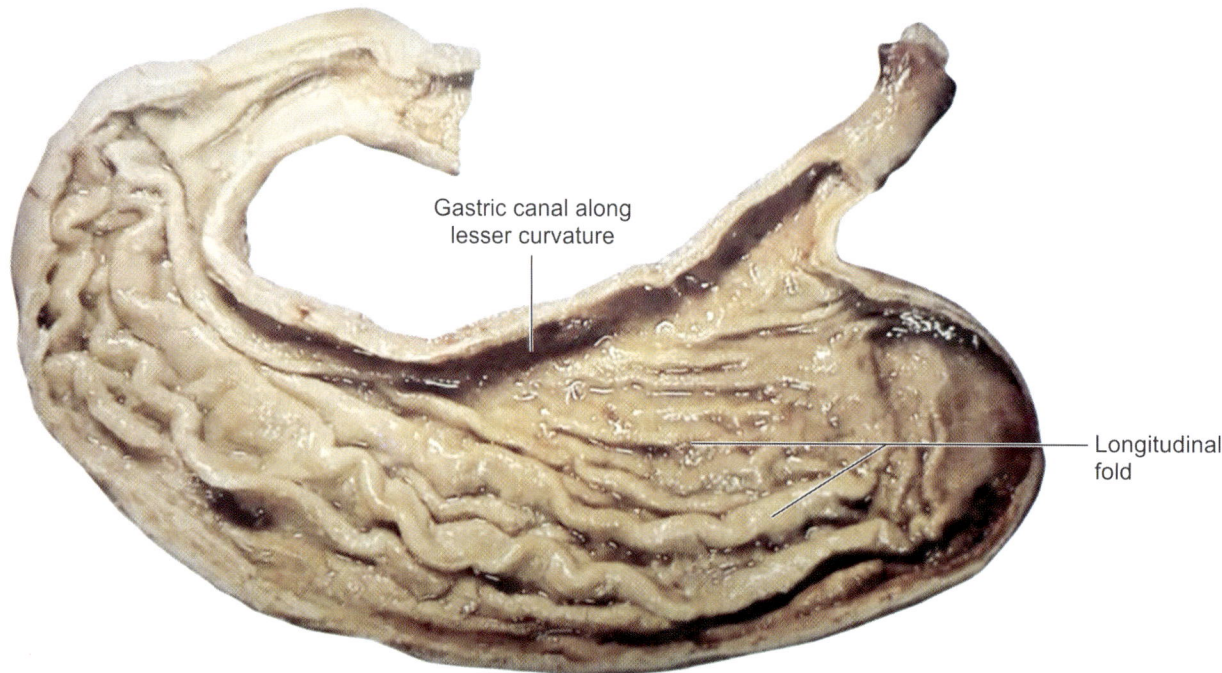

Fig. 29.4: Longitudinal folds of mucous membrane of stomach including the gastric canal

folds of mucous membrane (Fig. 29.4). Try to see the opening of gastric glands with the help of hand lens.

- Next strip the mucous membrane from one part to expose the internal muscle layer.

- Dissect the muscle coat, e.g. outer longitudinal, middle circular and inner oblique muscle fibres (Fig. 29.5). Feel the thickened pyloric sphincter.
- Identify gastric canal along the lesser curvature (Fig. 29.4). See that this canal is deficient in oblique fibres.

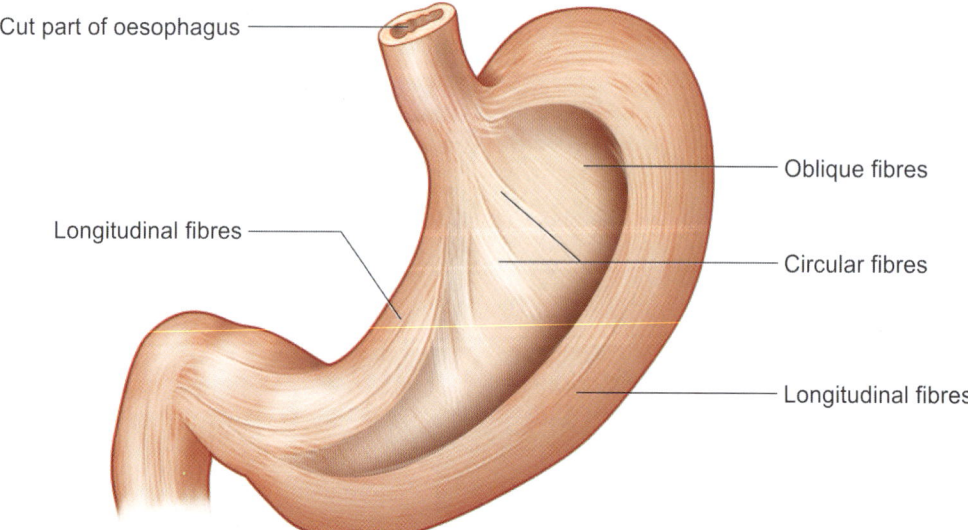

Fig. 29.5: Outer longitudinal middle circular and inner oblique muscle fibres

- Incise the beginning of duodenum and examine the duodenal and pyloric aspects of pyloric sphincter.

Lymphatic Drainage

- Identify the left gastric, coeliac, hepatic and right gastroepiploic lymph nodes along these respective arteries.
- Also identify pyloric lymph nodes inferior to pylorus and pancreatico-splenic nodes.
- Divide the stomach by a line into medial 2/3rd and lateral 1/3rd part which is further subdivided into upper 1/3rd and lower 2/3rd parts. Lymph from the various areas drain to the nearest lymph nodes.

Nerve Supply

The stomach is supplied by sympathetic and parasympathetic nerves.

The sympathetic nerves are derived from thoracic six to ten segments of the spinal cord, via the greater splanchnic nerves, coeliac and hepatic plexuses. These travel along the arteries supplying the stomach.

These nerves are:

a. Vasomotor

b. Motor to the pyloric sphincter, but inhibitory to the rest of the gastric musculature

c. The chief pathway for pain sensations from stomach The parasympathetic nerves are derived from the vagi, through the oesophageal plexus and gastric nerves. Parasympathetic nerves are motor and secretomotor to the stomach. Their stimulation causes increased motility of the stomach and secretion of gastric juice rich in pepsin and HCl.

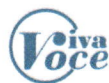 **Viva Voce**

- What veins anastomose at the lower end of oesophagus?
- Name the structures forming the stomach bed.
- Why is gastric ulcer common along the lesser curvature of stomach?
- How does one identify the pylorus?
- Name the lymph nodes draining the stomach.

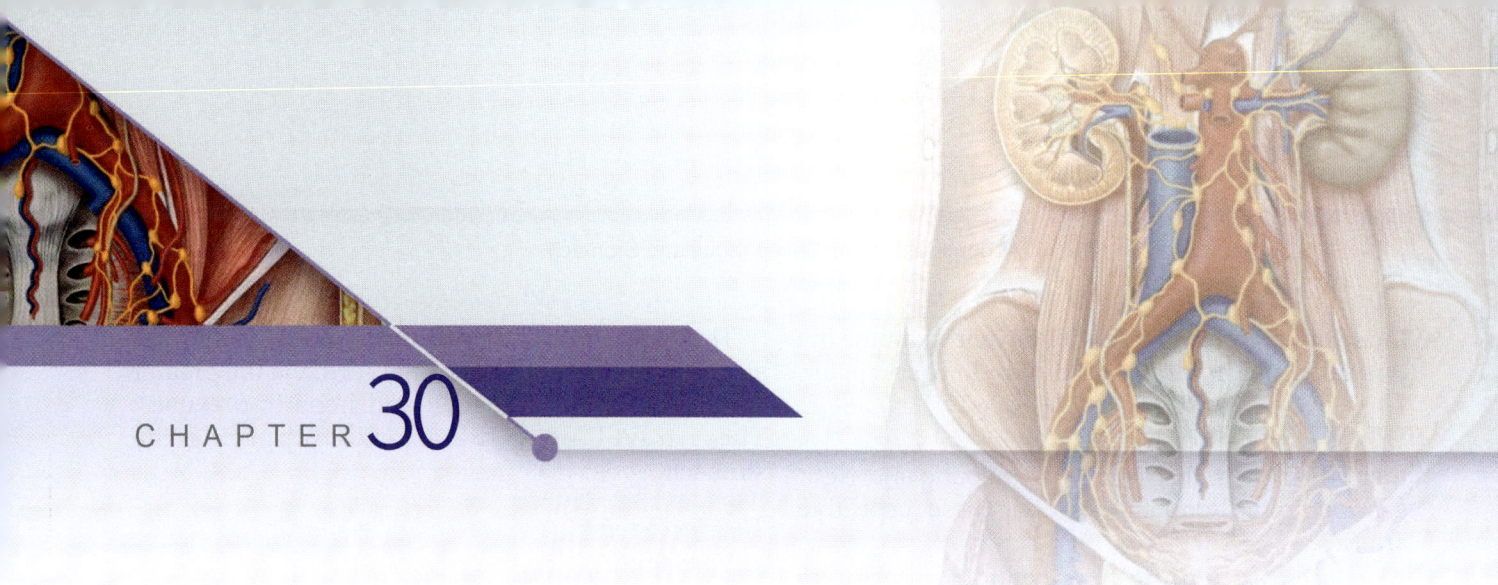

CHAPTER 30

Small and Large Intestines

Learning Objectives

One should be able to

1. Name the ducts opening into the 2nd part of duodenum.
2. Tabulate differences between small intestine and large intestine.
3. Enumerate contents of the root of the mesentery.
4. Enumerate the subdivisions of small intestine and large intestine.

OVERVIEW

Small intestine follows the pylorus of stomach. There are three subdivisions of small intestine. These are duodenum—25 cm, jejunum—approximately 2 metres and ileum—approximately 3 metres.

The small intestine is continuous with caecum, which is the blind beginning of large intestine. Its parts are caecum, vermiform appendix, ascending, transverse, descending, pelvic colons, rectum and anal canal.

Both the intestines are supplied mainly by superior and inferior mesenteric arteries, the 2nd and 3rd ventral branches of abdominal aorta.

Most of the small intestine is suspended by the obliquely placed mesentery of small intestine. But only parts of large intestine have mesentery. These parts are vermiform appendix, transverse colon and sigmoid colon.

Large intestine can be identified from small intestine by the presence of three taeniae, sacculations and appendices epiploicae.

Superior mesenteric vein carries the end products of digestion of food, e.g. amino acids, glucose, etc. It joins with the splenic vein to form an important portal vein which ends in the liver.

Competency achievement: The student should be able to:

AN 47.5 Describe and demonstrate major viscera of abdomen under following headings (anatomical position, external and internal features, important peritoneal and other relations, blood supply, nerve supply, lymphatic drainage and applied aspects) .

STEPS OF DISSECTION

Duodenum

- Examine the C-shaped duodenum with head of pancreas lying in its concavity (Fig. 30.1a and b).
- Cut through the lower wall of the 1st part. Extend the cut on the medial wall of 2nd and on the upper wall of 3rd part of duodenum to see the interior of duodenum.
- Carefully look for the longitudinal fold on the posteromedial wall below the middle of 2nd part. The longitudinal fold is often covered by a circular fold containing the orifice of the major duodenal papilla, which drains both the bile and pancreatic ducts (*see* Fig. 32.3).
- Identify and dissect the structures related to all the four parts of duodenum.
- Identify the suspensory muscle of duodenum at the duodeno-jejunal flexure.

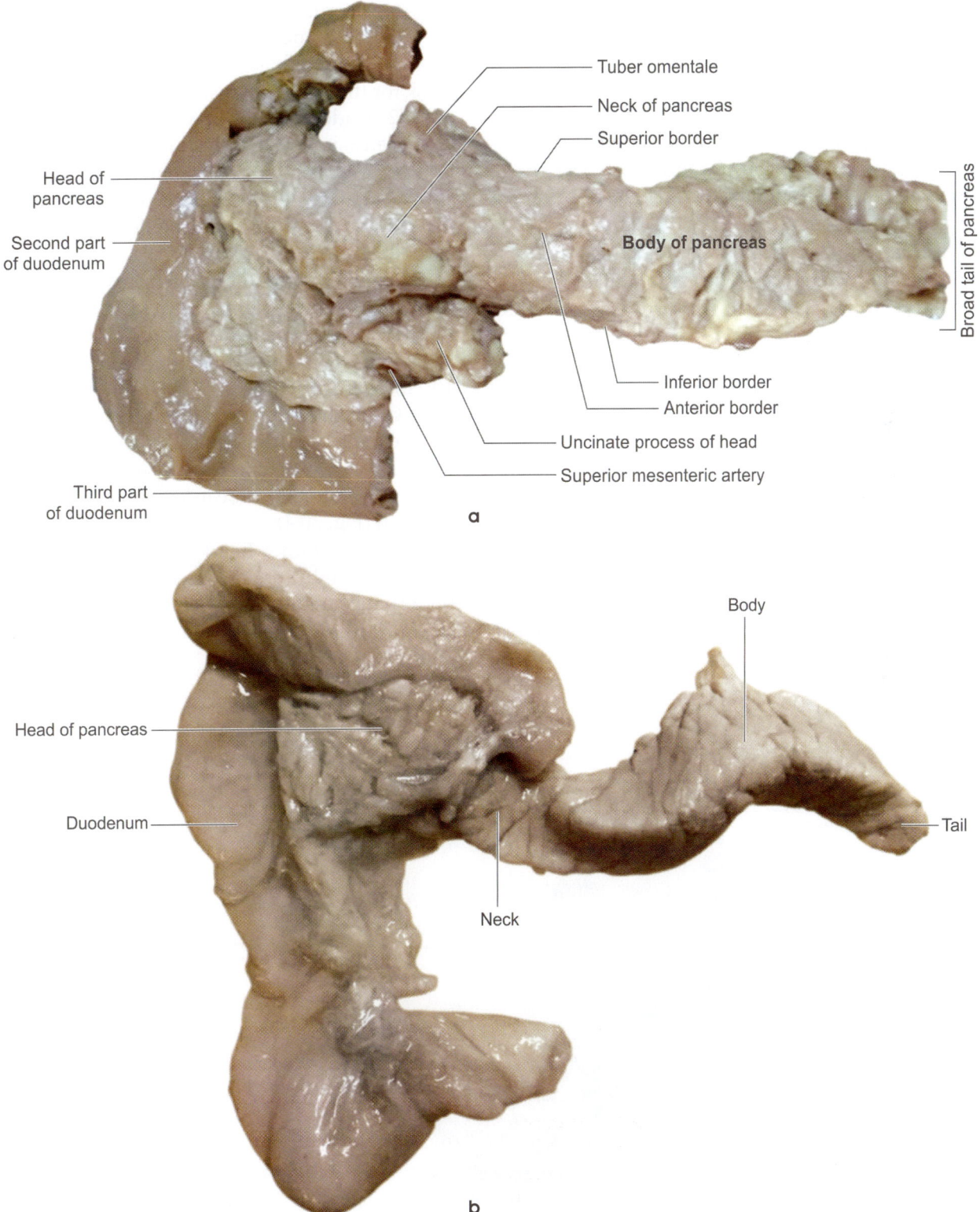

Tuber omentale

Neck of pancreas

Superior border

Head of pancreas

Body of pancreas

Second part of duodenum

Broad tail of pancreas

Inferior border

Anterior border

Uncinate process of head

Superior mesenteric artery

Third part of duodenum

a

Body

Head of pancreas

Duodenum

Tail

Neck

b

Fig. 30.1a and b: 'C' shaped duodenum with head of pancreas lying in its concavity

- Trace its attachment from right crus of diaphragm to posterior surface of duodeno-jejunal junction (flexure).
- Identify the arteries supplying the duodenum. These are anterior and posterior branches of both superior and inferior pancreaticoduodenal arteries.
- Close to duodeno-jejunal junction identify duodenal recesses with its folds. The recesses are:
  i. Superior duodeno-jejunal with orifice below
  ii. Inferior duodeno-jejunal with orifice above
  iii. Retroduodenal recess with orifice to the left
  iv. Paraduodenal recess. This recess contains inferior mesenteric vein, it drains into the splenic vein. Its orifice faces to the right.

At times internal hernia may take place in these recesses. Loop of intestine may get obstructed and strangulated.

Jejunum and Ileum

- The jejunum forms about 2 metres and ileum forms about 3 metres of small intestine. See that these parts are intraperitoneal.
- Identify the attached part of root of mesentery from upper left side of abdomen to lower right side of abdomen. Appreciate that it is narrower on left side and wider on right side. See the folding towards the free end of mesentery, which encloses the long small intestine (Fig. 30.2).
- Look for the arteries which show vasa recta. These are 1–2 arcades in jejunum with long vasa recta and 3–5 arcades in ileum with shorter vasa recta.
- To visualise the interior of jejunum and ileum, tie a pair of ligatures around the jejunum close to D-J flexure and a pair around the ileum close to the caecum.
- Cut through the small intestine between each pair of ligatures and remove it by dividing the mesentery close to the intestine.
- Wash intestine in running tap water. Remove 10 cm each of jejunum and ileum and open it longitudinally. Remove the peritoneal coat to expose the longitudinal muscle layer.
- Identify plicae circulares—the permanent folds of mucous membrane, more in jejunum (Fig. 30.3), less in ileum (Fig. 30.4).
- Identify villi with a hand lens. Remove only the mucous membrane and submucosal to see the underlying circular and longitudinal muscle coats.
- Examine the differences between jejunum and ileum.

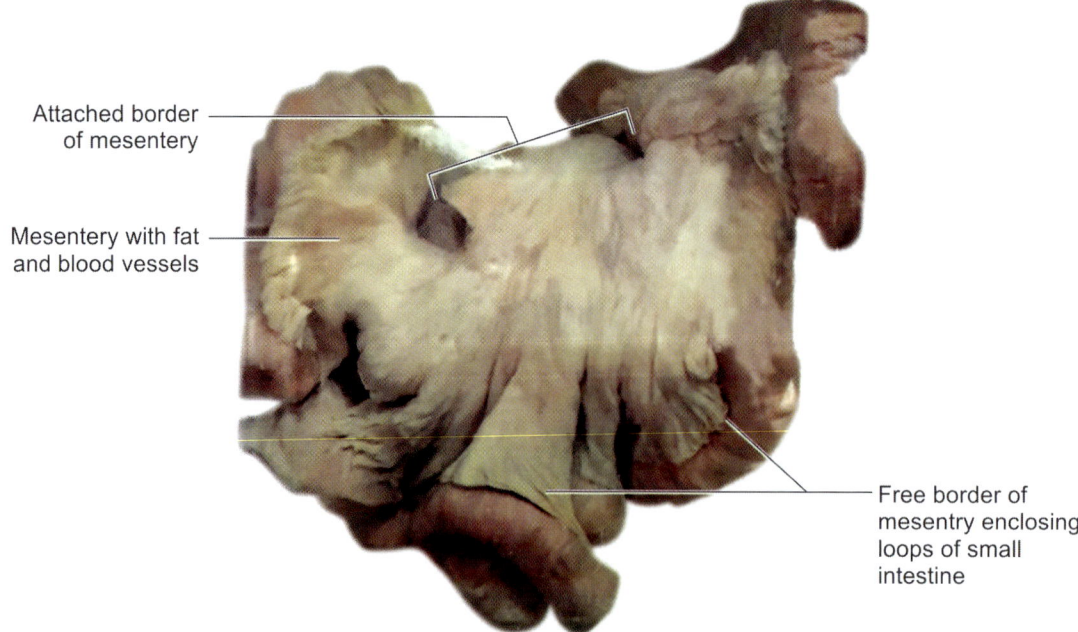

Fig. 30.2: Mesentery of jejunum and ileum (small intestine)

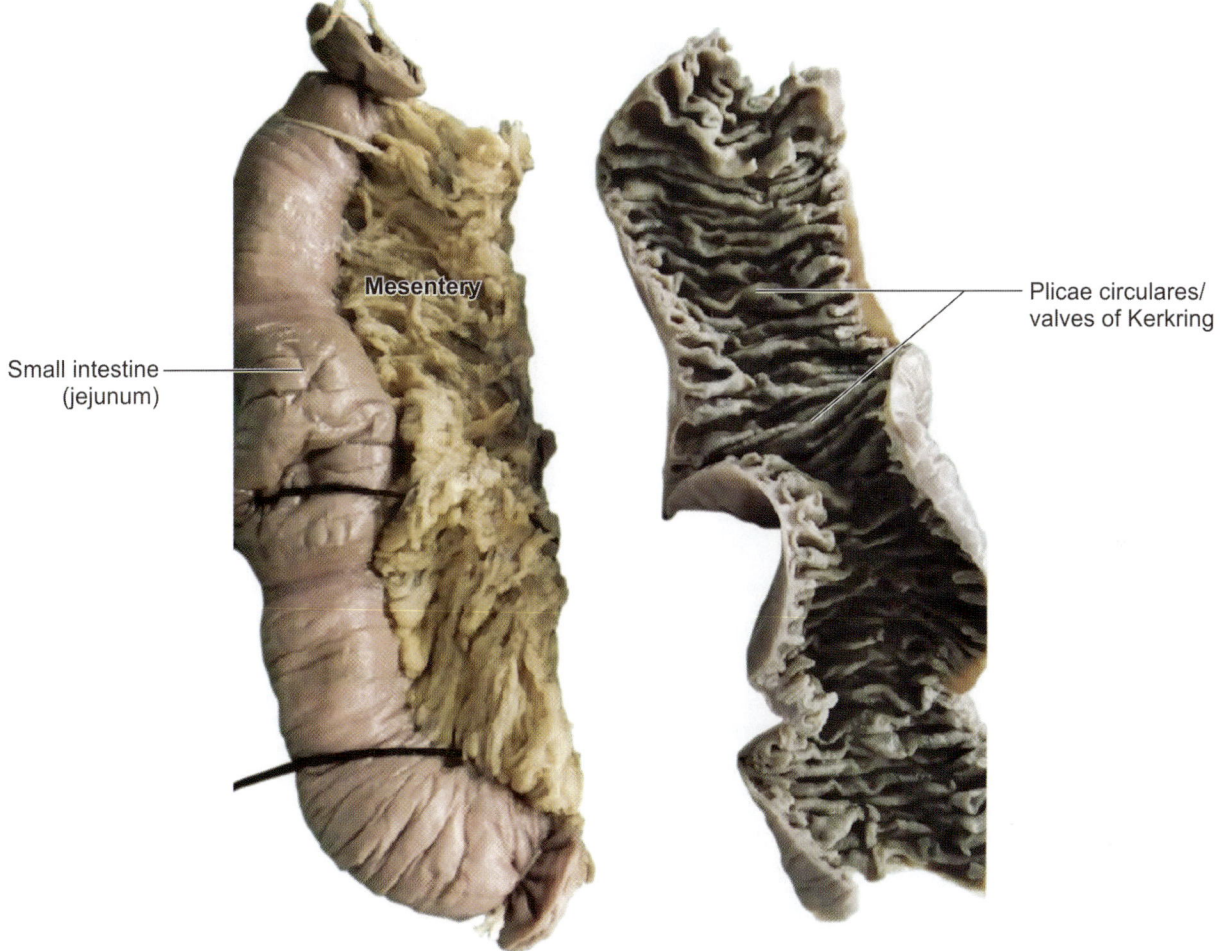

Fig. 30.3: Jejunum with mesentery. Opened up jejunum showing abundant plicae circulares

- Look at Meckel's diverticulum if present. It is 5 cm long, 60 cm proximal to ileocecal valve and attached to antimesenteric border of the ileum.

Large Intestine

Large intestine is called 'large' as it is capable of more distension than the small intestine. It lies at the periphery of the abdominal cavity. The beginning of the large intestine is a blind tube known as caecum. The ileum opens on the medial side of caecum. Below the ileocaecal orifice is the appendicular orifice (Fig. 30.5).

Caecum continues up on the right side of abdomen as ascending colon till the right lobe of liver, where it bends and twists to form the transverse colon (*see* Fig 28.7).

Transverse colon continues across the abdomen from right to left sides. It is seen to descend down between the two ends. It reaches the left side of abdomen till the spleen, where the colon bends at the splenic flexure. Then it continues as descending colon till the left iliac fossa (*see* Fig. 28.7).

Now the descending colon continues as sigmoid (S-shaped) colon or pelvic colon into the pelvis till sacral 3 vertebra where the last part, i.e. rectum starts. Rectum continues as anal canal which ends in an opening, the anus (*see* Fig. 28.7)

- Locate the various parts of the large intestine, beginning from caecum, vermiform appendix, ascending, transverse, descending and sigmoid colons and ending with the rectum and anal canal.
- Identify the taenia, haustrations and appendices epiploicae. Trace the taenia from the root of the

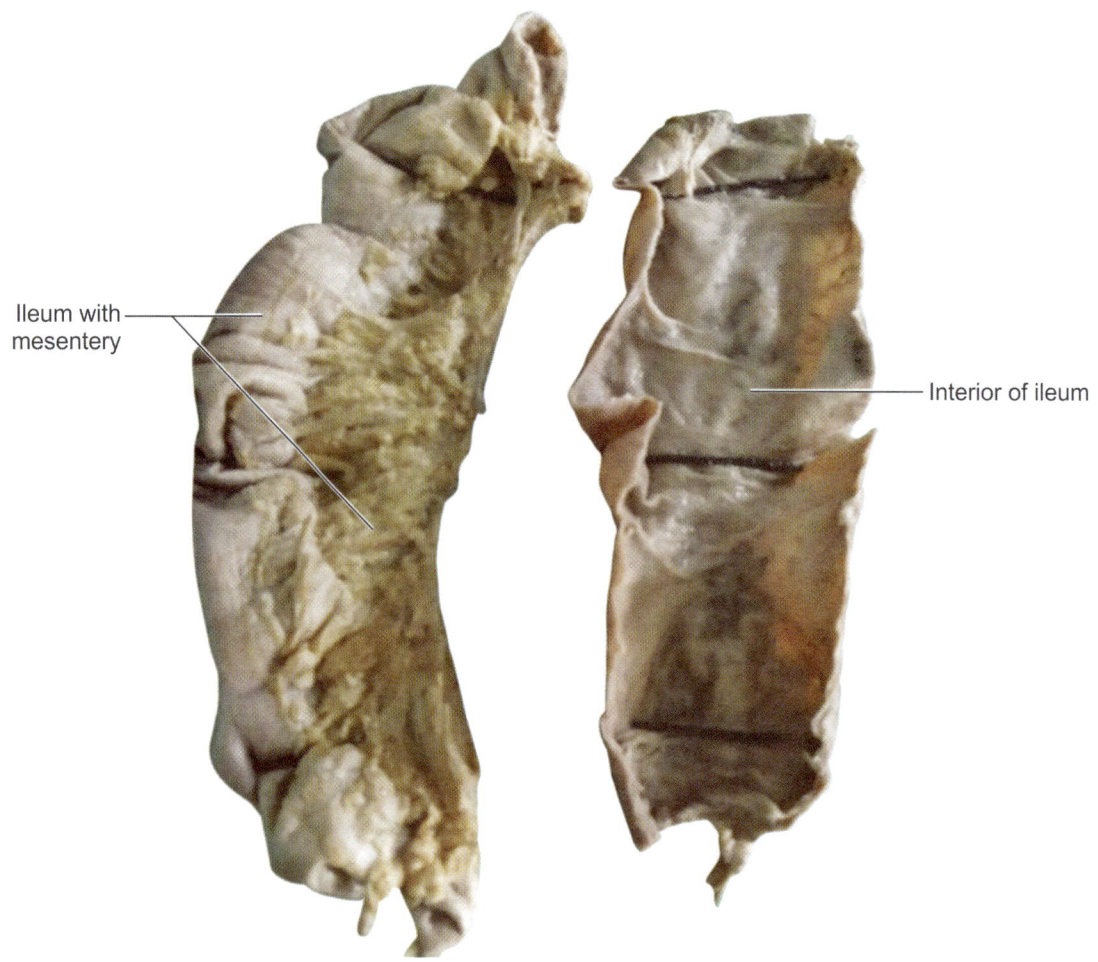

Ileum with mesentery

Interior of ileum

Fig. 30.4: Ileum with mesentery. Opened up ileum with sparse plicae circulares

vermiform appendix through the ascending to the transverse colon and note the change in their respective positions (*see* Fig. 28.7).

Ascending colon	*Transverse colon*
Anterior taenia	Taenia libera
Posteromedial taenia	Taenia mesocolica (posterior)
Posterolateral taenia	Taenia omentalis (superior)

Caecum

- Turn the caecum upwards and identify its posterior relations. These are right psoas major, with the genitofemoral nerve on its anterior surface; lateral cutaneous nerve of thigh and femoral nerve along the lateral border of psoas major muscle. Look for part of external iliac artery also behind the caecum.

- Locate the ileocaecal orifice (Fig. 30.6) and its associated valve. See that this valve has two lips and two frenula. Upper lip is horizontal lying at ileocolic junction whereas lower lip is longer and concave and lies at the ileocaecal junction. Ends of the two valves join to form an anterior and a posterior frenula.

Since the partially digested food stays at the ileocaecal junction for a long time, tuberculosis of ileocaecal junction is very common.

- Identify appendicular orifice 2 cm below the ileocaecal orifice on posteromedial aspect of the caecum (Fig. 30.5).

- Identify the appendicular valve, if present at the appendicular orifice.

- Look for a small triangular fold of peritoneum called mesoappendix (Fig. 30.5). Look for the

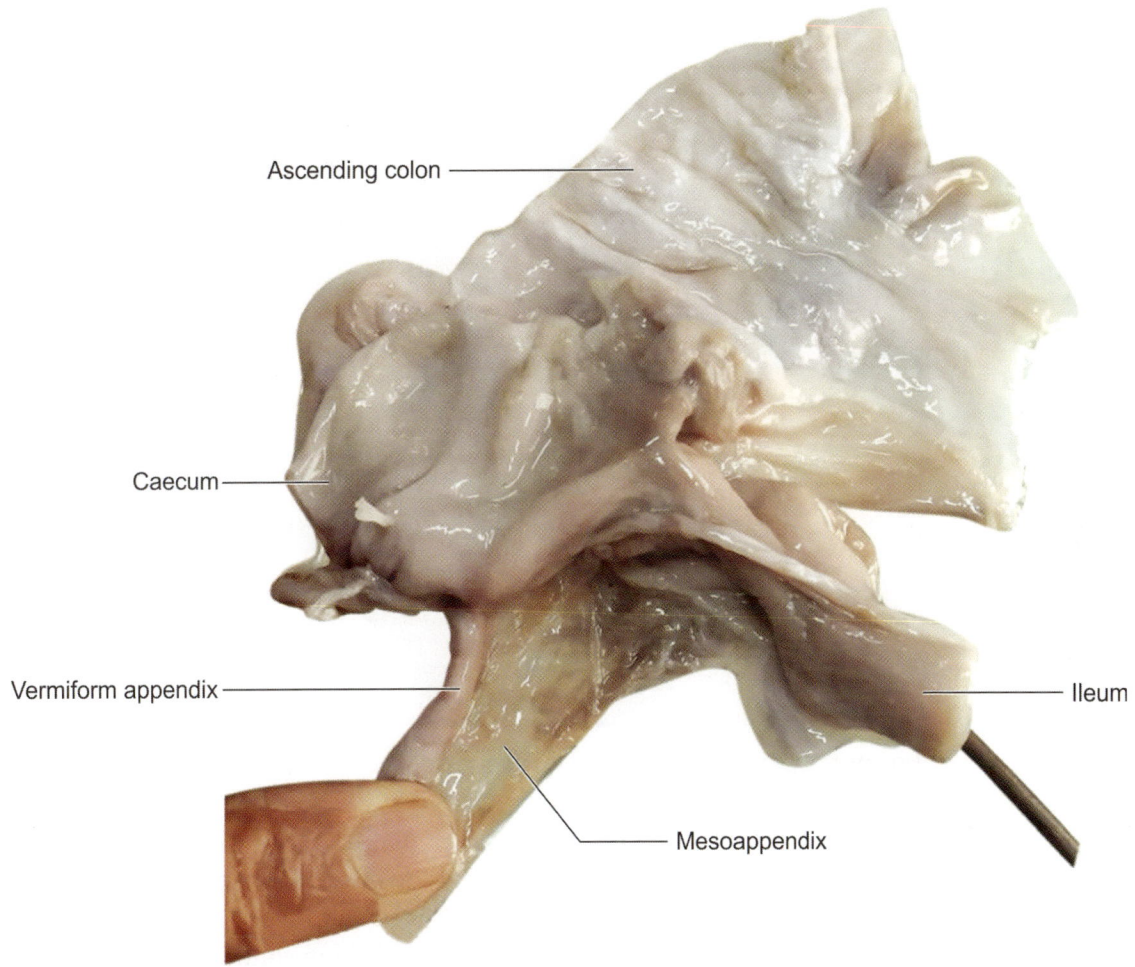

Fig. 30.5: Caecum with ileum, vermiform appendix and ascending colon

appendicular artery running in free border of mesoappendix.

- Look for the position of appendix
  i. Most common is retrocolic—65%
  ii. Less common is pelvic—31%
  iii. Still less common is midinguinal or paracolic—each 2%
- Identify peritoneal recesses at the ileocaecal junction. Above the ileum are superior vascular ileocaecal fold and a recess with a branch of ileocolic artery.
- Identify inferior ileocaecal fold with another recess, but there is no blood vessel in this fold.

Ascending Colon

The upward continuation of caecum is ascending colon. This colon bends to continue as transverse colon on the inferior surface of liver. The area of bend and twist is called hepatic/right colic flexure.

- See that the ascending colon is covered on three sides by peritoneum. It is not mobile.
- On its lateral side look for paracolic gutter.

Transverse Colon

See that the transverse colon is enclosed by a peritoneal fold, the transverse mesocolon, and so is mobile. The colon ascends to the left to reach the spleen and bends there. This bend is known as splenic flexure/left colic flexure (*see* Fig. 28.7).

Descending Colon

- See that the descending colon extends between the left colic flexure and the sigmoid colon.

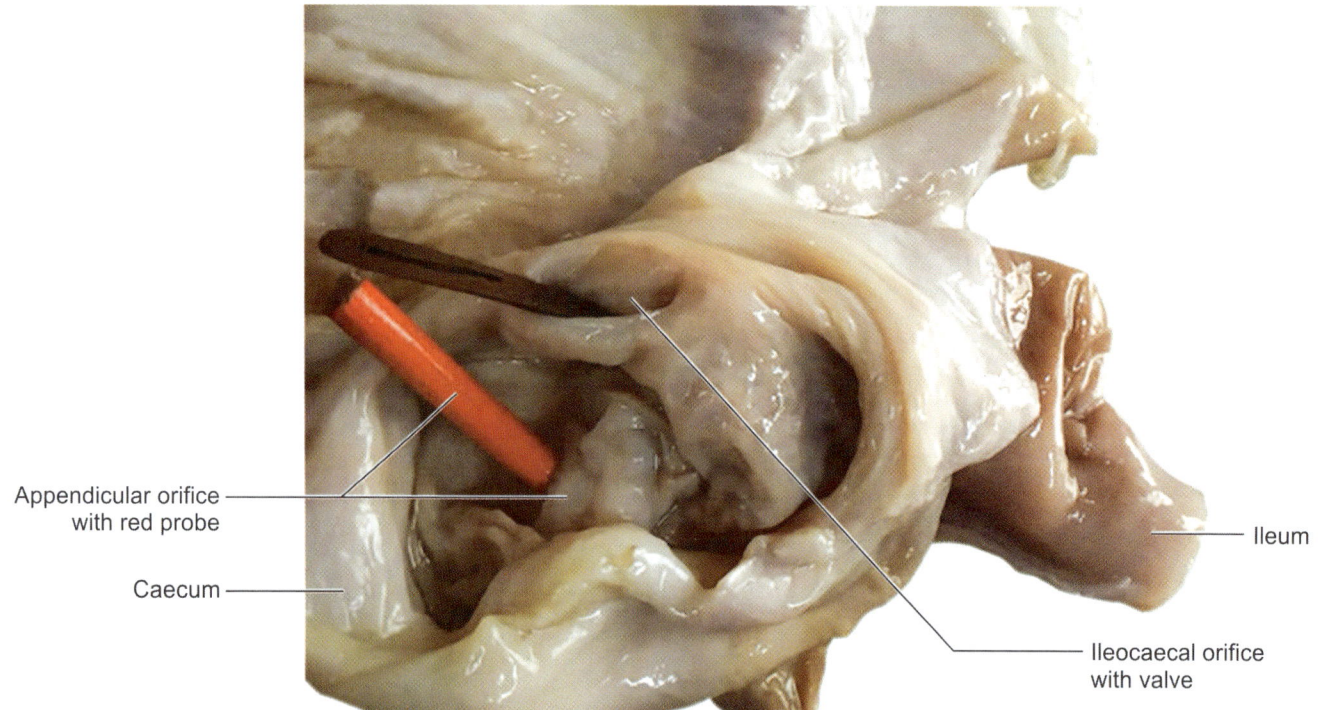

Appendicular orifice with red probe

Caecum

Ileum

Ileocaecal orifice with valve

Fig. 30.6: Openings of ileum and vermiform appendix in caecum

- See that it descends till the iliac crest to incline medially on iliacus and psoas muscles where it continues as sigmoid colon.
- Appreciate that the descending colon is covered on three sides by peritoneum. It is not mobile (*see* Fig. 28.7).

Sigmoid Colon

- See the sigmoid colon lying between the left side of pelvic brim and S3 vertebra. Between these two areas it makes 'S' shaped loop.

- Observe that it is enclosed in sigmoid mesocolon, which is inverted 'V' shaped. Look for the ureter at the apex of 'V' of the sigmoid colon.
- The sigmoid colon continues as rectum.
- Appreciate the differences between the small and large intestines. Macroscopic differences are presence of taenia, sacculations and appendices epiploicae in the large intestine. All these are typically absent in the small intestine.

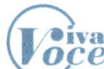

- Name the parts of small intestine.
- Name the parts of large intestine.
- Name the various positions of vermiform appendix.
- What is the relation of superior mesenteric artery to third part of duodenum?

- Where is the pain of early appendicitis referred to and why?
- What is McBurney's point?

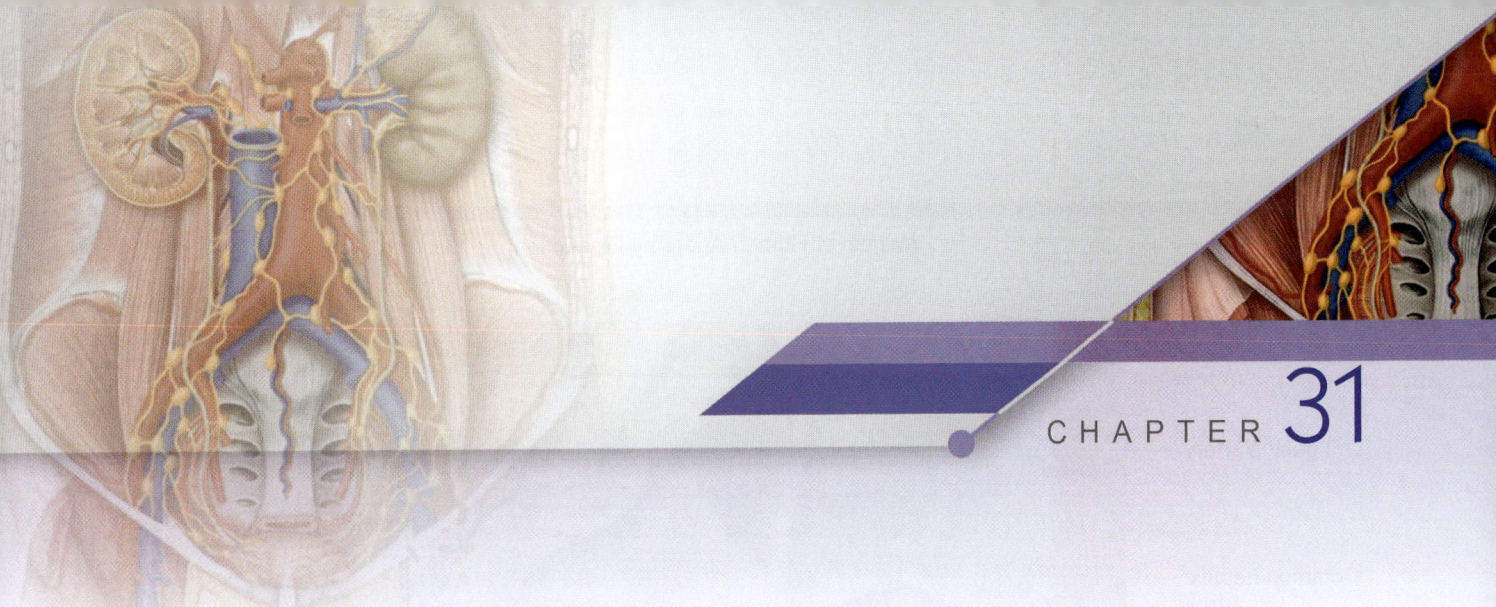

CHAPTER 31

Large Blood Vessels of the Gut

Learning Objectives

One should be able to

1. Enumerate main branches of coeliac axis, superior mesenteric and inferior mesenteric arteries.

2. Mention formation, tributaries and branches of portal vein.

3. Enumerate sites of portosystemic anastomoses and their clinical importance.

The gastrointestinal tract is supplied by three branches of abdominal aorta. These are coeliac axis/coeliac trunk; superior and inferior mesenteric arteries. The branches of these arteries anastomose with each other.

The venous drainage of the gastrointestinal tract finally drains into the portal vein. There is no coeliac vein, the blood from the stomach drains directly into the portal vein. The superior mesenteric vein joins with splenic vein to form portal vein. Inferior mesenteric vein drains into splenic vein, thus the whole venous blood enters into portal vein which ends in the liver.

Competency achievement: The student should be able to:

AN 47.9 Describe and identify the origin, course, important relations and branches of abdominal aorta, coeliac trunk, superior mesenteric, Inferior mesenteric and common iliac artery.

STEPS OF DISSECTION

- Identify the short trunk of coeliac axis artery at the level of the intervertebral disc between T12 and L1 vertebrae arising from the descending abdominal aorta (Fig. 31.1).
- Dissect its relations. These are:

1. Coeliac plexus of nerves
2. Lesser omentum anteriorly
3. Right crus of diaphragm and right coeliac ganglion on right side
4. Left crus of diaphragm and left coeliac ganglion on left side
5. Body of pancreas and splenic vein inferiorly
- Identify and trace the course of the three branches of coeliac axis artery. They are the left gastric artery, splenic artery and common hepatic artery (Fig. 31.1). Since the arteries and their branches are given off behind the peritoneum, these have to run for some distance, turn forwards to enter the peritoneal fold/ligament and reach the viscera.

Left Gastric Artery

- Identify left gastric artery as the smallest branch of coeliac trunk.
- See it running upwards to the left behind the lesser sac to the cardiac end of stomach, where it turns forwards to enter the lesser omentum and lies along the lesser curvature of stomach.
- See its branches to the oesophagus and cardiac end of stomach.

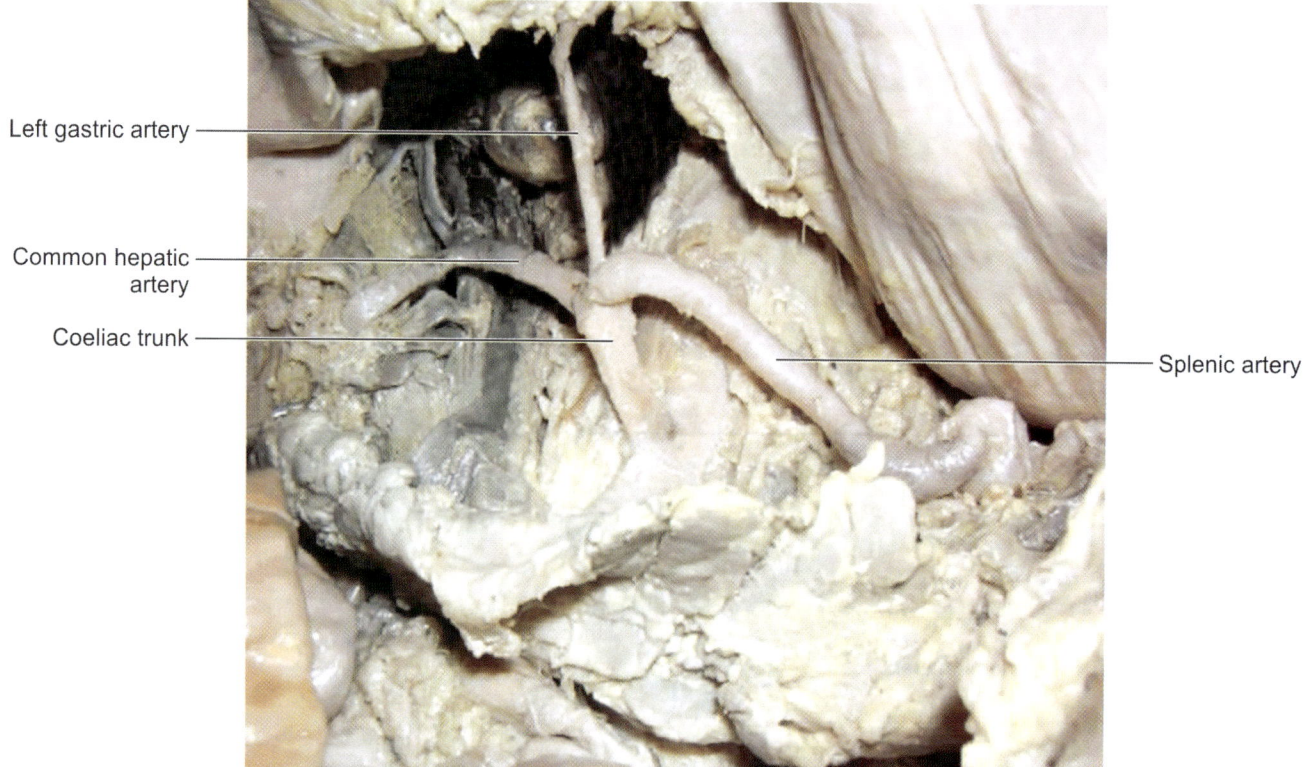

Left gastric artery

Common hepatic artery

Coeliac trunk

Splenic artery

Fig. 31.1: Coeliac axis artery/coeliac trunk with its main branches

- Identify and clean the gastric branches along the lesser curvature of stomach.

Common Hepatic Artery

- Identify the common hepatic (CHA) artery arising from coeliac trunk. See it passing downwards forwards and to the right behind the lesser sac to reach upper border of 1st part of duodenum where it enters the lesser omentum. Here it gives gastroduodenal artery.
- Trace the artery now named proper hepatic artery in the right free margin of lesser omentum anterior to portal vein and to the left of bile duct. As it reaches porta hepatis it ends by dividing into right and left hepatic arteries.
- Identify its branches (CHA). These are gastro-duodenal artery and right gastric artery.

Splenic Artery

- Identify the splenic artery which is the largest branch of coeliac axis artery (Fig. 31.1).

- Note that it has a tortuous course as it runs along the upper border of pancreas. Near the tail of pancreas, it enters lienorenal ligament to reach the hilum of spleen.
- *Identify the following branches:*
  i. Numerous pancreatic branches
  ii. 5–7 short gastric branches for the fundus of stomach
  iii. Left gastroepiploic, which lies along the greater curvature of stomach
  iv. 5–7 splenic branches

SUPERIOR MESENTERIC ARTERY

Superior mesenteric artery is the artery of the midgut. So it supplies distal 2½ parts of duodenum, jejunum and ileum of small intestine. In addition the artery supplies caecum, vermiform appendix, ascending colon and right 2/3rd of transverse colon. This artery is given off retroperitoneally from the descending abdominal aorta behind the body of pancreas. Then it lies anterior to uncinate process of head of pancreas to reach anterior to 3rd part of duodenum. At that point it enters root of mesentery to run between two layers of root of mesentery to reach the right iliac fossa.

Steps of Dissection

- Identify the superior mesenteric artery by shifting loops of small intestine to the left and lifting body of pancreas (Fig. 31.2).
- See the right concave side and left convex side of the artery.
- See the artery lying anterior to the uncinate process of pancreas and anterior to 3rd part of duodenum and then on the right psoas major muscle.
- Identify its branches both from right and left sides.

Branches from the Right Side

- See inferior pancreaticoduodenal supplying both pancreas and duodenum.
- See middle colic as it enters transverse mesocolon and divides into left and right branches (Fig. 31.2).
- Look for right colic which lies first behind the peritoneum to reach the ascending colon and then divides into upper ascending branch and lower descending branch.
- Trace ileocolic artery (Fig. 31.2). It is the last branch from right side. It divides into superior and inferior branches. See the inferior branch supplying the caecum and vermiform appendix.

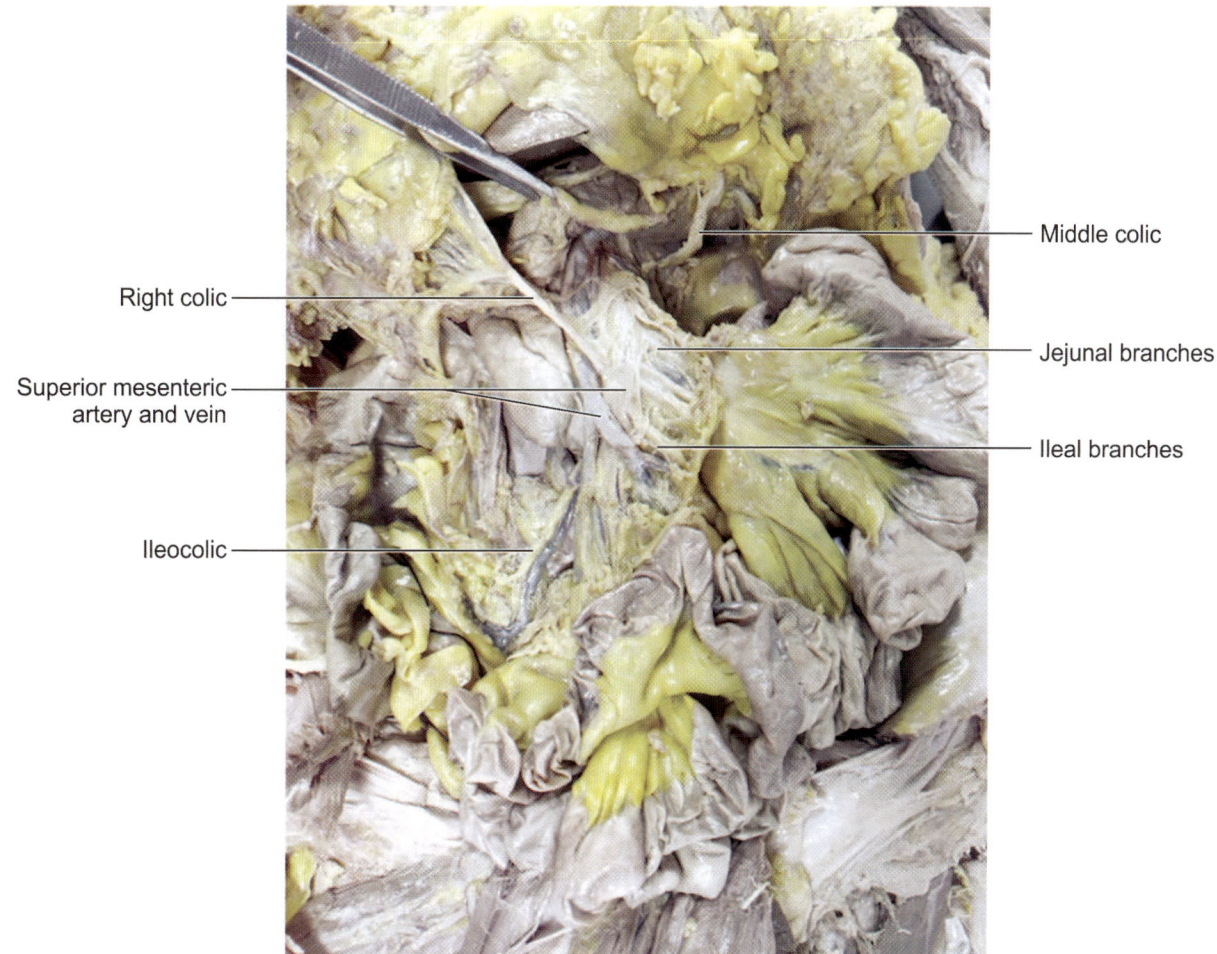

Fig. 31.2: Superior mesenteric artery and vein with its branches and tributaries

Branches from the Left Side

- 12–15 jejunal and ileal branches. These arteries form arcades which have to be identified in the depth of the mesentery. The arcades then give vasa recta (Fig. 31.2).
- Appreciate that the arcades are 1–2 in jejunum and 3–5 in ileum. So vasa recta are longer in jejunum than in ileum.
- To see these arteries one has to remove one layer of mesentery and fat.
- Look for the superior mesenteric vein running on right side of the artery.
- See it running up to neck of pancreas where it joins the splenic vein to form the portal vein.

INFERIOR MESENTERIC ARTERY

The inferior mesenteric artery is the artery of the hindgut (Fig. 31.3). So, it supplies left 1/3rd of transverse colon, splenic flexure, descending and pelvic colons, rectum and proximal part of anal canal.

This artery arises from the abdominal aorta at the level of L3 vertebra. See its short course in the abdomen. It then enters the medial limb of pelvic mesocolon. This artery ends by changing its name to superior rectal artery.

Steps of Dissection

- Clean the lower part of descending abdominal aorta and identify inferior mesenteric artery (Fig. 31.3).

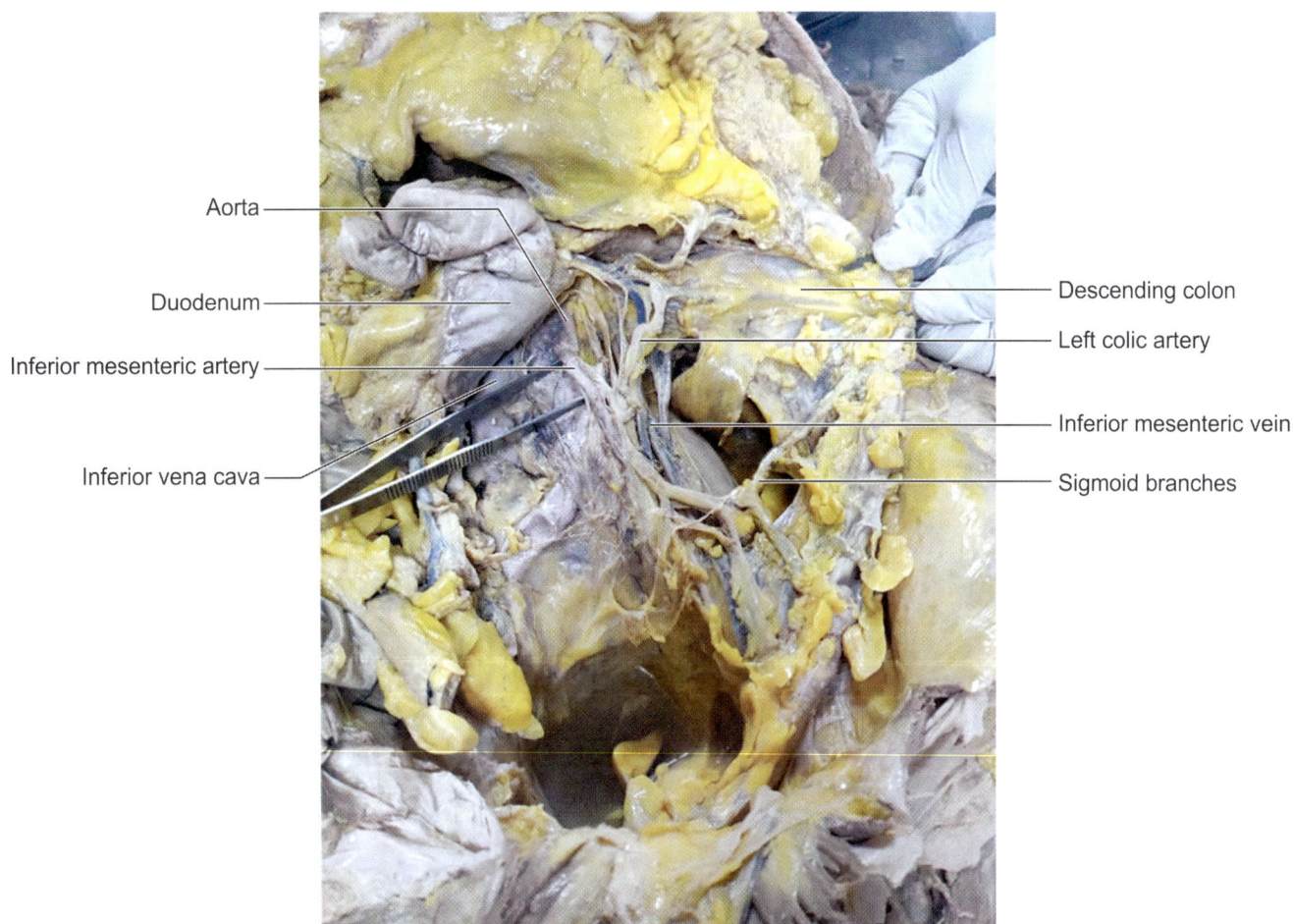

Fig. 31.3: Inferior mesenteric artery and vein and its branches and tributaries

- Trace it as it crosses the left common iliac artery to enter the pelvic cavity as superior rectal artery.
- Clean its few branches. These are: (i) Left colic which runs to left side and divides into ascending and descending branches (Fig. 31.3). (ii) 3–4 sigmoid branches for sigmoid/pelvic colon. All the colic arteries from superior mesenteric and inferior mesenteric artery anastomose with each other to form a marginal artery (Figs 31.4 and 31.5).
- Inferior mesenteric vein is longer than inferior mesenteric artery. See the vein ascending up to left of inferior mesenteric artery, lying in paraduodenal fold of peritoneum at duodenojejunal junction to drain into the splenic vein.
- In addition it receives tributaries from sigmoid colon and descending colon.

Competency achievement: The student should be able to:
AN 47.8 Describe and identify the formation, course relations and tributaries of portal vein, inferior vena cava and renal vein.

PORTAL VEIN

Portal vein is formed by union of superior mesenteric vein and splenic vein. Since nutrients are absorbed in small intestine, portal vein carries them and stores them in the liver till they are needed by the body.

Portal vein is 8 cm long. Its parts are infraduodenal (retropancreatic), retroduodenal and supraduodenal. The supraduodenal part lies in the free margin of lesser omentum.

Identify the portal vein lying posteriorly and bile duct and proper hepatic artery lying anteriorly in the free margin of lesser omentum.

Steps of Dissection

- Trace the superior mesenteric vein from right iliac fossa to right of superior mesenteric artery, anterior to 3rd part of duodenum and uncinate process of pancreas to reach the neck of pancreas.
- Identify splenic vein coming from left side to join superior mesenteric vein thereby forming the portal vein.

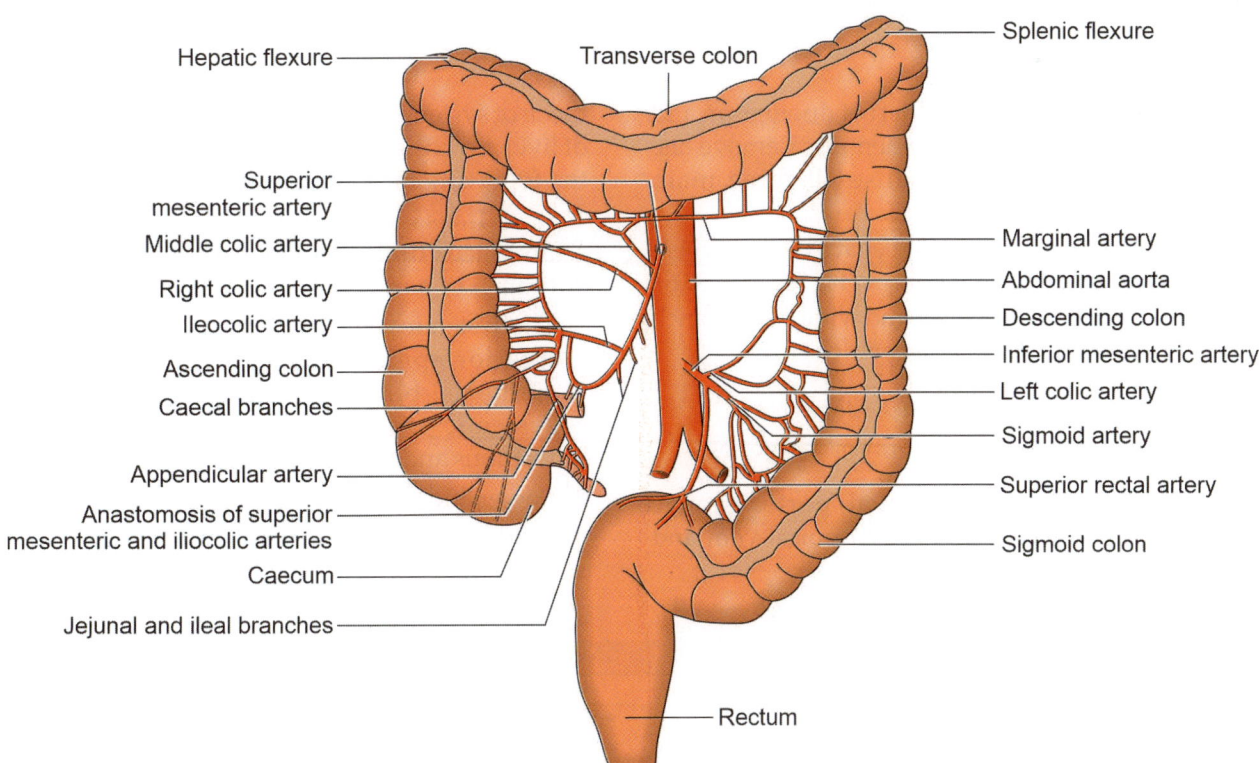

Fig. 31.4: Branches of superior and inferior mesenteric arteries forming marginal artery

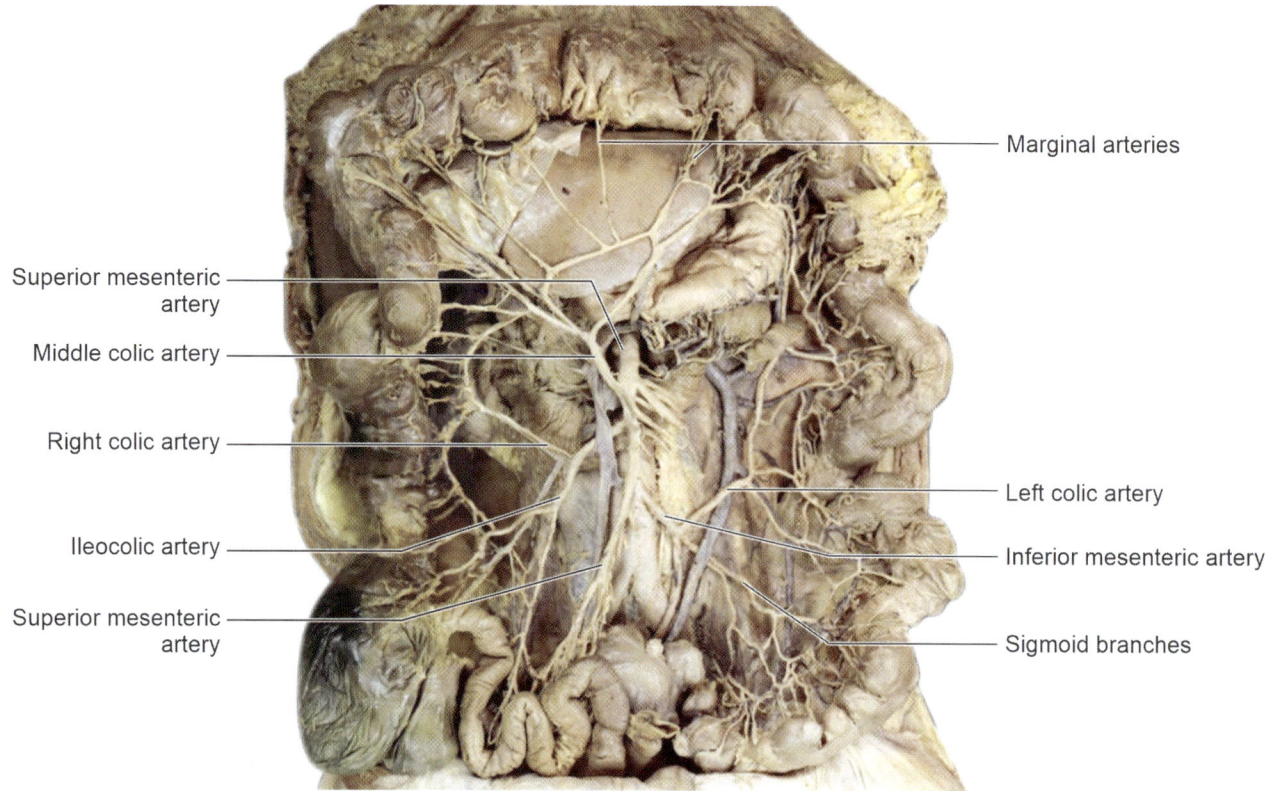

Fig. 31.5: Branches of superior and inferior mesenteric arteries

- Trace it upwards behind 1st part of duodenum and then in free margin of lesser omentum. Remove one layer of omentum to visualise all three main structures there.
- Further trace the vein to porta hepatis of liver where it lies as most posterior structure (*see* Fig 32.1 and 33.6).
- Portal vein divides into short and wide right branch and longer and narrower left branch.

Competency achievement: The student should be able to:

AN 47.10 Enumerate the sites of portosystemic anastomosis.

- Identify the sites of portocaval/portosystemic anastomoses where tributaries of portal vein and those of systemic or caval veins anastomose. In case of liver cirrhosis these sites acquire importance. See the following important sites:

1. *Umbilicus:* Few paraumbilical veins from umbilicus drain via ligamentum teres into left branch of portal vein.

   The systemic veins are tributaries of superior and inferior epigastric arteries. In case of liver cirrhosis, blood from liver is returned via systemic veins. These veins get dilated and tortuous and the site is called "Caput Medusae".

2. Lower end of oesophagus—oesophageal varices
3. Anal canal—haemorrhoids/piles

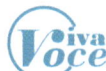

- Name the branches of coeliac trunk.
- Name the branches of superior mesenteric artery from the right side.
- Name the branches of inferior mesenteric artery.

- Where and how is the portal vein formed?
- What is the importance of portosystemic anastomoses at the lower end of oesophagus and anal canal?

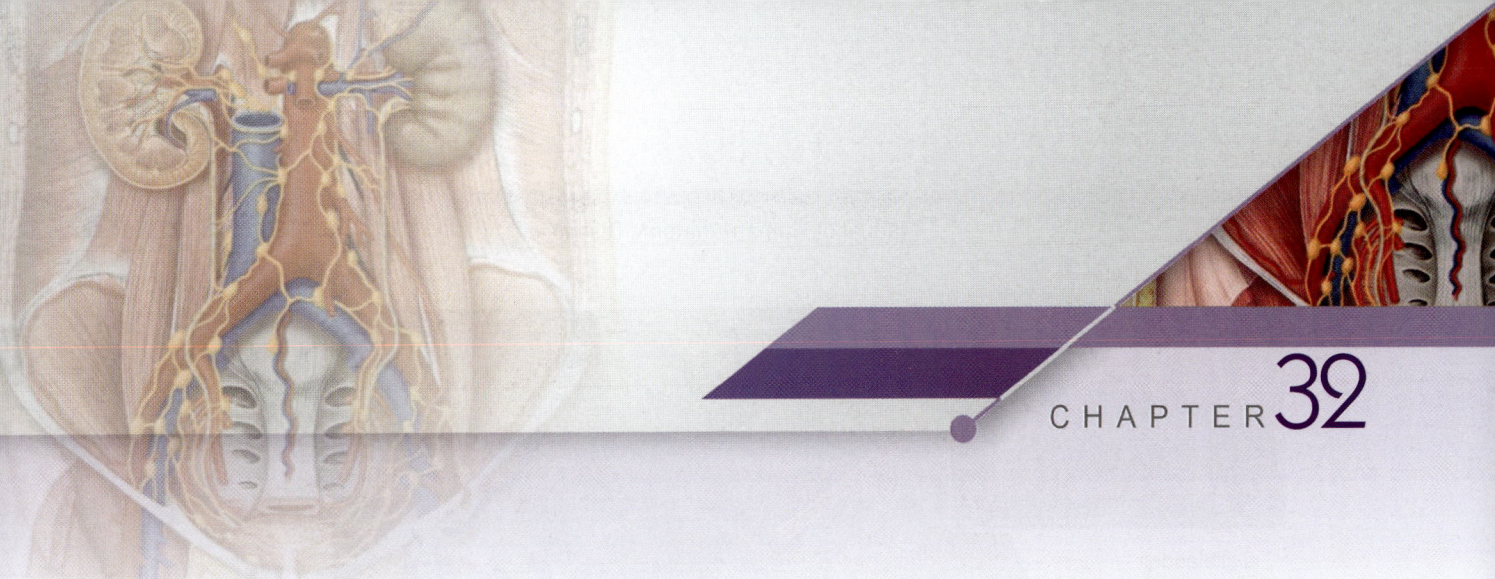

CHAPTER 32

Extrahepatic Biliary Apparatus

Learning Objectives

One should be able to

1. Mark the course of bile duct from porta hepatis of liver to 2nd part of duodenum.
2. Name the sphincters present in relation to the ducts.
3. Name the boundaries and contents of Calot's triangle

OVERVIEW

Bile formed in the liver is carried and stored in ducts and viscera before it is secreted into the 2nd part of duodenum. These ducts and viscera are collectively called extrahepatic biliary apparatus. Its components are right and left hepatic ducts, common hepatic duct, gallbladder with cystic duct and bile duct.

Bile is stored and concentrated to 1/10th amount in the gallbladder. That is why gallbladder is a site of formation of gallstones. Bile gets concentrated and its cholesterol may get precipitated to form gallstones. Pain of inflammation of gallbladder due to stones may be referred to tip of right shoulder, epigastric region or inferior angle of right scapula.

STEPS OF DISSECTION

- Locate the porta hepatis on the inferior surface of liver (Fig. 32.1).
- Look for two hepatic ducts there. Follow them till these join to form common hepatic duct.
- Identify cystic duct and usually green-coloured gallbladder.

- See the point of junction of cystic duct with common hepatic duct and the formation of bile duct.
- Trace the bile duct in relation to the duodenum.
- Trace the cystic artery supplying gallbladder, cystic duct, hepatic ducts and upper part of bile duct.
- Identify and clean the various parts of gallbladder (Fig. 32.2). These are:
  i. *Fundus:* Part projecting beyond the inferior border of liver
  ii. *Body:* Part lying in the fossa for gallbladder
  iii. *Neck:* Upper end of gallbladder which curves to become cystic duct
  iv. *Cystic duct:* It is 3–4 cm long. It joins common hepatic duct to form bile duct.
- Now trace the bile duct. It is closely related to the duodenum. See its parts as:
  i. Supraduodenal part lies in free margin of lesser omentum with proper hepatic artery to its left and portal vein posteriorly.
  ii. Retroduodenal part lies behind the 1st part of duodenum. Identify inferior vena cava behind bile duct and gastroduodenal artery to left of bile duct.

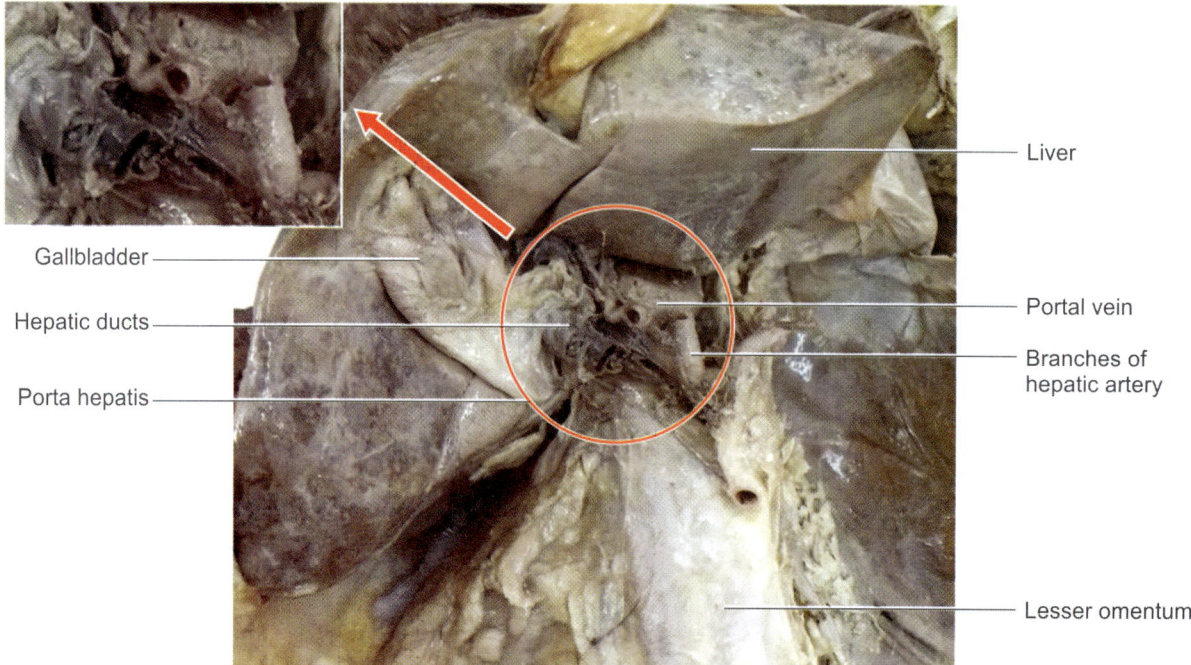

Liver

Portal vein

Branches of hepatic artery

Lesser omentum

Gallbladder

Hepatic ducts

Porta hepatis

Fig. 32.1: Structures in the porta hepatis

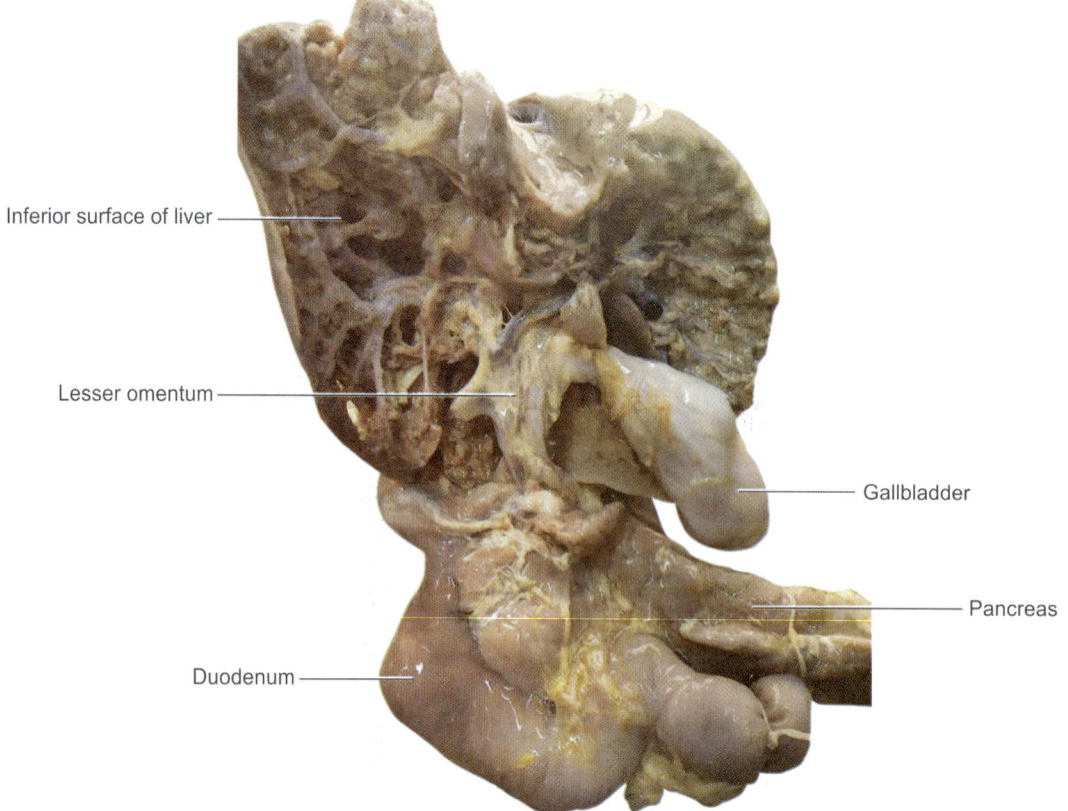

Inferior surface of liver

Lesser omentum

Duodenum

Gallbladder

Pancreas

Fig. 32.2: Gallbladder seen on inferior surface of liver

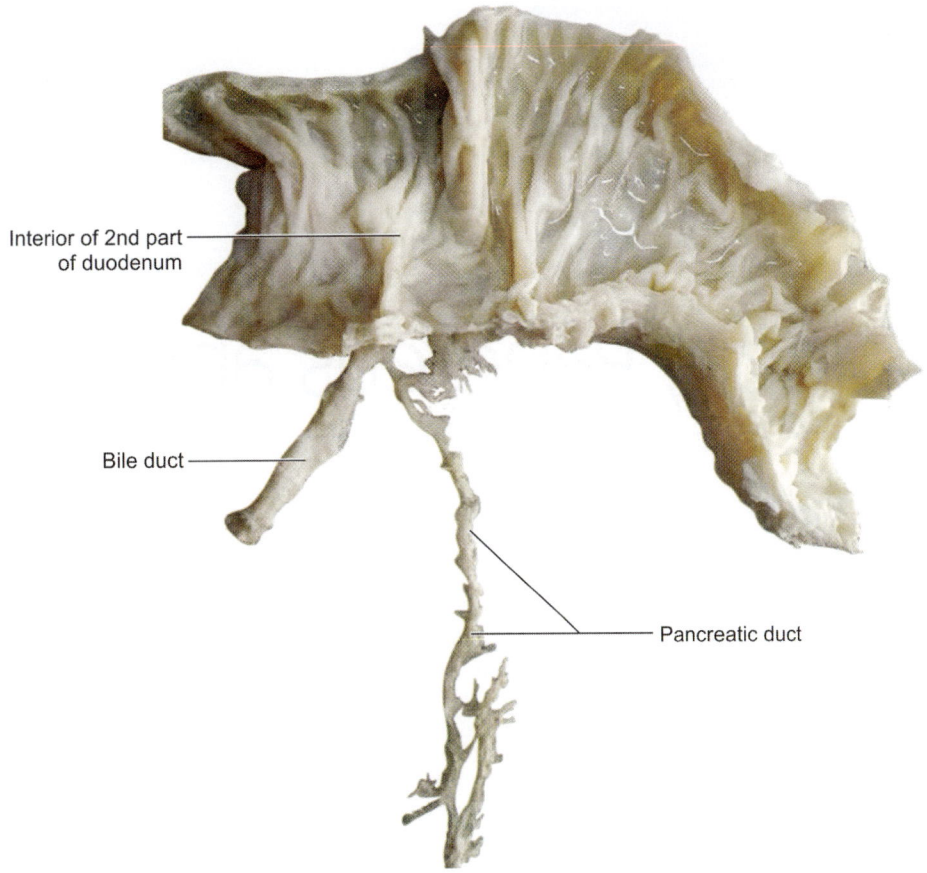

Interior of 2nd part of duodenum

Bile duct

Pancreatic duct

Fig. 32.3: Bile and pancreatic ducts opening in 2nd part of duodenum

iii. Infraduodenal part lies in a groove in the upper and lateral part of posterior surface of head of pancreas. Inferior vena cava is seen posterior to the pancreas.

iv. Intraduodenal part opens into 2nd part of duodenum (Fig. 32.3).

- See that the bile duct is joined by main pancreatic duct from head of pancreas (Fig. 32.3).
- Clean the area of duodenum and look for longitudinal fold at posteromedial wall of 2nd part of duodenum (Fig. 32.3). A papilla is situated at upper end of the fold where the two combined ducts open.

- This opening is surrounded by sphincters formed of smooth muscle fibres.
- Try to identify sphincter choledochus around bile duct, sphincter pancreaticus around pancreatic duct and sphincter of Oddi around common opening of bile duct and pancreatic duct.

Blood Supply

- The gallbladder and its duct are supplied by the cystic artery from right hepatic artery.
- Identify the cystic artery. The course of cystic artery and its relation to ducts may be variable. This has to be kept in mind during surgery of the region.

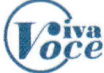

- Name the structures at porta hepatis in order.
- Name the 4 parts of the bile duct.
- Where is pain of gallbladder (cholecystitis) referred to?

- Why are gallstones not radio-opaque?
- Name the sphincters around bile duct, pancreatic duct and their common opening.

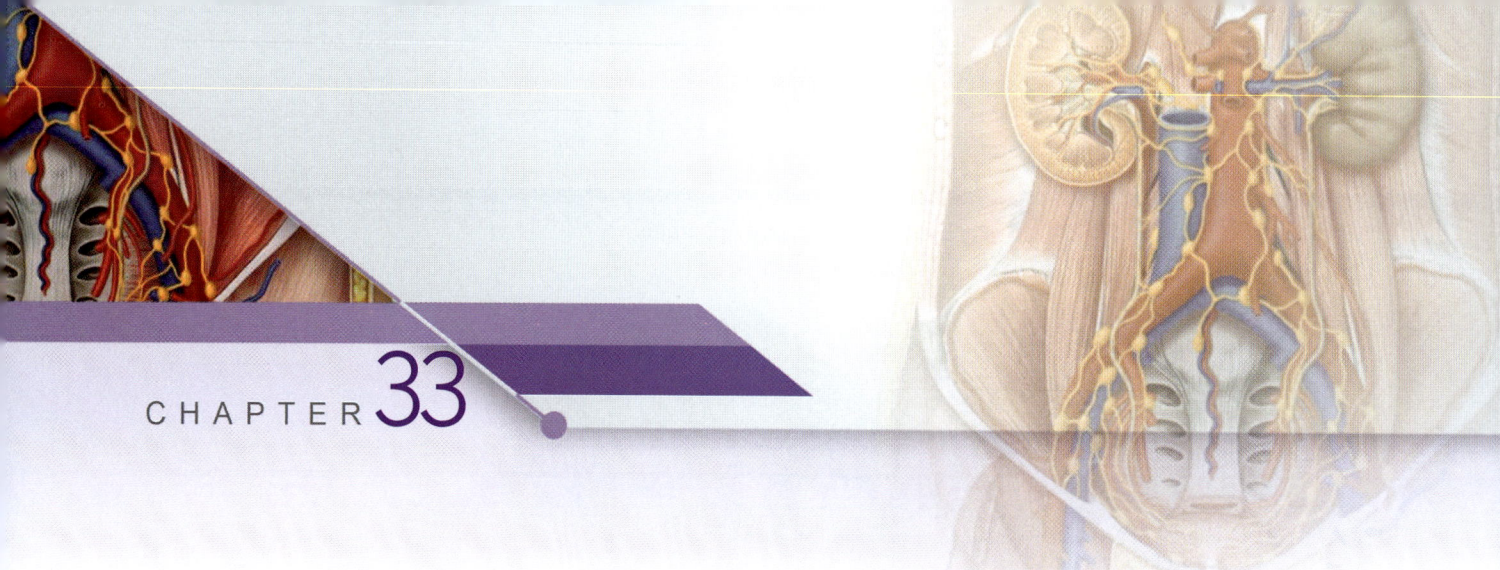

CHAPTER 33

Spleen, Pancreas and Liver

Learning Objectives

One should be able to
1. Show the visceral relations of the spleen
2. Trace the circulation of blood through spleen.
3. Trace the course of pancreatic and accessory pancreatic ducts.

4. What is relation of peritoneum to the pancreas.
5. Trace the course of bile duct from liver to the duodenum.

OVERVIEW

Spleen

Spleen is part of reticuloendothelial system, located in left hypochondrium behind the midaxillary line. Comprised of two ends—posterior and anterior; two surfaces-diaphragmatic and visceral; three borders—superior notched border, inferior border and an intermediate border. Viscera related to the spleen are left kidney, descending colon, stomach and pancreas. Arterial supply to spleen is by the splenic artery—the largest branch of coeliac axis artery. Histologically spleen is comprised of red pulp and white pulp with no differentiation into cortex or medulla. Spleen enlarges considerably in malaria.

PANCREAS

Pancreas is an obliquely placed gland along the posterior abdominal wall with both exocrine (pancreatic juice) and endocrine (insulin and glucagon) secretions. Pancreas comprises a head, a small neck, triangular body and a tail reaching till the spleen. Pancreas gets its arterial supply from the

tortuous splenic artery running along its upper border.

The exocrine secretion of the gland is poured in the pancreatic duct which runs towards its head. There it joins the bile duct and the two together open at the major duodenal papilla situated in the descending/2nd part of the duodenum.

Endocrine secretion is insulin and glucagon. Insufficient levels of insulin may result in diabetes mellitus.

LIVER

Overview

Liver is the brownish largest gland of the body capable of doing numerous functions. It is situated chiefly in right hypochondrium, epigastrium and right lumbar regions. It is comprised of:
- Two main lobes—the right and left
- Two small lobes—the caudate and quadrate lobes

Gateway to the liver is the porta hepatis, which contains bile duct, proper hepatic artery and portal vein.

Liver is protected by the right side of thoracic cage. It extends till 5th rib.

The inferior surface of liver is related to oesophagus, stomach, part of duodenum, hepatic flexure of colon and right kidney with right suprarenal.

Liver is kept in position by intra-abdominal pressure, hepatic veins draining into the well supported inferior vena cava.

Liver is subdivided into eight segments.

Liver biopsy is done to estimate the extent of disease especially cirrhosis of liver.

STEPS OF DISSECTION

- Locate the spleen situated deep in the left hypochondrium.
- The gastrophrenic ligament has already been cut during removal of stomach.
- Now cut through posteriorly placed lienorenal ligament taking care of the splenic vessels and tail of pancreas present in the ligament.
- See the close relation of spleen to the costo-diaphragmatic recess, the left lung and 9th–11th ribs.

- Identify the four viscera related to spleen (Fig. 33.1). The gastric area is the largest and is occupied by fundus of stomach.
- Colic area is the junction of transverse colon and descending colon/the splenic flexure. Pancreatic area is small area close to the hilum of spleen.
- Renal area is the posterior part and is related to anterior surface of left kidney.
- Separate the viscera and trace the tortuous splenic artery towards the hilum of spleen. See it dividing into 5–6 branches at the hilum.
- Now cut the phrenicocolic ligament of peritoneum extending between left colic flexure and the diaphragm. Take the spleen out of the abdominal cavity.
- Study the gross features (Figs 33.1 and 33.2). These are:
  a. *2 ends*
     – Anterior or lateral wide end
     – Posterior rounded end

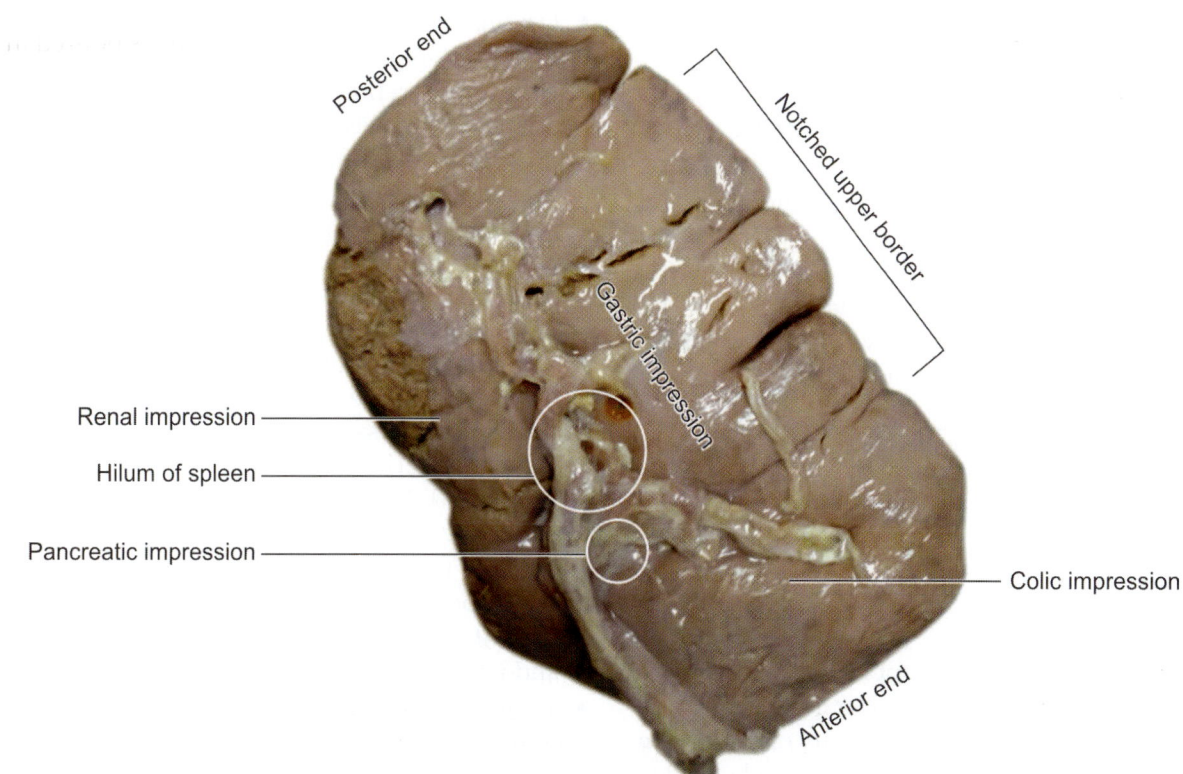

Fig. 33.1: Visceral surface of spleen

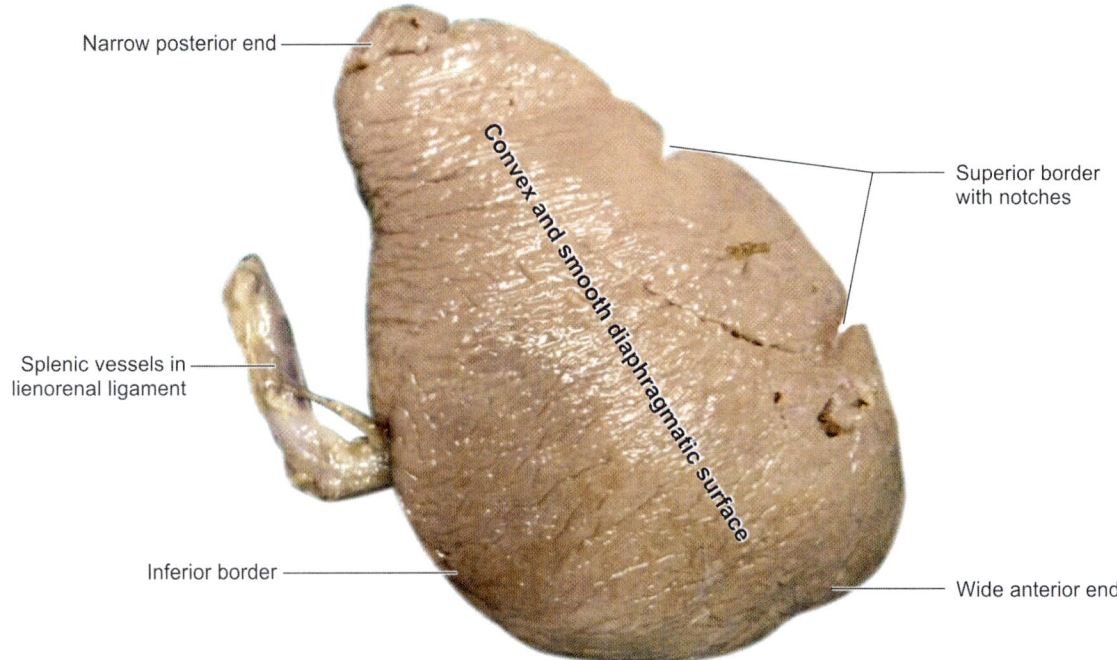

Fig. 33.2: Gross features of spleen

b. *3 borders*
   – Superior border, usually notched
   – Inferior rounded border
   – Intermediate border also rounded
c. *2 surfaces*
   – Diaphragmatic—convex and smooth
   – Concave and irregular
- Hilum lies between superior and intermediate borders. See and clean the branches of splenic artery and tributaries of splenic vein, nerve plexus, lymphatic vessels and areolar tissue at the hilum (Fig. 33.1).
  Spleen is enlarged most commonly in malaria. Enlarged spleen projects diagonally towards the right iliac fossa.

PANCREAS

Steps of Dissection

- Identify the pancreas, a retroperitoneal organ lying horizontally across the posterior abdominal wall.
- Head is identifiable in the concavity of duodenum. Uncinate process of the head is the part behind the upper part of superior mesenteric artery (*see* Fig. 30.1).
- *Identify:*
   i. 3 borders of head—superior, right lateral and inferior, related to 1st, 2nd and 3rd parts of duodenum respectively.
   ii. 2 surfaces—anterior and posterior
   iii. 1 process—uncinate process
- Between the head of pancreas and 1st, 2nd and 3rd parts of duodenum locate superior and inferior pancreaticoduodenal vessels.
- See that the superior mesenteric artery arises from abdominal aorta behind the body of pancreas. Then it descends to the right to lie on anterior surface of uncinate process of pancreas. It further descends to lie on anterior surface of 3rd part of duodenum.
- Trace the bile duct lying posterior to the head of pancreas.
- Identify the neck of pancreas as the part behind which portal vein is formed.
- Rest of the part extending to the left is the body and tail which reaches till the hilum of spleen.
- Turn the descending part of duodenum and the head of pancreas to the left. Look for the posterior pancreaticoduodenal vessels and the bile duct on the pancreas again.

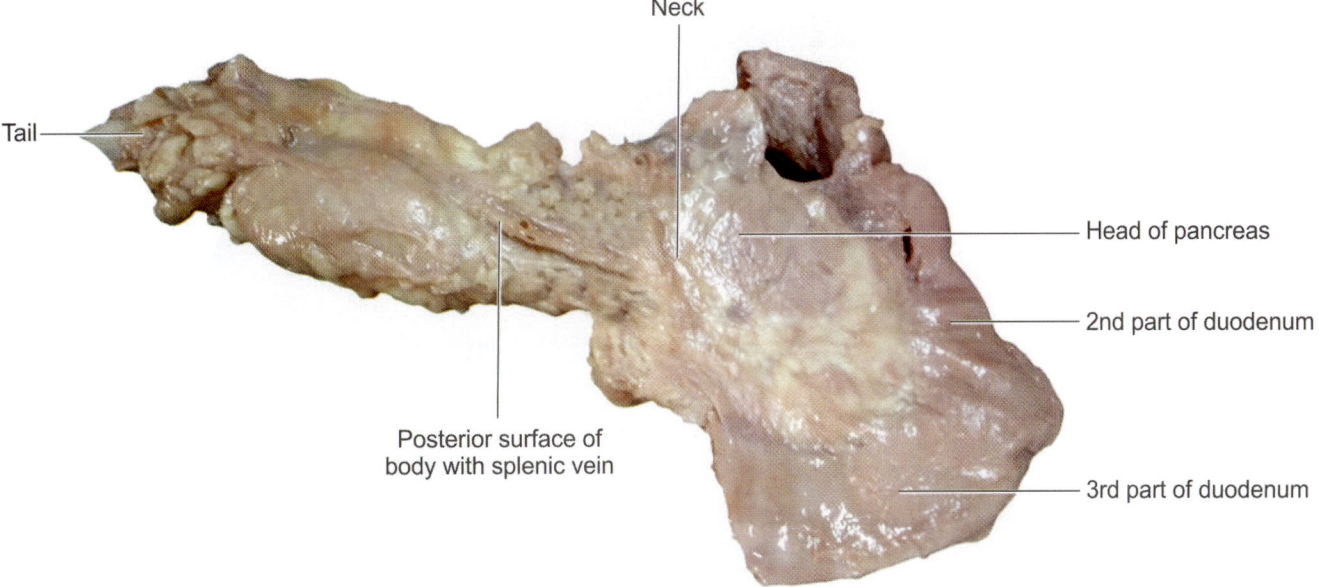

Fig. 33.3: Posterior surface of pancreas with splenic vein

- Expose the structures posterior to pancreas.
- Turn the tail and body of pancreas to the right stripping the splenic artery and vein from its posterior surface (Fig. 33.3).
- Identify branches of tortuous splenic artery passing to the gland.
- On the posterior surface of pancreas, make cut into the gland parallel to and close to the superior and inferior margins of the body.
- Pick away the lobules of the gland between the cuts to expose the greyish white duct and the interlobular ducts draining into the main duct (*see* Fig. 32.3).

LIVER

Steps of Dissection

- Pull the liver downwards (Fig. 33.4). Identify the falciform ligament.
- As the ligament reaches the anterosuperior surface of liver, it separates into right and left layers.
- The right layer covers the right side of liver and forms superior layer of coronary ligament. Covering the posteroinferior surface of right lobe is the inferior layer of coronary ligament.
- Trace these two layers to right where these form the right triangular ligament which reaches till the diaphragm.

- Note and identify a part of liver between the superior and inferior layers of coronary ligaments. This area is not covered by visceral peritoneum and is called "the bare area of the liver" (Fig. 33.5). Understand that the bare area is only in relation to right lobe as right lobe is massive. As the left lobe is much smaller, the two layers come together to form left triangular ligament; there are no coronary ligaments on the left side of liver.
- Identify the porta hepatis on the inferior surface and two layers of peritoneum attached to its two borders. These get continuous with each other along the right margin of porta hepatis. Along the left margin of porta hepatis, the two layers remain separate as they line the fissure for the ligamentum venosum.

Identify the bare area of liver:

i. The bare area between two layers of coronary ligaments. See that this area is one of the sites of portosystemic anastomosis.

ii. Area of porta hepatis containing hepatic ducts, cystic duct, bile duct, branches of proper hepatic artery and portal vein (Fig. 33.6).

iii. Area of fissure for ligamentum venosum and for attachment of lesser omentum

iv. Fossa for gallbladder

v. Groove for inferior vena cava

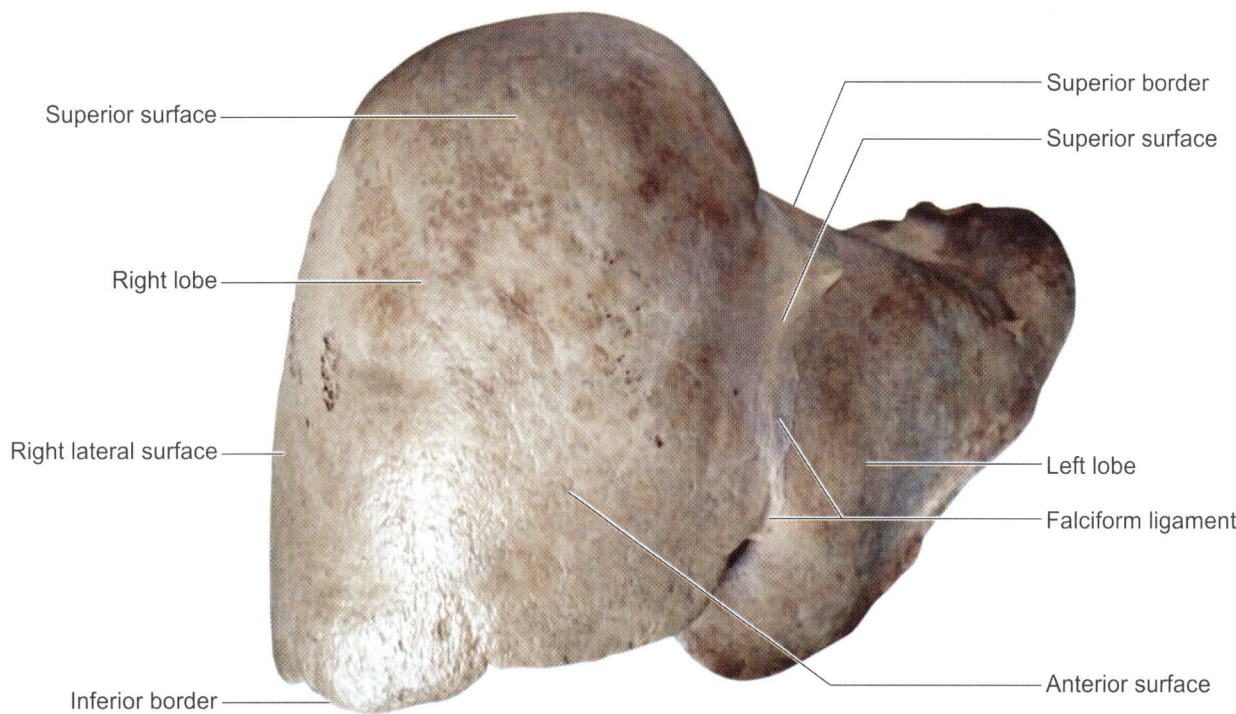

Superior surface

Right lobe

Right lateral surface

Inferior border

Superior border

Superior surface

Left lobe

Falciform ligament

Anterior surface

Fig. 33.4: Surfaces of liver

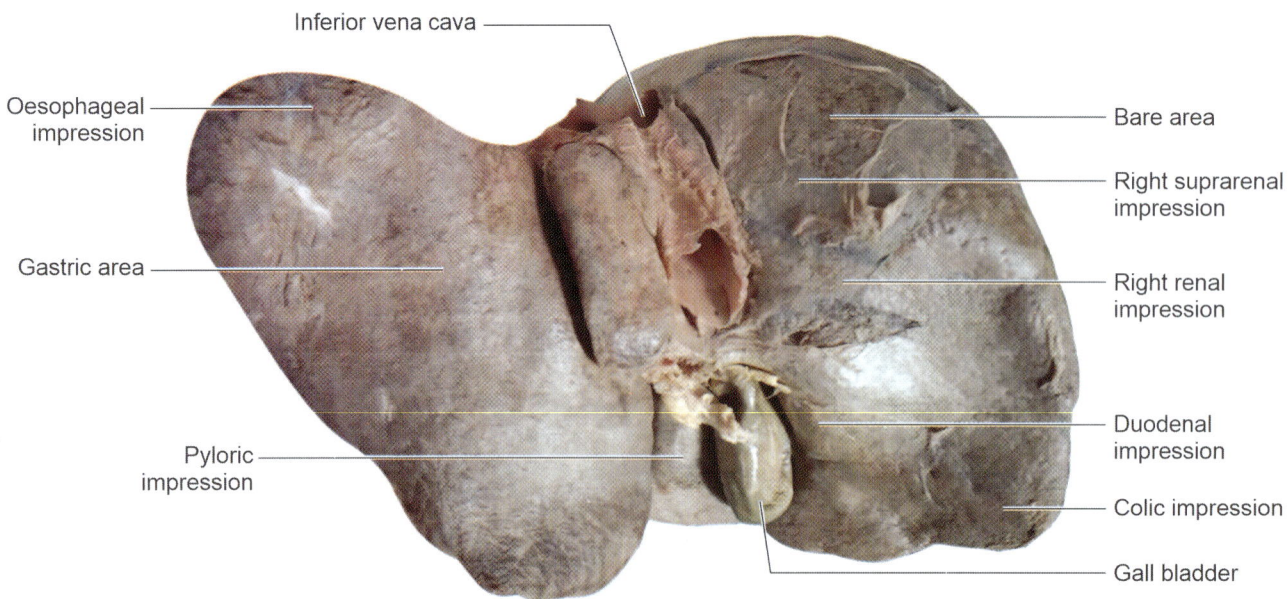

Inferior vena cava

Oesophageal impression

Gastric area

Pyloric impression

Bare area

Right suprarenal impression

Right renal impression

Duodenal impression

Colic impression

Gall bladder

Fig. 33.5: Impressions on the visceral surface of liver including "the bare area"

- Identify the inferior vena cava between the liver and diaphragm. Separate the liver downwards from inferior vena cava.
- If the inferior vena cava happens to be deeply buried in the liver, divide it and remove a segment with the liver (Fig. 33.6).
- Expose the three main structures in the porta hepatis and follow them to their entry into the liver.
- Identify the visceral impressions related to inferior surface of liver. These are:
  i. Gastric impression area on the inferior surface of left lobe (Fig. 33.5).
  ii. Fissure for ligamentum teres (Fig. 33.6)
- Identify the quadrate lobe between porta hepatis, inferior border of liver, fissure for ligamentum teres and gallbladder (Fig. 33.5). See that quadrate lobe is related to pylorus and 1st part of duodenum.
- Look at fossa for body of gallbladder to right of quadrate lobe (Fig. 33.6)
- On the inferior surface of the big right lobe the impressions are:
  i. Hepatic flexure of colon
  ii. Junction of 1st and 2nd parts of duodenum
  iii. Right kidney and right suprarenal gland (Fig. 33.5)
- Explore the extent of the right and left pleural cavities and pericardium related to the superior and anterior surfaces of liver, though separated from it by the diaphragm.
  i. The upper 1/3rd of right surface is related to diaphragm, the pleura and right lung
  ii. Middle 1/3rd is related to diaphragm and costodiaphragmatic recess of the pleura.
  iii. Lower 1/3rd is related only to the diaphragm.
- Cut the structures close to the porta hepatis and separate all the peritoneal ligaments and folds of the liver.
- Remove the liver from the body. Identify various lobes, borders, surfaces, etc. Surfaces of the liver are:
  i. Anterior (Fig. 33.4)
  ii. Posterior
  iii. Superior
  iv. Right
  v. Inferior

These are continuous with each other. Inferior surface is separated from anterior and superior surfaces by a prominent inferior border.

- Identify two lobes of liver. Liver comprises big right and small left lobe by the attachment of falciform ligament. The right lobe in addition reveals quadrate lobe anteriorly and a caudate lobe posteriorly.

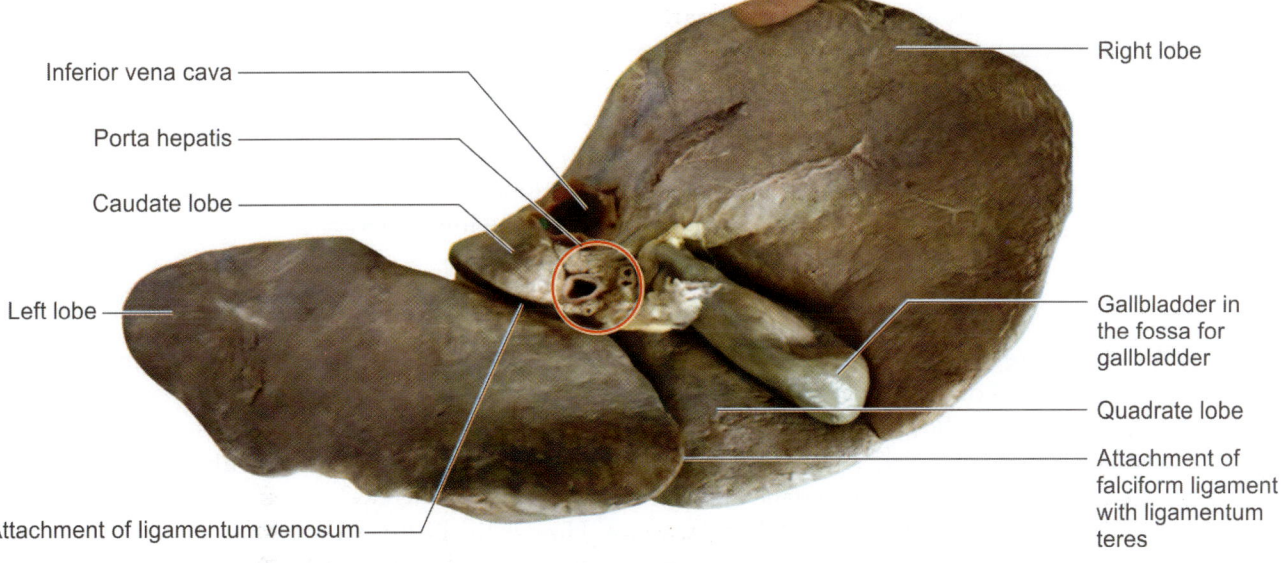

Fig. 33.6: Porta hepatis and few related structures

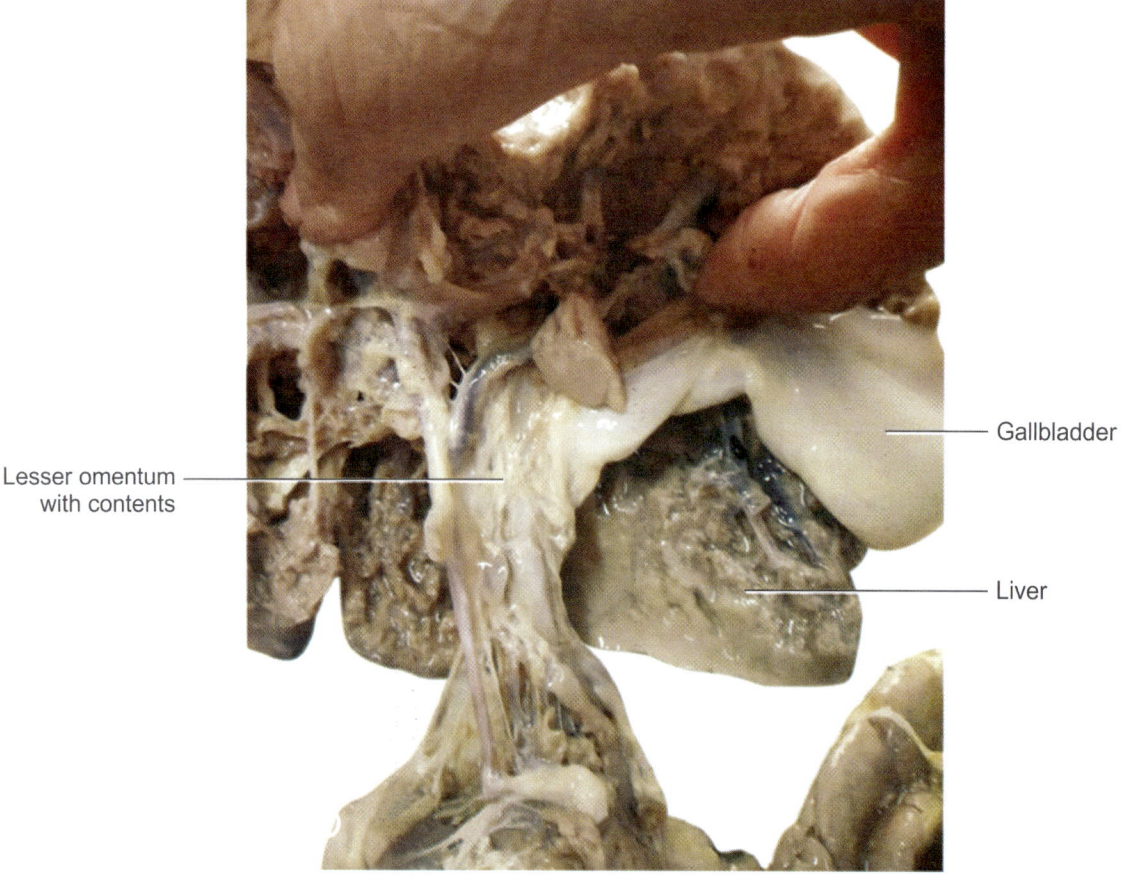

Fig. 33.7: Contents of lesser omentum

- On the inferior surface look for deep porta hepatis with hepatic ducts anteriorly, hepatic arteries in between and branches of portal vein posteriorly.
- See that the posterior surface is marked by following impressions from right to left side:
  i. The bare area
  ii. Groove for inferior vena cava
  iii. Caudate lobe
  iv. Fissure for ligamentum venosum
  v. Impression for the oesophagus
- See that both proper hepatic artery and portal vein supply blood to the liver. Hepatic artery provides 20% oxygenated blood while portal vein gives 80% of blood laden with nutrients which are absorbed from the intestines.

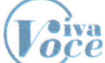

- Name the visceral relations of spleen.
- What are the contents of lienorenal ligament?
- Which border of spleen shows notches and why?
- What are the parts of pancreas?
- Which vessels lie behind the body of pancreas and anterior to its uncinate process and why?
- Which part of pancreas has maximum islets?
- What are the relations of visceral surface of liver?
- How much blood does the portal vein supply to the liver?
- How much blood hepatic artery supply to the liver?
- Why is jaundice associated with malignant growth of head of pancreas?
- How is liver biopsy done?
- In which directions do the enlarged spleen and liver point?

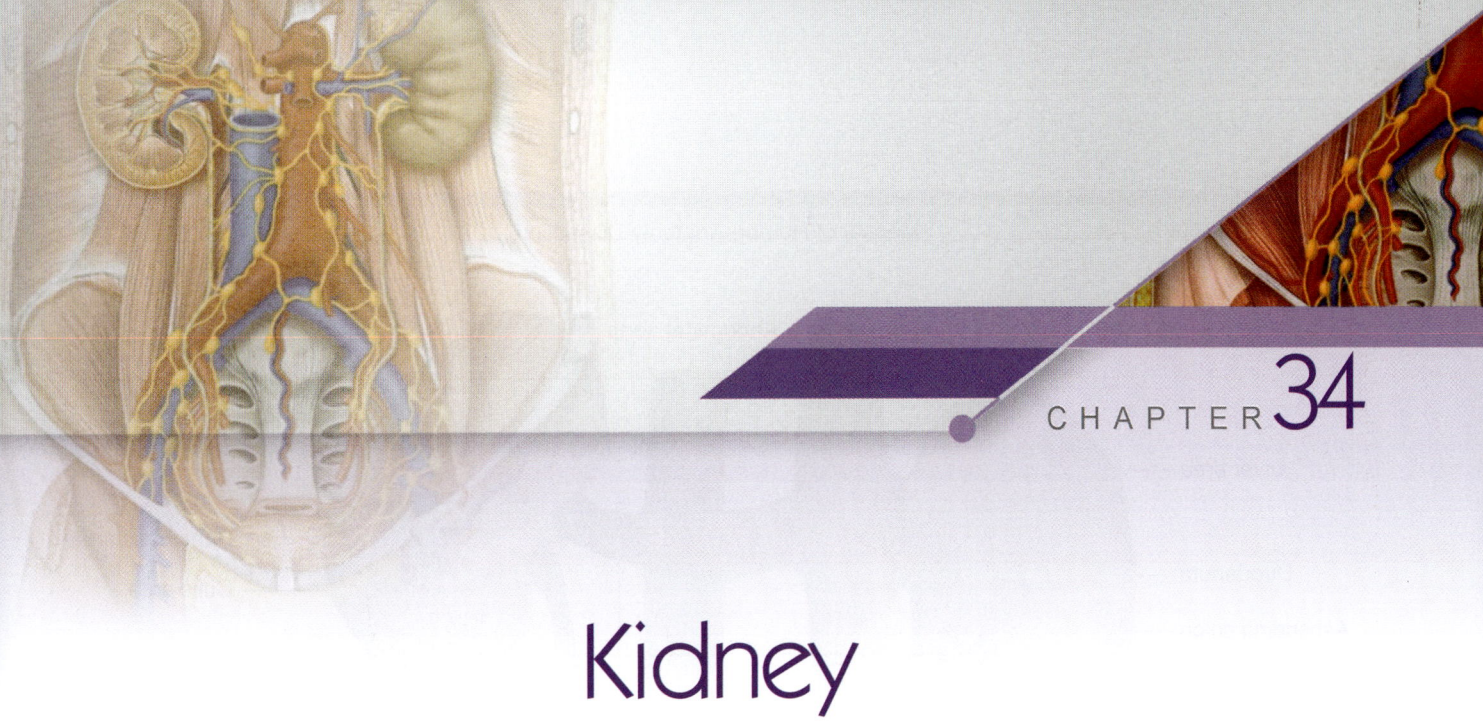

CHAPTER 34

Kidney

Learning Objectives

One should be able to
1. Discuss genesis of formation of renal and ureteric stones
2. Mention relations of posterior surface of two kidneys
3. Enumerate relations of anterior surface of left kidney
4. Mention positions of the ureteric constrictions and their importance.

OVERVIEW

The kidneys are retroperitoneal organs which are instrumental for filtering the blood and forming urine.

The posterior surface of kidney is related to diaphragm and muscles of posterior abdominal wall. Relations of the anterior surface are different on the right and left sides.

The hilum contains the following structures from before backwards:
- Renal vein
- Renal artery
- Pelvis of ureter

Kidney is very richly supplied by the renal artery—a branch of abdominal aorta at level of L2 vertebra.

Kidneys are supported by intra-abdominal pressure, renal capsule, renal fascia, perirenal and pararenal fat.

Ureter

The ureter exits from the hilum as pelvis of ureter. Then it narrows and continues as ureter partly in posterior abdominal wall and partly in the pelvis. There are five normal constrictions in the ureter: At pelvi-ureteric junction, at brim of the pelvis, point of crossing of ureter by ductus deferens, through its passage in the wall of urinary bladder and at its opening in the trigone of urinary bladder.

Ureter is supplied by blood from the medial side in abdominal part and from lateral side in the true pelvis.

STEPS OF DISSECTION

- Remove the fat and fascia from the anterior surface of left and right kidneys and suprarenal glands.
- Identify the structures related to the anterior surface of both the kidneys (Fig. 34.1). These structure on the right kidney are:
  i. Right suprarenal
  ii. Big hepatic area
  iii. Duodenum near the hilum
  iv. Ascending colon along the convex border
  v. Coils of intestine in the remaining area.
- Identify the structures related to the anterior surface of the left kidney. These are:
  i. Left suprarenal
  ii. Spleen
  iii. Part of stomach

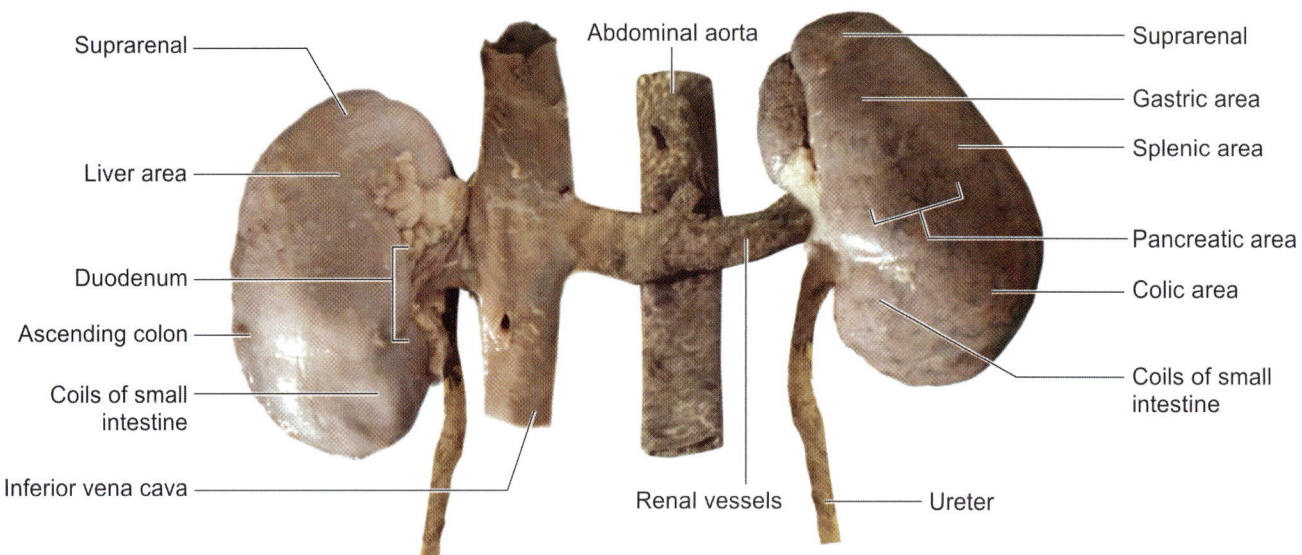

Fig. 34.1: Anterior relations of right and left kidneys

iv. Pancreas

v. Descending colon along left convex border

vi. Coils of small intestine in the remaining area

- Turn the left kidney medially to expose the posterior surface. The structures related are:

  i. Diaphragm in upper half (Fig. 34.2)

  ii. Psoas major in medial area of lower half

  iii. Quadratus lumborum in middle of lower half

  iv. Transversus abdominis in lateral area of lower half

  v. 11th and 12th ribs

  vi. Subcostal nerve and vessels

- Turn the right kidney medially and examine the relations of posterior surface. These happen to be same as that of the left kidney. The difference is that right kidney is related only to 12th rib as it is lower than the left kidney.

- Find the left suprarenal vein and left testicular/ovarian vein and trace both these to the left renal vein.

- Follow this vein from the left kidney to inferior vena cava and see that two veins, i.e. left suprarenal vein and left testicular/ovarian vein are its tributaries. Displace the vein and expose left renal artery. Follow its branches to kidney, left suprarenal and left ureter.

- Trace the ureter from the kidney on posterior abdominal wall.

- Now follow the right renal vein. It is smaller than left renal vein. The right renal vein drains into inferior vena cava. The right suprarenal and right testicular/ovarian veins also drain directly into the inferior vena cava.

- Note that the right renal artery is longer than the left whereas the right renal vein is shorter than left renal vein.

- The right ureter starts from the renal sinus as pelvis of ureter and narrows down at the lower end of the kidney.

Now the structures at the hilum have to be cut and fat and fascia cleaned to remove the kidneys from the abdominal cavity.

Examine the delivered kidney to see:

- 2 poles—upper broad pole and lower pointed pole (Fig. 34.3)

- 2 surfaces—irregular anterior surface and smooth posterior surface

- 2 borders—lateral convex border and medial border showing a depression in its middle part

- 1 hilum—the gateway to the kidney is the hilum. It contains from anterior to posterior:

  a. Renal vein

  b. Renal artery

  c. Renal pelvis—the upper expanded end of the ureter.

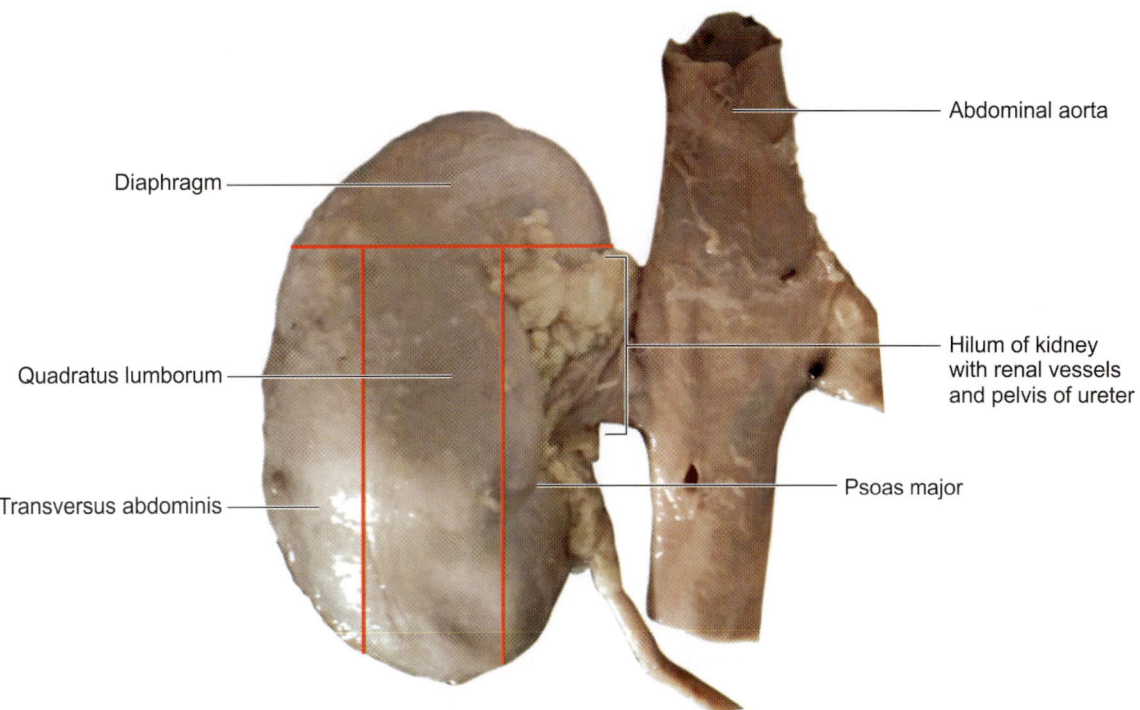

Diaphragm

Quadratus lumborum

Transversus abdominis

Abdominal aorta

Hilum of kidney
with renal vessels
and pelvis of ureter

Psoas major

Fig. 34.2: Relations of posterior surface of left kidney

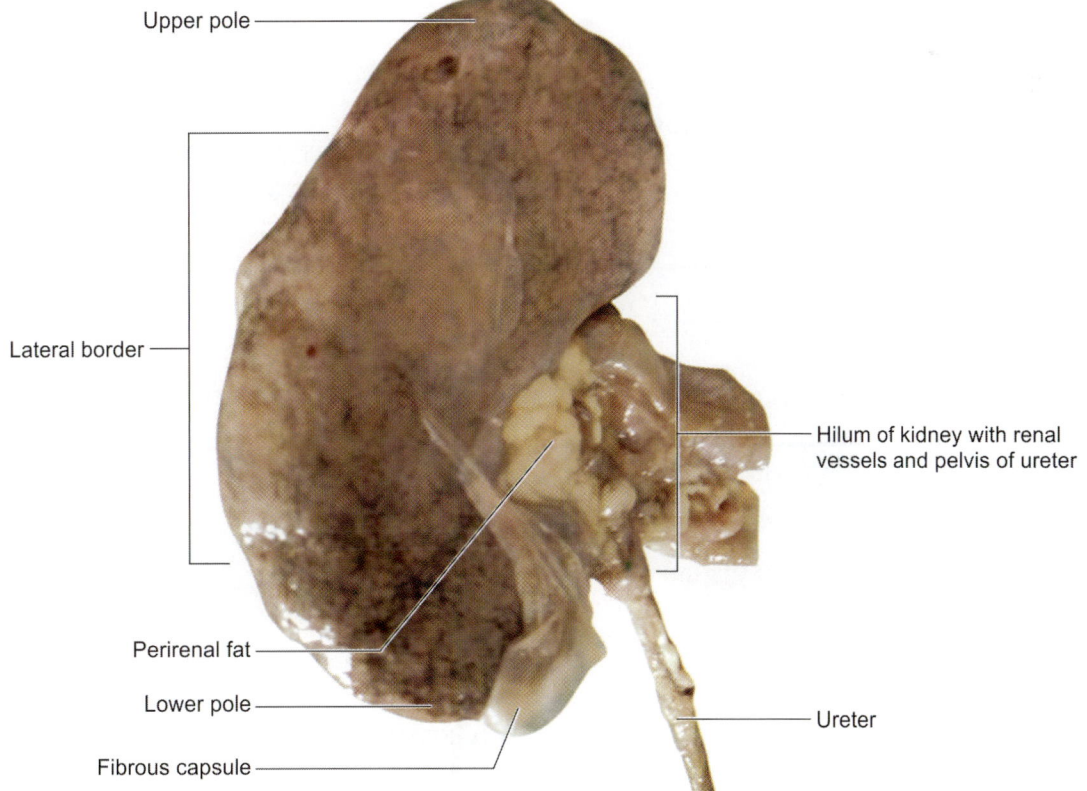

Upper pole

Lateral border

Perirenal fat

Lower pole

Fibrous capsule

Hilum of kidney with renal
vessels and pelvis of ureter

Ureter

Fig. 34.3: Gross features of the kidney

- Cut through the convex border of the kidney till the hilus. Identify the structures in its interior (Fig. 34.4). The structures are:
  - Outer peripheral reddish brown cortex
  - Inner pale medulla
  - Innermost renal sinuses

The medulla is made up of 10 pyramidal masses— the pyramids. The apex of a pyramid forms the renal papilla which indents a minor calyx.

Cortex is in two parts:

- Outer peripheral cortex
- Renal columns which dip in between the pyramids.

Innermost renal sinus contains:

- Branches of renal artery
- Tributaries of renal vein
- Renal pelvis which divides into 2 major calyces which in turn divides into 7–13 minor calyces.

Vascular segments: According to the arterial supply, there are 5 renal segments in each kidney with independent blood supply. Segments are apical, upper, middle, lower and posterior. Thus segmental resection is possible if need arises.

Arterial supply: Each kidney is supplied by wide renal artery which arises from the abdominal aorta at right angle.

THE URETER

Each ureter is 25 cm long and 3 mm in diameter (Fig. 34.5). The upper half of ureter lies in abdomen whereas lower half is placed in the pelvis. Notice that it starts from upper part of posterior abdominal wall and ends in the lower part of anterior abdominal wall.

Since the ureter is narrow, the renal calculi may obstruct the flow of urine. This gives rise to ureteric colic. The ureter is further narrowed at 5 places:

  i. At the pelviureteric junction

 ii. At the brim of pelvis

iii. At the crossing of ureter by ductus deferens or broad ligament of uterus

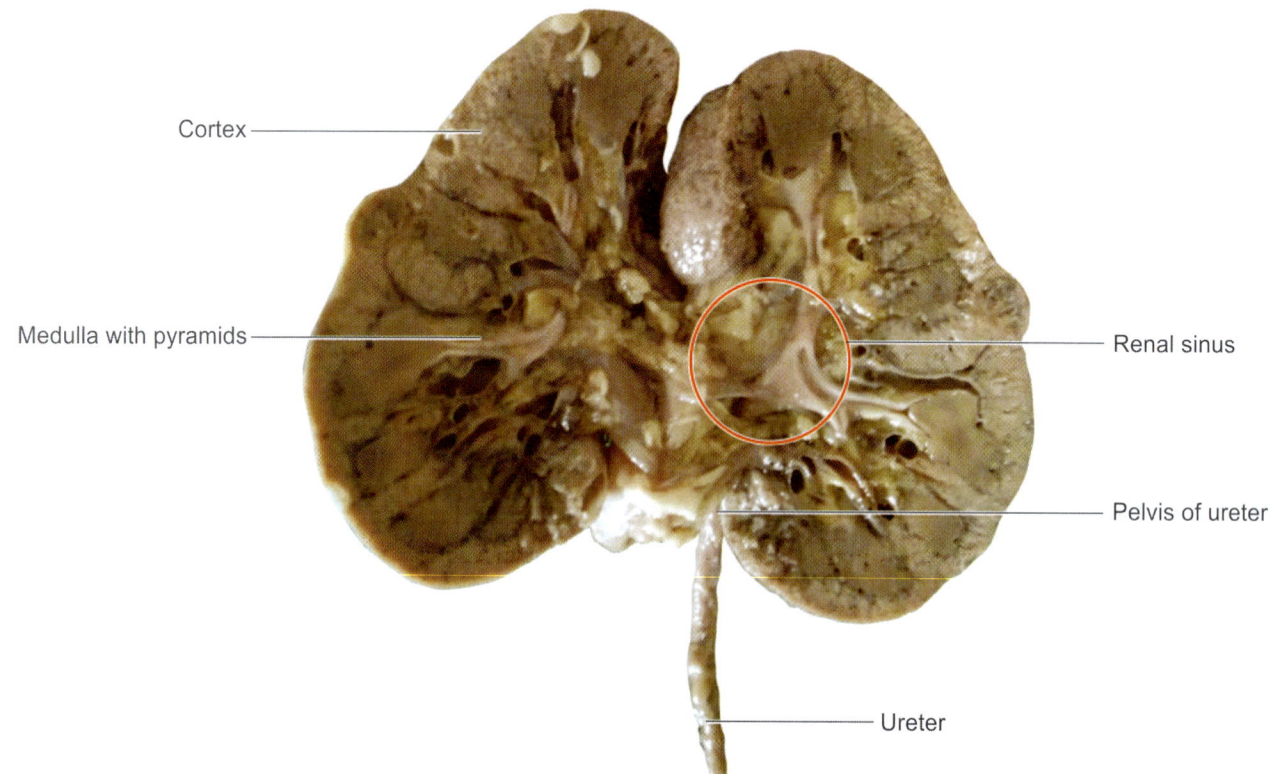

Fig. 34.4: Cut section of the kidney

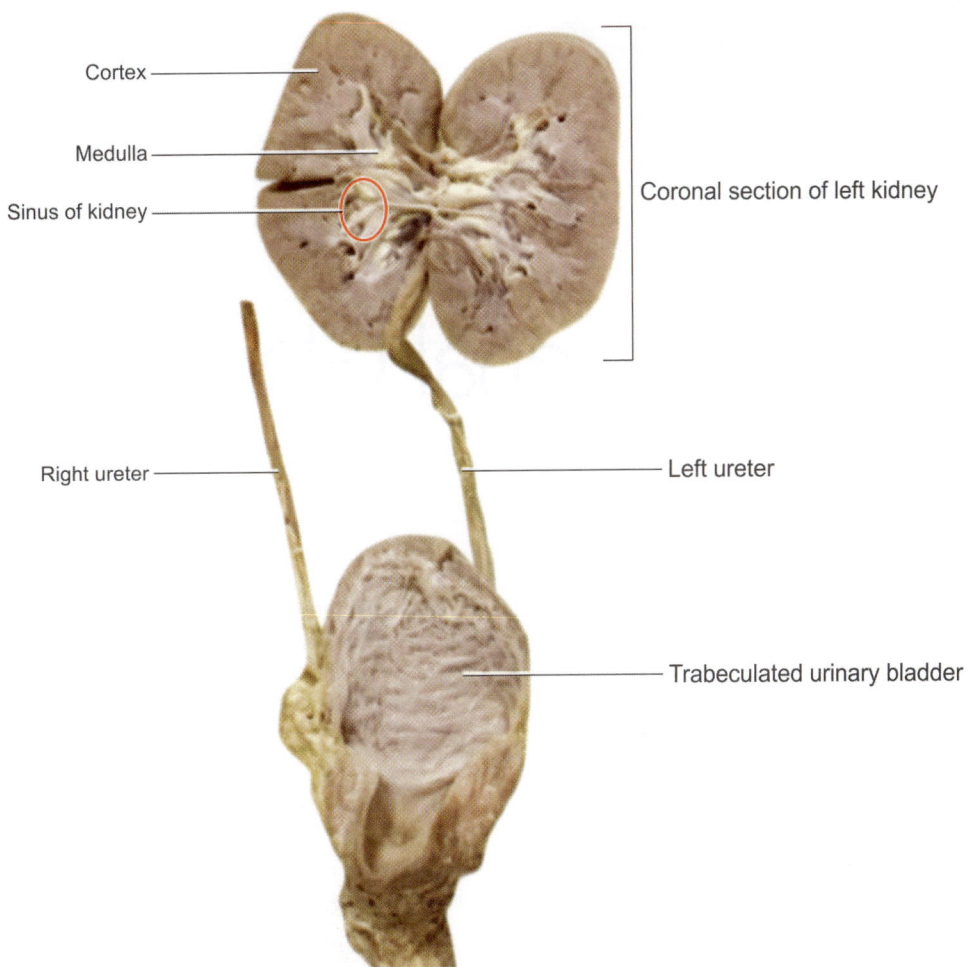

Cortex

Medulla

Sinus of kidney

Coronal section of left kidney

Right ureter

Left ureter

Trabeculated urinary bladder

Fig. 34.5: Ureters opening in urinary bladder

iv. During its oblique passage through the bladder wall (Fig. 34.5)

v. At its opening into the lateral angle of trigone of the bladder

Steps of Dissection

Follow the ureters from the renal pelvis in the abdomen, then in the pelvic cavity and lastly through the wall of the urinary bladder.

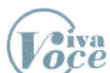

- Name the structures present at the hilum of kidney 'in order'.
- Name the relations of posterior surface of the kidneys.
- Which kidney is at a lower level and why?
- Name the relations of anterior surface of right kidney.
- Name the sites of normal constrictions of the ureter.

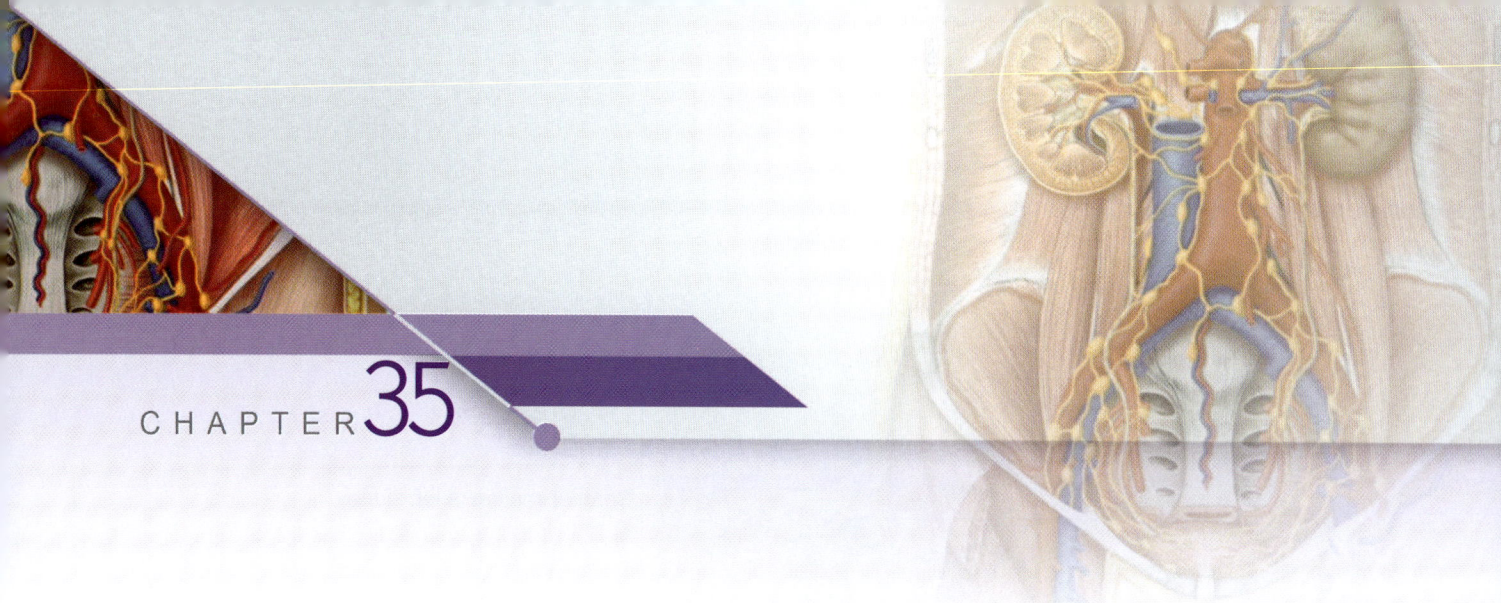

CHAPTER 35

Suprarenal Gland

Learning Objectives

One should be able to

1. Recapitulate origin of three arteries which supply the suprarenal gland.
2. Mention the venous drainage of the gland
3. Name the three zones of suprarenal cortex.
4. Discuss the importance of suprarenal gland for our body.

OVERVIEW

Suprarenal glands are endocrine glands of great importance. The gland comprises an outer cortex of mesodermal origin and an inner medulla of neural crest origin.

The gland caps the upper pole of kidneys. Hence these are called suprarenal. These glands are retroperitoneal organs like the kidneys, ureter, duodenum and pancreas.

The suprarenal gland is much smaller than the kidney. The right gland is triangular while the left is semilunar in shape. These glands are richly supplied by three arteries each.

STEPS OF DISSECTION

- Locate the suprarenal glands along the upper pole and medial border of the two kidneys. See that the posterior surfaces of the glands are related to respective crus of diaphragm and the kidneys.
- Identify the right triangular gland (Fig. 35.1). Its anterior relations are to the liver in the right half and to inferior vena cava in left half.
- Identify and see the left semilunar gland (Fig. 35.1). Its anterior relations are to the pancreas on medial side and to stomach on left side.
- Clean and identify the middle suprarenal arteries to each of the gland. This is its own artery.
- See that it also receives a descending branch from inferior phrenic artery of abdominal aorta.
- Identify and ascending branch to the gland from the renal artery.
- Look for a single vein only from each gland.
- Left vein drains into left renal vein which further drains into inferior vena cava.
- Right vein drains directly into inferior vena cava.

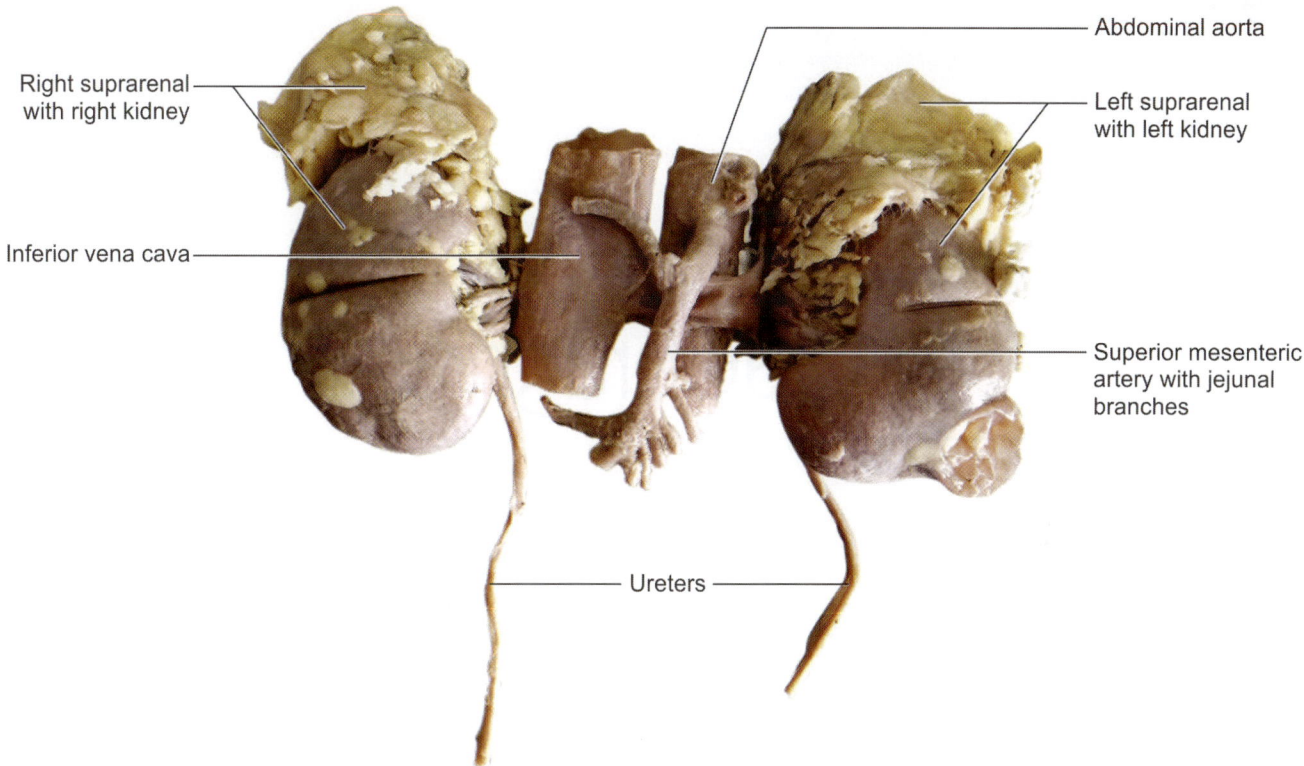

Right suprarenal with right kidney

Inferior vena cava

Abdominal aorta

Left suprarenal with left kidney

Superior mesenteric artery with jejunal branches

Ureters

Fig. 35.1: Right and left suprarenal glands

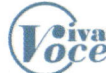

- What are the developmental components of the suprarenal gland?
- Name the anterior relations of left suprarenal gland.
- Where does left suprarenal vein drain?
- Name the arteries supplying the suprarenal gland.

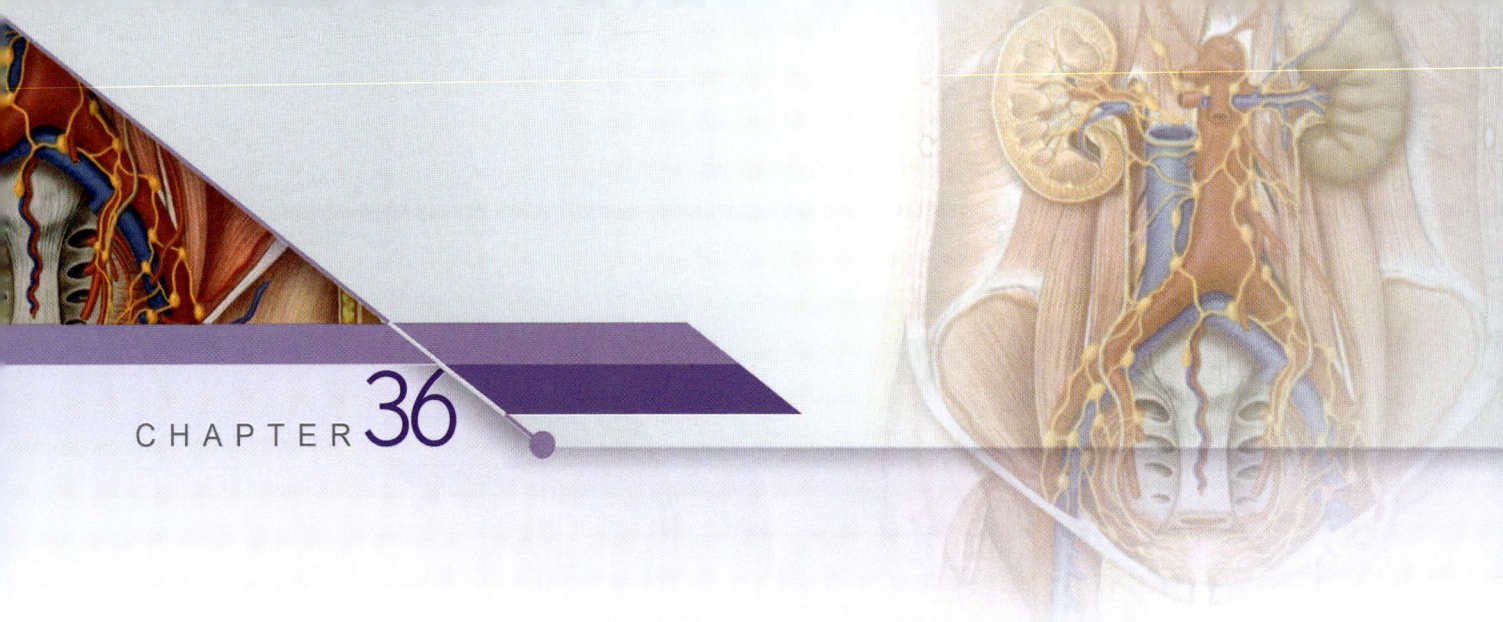

Diaphragm

Learning Objectives

One should be able to
1. Name the major openings in the diaphragm.
2. What structures pass through these openings?

3. What is the basis of sliding and rolling hernia?

OVERVIEW

Diaphragm is a muscular dome-shaped partition between thoracic and abdominal cavities (Fig. 36.1). It is the chief muscle of respiration. In addition it permits some structures to pass up and down between abdomen and the thorax. It arises from:
  i. Back of xiphoid process (sternum)
 ii. *Costal:* Inner aspects of cartilages and adjacent parts of 7th–12th ribs
iii. Lumbar part from right crus arising from L1 to L3 vertebra and from left crus arising from L1 to L2 vertebra; median arcuate, medial arcuate and lateral arcuate ligaments.

It gets inserted into a triangular leaf like structure, the central tendon (Fig. 36.1).

Diaphragm contains many orifices. The main ones are aortic opening (T12); oesophageal opening (T10) and inferior vena caval opening (T8). There are number of minor orifices for the passage of intercostal nerves, vessels and splanchnic nerves, etc.

Diaphragm develops from diverse components. If these do not fuse in the orderly manner, it remains weak or missing. Hernia may protrude from these undeveloped spaces.

Competency achievement: The student should be able to:

AN 47.14 Describe the abnormal openings of thoracoabdominal diaphragm and diaphragmatic hernia.

STEPS OF DISSECTION

- Strip the peritoneum from the under aspect of the diaphragm and expose its crura on the anterior surfaces of upper three lumbar vertebrae on right side and upper two lumbar vertebrae on left side.
- Dissect the median, medial and lateral arcuate ligaments.

Median arcuate ligament is a tendinous arch which connects the right and left crus across the midline. Medial arcuate ligament is attached medially to the sides of L1–L2 vertebra extending laterally to the transverse process of L1 vertebra.

Lateral arcuate ligament is attached medially to transverse process of L1 vertebra and laterally to 12th rib. The fibres of diaphragm arise from all these five ligaments.

- Expose the slips of diaphragm arising from the internal surfaces of 7–12 costal cartilages.
- Identify the intercostal vessels and nerves entering the abdominal wall between them.

262

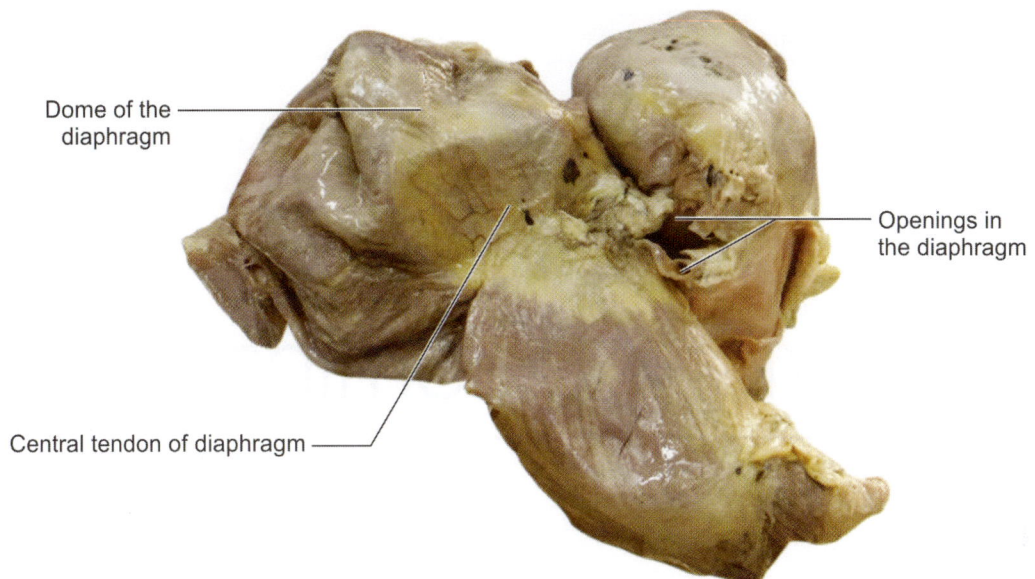

Dome of the diaphragm

Openings in the diaphragm

Central tendon of diaphragm

Fig. 36.1: Parts of the diaphragm

- Trace the phrenic nerves (C4), arising from the cervical plexus, downwards into the thoracic cavity on the surface of fibrous pericardium on each side. The nerve pierces the diaphragm and innervates each dome of diaphragm from the abdominal side.
  Phrenic nerve also carries sensory fibres from central part of diaphragm, fibrous pericardium and parietal layers of serous pericardium and mediastinal pleura.
- Identify the artery-pericardiacophrenic artery (branch of internal thoracic) and vein accompanying the nerve.
- Locate the main openings of the diaphragm. These are:
  i. Caval opening at T8 and transmits inferior vena cava and branches of right phrenic nerve.
  ii. Oesophageal opening at level of T10 vertebra. It transmits oesophagus, right and left gastric nerves and oesophageal branches of left gastric artery.
  iii. Aortic opening at level of T12 vertebra. It transmits aorta, thoracic duct and vena azygos.

Minor Openings of the Diaphragm

1. Right and left crus of diaphragm are pierced by greater splanchnic nerve formed by branches from T5–T9 ganglia and by lesser splanchnic (visceral) nerve formed by branches of T10–T11 ganglia.
2. Sympathetic trunk travelling behind medial arcuate ligament from thorax to abdomen.
3. Subcostal nerve and vessels pass behind the lateral arcuate ligament.
4. Superior epigastric vessels pass between the sternal and 7th costal cartilaginous origin of diaphragm.
5. Musculophrenic vessels pass out at the level of 9th costal cartilage.
6. Lower intercostal nerves pass in between the slips of origin of transversus abdominis and the diaphragm
   - See that right dome of diaphragm is related to liver, kidney and suprarenal gland.
   - Identify structures related to left dome of diaphragm. These are fundus of stomach, spleen, kidney and suprarenal gland.

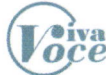
Viva Voce

- What are the functions of thoracoabdominal diaphragm?
- Name the major openings present in the diaphragm. What structures pass through these openings?
- What is the motor nerve supply of the diaphragm and what is its root value?
- Which crus of diaphragm is longer and why?

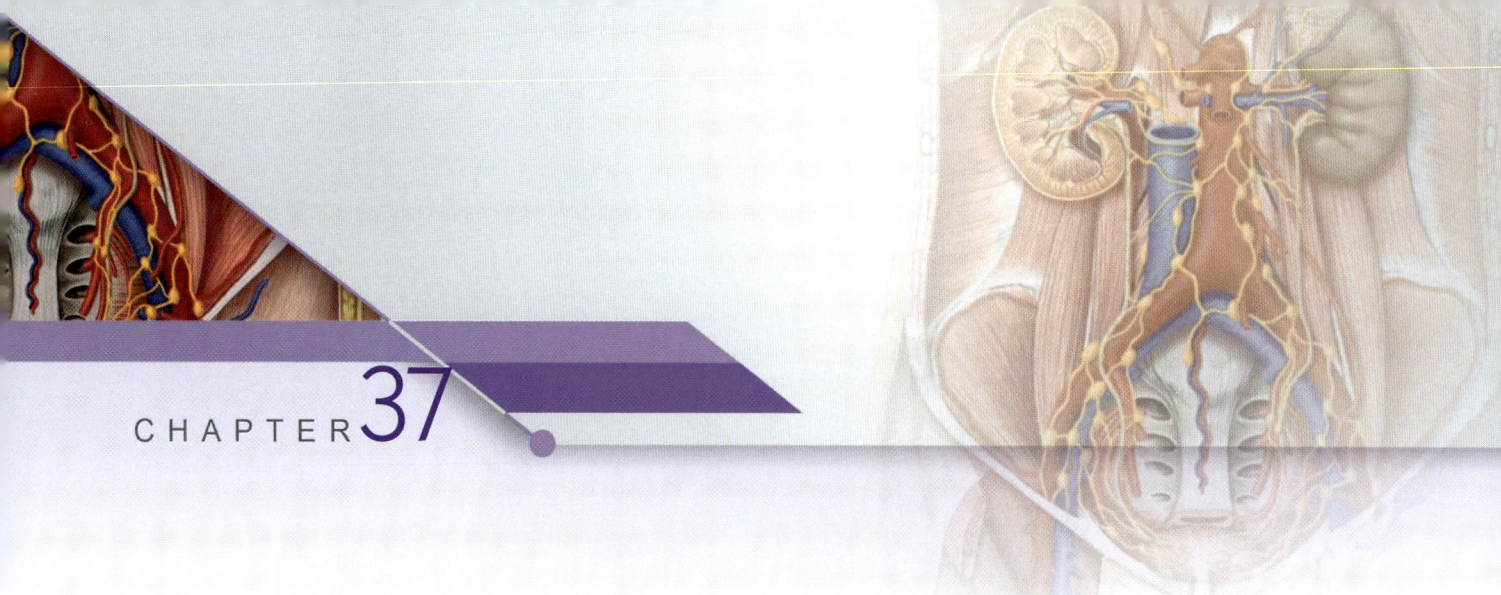

CHAPTER 37

Posterior Abdominal Wall

Learning Objectives

One should be able to

1. Enumerate visceral/anterior branches of abdominal aorta.
2. Enumerate tributaries of inferior vena cava.
3. Name the muscles of posterior abdominal wall

OVERVIEW

The posterior abdominal wall comprises:

i. The muscles, e.g. psoas major, quadratus lumborum, transversus abdominis and thoraco-abdominal diaphragm.

ii. Large blood vessels like abdominal aorta and inferior vena cava.

iii. Lumbar plexus embedded within the psoas major muscle. Sympathetic and parasympathetic nerve plexuses are also present.

iv. Lymph nodes and lymph vessels

v. Abdominal parts of azygos vein on right side and hemiazygos vein on the left side.

Abdominal aorta gives numerous branches and inferior vena cava receives numerous tributaries.

STEPS OF DISSECTION

• Expose the centrally placed abdominal aorta and inferior vena cava to the right of aorta (Fig. 37.1).

• Trace the ventral, lateral, posterior and terminal branches of abdominal aorta and the respective tributaries of inferior vena cava.

• Look for the branches of abdominal aorta (Figs 37.2 and 37.3). These are:

i. *Ventral branches:* Coeliac axis, superior mesenteric and inferior mesenteric

ii. *Lateral branches:* Inferior phrenic, suprarenal, renal and gonadal (testicular/ovarian)

iii. *Posterior branches:* Four pairs of lumbar arteries and median sacral artery

iv. *Terminal branches* at level of L4 vertebra: Right and left common iliac arteries

Inferior vena cava is formed at level of L5 by union of longer left common iliac and shorter right common iliac veins.

Inferior vena cava lies to right of median plane. Its tributaries are numerous.

It passes through an opening in the diaphragm to open into right atrium of the heart.

• Trace right and left common iliac veins uniting to form inferior vena cava.

• Trace the tributaries of inferior vena cava. These are:

i. 3rd and 4th lumbar veins of both sides

ii. Testicular/ovarian veins of both sides

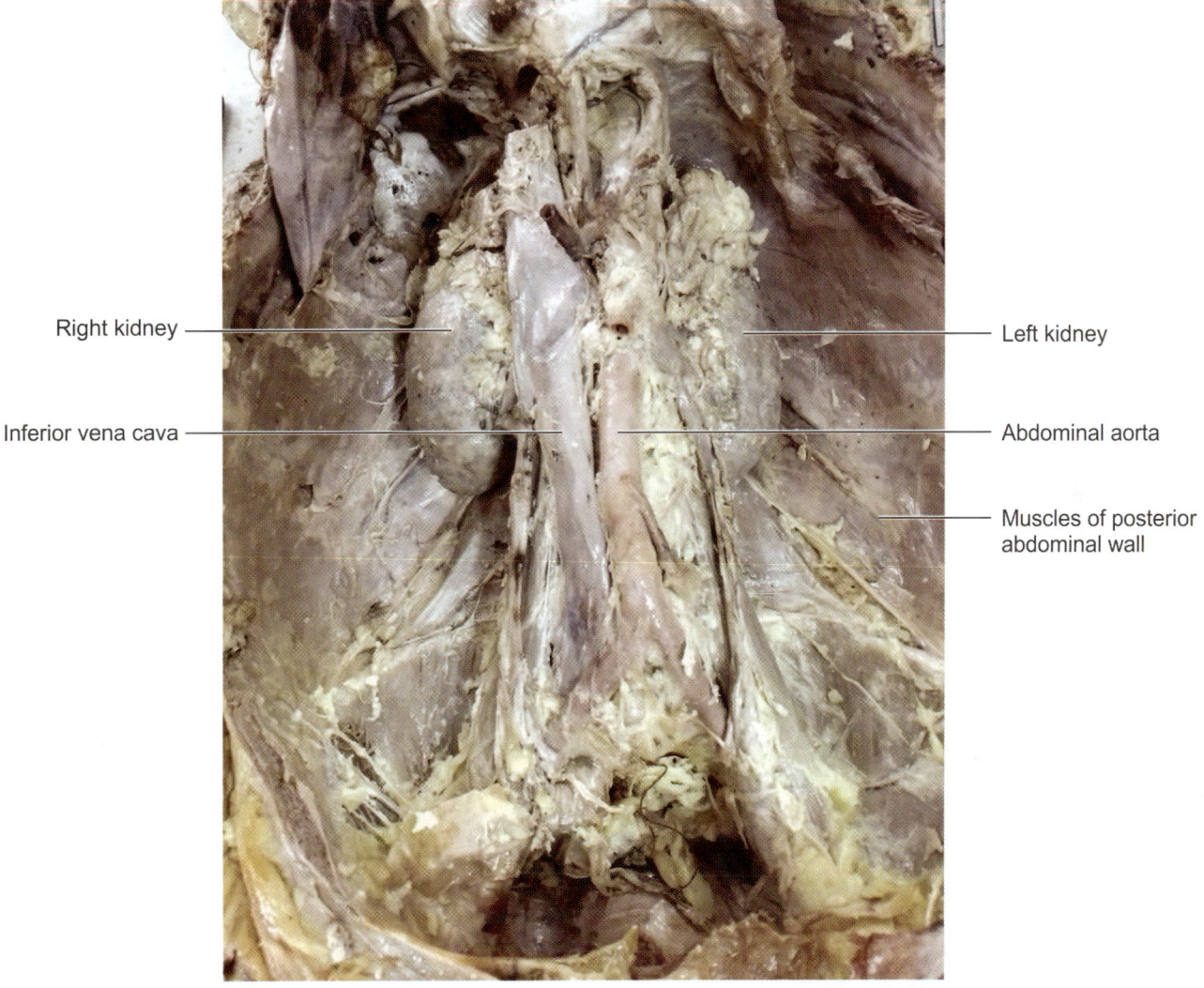

Right kidney — Left kidney

Inferior vena cava — Abdominal aorta

— Muscles of posterior abdominal wall

Fig. 37.1: Some structures in the posterior abdominal cavity wall

iii. Renal veins of both sides. Left renal vein receives left suprarenal and left testicular before it ends in inferior vena cava

iv. Right suprarenal vein

v. 3–4 hepatic veins

- See azygos vein arising commonly from back of inferior vena cava
- See hemiazygos arising from back of left renal vein

Lymph Nodes

Identify external iliac group of lymph nodes. These receive afferents from inguinal lymph nodes, glans penis, prostate, urinary bladder and cervix and part of vagina. Their efferents go to common iliac lymph nodes. Efferents from common iliac lymph nodes reach the lumbar/aortic lymph nodes.

Autonomic Plexuses

Coeliac, aortic, superior mesenteric, inferior mesenteric, superior hypogastric, right and left inferior hypogastric plexuses.

Competency achievement: The student should be able to:

AN 45.3 Mention the major subgroups of back muscles, nerve supply and action.

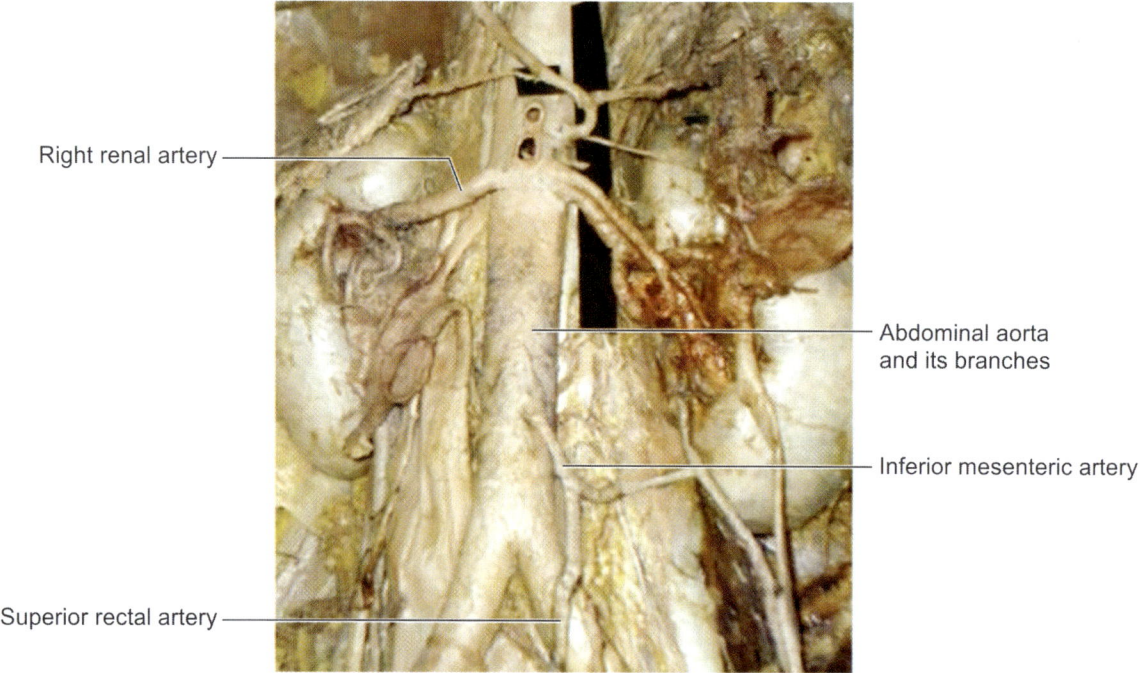

Right renal artery

Abdominal aorta and its branches

Inferior mesenteric artery

Superior rectal artery

Fig. 37.2: Abdominal aorta and some of its branches

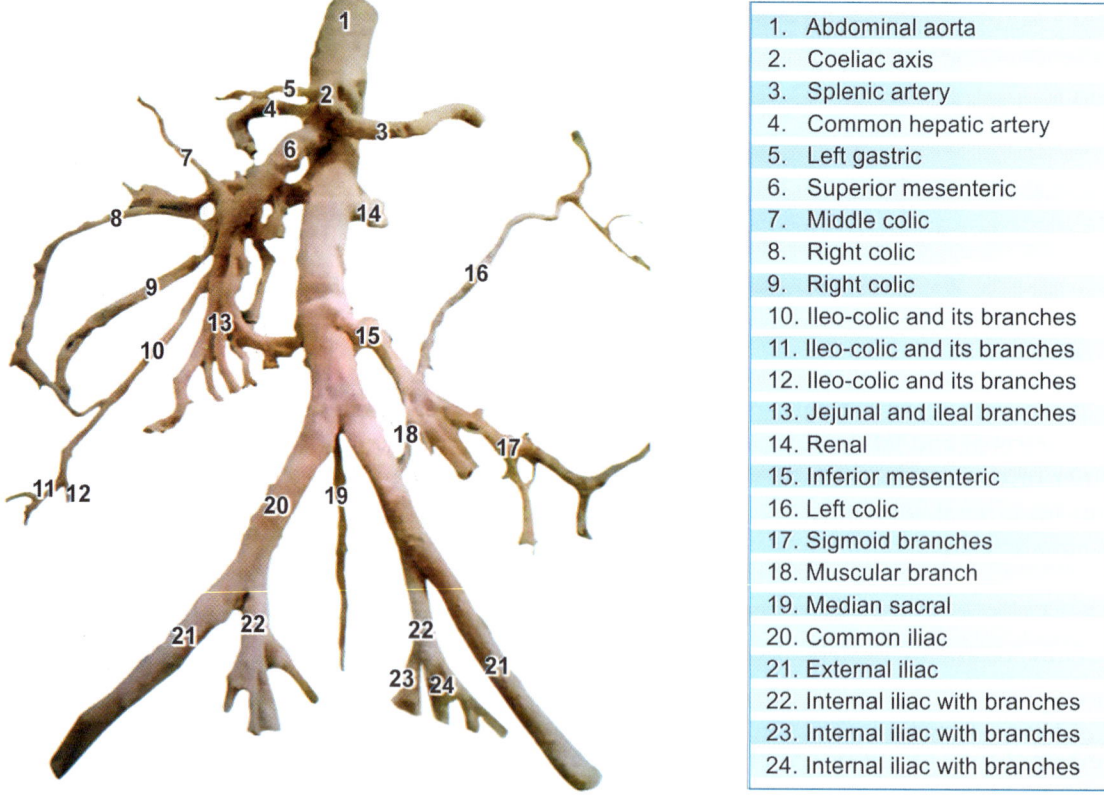

1.	Abdominal aorta
2.	Coeliac axis
3.	Splenic artery
4.	Common hepatic artery
5.	Left gastric
6.	Superior mesenteric
7.	Middle colic
8.	Right colic
9.	Right colic
10.	Ileo-colic and its branches
11.	Ileo-colic and its branches
12.	Ileo-colic and its branches
13.	Jejunal and ileal branches
14.	Renal
15.	Inferior mesenteric
16.	Left colic
17.	Sigmoid branches
18.	Muscular branch
19.	Median sacral
20.	Common iliac
21.	External iliac
22.	Internal iliac with branches
23.	Internal iliac with branches
24.	Internal iliac with branches

Fig. 37.3: Branches of abdominal aorta

Muscles of Posterior Abdominal Wall

- Identify psoas major muscle arising from lateral surface of bodies of T12–L5 vertebrae, from transverse processes of lumbar vertebrae and intervertebral discs between T12–L5 vertebrae.
- It courses through posterior abdominal wall, skirts the margin of the lesser pelvis, passes under inguinal ligament to be inserted into lesser trochanter of femur (*see* Fig. 25.2a).
- See and identify nerves present in relation to its medial, anterior and lateral surfaces. Along the medial border emerges obturator nerve and lumbosacral trunk. On the anterior surface emerges the genitofemoral nerve. Along the lateral border the nerves are iliohypogastric, ilioinguinal, lateral cutaneous nerve of thigh and femoral nerves.
- Identify quadratus lumborum arising from transverse process of L5 vertebra, iliolumbar ligament and posterior part of iliac crest. The muscle passes upwards and is inserted by slips into transverse processes of L1–L4 vertebrae including the anterior surface of 12th rib.
- Look for iliacus in the iliac fossa, arising from upper 2/3rd of iliac fossa and ventral sacroiliac ligament (*see* Fig. 25.1b).

- It also passes downwards deep to inguinal ligament to be inserted with psoas major into the lesser trochanter of femur (*see* Fig. 25.2b).

Competency achievement: The student should be able to:

AN 45.1 Describe thoracolumbar fascia.

Thoracolumbar Fascia

- Identify thoracolumbar fascia as it encloses muscles of the back.
- See that it is made up of three layers—posterior, middle and anterior layers. Posterior layer is thickest and extensive. See its attachments to tips of lumbar and sacral spines. Between posterior and middle layers is enclosed erector spinae/sacrospinalis muscle.
- See that latissimus dorsi (part) and serratus posterior inferior arise from posterior layer.
- Note that the middle layer is attached to tips of lumbar transverse processes.
- Between the middle and anterior layer is enclosed quadratus lumborum muscle.
- Parts of internal oblique and transversus abdominis arise from the fused parts of middle and anterior layers of thoracolumbar fascia.
- Anterior layer is the thinnest and forms anterior sheath which encloses quadratus lumborum muscle.

- How do you classify the branches of the abdominal aorta?
- Name the tributaries of the cisterna chyli.
- Name the muscles of posterior abdominal wall.

- Trace the course of psoas abscess.
- What is the root value of pelvic splanchnic nerve?
- Name the largest and widest vein of the body. Name its tributaries.

Perineum

OVERVIEW

Perineum is the area between upper medial sides of two thighs. In this area there are three openings in the female, e.g. anal canal, vagina and urethra and two openings in the male, e.g. anal canal and urethra. Urethra in the male carries the urine and semen according to the need of the body.

The centre of perineum contains a muscular perineal body made up of many muscles, which support anal canal and vagina.

Perineum is divided into a posterior anal region and an anterior urogenital region. Anal canal is same in male and female. It is divided into a central part known as anal canal and ischioanal fossae on each side.

Urogenital region comprises a superficial perineal space/pouch and a thin deep perineal space. Main difference between male and female urogenital regions is the difference in nomenclature of nerves and vessels.

Most important is the presence of an additional opening—the vagina. Another difference is the absence of erectile body—corpus spongiosum in females.

Males have three erectile bodies—two corpus cavernosa and one corpus spongiosum containing the urethra. In females instead of corpus spongiosum there are two bulbs of vestibule on each side of the orifices of urethra and vagina. These two bulbs of vestibule unite and get attached to the glans clitoridis.

The deep perineal space/pouch is thin in male and the urethral sphincter is within wall of urethra and not outside.

In female also the sphincter is within wall of urethra; there are two additional muscles, e.g. compressor urethrae and sphincter urethrovaginalis.

Pudendal nerve with internal pudendal vessels enter the gluteal region from the pelvis, through the greater sciatic notch and exit gluteal region through lesser sciatic notch to enter pudendal canal in the lateral wall of ischioanal fossa where inferior rectal branch is given off. Then these traverse through the deep perineal space into the superficial perineal space. The pudendal neurovascular bundle gives many branches for the sphincter ani externus, muscles of both the deep and superficial perineal spaces including overlying skin.

STEPS OF DISSECTION

- Put the cadaver in lithotomy position if lower limbs are intact.
- Make the following incisions:
  a. In the male, a median incision from the coccyx to the root of penis.
  b. In the female, a median incision from the coccyx to mons pubis encircling the anus and pudendal cleft.
  c. Horizontal incision from anterior part of right ischial tuberosity to the anterior part of left ischial tuberosity.
- Reflect the four flaps.
- See that two posterior flaps cover the anal region. The anterior two flaps cover the urogenital region.
- Pass a forceps downwards and backwards deep to the membranous layer of superficial fascia of the anterior abdominal wall.
- In the male, expose the membranous layer in the perineum.
- In the female, remove the fat from labium majus and expose the membranous layer.

Anal Region

- The gluteal region is already dissected in the cadaver. If not, make the incisions according to chapter on gluteal region and reflect gluteus maximus muscle.
- Clean the sacrotuberous and sacrospinous ligaments. Identify coccyx in the midline posteriorly and locate ischial tuberosities.

- Define the ischiopubic rami till the lower margins of pubic symphysis anteriorly.

Competency achievement: The student should be able to:

AN 49.2 Describe and identify perineal body.

If the cadaver is female

- Identify the openings of anal canal and vagina.
- Define perineal body in the centre of perineum between anus and vagina (Fig. 38.1). It is very important muscular body for support of female genital organs. There are ten muscles attached to this body. These are:
  i. 2 levator ani
  ii. 2 deep transversus perinei
  iii. 2 superficial transversus perinei
  iv. 2 bulbospongiosus
  v. 1 sphincter ani externus
  vi. 1 longitudinal muscle coat of rectum

  If cadaver is male the perineal body is situated between anal orifice and root of penis. The same muscles are attached to this body.

- Examine the muscular sphincter surrounding the anal canal. This is known as sphincter ani externus.
- See that there are three ill defined parts of this muscle. Subcutaneous part surrounds the anal orifice, superficial part encircles the middle part of anal canal and extends from perineal body in front to anococcygeal body. Deep part encircles the upper part of anal canal.

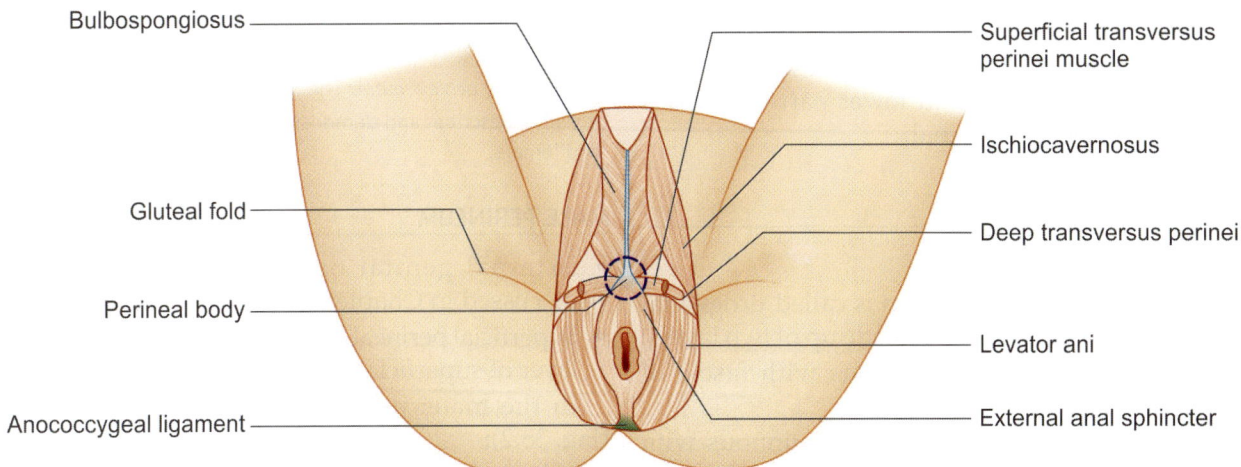

Fig. 38.1: Perineal body

- Look for the nerves supplying sphincter ani externus. These are branches of inferior rectal nerve and perineal branch of S4. Sphincter ani externus surrounds whole anal canal.
- The upper 3/4th of anal canal is surrounded by smooth sphincter ani internus muscle. At the anorectal junction see "U" shaped fibres of puborectalis which keep anorectal junction pulled forwards.
- Look for anococcygeal body situated posteriorly between anal orifice and perineal body.
- See the interior of anal canal by opening the anal canal from posterior aspect.

Competency achievement: The student should be able to:

AN 49.4 Describe and demonstrate boundaries, content and applied anatomy of ischiorectal fossa.

Ischio-anal/Ischio-rectal Fossa

- The ischio-anal fossa. It is a wedge shaped area.
- Lateral wall is formed by ischium and obturator internus covered by fascia.
- Medial wall is the anal canal covered by sphincters.
- Roof is the small area which is meeting point of levator ani and obturator internus muscles.
- Floor: Skin of buttock.
- Anterior wall: The fossa is limited by posterior border of perineal membrane.
- Posterior wall formed by sacrotuberous ligament and gluteus maximus muscle.
- Remove the fat of ischioanal fossa. Look for pudendal canal on the inner surface of obturator internus.
- Identify the inferior rectal nerve given off by pudendal nerve in ischioanal fossa. It supplies skin, sphincter ani externus and lower part of mucous membrane of the anal canal.

UROGENITAL REGION

Overview

The anterior region of perineum is called urogenital region. The superficial fascia is made up of two layers:

1. *Superficial layer*: It is continuous with fascia of surrounding organs
2. *Membranous layer:* This fascia is continuous with membranous layer of fascia of anterior abdominal wall and with fascia of scrotum and penis.

The deep fascia gets modified to form perineal membrane. Between membranous layer of superficial fascia and perineal membrane is the superficial perineal pouch/space.

Competency achievement: The student should be able to:

AN 49.1 Describe and demonstrate the superficial and deep perineal pouch (boundaries and contents).

Steps of Dissection

- Cut through the membranous layer of superficial fascia attached to ischiopubic rami.
- Now the superficial perineal space in male is opened.
- Identify ischiocavernosus muscles attached to ischiopubic rami. Also identify bulbospongiosus muscles in the centre, the muscles of two sides are united by a raphe.
- Posteriorly are two small superficial transversus perinei muscles.
- Identify the nerves supplying all the three muscles on each side. These are branches of perineal nerve.
- After the study of these three muscles on each side, trace two corpora cavernosa backwards as crura to be attached to ischiopubic rami. Identify single corpus spongiosum passing backwards to perineal membrane, where it expands as the bulb of penis.
- Detach both crus (crura) from ischiopubic rami and bulb from perineal membrane.
- Clean the perineal membrane. See the perineal membrane being pierced by the urethra which now enters the bulb of penis.
- Identify strong perineal body just behind the centre of perineal membrane.

Competency achievement: The student should be able to:

AN 49.3 Describe and demonstrate perineal membrane in male and female.

MALE PERINEUM

- External genital organs of males have been discussed in Chapter 27.
- Superficial perineal space lies between membranous layer of superficial fascia and perineal membrane.

In the male, perineal membrane is pierced by (Fig. 38.2):

  i. Urethra single. Rest in paris

  ii. Duct of bulbourethral gland and artery to bulb

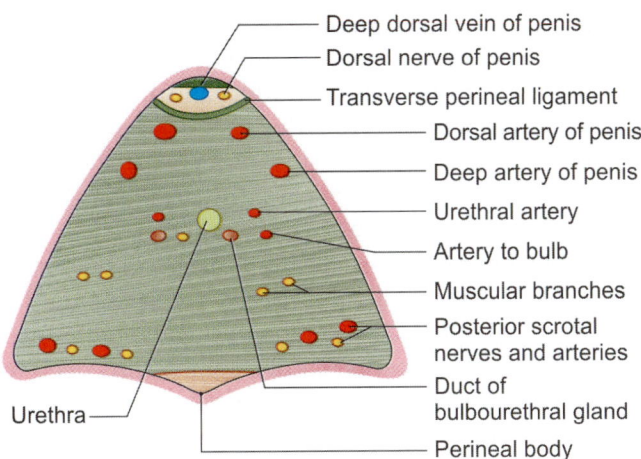

Fig. 38.2: Structures piercing perineal membrane in male

iii. Deep artery of penis

iv. Urethral artery

v. Dorsal artery of penis

vi. Muscular branches

vii. Dorsal nerve of penis

viii. Posterior scrotal vessels and nerves

Identify structures in deep perineal space in male

  i. Membranous part of urethra

  ii. Sphincter urethrae within wall of urethra

  iii. Deep transversus perinei muscles

  iv. Bulbourethral glands

  v. Dorsal nerve of penis

  vi. Origin of artery to the bulb of penis

  vii. Urethral artery and deep artery of penis

  viii. Dorsal artery of penis

FEMALE PERINEUM

External genital organs/pudendum/vulva.

Following are the external genital organs in the female:

1. Mons pubis

2. Labia majora

3. Labia minora

4. Clitoris

5. Vestibule of vagina

6. Bulbs of vestibule

7. Greater vestibular glands

Superficial Perineal Space in Female

The most important difference between the superficial perineal spaces of male and female is the passage of an additional tube, the vagina.

- Remove the skin from the sides of the vestibule. Trace the two crura of clitoris attached to ischiopubic ramus of each side.

- Identify ischiocavernosus muscles covering each crus.

- In the centre of vestibule see the two openings, one of urethra anteriorly and other bigger opening of vagina.

- See the bulbs of vestibule on each side of these two openings. Behind these bulbs identify greater vestibular glands. These bulbs are also covered by the bulbospongiosus muscles. These appear to join the ischiocavernosus muscles near the clitoris.

- Identify the superficial transversus perinei between perineal body and ischiopubic rami.

- See that all these three pairs of muscles get innervated by branches of perineal nerve as in male perineum.

- Perineal membrane is triangular. Its anterior part near pubic symphysis is narrow while its posterior part is broad.

In the female, perineal membrane is pierced by (Fig. 38.3):

  i. Urethra–single

  ii. Vagina behind urethra–single. Rest in pairs

  iii. Deep artery of clitoris

  iv. Dorsal artery of clitoris

  v. Artery to bulb of vestibule

  vi. Muscular branches

  vii. Dorsal nerve of clitoris

  viii. Posterior labial vessels and nerves

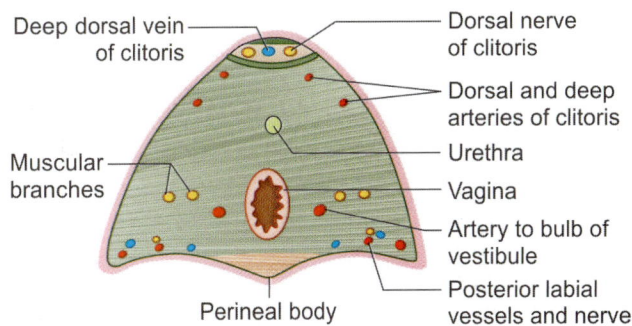

Fig. 38.3: Structures piercing perineal membrane in female

Identify the contents of deep perineal space in female

   i. Urethra

  ii. Vagina

 iii. Sphincter urethrae within wall of urethra

 iv. Compressor urethra

  v. Sphincter urethrovaginalis

 vi. Muscular branches of perineal nerve

 vii. Artery of clitoris

viii. Stems of origin of artery to bulb of vestibule

 ix. Urethral artery

  x. Deep artery of clitoris

 xi. Dorsal artery of clitoris

- Trace internal pudendal artery from lateral wall of ischioanal fossa into thin open deep perineal space.

- See that the artery gives branches which pierce the perineal membrane to reach their destinations. These are—artery to the bulb, deep artery and dorsal arteries. Deep artery is seen to enter corpus spongiosum, dorsal artery runs on the surface of penis/clitoris.

- See pudendal nerve entering the deep space from ischioanal fossa. Identify its branches.

Perineal nerve innervates all muscles of deep and superficial spaces. It also gives posterior/labial branches, which also pierce the perineal membrane.

Dorsal nerve of penis/clitoris which runs deep to the skin, lateral to dorsal artery of penis.

- See and find structures on dorsum of penis. These are one deep dorsal vein of penis, dorsal artery one on each side of vein and dorsal nerve one on each side of artery.

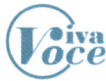 **Viva Voce**

- Name the boundaries of perineum.
- Name the muscles attached to perineal body.
- What are the boundaries of ischioanal fossa?
- Name the contents of pudendal canal.
- Name the structures piercing perineal membrane in male.
- Name the structures piercing perineal membrane in female.
- What is the main difference between penis of male and clitoris of female?
- Name the components of spincter ani externus.

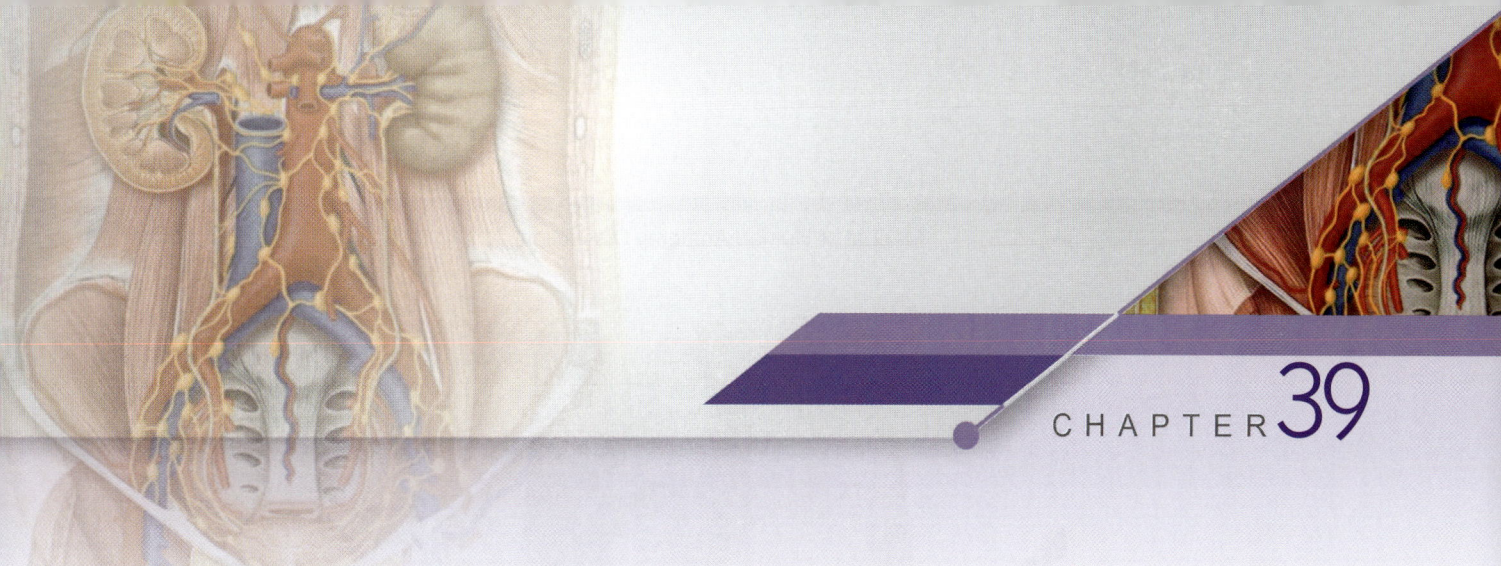

CHAPTER 39

Boundaries and Contents of Pelvis

Learning Objectives

One should be able to

1. Enumerate the structures crossing the inlet at the level of S1 vertebra.

2. Enumerate the structures crossing the inlet only on the left side.

3. Enumerate the structures crossing the inlet of pelvis only in the female.

OVERVIEW

Pelvis is formed by articulation of the two hip bones with the sacrum behind and with each other in front.

Pelvis is divided by the plane of pelvic inlet/pelvic brim into a greater or false pelvis lodging the abdominal viscera and a lower/lesser or true pelvis for the pelvic viscera. The junction of greater pelvis and lesser pelvis is the brim of the pelvis. This brim is crossed by many structures. Walls of lesser pelvis are formed by bones, ligaments, membranes and muscles.

Pelvic inlet is an oblique plane making an angle of 50°–60° with the horizontal plane. Pelvic floor is formed by gutter shaped levator ani muscles. Space between pelvic inlet and pelvic outlet is the pelvic cavity. Axis of the pelvic cavity follows the shape of letter "J".

True pelvis comprises:
- Pelvic inlet or brim of pelvis
- Pelvic cavity
- Pelvic outlet

STEPS OF DISSECTION

- *Identify the contents of pelvic cavity* (Fig. 39.1):
  i. Sigmoid colon and rectum in posterior part
  ii. Urinary bladder anteriorly behind symphysis pubis
  iii. In between rectum and urinary bladder lies the genital organs which are different in male and female
- *Identify structures crossing the pelvic brim:*
  i. Muscles in pelvis
     - Piriformis at the back
     - Obturator internus on the sides
     - Levator ani in the floor
  ii. Ligaments in pelvis
     - Sacrotuberous ligament
     - Sacrospinous ligament
     - Inferior pubic ligament
  iii. Membrane
     - Obturator membrane
     - Identify the peritoneal reflection in the pelvis

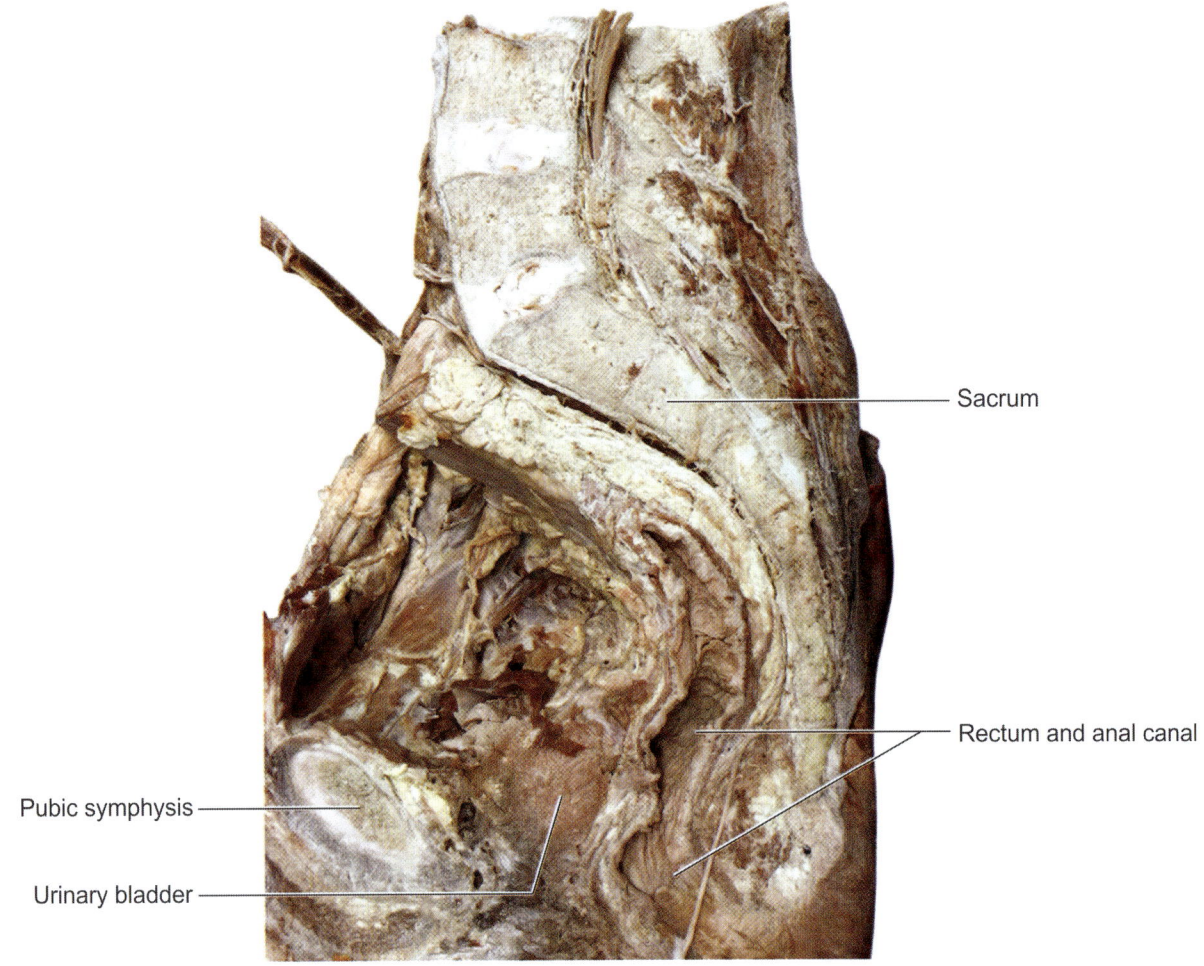

Fig. 39.1: Contents of pelvic cavity

- Trace the peritoneum from posterior aspect of anterior abdominal wall to the superior surface of urinary bladder. This loose attachment as peritoneum gets reflected from bladder as and when it gets filled.
- From superior surface it is reflected over the upper part of the posterior surface of urinary bladder.
- Then onwards the reflection is different in male and female.
  In the male, peritoneum is reflected backwards to the middle third of rectum. This pouch between bladder and rectum is known as rectovesical pouch (*see* Fig. 28.8a).
- In relation to urinary bladder identify the ductus deferens from deep inguinal ring reaching its posterior surface, close to median plane

- Identify the ureter from posterior abdominal wall reaching the posterolateral angles of the bladder and then piercing its wall to enter trigone of the bladder.
- See the peritoneal folds of ductus deferens and ureter crossing each other.
  In female, the peritoneum passes from the bladder to the anterior surface of uterus. Thus it forms a shallow vesicouterine pouch. Then it covers the fundus of uterus and its posterior surface. It descends down to cover upper part of vagina. From there it is reflected to anterior surface of middle 1/3rd of rectum. This deep pouch is called rectouterine pouch/pouch of Douglas (*see* Fig. 28.8b).
- The peritoneum from anterior and posterior surfaces of uterus form a fold on either side. This fold of peritoneum is known as broad ligament.

- Identify the structures in the broad ligament. They are:
  - i. Fallopian tube
  - ii. Ovary
  - iii. Ligament of ovary
  - iv. Round ligament of uterus
  - v. Uterine vessels lie between two layers close to the uterus
  - vi. Ovarian vessels
  - vii. Remnants of mesonephric ducts and tubules
- See ureter lying inferior to the broad ligament. It is crossed superiorly by the uterine artery.
- Structures crossing the pelvic inlet of the pelvis
  - Median sacral vessels
  - Sympathetic trunk
  - Lumbosacral trunk
  - Iliolumbar artery
  - Obturator nerve
  - Internal iliac vessels
  - Medial limb of sigmoid mesocolon with superior rectal vessles (on left side only)
  - Ureter
  - Sigmoid colon (only on left side)
  - Ovarian vessels (only in female)
  - Ductus deferens/round ligament of uterus
  - Lateral umbilical ligament
  - Median umbilical ligament
  - Autonomic nerve plexuses
  - Coils of intestine
  - Pregnant uterus
  - Full urinary bladder

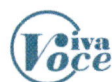

- How much is the angle between plane of outlet of pelvis and the horizontal plane?
- How much is the angle between plane of inlet of pelvis and the horizontal plane?
- Name the structures crossing the brim of pelvis.
- Which structures, though not bilateral, cross the brim of pelvis?

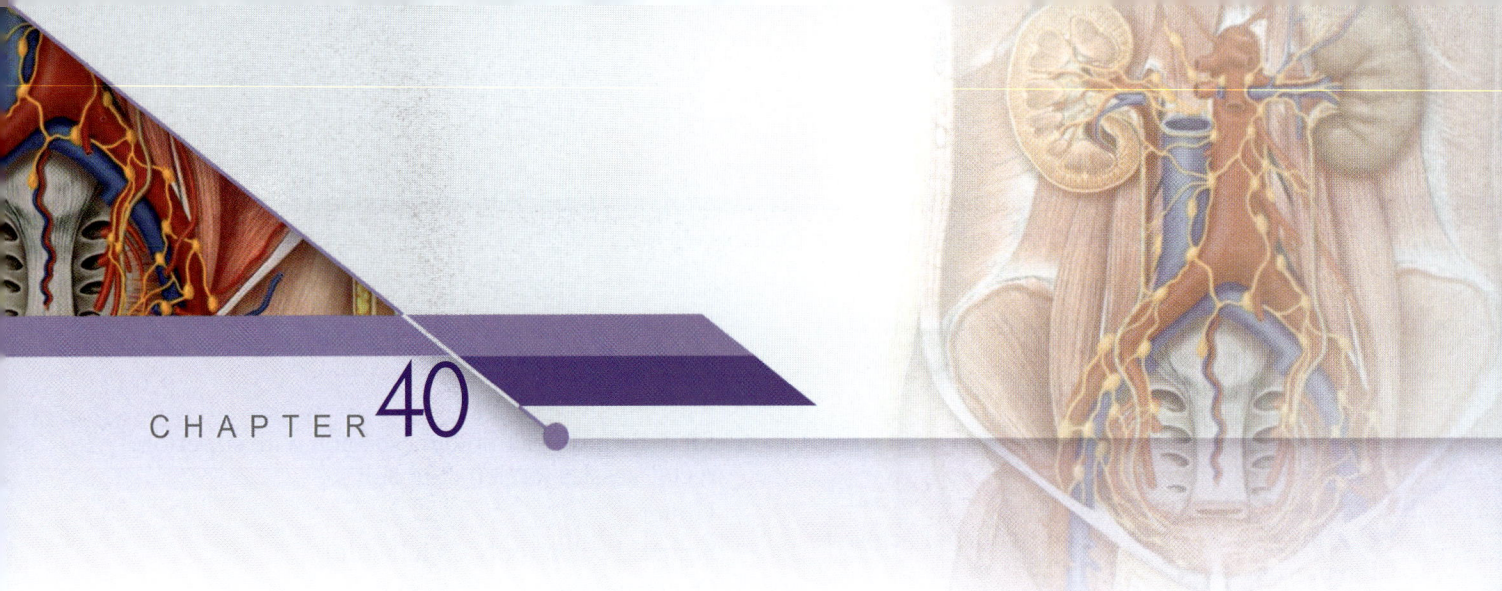

CHAPTER 40

Urinary Bladder and Urethra

Learning Objectives

One should be able to

1. Mention the areas of perineum which get full of urine in case of injury to the penile urethra.
2. To identify structures opening into prostatic part of urethra.
3. Where does urine collect if there is rupture of the membranous urethra.
4. Name the openings in the trigone of urinary bladder.

OVERVIEW

Urinary bladder is a temporary muscular storehouse of urine. It comprises an apex, base or fundus, neck, three surfaces and four borders.

Neck is the lowest and most fixed part of the bladder, pierced by the internal urethral orifice. The true ligamentous support is provided by lateral true ligament, lateral puboprostatic ligament, medial puboprostatic ligament, posterior ligament of bladder and median umbilical ligament—a remnant of urachus.

Interior of bladder can be examined via a cystoscope. Lower part of base of bladder shows a trigone with three openings—two of ureters and one of internal urethral orifice.

Nerve supply: Parasympathetic nerve supply is from S2–S4. These are motor to the muscle, e.g. detrusor muscle of the urinary bladder. The sympathetic nerve supply is from T11–L2 segments and is motor to preprostatic sphincter mechanism. Somatic nerves are from pudendal nerve (S2–S4).

Male urethra comprises short posterior and long anterior part. Short posterior part is subdivided into preprostatic, prostatic and membranous parts. The long anterior part is subdivided into bulbar/perineal part and penile part.

Preprostatic sphincter innervated by sympathetic fibres surround the preprostatic part of urethra.

Prostatic part shows urethral crest, prostatic sinuses, verumontanum with openings of the two ejaculatory ducts and a single prostatic utricle.

Membranous part contains distal urethral sphincter.

Bulbar urethra is the anterior part of urethra surrounded by bulbospongiosus muscle.

Longest penile part lies in penis and opens by a narrowest external urethral orifice.

Female urethra is only 4 cm long. Its proximal part is embedded in anterior wall of vagina. It pierces perineal membrane and ends at external urethral orifice between the glans clitoridis and vaginal orifice.

STEPS OF DISSECTION

- Identify urinary bladder just behind the pubic symphysis.

- Identify the levator ani muscles in the pelvic floor and obturator internus in the lateral wall of the pelvis.
- See that the ligaments are median and medial umbilical ligaments.
- Define surfaces and blunt borders of urinary bladder.

The surfaces are superior; right and left inferolateral.

Borders are two lateral, one anterior and one posterior.

Apex is directed forwards. It is continuous with median umbilical ligament.

Neck is the lowest and most fixed part of the bladder.

Base or fundus is directed backwards. It is related to ampulla of ductus deferens close to median plane and to seminal vesicles laterally.

- See that the fascia around the neck is condensed to form medial and lateral puboprostatic ligaments.
- Also identify two lateral ligaments and two posterior ligaments.

Interior of Bladder

- Make the incision through the bladder along the junction of superior and inferolateral surface on both sides. Extend these incisions till the lateral extremities of the base. Incise the superior wall of the bladder to be able to visualise its interior.

- See that the mucosa of most of the bladder is thrown in irregular folds (Fig. 40.1).
- Identify the trigone—a small triangular area over lower part of the base. The mucosa here is smooth. The ureters open at the posterolateral angles of the trigone (*see* Fig. 34.5). The apex of trigone is downwards and this is called the internal urethral orifice.
- Appreciate the differences in male and female urinary bladder.

Male

i. 2 medial and 2 lateral puboprostatic ligaments
ii. Base related to ampullae of ductus deferens and seminal vesicles.
iii. At the neck is present preprostatic sphincter
iv. Peritoneum forms rectovesical pouch
v. Arterial supply from superior and inferior vesical arteries.
vi. Median lobe of prostate may produce an elevation just posterior to urethral orifice. It is known as uvular vesicae.

Female

i. Only 2 pubovesical ligaments
ii. Base related to cervix of uterus and vagina
iii. Neck is related to pelvic fascia only, sphincter is not present.
iv. Peritoneum forms vesicouterine pouch

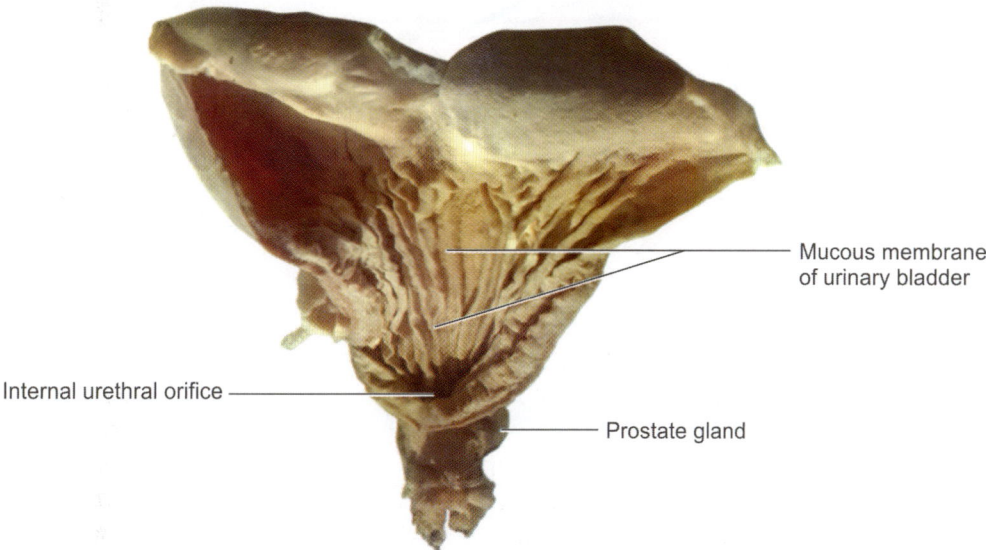

Internal urethral orifice

Mucous membrane of urinary bladder

Prostate gland

Fig. 40.1: Mucosal folds of urinary bladder

v. Arterial supply from superior vesical, vaginal arteries.

vi. Inferior vesical is replaced by vaginal arteries. No such structure as median lobe of prostate.

Urethra

Urethra connects the internal urethral meatus of urinary bladder to the external urethral meatus at the end of urethra.

Urethra is entirely different in male and female. In male, urethra carries both urine and semen at different times. In female, urethra and vagina are separate openings.

Male Urethra

Male urethra is 18–20 cm.
- Identify its parts (Fig. 40.2). They are:
  1. Short posterior part—4–5 cm. Its three segments are:
     i. Preprostatic segment—1–1.5 cm
     ii. Prostatic segment—3–4 cm
     iii. Membranous segment—1.5 cm

2. Long anterior part—16 cm. Its two segments are-
   i. Perineal segment—1.5–2 cm
   ii. Penile segment—14–15 cm

Penile part of urethra is longest. It is dilated at its termination within the glans penis. The dilatation is called navicular fossa. External urethral meatus is the narrowest part of urethra.

Catheterisation is difficult in males as urethra is long and curved.

Female Urethra

Female urethra is only 4 cm long.
- See that it starts at internal urethral orifice of bladder (see Fig. 28.8b).
- See that it is embedded in anterior wall of vagina, it pierces the perineal membrane and ends as an opening in the vestibule (between right and left labia minora), 2.5 cm behind the clitoris.

Catheterisation is easier in females.

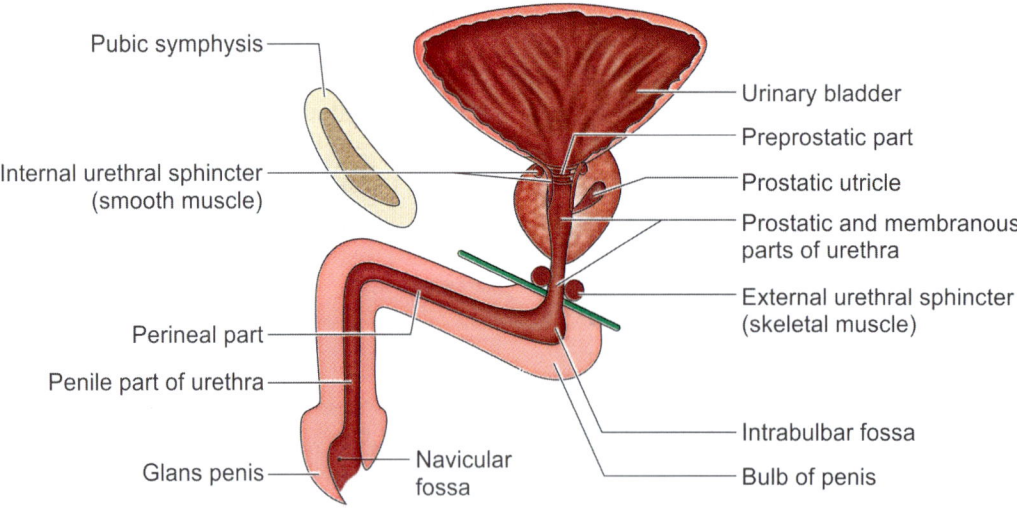

Fig. 40.2: Parts of male urethra

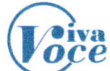

- Name the pouches between rectum, uterus and urinary bladder in female. Which is the deepest pouch and how deep is it from skin of perineum?
- Name the parts of male urethra.

- Name the pouch between rectum and urinary bladder in male. How deep is it from skin of perineum.
- What are the openings in prostatic urethra?

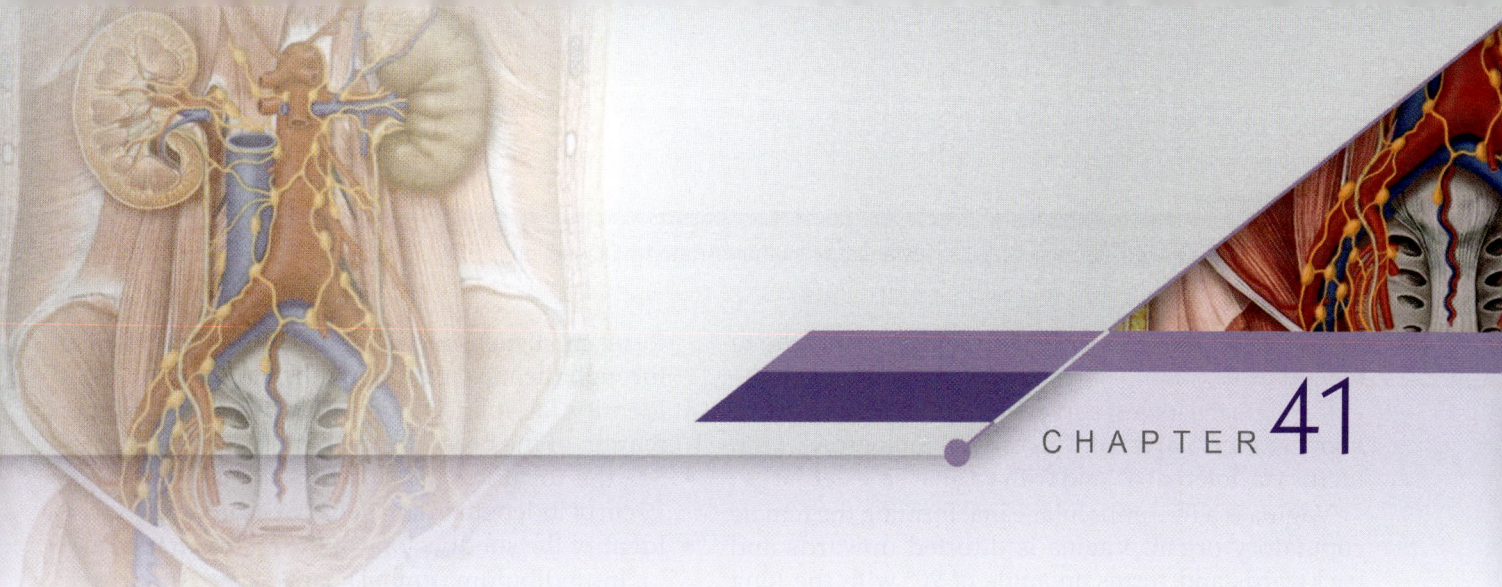

CHAPTER 41

Female Reproductive Organs

Learning Objectives

One should be able to

1. Explain per vaginal examination (P/V) and which organs are palpable by P/V
2. Enumerate the parts of levator ani and muscles inserted into perineal body.
3. Identify structures in the broad ligament.
4. Learn clinical importance of uterine artery crossing over the ureter.

OVERVIEW

Female reproductive organs are both external and internal. External genital organs are mons pubis, labia majora, labia minora, clitoris, vestibule of the vagina, bulbs of vestibule and greater vestibular glands. Internal genital organs are a pair of ovaries, pair of oviducts, single uterus and vagina.

Ovary: It lies in the lateral wall of pelvis in the ovarian fossa bounded by the ureter and obliterated umbilical artery. It is almost covered by peritoneum. Ovary is mostly related to the fallopian tube. Only lower pole and lateral surface are not related to uterine tube. Remaining two borders, upper pole and medial surface are related to the tube.

Lateral part of the broad ligament forms suspensory ligament of ovary. It contains the ovarian vessels. Ovary undergoes cyclical changes and produces oestrogen and progesterone hormone according to the stage of the cycle.

Uterine tubes: These are tortuous 10 cm long ducts conveying oocyte from the ovary to the uterus. Its parts are infundibulum, ampulla, isthmus and intramural. Blood supply is partly from ovarian and partly from uterine artery.

Uterus: Uterus/hystera is a child-bearing organ in females situated between bladder and rectum. It is 7.5 × 5 × 2.5 cm in size. It comprises fundus, body and cervix. Angle of anteversion is between long axis of vagina and long axis of uterus and is 90°. Angle of anteflexion is between long axis of cervix and that of uterus and is 170°. The uterine arteries, branches of internal iliac arteries, supply the uterus, in addition to ovarian arteries. Uterine artery crosses the ureter anteriorly (from lateral side to medial side) as it bends to reach the lateral side of uterus where it runs tortuously. Uterus is supported by muscular, fibromuscular and peritoneal supports. Muscular supports are pelvic diaphragm—the levator ani, perineal body with ten muscular slips and distal urethral sphincter mechanism.

Fibromuscular supports are transverse cervical, pubocervical and uterosacral ligaments.

Uterine axis forming an angle of 90° is also a support preventing prolapse of the uterus. Peritoneal ligaments like broad ligament form weak support. The uterus undergoes cyclical changes from menarche to menopause.

Cervix is the lowest part of uterus. It contains a canal known as cervical canal. This canal communicates with uterus via 'internal os' and with vagina via 'external os'.

Vagina is a fibromuscular canal forming the female copulatory organ. Vagina is directed upwards and backwards and forms an angle of 90° with the long axis of uterus. There are four fornices of vagina in relation to protruding cervix. The posterior fornix is deepest. The peritoneum of rectouterine pouch covers the posterior fornix. Vagina is supplied by the vaginal branch of internal iliac artery and a cervicovaginal branch of the uterine artery.

Competency achievement: The student should be able to:

AN 48.2 Describe and demonstrate the (position, features, important peritoneal and other relations, blood supply, nerve supply, lymphatic drainage and clinical aspects of) important male and female pelvic viscera.

STEPS OF DISSECTION

- Cut through the pubic symphysis with a knife in the median plane and extend the incision into the urethra. Make a median dorsal cut with a saw through the 4th and 5th lumbar vertebrae, the sacrum and coccyx to meet the knife. Cut through the soft tissues. Separate the two halves of the pelvis and examine the surface of all the tissues.
- Locate the ovary on the lateral wall of pelvis in the female cadaver.
- Identify the upper or tubal pole, as it is related to the fallopian tube.
- See the lower pole close to the pelvic floor. The ligament of ovary connects the lower pole to the lateral angle of the uterus. See its anterior mesovarian border. It is related to uterine tube. It is like hilum of ovary.
- See that the posterior border is free.
- The lateral surface is related to ovarian fossa and is lined by parietal peritoneum. Medial surface is also related to uterine/fallopian tube.
- Appreciate that the fallopian tube is related to anterior and posterior borders, upper pole and medial surface of the ovary (Fig. 41.1).
- Trace the ovarian artery from lateral surface of abdominal aorta across posterior abdominal wall

to reach suspensory ligament of ovary and then through the mesovarian to the ovary.
- Identify fallopian tube present in the free upper margin of the broad ligament of the pelvis.
- See the tortuosity of this tube, to accommodate 10 cm of its length in smaller 5 cm of broad ligament.
- Identify the subdivisions of the fallopian tube as:
  i. Infundibulum (funnel shaped) with fimbriae is the most lateral part
  ii. Medial to it is ampulla—6–7 cm
  iii. Isthmus is the narrow part of the tube
  iv. Intramural or uterine part 1 cm long and lies in the wall of the uterus.
- Identify the parts of broad ligament. These are:
  i. Mesosalpinx is the upper part of broad ligament between fallopian tube and the mesovarium.
  ii. Mesovarium is a small fold of peritoneum on the posterior layer of broad ligament carrying ovarian vessels to the ovary.
  iii. Suspensory ligament is the most superolateral part of ovary between lateral pelvic wall and the fallopian tube.
  iv. Mesometrium is the fold of broad ligament close to the uterus. The tortuous uterine artery and vein run in this fold.
  v. Identify the arteries supplying the tube. Trace the uterine artery from medial side and ovarian artery from lateral side giving branches to the uterine tube. See that the two arteries anastomose with each other.
- See carefully that uterine artery crosses the ureter as the artery ascends between two layers of broad ligament.

Uterus

- Identify the muscular firm, pyriform shaped uterus between the broad ligament of the two sides (Fig. 41.1). The uterus is 7.5 × 5 × 2.5 cm in size.
- See its parts:
  i. Fundus—part above opening of fallopian tube
  ii. Body—upper expanded part
  iii. Cervix—lower cylindrical part
     Normally fundus and body are 2/3rd part whereas cervix (neck) is 1/3rd part and its external opening, the external os is the mouth.
- Identify the superolateral angle present at the junction of fundus and body. See that the ligament

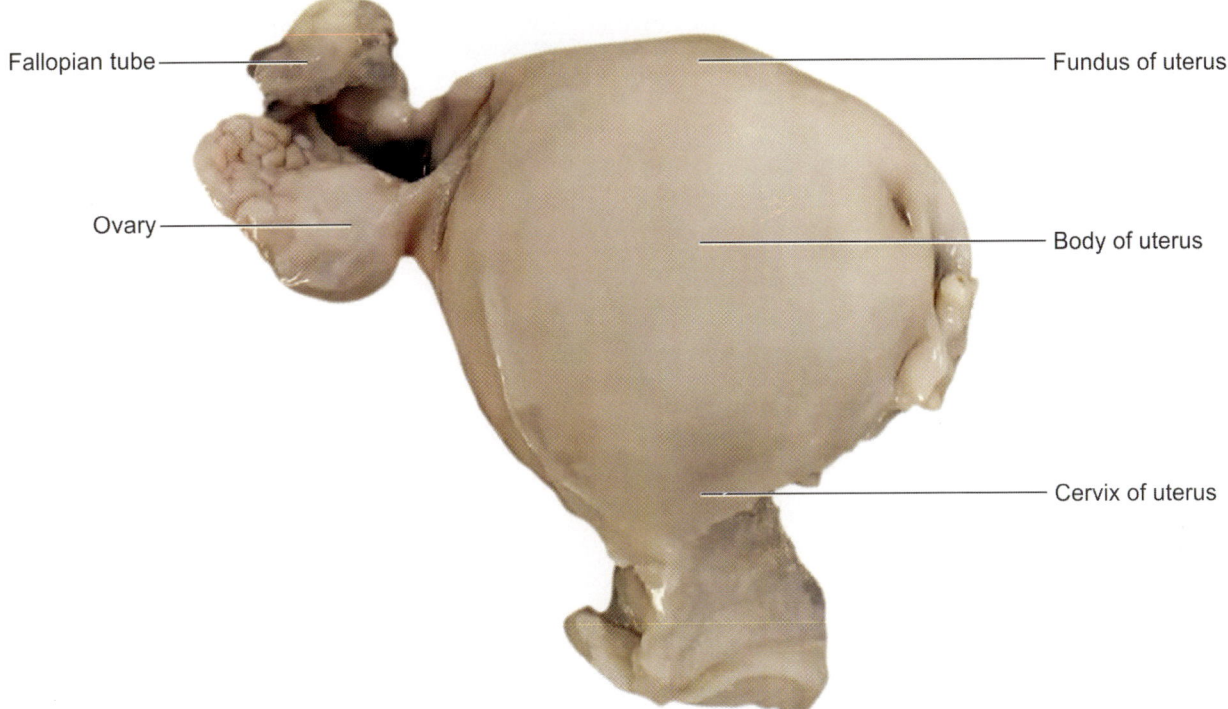

Fallopian tube

Ovary

Fundus of uterus

Body of uterus

Cervix of uterus

Fig. 41.1: Parts of female reproductive system

of ovary, uterine tube and round ligament of uterus are attached to this angle, close to each other.

Angulations of Uterus

Understand that the long axis of uterus and long axis of vagina are almost at right angle to each other. This angle is known as angle of anteversion.

The long axis of cervix makes an angle of 170° with the long angle of uterus. This is known as angle of anteflexion.

- *Cervix comprises:*
  - Supravaginal part—anteriorly related to urinary bladder and to intestines posteriorly. See its relations laterally to ureter and uterine artery. Tortuous uterine artery crosses the ureter anteriorly to ascend along the lateral border of the uterus. It supplies vagina, cervix, body, fundus of uterus and medial part of fallopian tube.
  - Vaginal part of cervix projecting into the anterior wall of vagina. Feel the spaces between cervix and vagina. These are the fornices, named anterior, posterior, right lateral and left lateral fornices. The posterior vaginal fornix is the deepest.

- Incise the cervix to see cervical canal with its internal os/upper opening in uterus and external os/lower opening into the vagina (Fig. 41.2).
- Carry the incision up to open up the uterus. See the inner endometrium, middle thick myometrium and outer thin layer of peritoneum.
- Confirm the peritoneal spaces—shallow uterovesical pouch of peritoneum and deep rectouterine pouch/pouch of Douglas.
- Clean the various ligaments of uterus. These are:
  - Most important ligament of uterus providing adequate support is the transverse cervical ligament.
  - Other ligaments are pubocervical ligament and uterosacral ligaments.

Vagina

Vagina (sheath) is a fibromuscular sheath forming the female copulatory organ. See vagina is directed upwards and backwards in erect posture. Long axis of vagina and long axis of uterus shows an angle of anteversion (90°) to each other (Fig. 41.3).

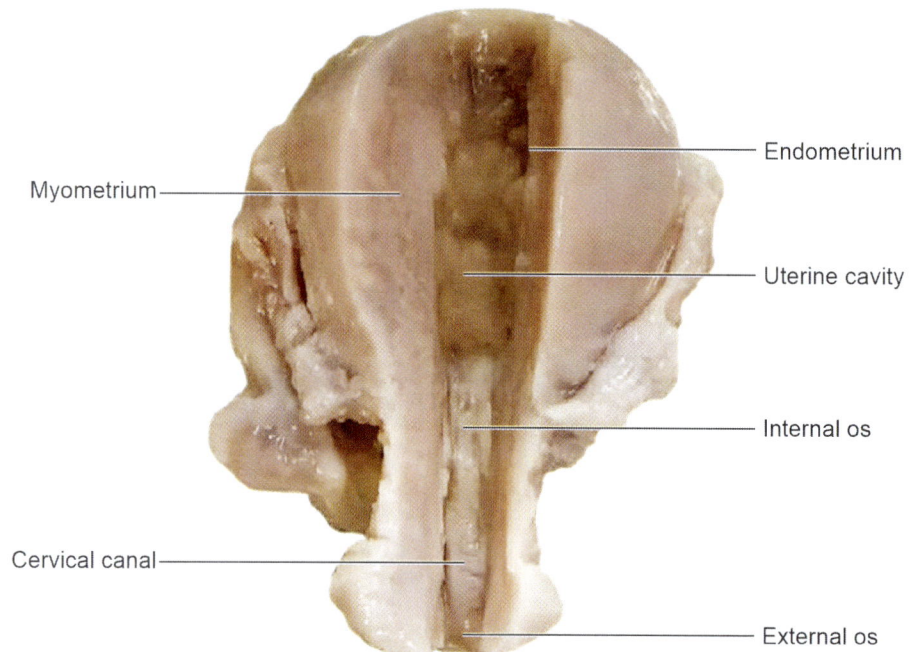

Fig. 41.2: Cut section through uterus and cervix

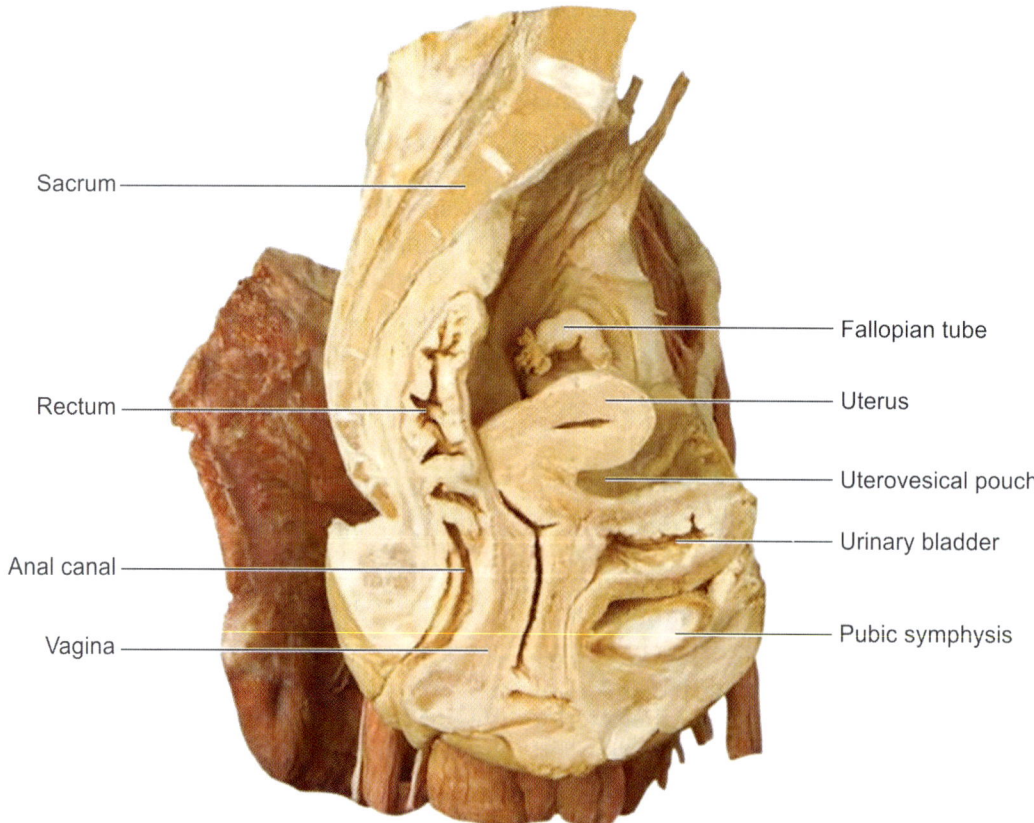

Fig. 41.3: Section through female pelvis

- Identify transverse cervical ligament attached to upper 1/3rd of vagina.
- Lower 1/3rd of vagina pierces the perineal membrane to lie in superficial perineal space. It is related on each side to bulb of vestibule, bulbo-spongiosus muscle and greater vestibular gland.
- Trace the vaginal artery from anterior division of internal iliac artery till the vagina. See that this artery anastomoses with cervicovaginal branch of uterine artery.
- Do a P/V or per vaginal examination in an intact female cadaver, if available. For this introduce two gloved fingers of right hand in the vagina. Put the left hand on lower abdominal wall. Feel the size, position of uterus, pouch of Douglas, urethra and enlarged ovaries between the two hands.

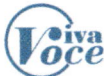 **Viva Voce**

- Which surface and which pole of ovary are not related to the fallopian tube?
- Name the parts of fallopian tube.
- In which part of fallopian tube, does the fertilization take place?
- Name the supports of uterus.
- What is anteversion and anteflexion of uterus?
- Which is the deepest fornix of vagina?
- What is the relation of uterine artery and ureter near lateral fornix of vagina?
- What is episiotomy and what muscles are incised?

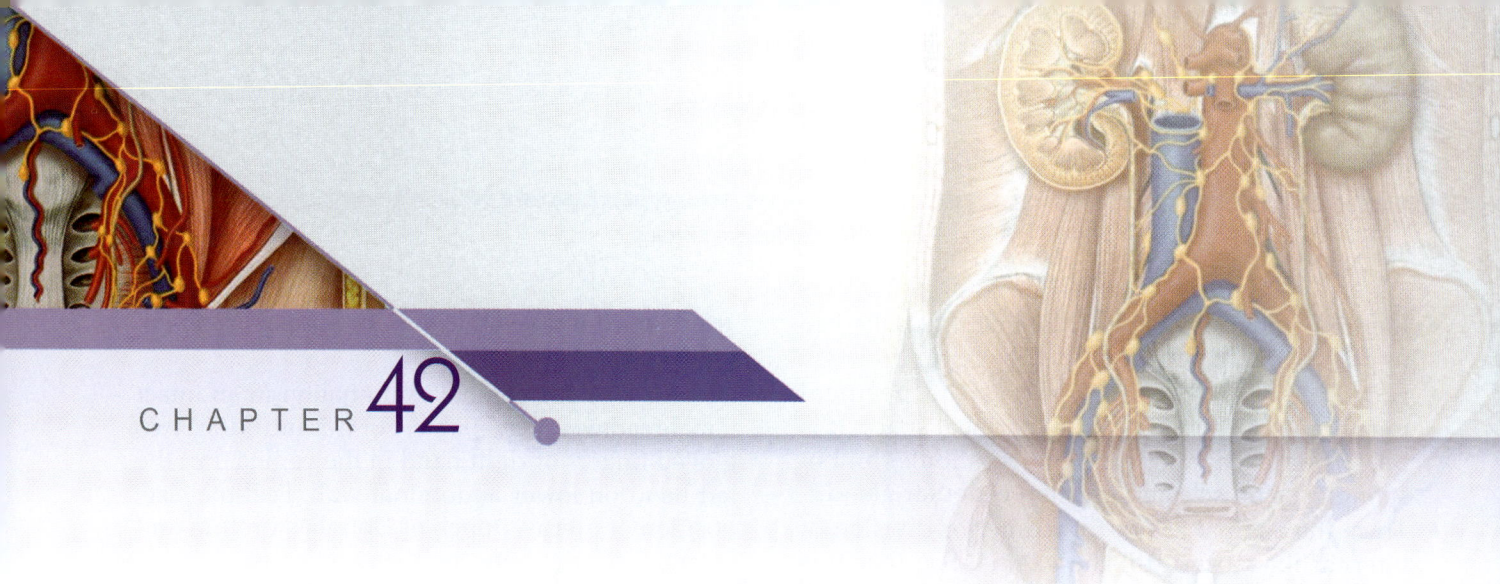

CHAPTER 42

Male Internal Genital Organs

Learning Objectives

One should be able to
1. Identify the organs felt by per rectal (P/R) examination
2. Know the position of prostatic venous plexus in relation to its capsule. What is the clinical importance of this fact?
3. Learn the formation of ejaculatory duct and its opening in the prostatic urethra.
4. Explain the pathway of cancer cells from the prostate gland till the cranial cavity.

OVERVIEW

Male Internal Genital Organs

Male internal genital organs comprise ductus deferens, seminal vesicles and prostate. Testis and epididymis are also genital organs, but are described as external genital organs as these are placed inside the scrotal sac outside the abdominal cavity.

Ductus deferens is the continuation of tail of epididymis. It courses through scrotal sac, spermatic cord, false pelvis and true pelvis. In the true pelvis in relation to base of urinary bladder, dilated part of ductus deferens lie medial to seminal vesicle. Ductus deferens joins the duct of seminal vesicle to form ejaculatory duct which opens in the prostatic urethra.

Seminal vesicles are two sacs like glands lying lateral to ampulla of ductus deferens (Fig. 42.1). Its secretions add to the quantity of seminal fluid.

Prostate is a fibromuscular glandular organ enveloping the neck of urinary bladder (Fig. 42.1). Its secretions also add to the seminal fluid. Prostate comprises base above and apex below, with five lobes; one each anterior, posterior and median and two lateral lobes. This gland contains mucosal and submucosal glands prone to benign hypertrophy. The outer peripheral glands are vulnerable to malignancy.

INTERNAL GENITAL ORGANS

Steps of Dissection

- The ductus deferens has been seen till the deep inguinal ring in the lowest part of the anterior abdominal wall.
- Trace it from there as it hooks around the lateral side of inferior epigastric artery to pass backwards and medially across the external iliac vessels to enter into the lesser pelvis.
- See it reaching close to the urinary bladder where it crosses the ureter anteriorly to lie on the posterior surface of urinary bladder medial to the seminal vesicle.
- Identify this part of ductus deferens as dilated part and is called the ampulla of ductus deferens.
- Remove the fascia from this tube and clean its whole course.
- Try to separate ductus from its neighbour, the seminal vesicle.

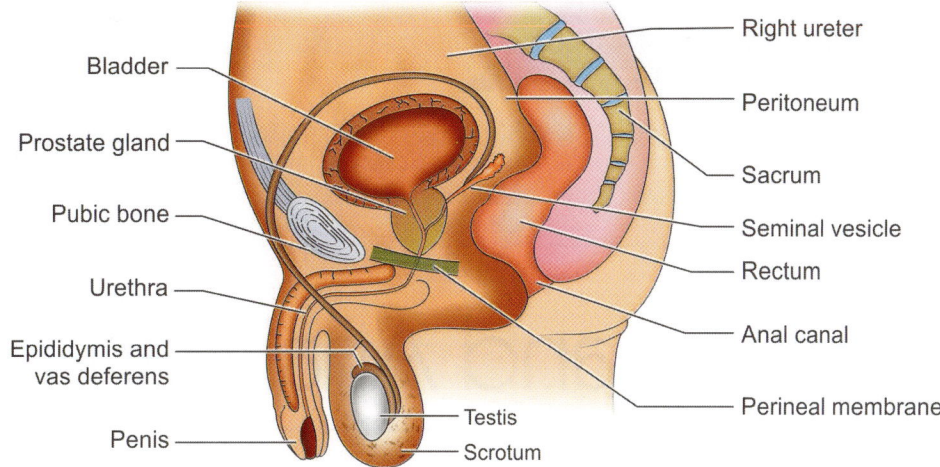

Fig. 42.1: Parts of male reproductive system

- Trace the ductus joining the duct of seminal vesicle to form the ejaculatory duct.
- Identify the two lobulated sac like structures. These are the seminal vesicles. Its lower narrow end forms the duct of seminal vesicle which joins with the ductus deferens to form the ejaculatory duct (Fig. 42.1).

Prostate

- Identify and feel the fibromuscular glandular organ below the neck of the urinary bladder (Fig. 42.1). It is situated behind the lower part of pubic symphysis. Normal size is 4 cm wide, 3 cm long and 2 cm thick.
- Feel the base of prostate gland upwards and apex downwards.

Surfaces

- Feel the anterior narrow surface behind pubic symphysis. Puboprostatic ligaments connect this surface to pubic symphysis. Urethra emerges from this surface above its apex.

- Feel the posterior surface which is convex by a P/R (per rectal) examination. By this examination one can feel enlarged prostate, irregularity of the surfaces, any nodules and hardness of the gland. Some pathologies of anal canal can also be felt. In addition feel the two inferolateral surfaces.

- Cut through the prostate gland to see its interior. Structures inside the prostatic urethra are:

  i. Urethral crest
  ii. 2 ejaculatory ducts on each side of prostatic utricle.
  iii. Prostatic utricle is in the centre and prostatic sinus with openings of prostatic ducts.

Cancer of the prostate gland is the commonest malignancy in the male.

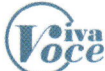

- Which is the common site for doing vasectomy?
- How is ejaculatory duct formed and where does it open?
- Which lobe is vulnerable for cancer of prostate?

- Where is prostatic venous plexus in relation to the capsules of the prostate?
- How do secondaries of prostatic cancer reach the cranial cavity?

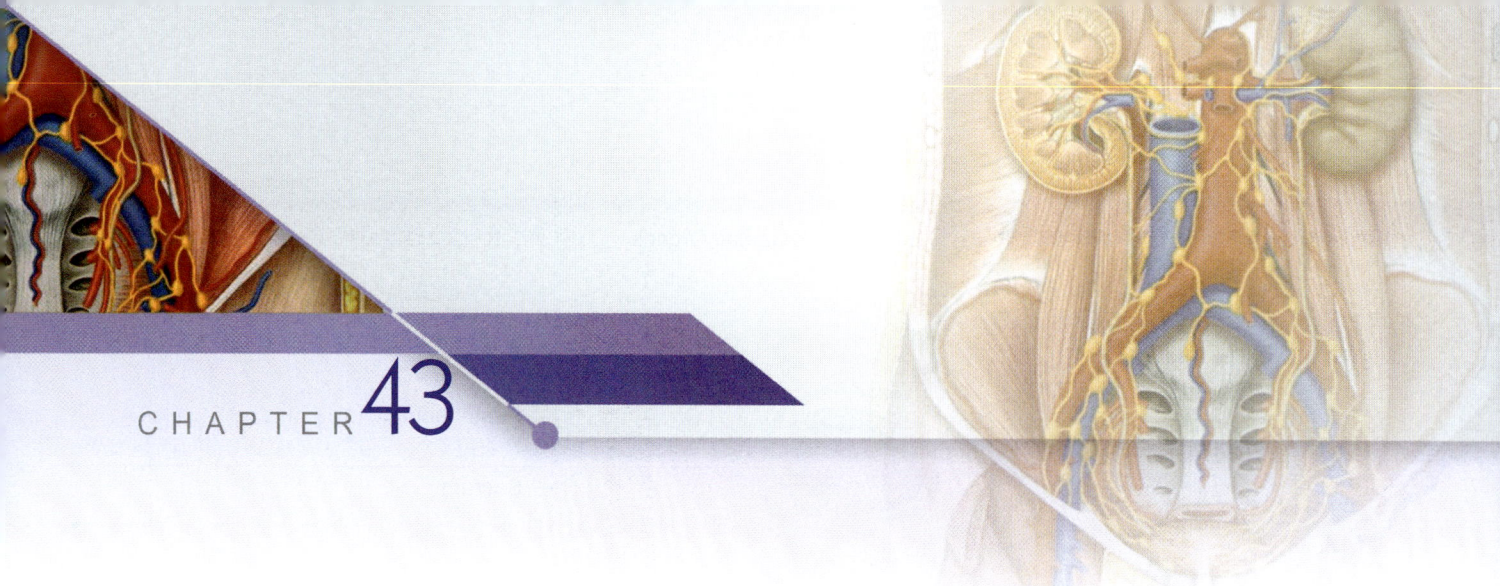

CHAPTER 43

Rectum and Anal Canal

Learning Objectives

One should be able to
1. Enumerate the nerves innervating the internal and external anal sphincters.
2. Name the main artery of anal canal.
3. Learn veins forming portosystemic anastomoses in anal canal. Name other such sites.

OVERVIEW

Rectum

Rectum lies between sigmoid/pelvic colon and the anal canal. It shows a concave sacral curve and perineal convex curve. It further reveals upper convexity to right, middle convexity to left and lower convexity again to right. Its upper 1/3rd is covered by peritoneum on three sides, middle 1/3rd on one side and lower 1/3rd is below level of peritoneum. Its main blood supply is from superior rectal artery, which is the continuation of inferior mesenteric artery. It also receives blood supply from middle rectal arteries—branches of internal iliac and from inferior rectal artery—branch of pudendal artery and also from median sacral artery. Veins drain into the respective veins.

Rectum is supported by levator ani, perineal body, fascia of Waldeyer and peritoneum.

Anal canal is the lowest 38 mm of the gastrointestinal tract. Upper 15 mm develops from endoderm of cloaca and middle 15 mm plus lowest 8 mm develop from the proctodaeum (ectoderm). Arterial supply of upper segment is from superior rectal artery while of middle and lower segments is from inferior rectal artery. Anal canal is an important site of portosystemic anastomosis.

Anal canal is surrounded in its upper 30 mm length by internal sphincter, made up of smooth muscle, and in its entire length by external sphincter, made up of skeletal muscle fibres. It is under voluntary control. It comprises upper, middle and lower parts. Only the middle fibres have bony attachment.

There are three primary positions of veins present at 3, 7 and 11 o'clock position. These are the sites for primary piles. Increased venous pressure in the radicles of superior rectal vein results in formation of piles. The mucus membrane of upper 15 mm of anal canal shows longitudinal anal columns and anal valves joining the ends of these columns.

Anal canal is subjected to lots of maladies due to improper dietary habits and improper timings of defaecation, etc.

STEPS OF DISSECTION (RECTUM)

- Identify and clean the rectum of any fat/fasciae. See it starts at the 3rd piece of sacrum and coccyx, as the continuation of sigmoid colon. Then it ends at anorectal junction by continuing as the anal canal (Fig. 43.1).

- See the anteroposterior curvatures. These are sacral flexure, which is concave and perineal flexure which is backwards. Its most prominent lateral curvature is convex to the left. It also shows small upper right and lower right curvatures which are convex to the right.

Relations

Anterior

In the male:

a. Rectovesical pouch with coils of intestines in upper 2/3rd part

b. Base of urinary bladder, ends of ureter, seminal vesicles, ductus deferens and prostate gland in lower 1/3rd part.

In the female:

a. Rectouterine pouch with coils of intestine in upper 2/3rd part

b. Vagina in lower 1/3rd part

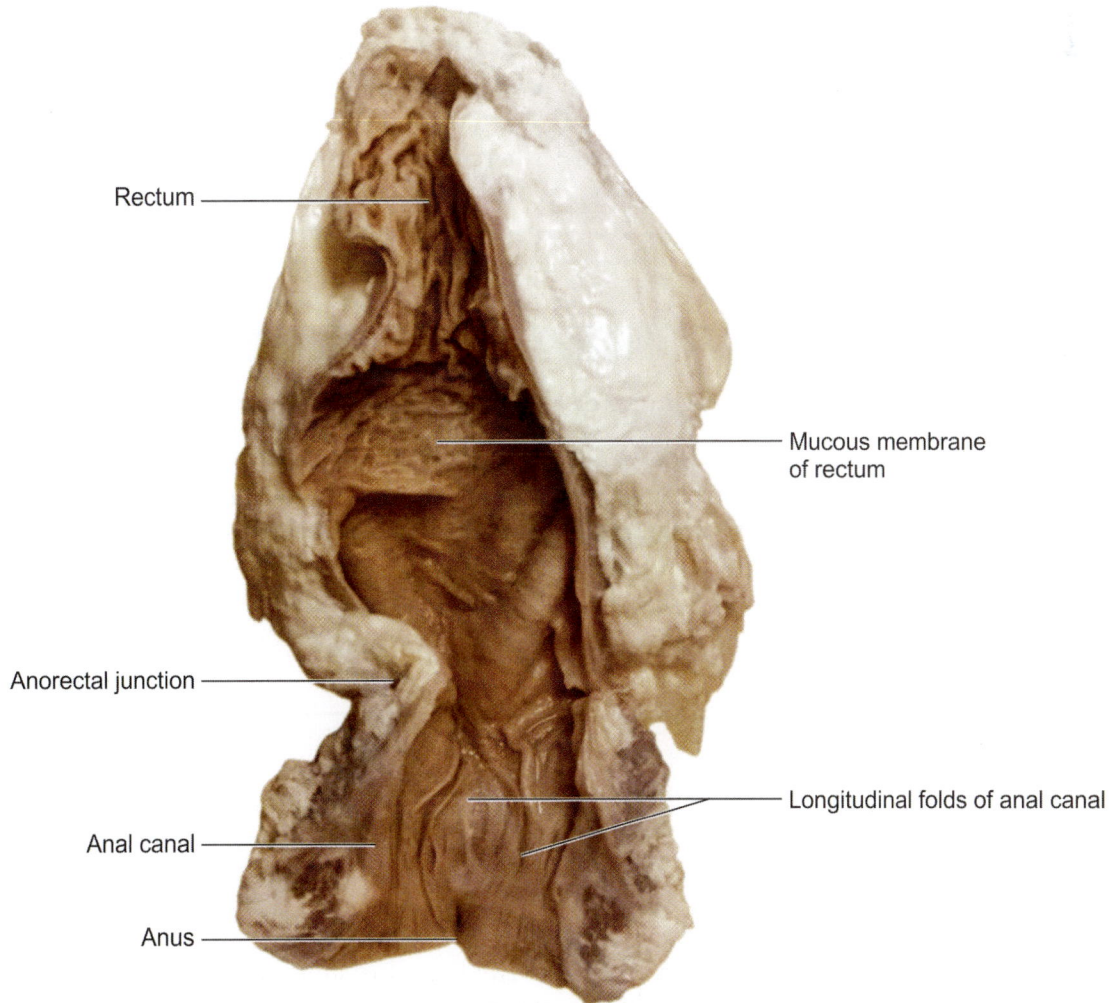

Fig. 43.1: Interior of rectum and anal canal

Posterior

- Sacrum, coccyx, anococcygeal ligament
- Piriformis, coccygeus and levator ani muscles
- Median sacral, superior rectal and lateral sacral vessels
- Two sympathetic chains getting fused to form ganglion impar, coccygeal plexus (S4, S5, Co1) and pelvic splanchnic nerves (parasympathetic nerves) fat, lymph nodes, lymphatics.
- Trace the superior rectal artery as the downward continuation of inferior mesenteric artery to the rectum where it divides into right and left branches. These branches then enter the walls of the rectum to supply its mucus membrane.
- Find and trace the middle rectal arteries from internal iliac artery.
- See the pelvic diaphragm formed by levator ani muscles.
- Dissect the lateral ligaments of rectum.
- Clean the perineal body between lower end of anal canal and vagina/root of scrotum.

STEPS OF DISSECTION (ANAL CANAL)

- The anal canal and rectum have already been taken out of the pelvis. Cut the anal canal in its centre. Clean the remains of faecal matter with wet cotton swabs.
- See longitudinal folds in upper 15 mm (Fig. 43.1). These are anal columns (8–10 in number). These are joined by anal valves.
- Middle 15 mm is transition zone and lies between pectinate line above and Hilton's line below.
- Distal 8 mm is lined by true skin.
- See the arteries in the anal canal. These are branches of superior rectal and inferior rectal arteries.
- Veins accompanying branches of superior rectal artery drain into portal venous system.
- Veins accompanying branches of inferior rectal artery drain into internal iliac vein, i.e. systemic circulation. Thus anal canal is an important site of portosystemic anastomoses.

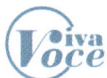

- Name the anteroposterior and lateral curvatures of the rectum.
- Name the arteries supplying the rectum.
- Which structures are felt by per rectal (PR) examination in male and female?

- What is the extent of the two anal sphincters?
- Why is anal canal a site of portosystemic anastomoses? Name these tributaries.
- Name the positions of the primary piles.
- What are the differences between upper 15 mm and middle 15 mm of anal canal?

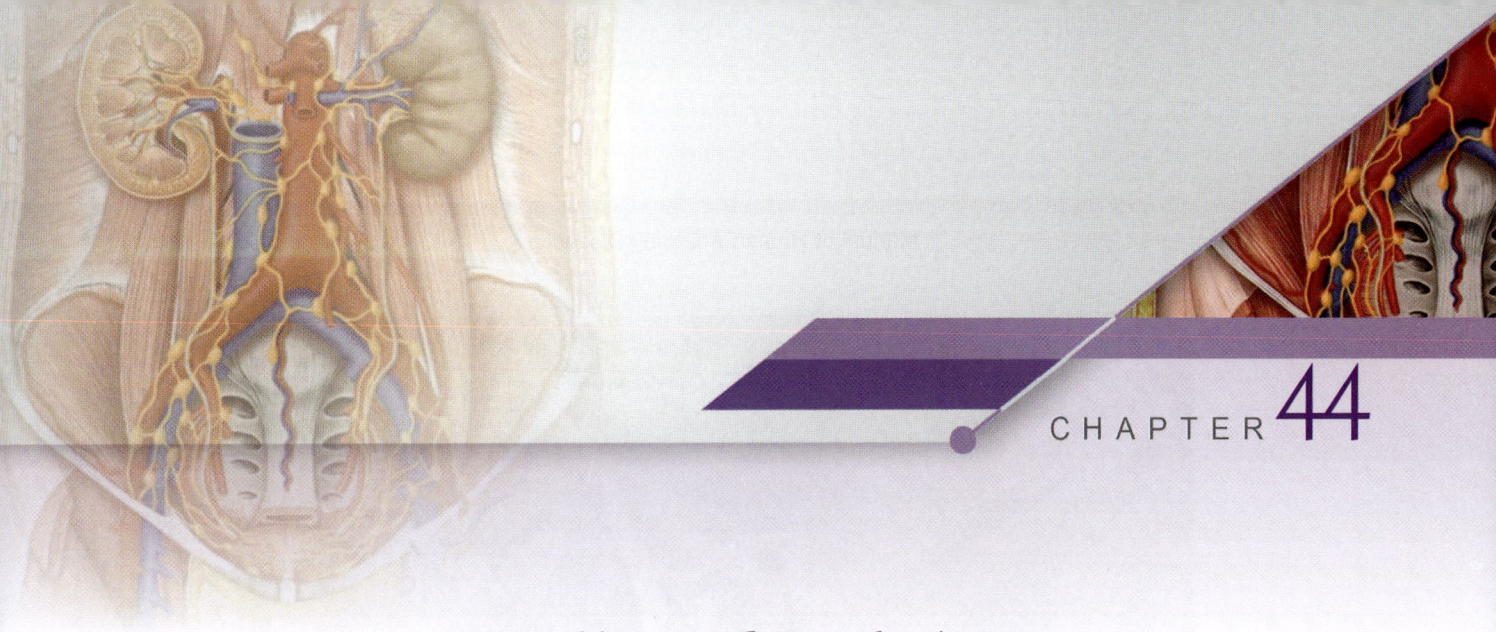

Walls of Pelvis

OVERVIEW

The pelvic viscera have been dissected and studied in the previous chapters. The walls of the pelvis, i.e. muscles, fascia, peritoneum, blood vessels, nerve both somatic and autonomic and joints will be studied in this chapter. Muscles of the pelvis are piriformis at the back, obturator internus on the lateral wall and pelvic diaphragm, i.e. levator ani in the floor.

Fascia is the pelvic fascia, which is comprised of parietal and visceral layers. Parietal layer covers the walls and the floor. The visceral layer is dense over non-distensible organs, e.g. prostate but is loosely attached over the distensible organs, e.g. urinary bladder.

Peritoneum has been discussed earlier with the concerned viscera.

Internal iliac artery is the main artery of the walls of the pelvis. This artery is a branch of common iliac artery and crosses the brim of the pelvis. It divides into number of branches which supply both the parietes and all the viscera of the pelvis.

Veins follow the arteries.

Nerves are both somatic and autonomic. Somatic nerve is the pudendal nerve S2,3,4. It gives branches to all the viscera of the pelvis.

The parasympathetic nerves also arise from S2,3,4 segments and form pelvic splanchnic nerves.

Competency achievement: The student should be able to:
AN 48.3 Describe and demonstrate the origin, course, important relations and branches of internal iliac artery.

Vessels of the Pelvis

- Remove the viscera from the pelvic cavity.
- Trace the internal iliac artery and its two divisions, anterior and posterior (Fig. 44.1).
- Follow the branches of each of its divisions to the position of the viscera and the parietes.
- Identify the branches of posterior division. These are all parietal branches. These are iliolumbar, lateral sacral and superior gluteal.
- The branches of anterior division are both parietal and visceral. The parietal branches are inferior gluteal and obturator.
- The visceral branches are superior vesical, middle rectal, inferior vesical (only in male), internal pudendal, vaginal and uterine (both only in female).
- Many veins follow the arteries. In some viscera like rectum, prostate and urinary bladder there are

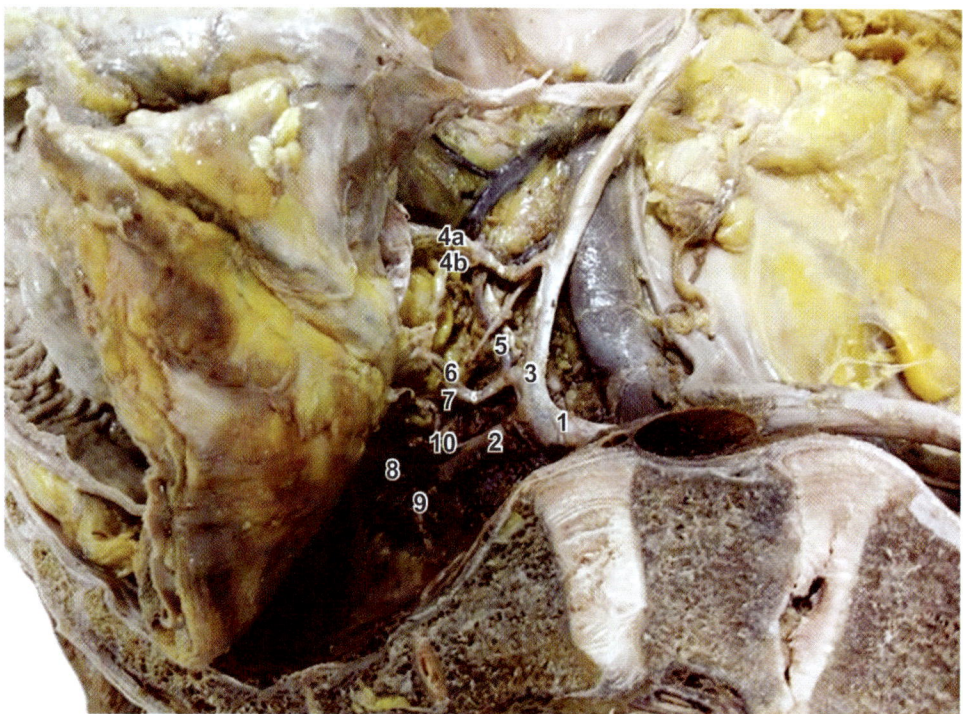

1. Internal iliac artery	6. Inferior vesicle
2. Posterior division	7. Superior vesicle
3. Anterior division	8. Lateral sacral
4a. Inferior gluteal	9. Superior gluteal
4b. Internal pudendal	10. Iliolumbar
5. Obturator	

Fig. 44.1: Branches of internal iliac arteries

venous plexuses which join to form veins and these follow the arteries.

Competency achievement: The student should be able to:

AN 48.4 Describe the branches of sacral plexus.

Nerves of the Pelvis

- Expose the lumbosacral trunk (L4,L5) in relation to ala of sacrum. Trace the ventral rami of S1, S2, S3 coming out from the ventral sacral foramina. All these nerves form the lumbosacral plexus. Identify the terminal branches of the plexus. These are the pudendal and the sciatic nerves.
- Identify and clean the nerves arising from the dorsal surface of the lumbosacral plexus. These are superior gluteal, inferior gluteal, perforating

cutaneous branch and perineal branch of 4th sacral nerve.

- Trace the sympathetic trunks in the pelvis till these terminate in a single ganglion impar (unpaired) on the coccyx.
- Trace the large grey rami communicantes from the ganglia to the ventral rami of sacral nerves.
- Find the inferior hypogastric plexus around the internal iliac vessels.
- In addition, trace the pelvic splanchnic nerves reaching the inferior hypogastric plexus from the ventral rami of S2,3,4 nerves.

Pelvic Muscles

- Identify the origin of piriformis from the ventral surface of the sacrum. Trace it through the greater sciatic foramen to its insertion into the upper border of greater trochanter of femur.

- Feel the ischial spine and trace the fibres of coccygeus and levator ani that arise from it. Trace the origin of levator ani from thickened fascia, i.e. tendinous arch over the middle of obturator internus muscle till the back of the body of the pubis. It is comprised of pubococcygeus, iliococcygeus and ischiococcygeus parts. Note that the right and left sheet like levator ani muscles are mostly united and the muscles are inserted into perineal body, anal canal and anococcygeal ligament. These muscles give space for passage of anal canal, urethra and vagina in female, and for urethra and anal canal in males.

- Detach the origin of levator ani from obturator fascia. While removing obturator fascia, identify pudendal canal with its contents in the lower part of the fascia.

- Trace the tendon of obturator internus muscle. This tendon along with superior and inferior gemelli muscles leaves through the lesser sciatic foramen to be inserted into the medial surface of the greater trochanter of femur.

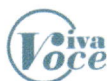

Viva Voce

- Name the branches of posterior division of internal iliac artery.
- Name the branches of anterior division of internal iliac artery.
- Name the two main branches of lumbosacral plexus.
- Name the axial artery of lower limb.
- Which nerve is called 'nervi furcalis' and why?

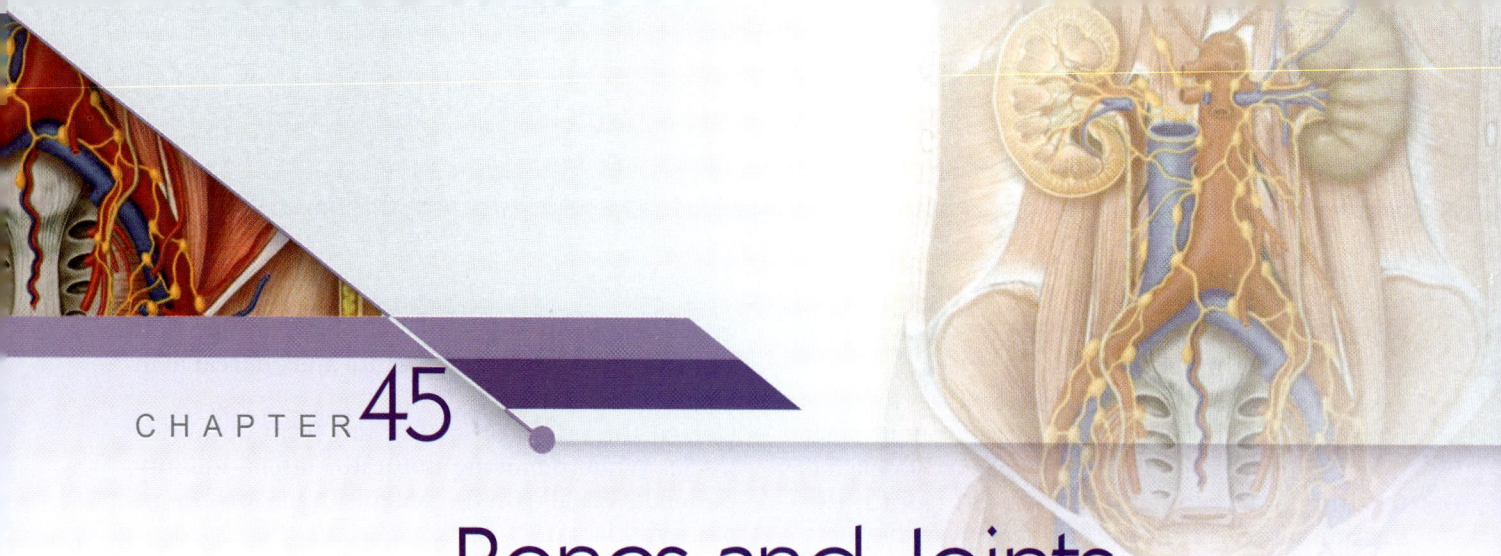

CHAPTER 45

Bones and Joints of Abdomen and Pelvis

Learning Objectives

One should be able to
- Name the ligaments of sacroiliac joint.
- Mention the degrees of subpubic angle in male and female.

Bones in the region of abdomen and pelvis are as follows:

1. 1–5 lumbar vertebrae (Fig. 45.1a to d)
2. Sacrum and coccyx (Fig. 45.2a and b)
3. Hip bones.

Each hip bone articulates with single sacrum on its right and left side to form sacroiliac joints (Fig. 45.3). Further, the pubic component of the hip bones articulate with each other in the anteroinferior part of abdomen to form a single joint—the pubic symphysis (Fig. 45.3). Both hip bones with sacrum form the pelvis (Fig. 45.3a and b).

Five lumbar vertebrae articulate with each other through the intervertebral discs.

1st lumbar vertebra articulates above with 12th thoracic vertebra.

5th lumbar vertebra articulates with 1st sacral vertebra to form limbosacral joint. Here the intervertebral disc is rather thick anteriorly and thin posteriorly, forming an angle of 120° posteriorly (Fig. 45.4a to c).

Sacroiliac Joints

Sacroiliac joints are joints of partly syndesmosis type posteriorly and partly synovial variety anteriorly with strong ligaments. These joints transmit the body weight from lumbar vertebrae to sacrum. The weight is divided into two parts. Each part reaches the respective sacroiliac joint and then through the hip bone to the hip joint from where it descends down to reach the ground.

The body weight tries to push the upper end of sacrum downwards and forwards. It is prevented by interosseous sacroiliac, iliolumbar and ventral sacroiliac ligaments (Fig. 45.5).

Further the lower end of sacrum has a tendency to be pushed backwards and upwards. This tendency is prevented by sacrotuberous and sacrospinous ligaments.

The ligaments of these joints relax during pregnancy to allow slight enlargement of the pelvic cavity during last trimester of pregnancy.

The pelvic cavity houses the male/female internal genital organs. Accordingly the bony pelvis shows features of male or female pelvis. In female pelvis the subpubic angle is more than in the male pelvis. Female pelvis is broad and shallow as compared to the male pelvis.

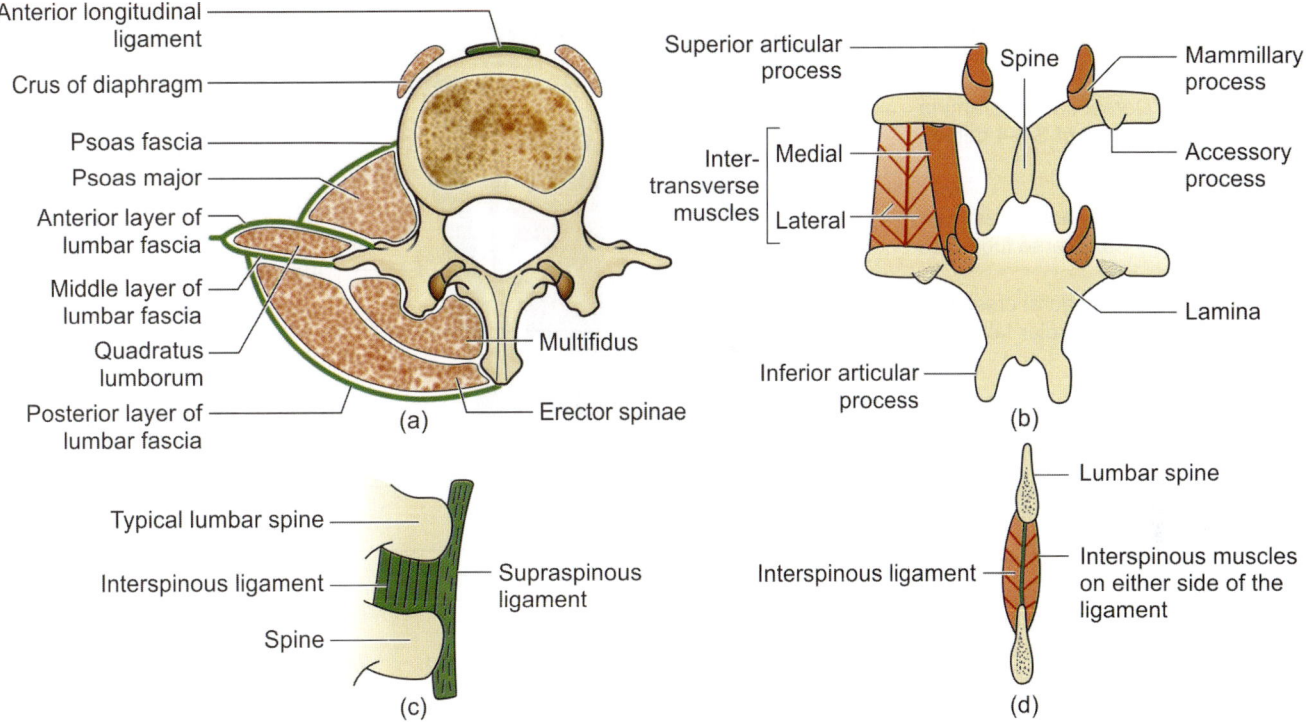

Fig. 45.1a to d: Attachments of the lumbar vertebra

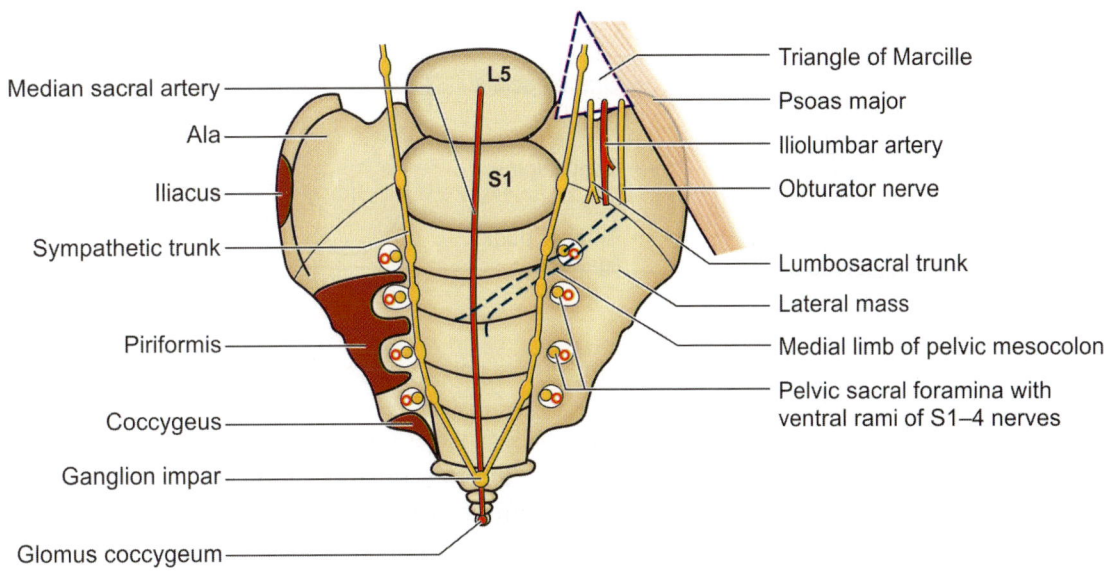

Fig. 45.2a: Anterior (pelvic) view of the sacrum and triangle of Marcille

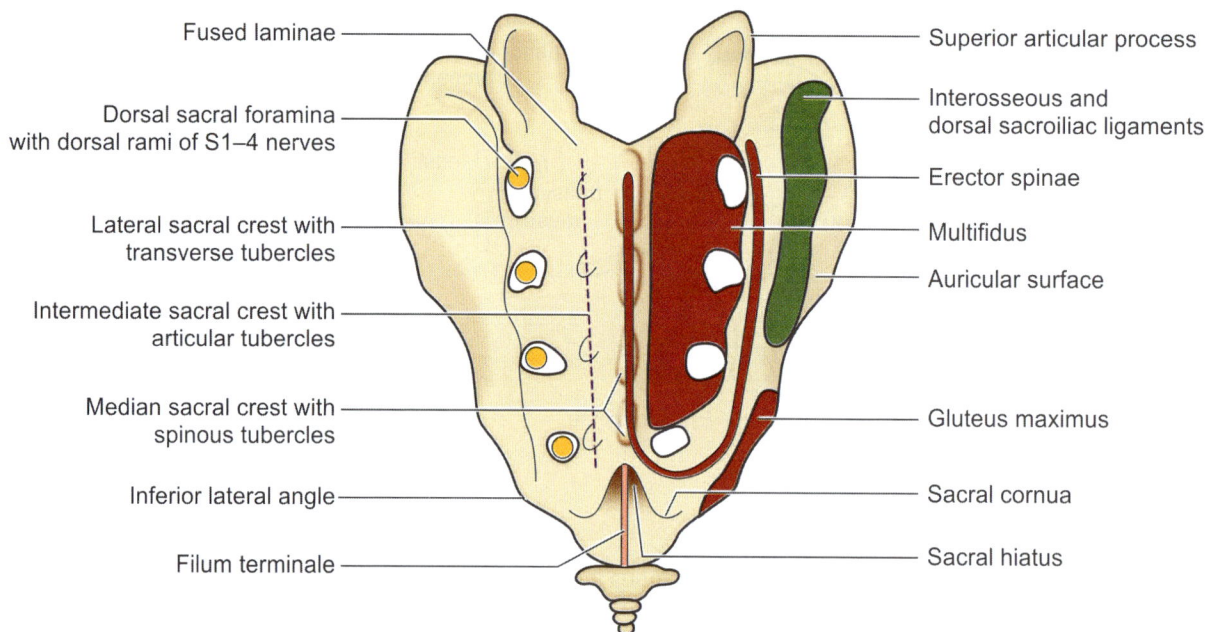

Fig. 45.2b: Posterior aspect of the sacrum

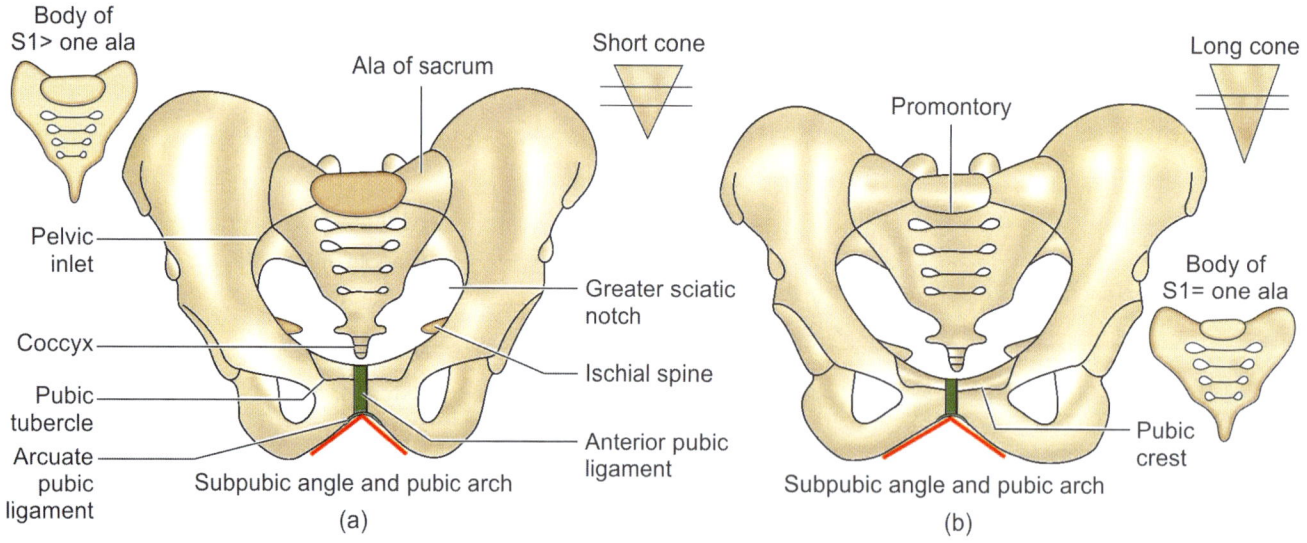

Fig. 45.3a and b: Anterior view: (a) A male pelvis, and (b) a female pelvis

Pubic Symphysis

Pubic symphysis is a secondary cartilaginous joint between the adjacent pubic bones. The ends of the bones are covered by hyaline cartilage with an intervening fibrocartilagenous disc. It is like the intervertebral joint presents between the bodies of the vertebrae. Ligaments of the pubic symphysis relax during last trimester of pregnancy to permit normal delivery. Sacrococcygeal joint is also united by the intervertebral disc.

Coccyx moves a little backwards during defaecation.

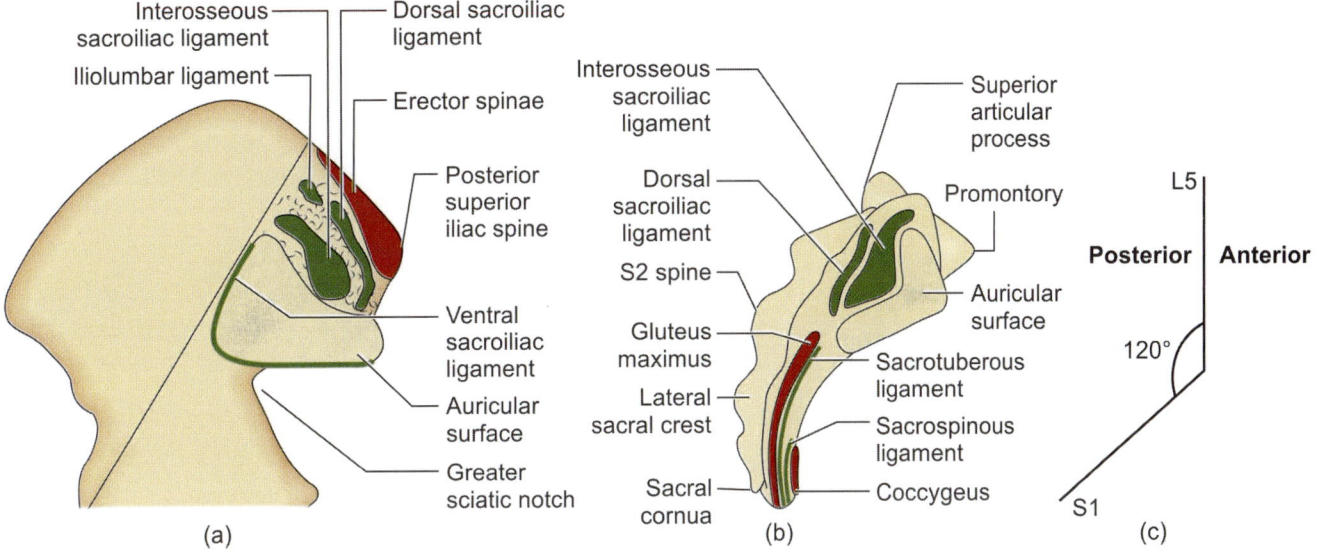

Fig. 45.4a to c: Articular surfaces of the right sacroiliac joint: (a) Medial view of the upper part of the right hip bone, (b) right lateral view of the sacrum, and (c) lumbosacral angle is 120° opening backwards

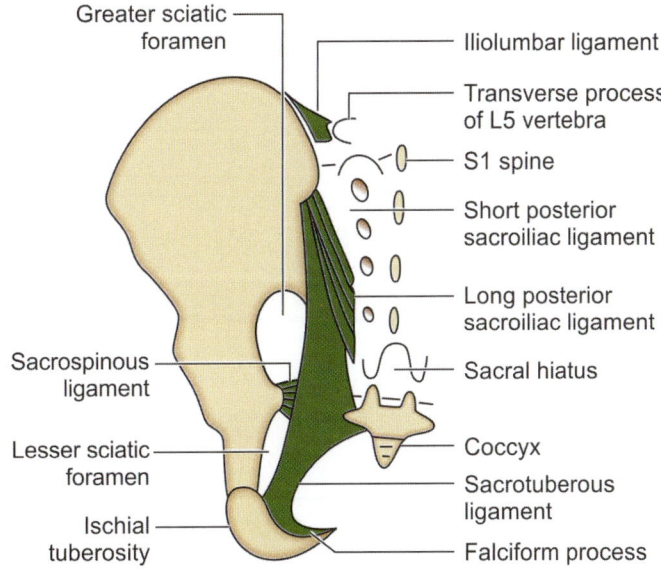

Fig. 45.5: Ligaments of the pelvis as seen from behind

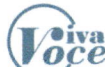

- How do you distinguish the lumbar from thoracic vertebra?
- What is sacralization of 5th lumbar vertebra?
- What is spondylolisthesis?

- What is disc prolapse?
- How much is the subpubic angle in male and in female pelvis?
- Which diameter is biggest at the outlet of true pelvis?

1. a. Name the highlighted structures.
    b. Where and how do these end?

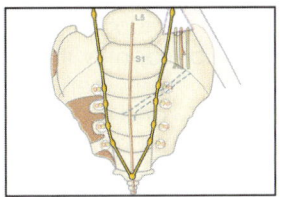

2. a. Identify the structure.
    b. What structures pass through it?

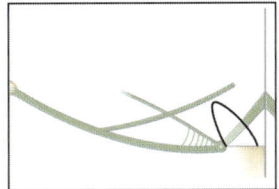

3. a. Name the venous plexus.
    b. Where does it drain on right and left sides?

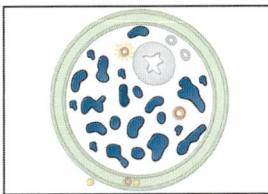

4. a. Identify the structure.
    b. What passes through it?

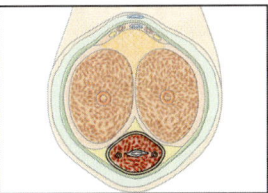

5. a. Identify the cell.
    b. Name its functions.

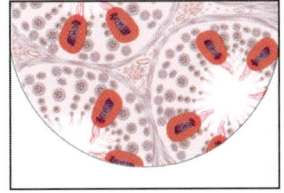

6. a. Identify the tortuous artery.
    b. Name its branches.

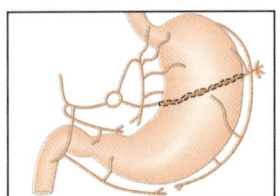

7. a. Name the pouch of peritoneum.
    b. What is its depth from skin of perineum?

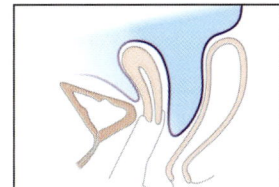

8. a. Identify the recess.
    b. What lies in its free margin?

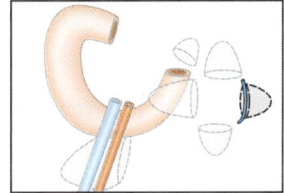

9. a. Where are these varices present.
    b. Name the veins participating.

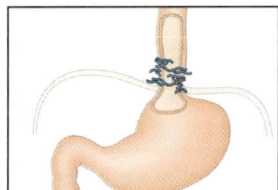

10. a. Identify the structure.
    b. Name its tributaries.

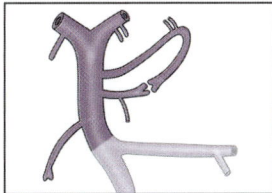

11. a. Identify the ligament.
    b. Name its constituents.

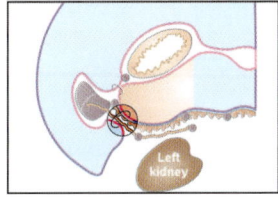

12. a. Name the organ.
    b. Name its segments.

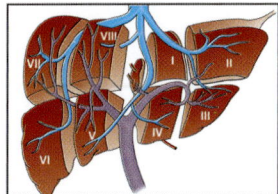

13. a. Identify the structure.
    b. Which veins take part in its formation?

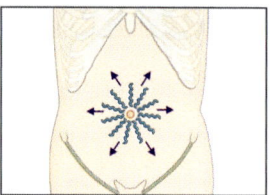

17. a. Identify the angle between vagina and uterus. How much is it.
    b. Identify the angle between cervix and uterus. How much is it?

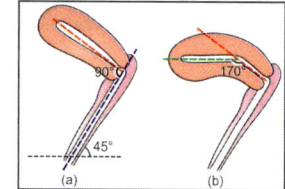

14. a. Identify the veins.
    b. Where do these drain?

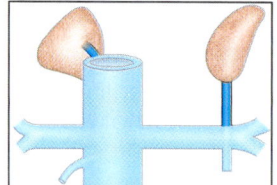

18. a. Name the venous plexus. Where does it drain?
    b. Identify the ligaments.

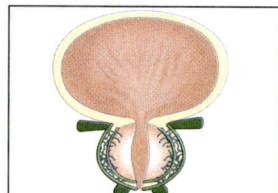

15. a. Identify the canal.
    b. Name the structures present in the canal.

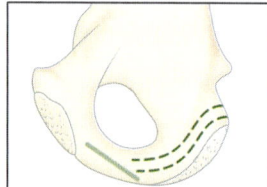

19. a. Identify the body.
    b. Name the muscles attached to it.

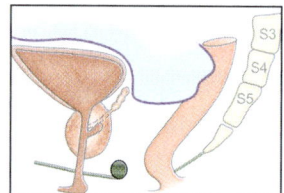

16. a. What does the figure show?
    b. What is its importance?

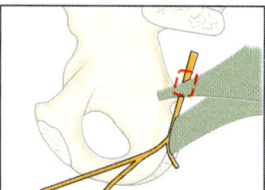

20. a. Name the main sites of portocaval anastomoses

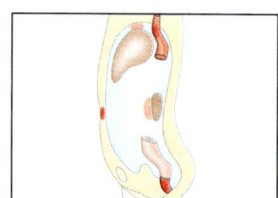

ANSWERS: ABDOMEN AND PELVIS

1. a. Sympathetic trunks lying medial to ventral sacral foramnia.
    b. Both the trunks fuse into a single ganglion impar (unpaired) anterior to the coccyx.

2. a. Superficial inguinal ring.
    b. The spermatic cord and ilioinguinal nerve exit from here

3. a. Pampiniform plexus from which one testicular vein arises.
    b. The testicular vein drains into left renal vein which drains into inferior vena cava. Right testicular vein drains directly into inferior vena cava.

4. a. The highlighted structure is corpus spongiosum presents in penis.
    b. Urethra passes through it.

5. a. Sertoli cell
    b. It gives protection and nourishment to the spermatogenic series of cells.

6. a. Tortuous artery is the splenic artery.
    b. It gives pancreatic branches, short gastric branches, left gastroepiploic branch and 5–7 splenic branches

7. a. Rectouterine pouch.
    b. It lies 7.5 cm deep to skin of perineum.

8. a. The marked recess is paraduodenal recess.
    b. Inferior mesenteric vein lies in its free margin.

9. a. Marked varices are oesophageal varies.
    b. The veins participating are: (i) Oesophageal veins draining through accessory hemiazygos into vena azygos and superior vena cana. (ii) Other veins are oesophageal veins draining into left gastric vein which end in the portal vein.

10. a. The structure is portal vein.
    b. Its tributaries are right and left gastric veins and superior pancreaticoduodenal vein.

11. a. Lineorenal ligament
    b. It contains the tail of pancreas, splenic vessels, autonomic nerves and lymph vessels.

12. a. Organ shown is liver.
    b. There are eight segments in the liver.
        i. Upper left medial
        ii. Upper left lateral
        iii. Lower left lateral
        iv. Lower left medial
        v. Upper right anterior
        vi. Upper right posterior
        vii. Lower right posterior
        viii. Lower right anterior

13. a. Caput medusae is shown.
    b. Veins participiting are paraumbilical veins running along ligamentum teres (ending in portal vein); lateral thoracic veins, superficial epigastric, superior and inferior epigastic veins (ending in systemic circulation).

14. a. Veins of suprarenal gland.
    b. Right vein ends in inferior vena cana. Left vein ends in left renal vein which also ends in inferior vena cava.

15. a. Pudendal canal is in the lateral wall of ischioanal fossa
    b. It lodges internal pudendal vessels and pudendal nerve.

16. a. Pudendal nerve block.
    b. It is given in vaginal operations. The drug is injected deep to ischial spine. It is also given during delivery to relieve pain.

17. a. Angle of anteversion. It lies between long axis of vagina and long axis of uterus and is 90°;
    b. Angle of anteflexion. It lies between long axis of cervix and long axis of uterus, and is 170°.

18. a. Prostatic venous plexus. It drains into internal iliac vein.
    b. Ligaments are medial and lateral puboprostatic ligaments.

19. a. Perineal body
    b. Gives attachment to 2 superficial and 2 deep transversus perenei, 2 bulbospongiosus, 2 levator ani, sphincter ani externus and longitudinal coat of rectum

20. a. Main sites of portocaval anastomoses are umbilicus, lower end of oesophagus and anal canal

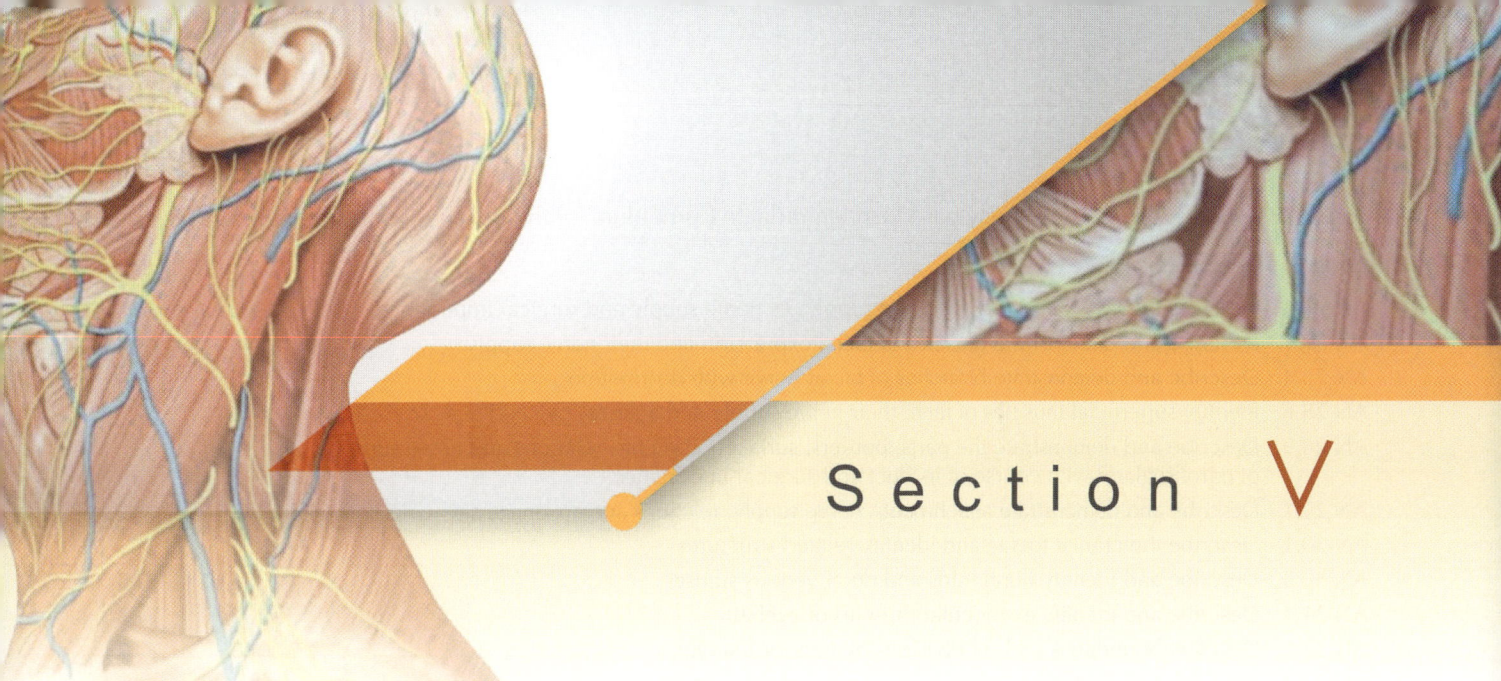

Section V

Head and Neck

CHAPTER 46

Scalp, Temple and Face

Learning Objectives

One should be able to

1. Name the arteries and nerves of the scalp.
2. Enumerate the layers in superficial temporal region.
3. Demarcate the dangerous area of face? Why is it so called?
4. Make a flowchart of the secretomotor supply of the lacrimal gland?

OVERVIEW

Scalp: The soft tissue covering the top of skull is known as the scalp. Its five layers are skin, rich in sebaceous glands, subcutaneous tissue with nerves and blood vessels, aponeurosis with emissary vein, loose connective tissue and pericranium.

There are four sensory nerves in front of ear and four sensory nerves behind the ear. Motor nerves in front and behind the ear are branches of facial nerve.

The only muscle is occipitofrontalis with its two occipital bellies innervated by posterior auricular branch of facial nerve and two frontal bellies supplied by temporal branches of facial nerve. The four bellies are united by epicranial aponeurosis.

Arteries of the scalp are supratrochlear, supraorbital, superficial temporal (palpable) in front of ear and posterior auricular and occipital arteries behind the ear.

The temple is the superficial temporal region lying in relation to the squamous part of temporal bone. This region contains the temporalis fascia and temporalis muscle instead of loose areolar tissue. So there are six layers, e.g. skin, subcutaneous tissue, thin extension of epicranial aponeurosis, temporal fascia, temporalis muscle and pericranium.

Face: It is the front of the skull extending from the hairline above to chin below and laterally from one ear to the other ear. The skin of face is innervated by all three branches of trigeminal nerve. Only the skin in front of ear (2 cm wide) is innervated by great auricular nerve (C2,3).

Muscles of the face are derived from 2nd pharyngeal arch and get inserted into the skin of the face. So these muscles are called muscles of facial expression. These get their nerve supply from various branches of facial (VII) nerve, injury to facial nerve (lower motor neuron paralysis) results in typical symptoms.

ARTERIAL SUPPLY

The arterial supply of face is mainly by tortuous facial artery, a branch of external carotid artery.

VEINS OF SCALP AND FACE

Superficial temporal vein from scalp and deep maxillary vein join to form a retromandibular vein lying in the parotid gland. This vein divides into a posterior and an anterior division. Posterior division joins the posterior auricular vein to form external jugular vein. The anterior division joins the facial vein from the face to common facial vein which drains into internal jugular vein. Facial vein gets connected to pterygoid venous plexus via the deep facial vein. This venous plexus is linked to cavernous venous sinus via an emissary vein. Infection from the face may travel via facial vein → deep facial vein → pterygoid venous plexus → emissary vein → cavernous sinus; leading to cavernous sinus thrombosis. So the area of the upper lip and adjoining parts of the cheeks is called "the dangerous area of the face".

EYELIDS

Eyelids/palpebrae are like curtains for the eyeball. The upper eyelid is bigger than the lower one. Each eyelid is made of skin, superficial fascia with palpebral part of orbicularis oculi muscle, palpebral fascia forming tarsal plate receiving the insertion of levator palpebrae superioris muscle and the smooth conjunctiva.

LACRIMAL APPARATUS

Structures concerned with formation, circulation and drainage of lacrimal fluid constitute the lacrimal apparatus. These are lacrimal gland with its multiple ducts, conjunctival sac, lacrimal puncta with lacrimal

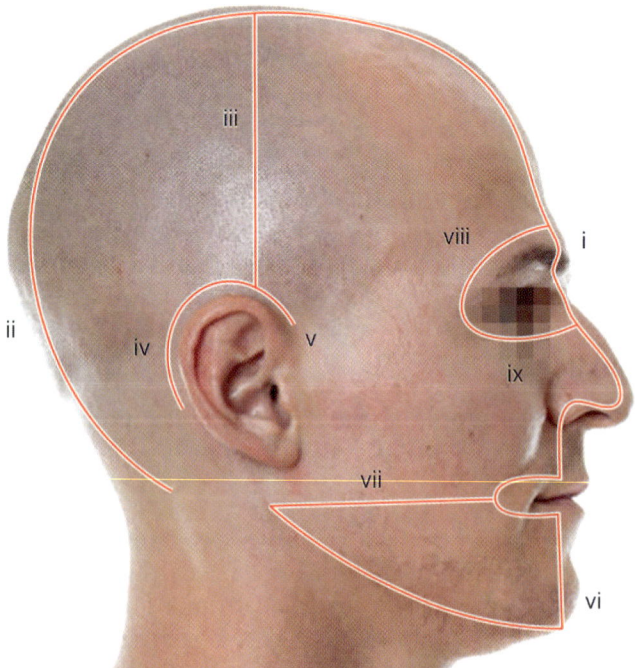

Fig. 46.1: Lines of incision

canaliculi, lacrimal sac and nasolacrimal duct with its fold.

Competency achievement: The student should be able to:

AN 27.1 Describe the layers of scalp, its blood supply, its nerve supply and surgical importance.

Steps of Dissection

- Place 2–3 wooden blocks under the head to raise it about 10–12 cm from the table.
- Figure 46.1 shows a median incision in the skin of scalp extending from root of the nose (i), to the prominent external occipital protuberance (ii). Give a coronal incision across the previous incision from root of one auricle to the other (iii). Extend curved incision from the auricle to the mastoid process posteriorly (iv), and to root of zygoma anteriorly (v). Reflect the skin in four flaps.
- Usually, the skin is so adherent to the subjacent connective tissue and aponeurotic layers that these all come off together. Dissect the layers, including the nerves, vessels, lymphatics and identify these structures in the cadaver.
- Examine the cut edge of the scalp and identify occipitofrontalis muscle. It is attached to the occipital bone and the epicranial aponeurosis. The superior attachment of the frontal belly is to the epicranial aponeurosis and its inferior attachment is to the skin of the forehead and the eyebrows. The layers of scalp are shown in Fig. 46.2.
- The anterior flap is pulled inferiorly to see the supraorbital margin. Identify supraorbital nerve (branch of frontal, a division of ophthalmic branch of trigeminal nerve) and supraorbital artery, a branch of ophthalmic artery. See that all the nerves and arteries enter the scalp from the periphery.
- Identify the temporalis muscle and fascia on the temporal region. Layers (1–6) of superficial temporal region are seen in Fig. 46.3.

Competency achievement: The student should be able to:

AN 28.1 Describe and demonstrate muscles of facial expression and their nerve supply.

Steps of Dissection of Face

- Give a median incision from the root of nose, across the dorsum of nose, centre of philtrum of upper lip, to centre of lower lip to chin (vi).

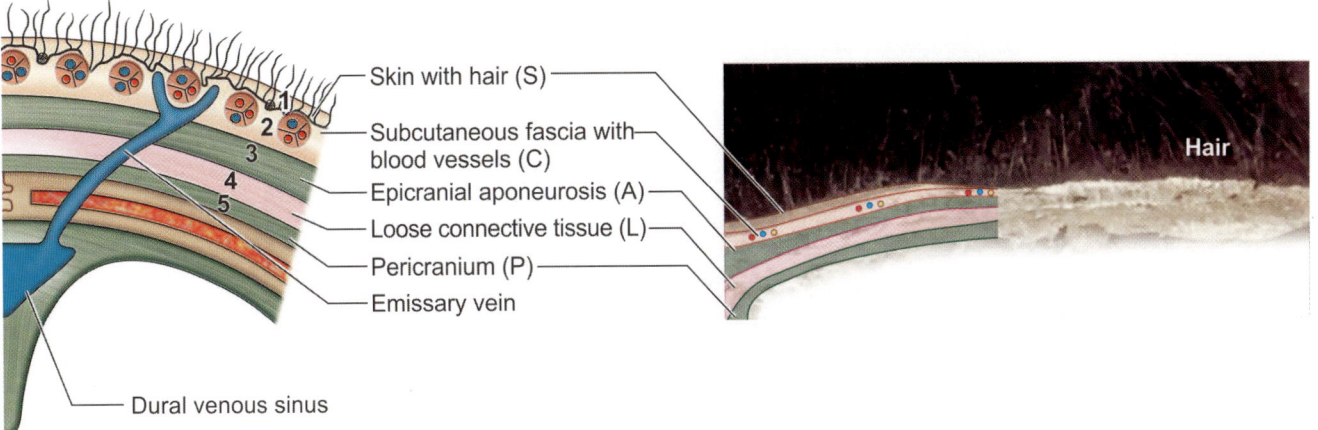

Fig. 46.2: Layers of scalp

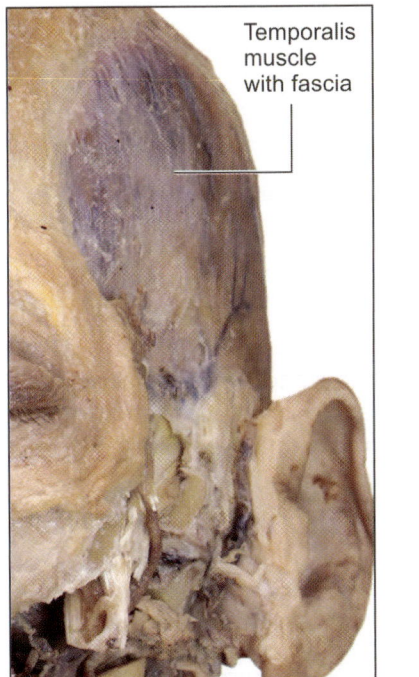

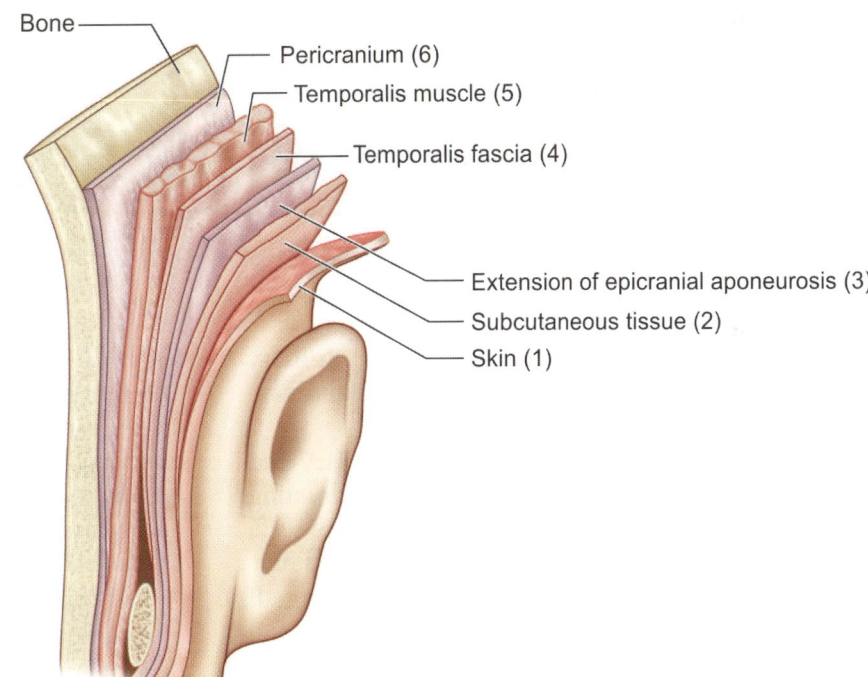

Fig. 46.3: (a) Temporalis muscle; (b) layers 1–6 of superficial temporal region

- Give a horizontal incision from the angle of the mouth to posterior border of the mandible (vii)
- Reflect the lower flap towards and up to the lower border of mandible (Fig. 46.1).
- Direct and reflect the upper flap till the auricle.
- Subjacent to the skin, the facial muscles are directly encountered as these are inserted in the skin. Identify the various functional groups of facial muscles (Fig. 46.4a and b).

Competency achievement: The student should be able to:

AN 28.4 Describe and demonstrate branches of facial nerve with distribution.

- Trace the various motor branches of facial nerve emerging from the anterior border of parotid gland to supply these muscles (Fig. 46.5).
- Amongst these motor branches on the face are the sensory branches of the three divisions of the

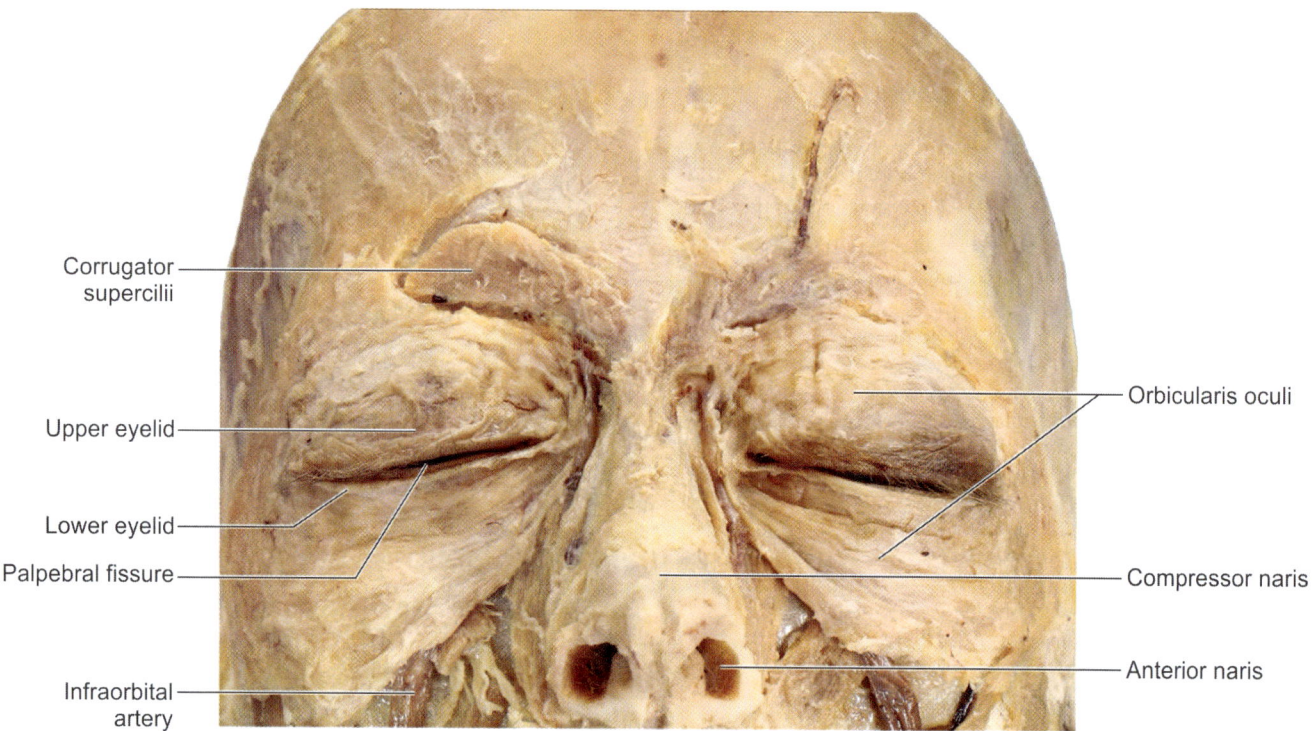

Fig. 46.4a: Some muscles of facial expression

trigeminal nerve (Fig. 46.5). Try to identify all these with the help of their course given in BD Chaurasia's *Human Anatomy*.

- Look for the branches of ophthalmic, maxillary and mandibular divisions of trigeminal nerve innervating most of the skin of the face. Great auricular nerve (C2, 3) innervates the skin, 2 cm wide, anterior to the pinna.
- Identify the branches of facial nerve supplying all the muscles of facial expressions.

Competency achievement: The student should be able to:

AN 28.6 Identify superficial muscles of face, their nerve supply and actions.

- Identify the muscles of facial expression. These are occipitofrontalis mentioned in the scalp, orbicularis oculi around the orbital margins, nasal muscles in relation to nose and its apertures, orbicularis oris around the orifice of mouth, platysma in the neck and vestigial auricular muscles. Some of these muscles are seen in Fig. 46.4b.
- Clean the buccal pad of fat and fascia anterior to masseter muscle.

- Identify the parotid duct emerging from the anterior border of the gland, running across the cheek on the masseter muscle, piercing the buccinator muscle to open into vestibule of mouth opposite 2nd upper molar tooth.
- Clean and dissect the branches of facial nerve on the face. These are:
  - Temporal branch crossing zygomatic arch
  - Zygomatic branch crossing the zygomatic bone
  - Two buccal branches across the cheek
  - Marginal mandibular along the inferior border of mandible
  - Cervical branch crosses the angle of mandible towards the neck where it innervates the platysma muscle (Fig. 46.5).
- Look, clean and identify the facial artery at the anteroinferior angle of masseter muscle at the lower border of mandible. Here it enters the face, runs up tortuously till 1.5 cm lateral to the angle of mouth, lateral to the nose till the medial angle of eye, where it ends by anastomosing with dorsal nasal branch of ophthalmic artery (Fig. 46.7a and b).

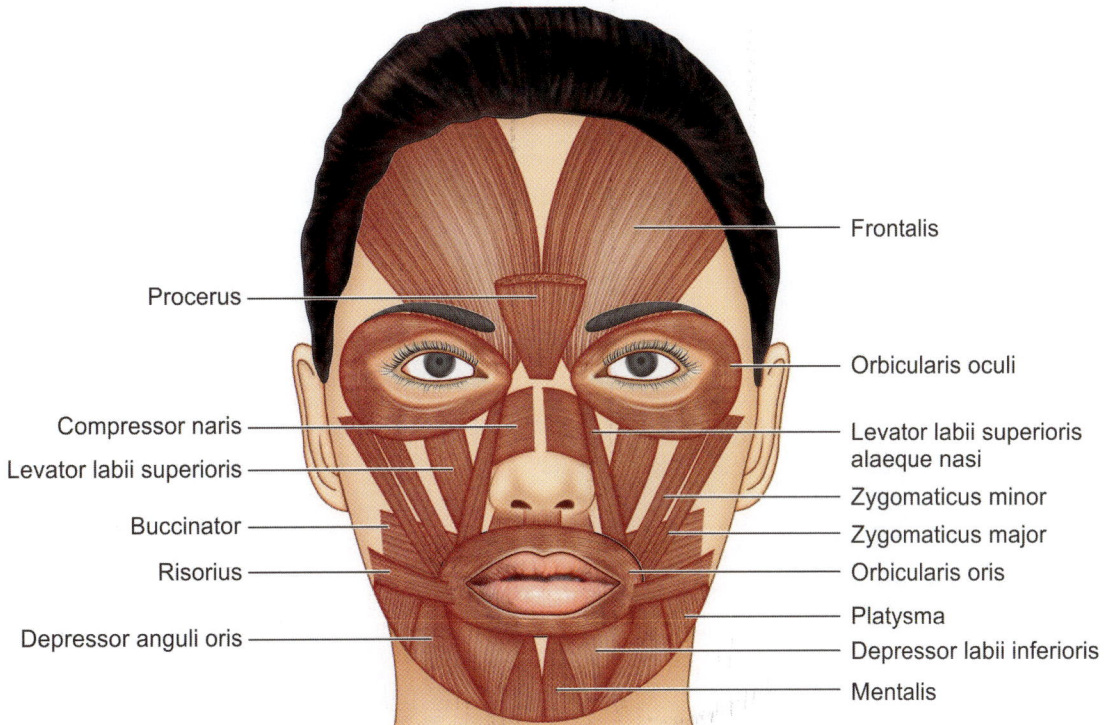

Fig. 46.4b: Some muscles of facial expression

Frontalis

Procerus

Orbicularis oculi

Compressor naris

Levator labii superioris alaeque nasi

Levator labii superioris

Zygomaticus minor

Buccinator

Zygomaticus major

Risorius

Orbicularis oris

Platysma

Depressor anguli oris

Depressor labii inferioris

Mentalis

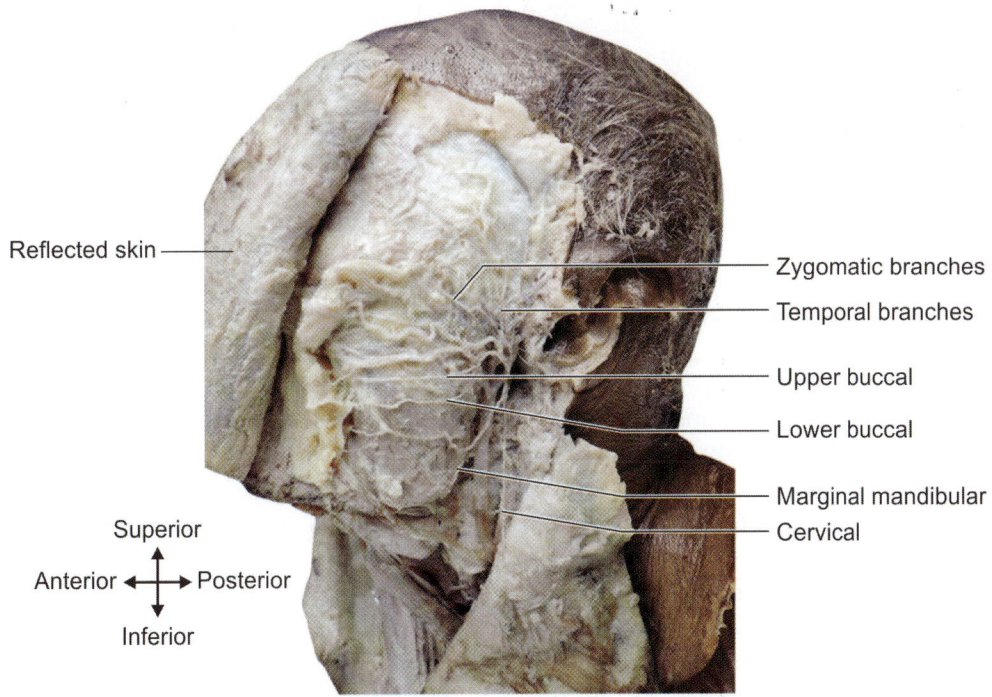

Fig. 46.5: Branches of facial nerve on the face

Reflected skin

Zygomatic branches

Temporal branches

Upper buccal

Lower buccal

Marginal mandibular

Cervical

Superior

Anterior ← → Posterior

Inferior

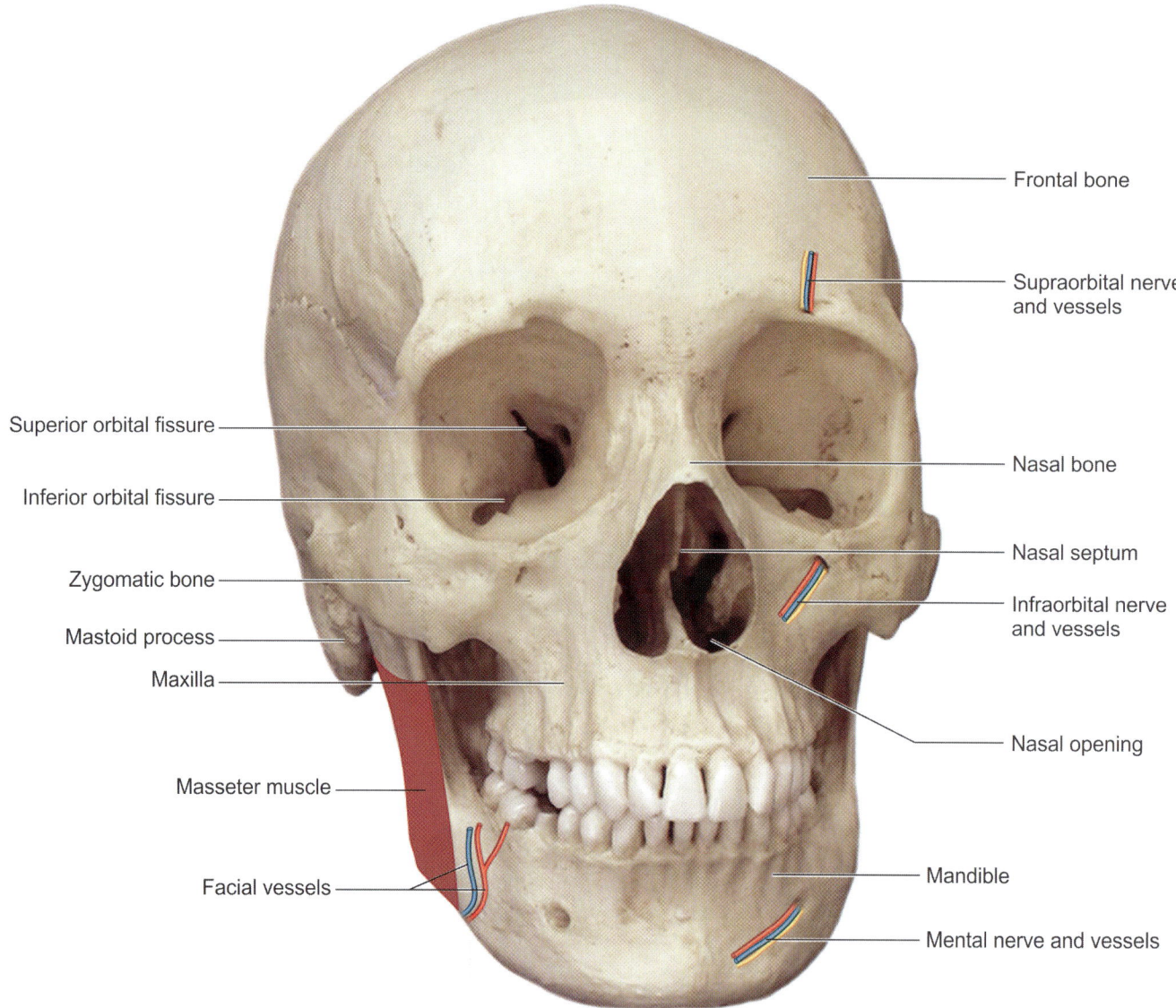

Fig. 46.6: Some branches of divisions of trigeminal nerve on the face and facial vessels

- Look for various muscular and cutaneous branches of the artery. The named branches are inferior labial, superior labial and lateral nasal branches.
- Look for another artery on the face, the transverse facial artery, a branch of superficial temporal running below the zygomatic arch.
- See that facial vein runs little posterior to the artery and joins anterior division of retromandibular vein to form common facial vein which drains into internal jugular vein (Fig. 46.8).

Steps of Dissection of Eyelids/Palpebrae and Lacrimal Apparatus

- Give a circular incision around the roots of eyelids (Fig. 46.1–viii and ix). This will separate the orbital part of orbicularis oculi from the palpebral parts.
- Carefully reflect the palpebral part towards the palpebral fissure.
- The upper and lower eyelids are movable curtains which protect the eyes from foreign bodies and

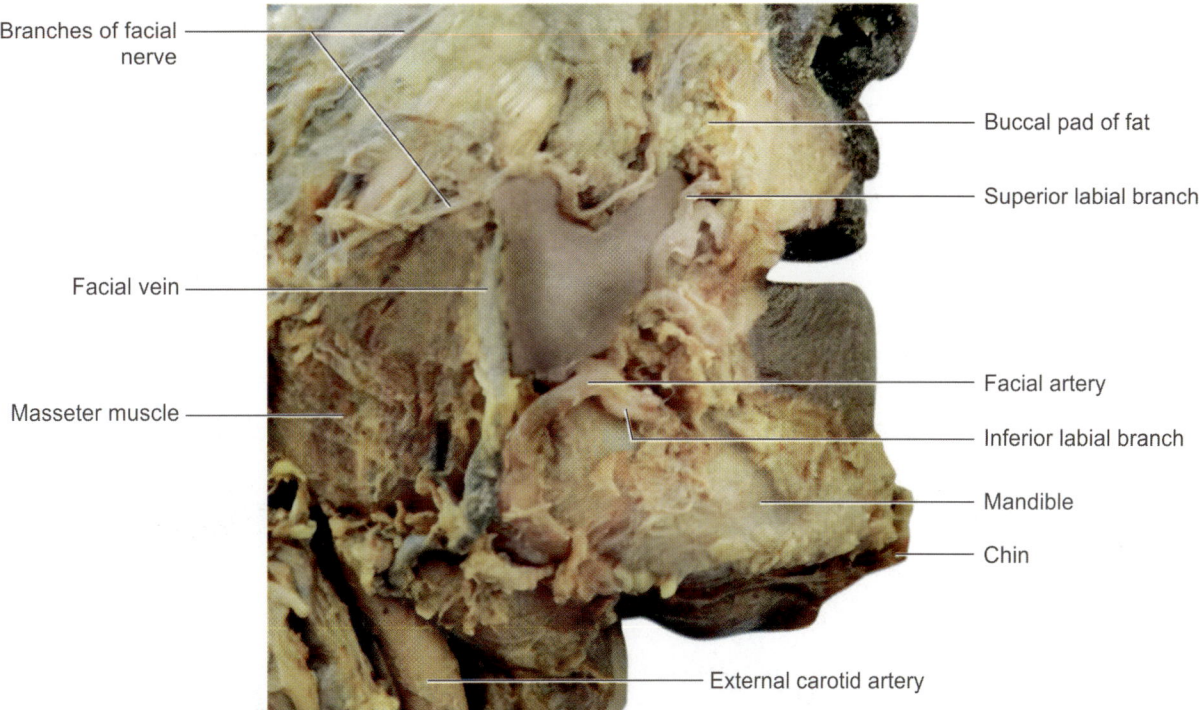

Branches of facial nerve

Buccal pad of fat

Superior labial branch

Facial vein

Facial artery

Inferior labial branch

Masseter muscle

Mandible

Chin

External carotid artery

Fig. 46.7a: Facial artery with its branches

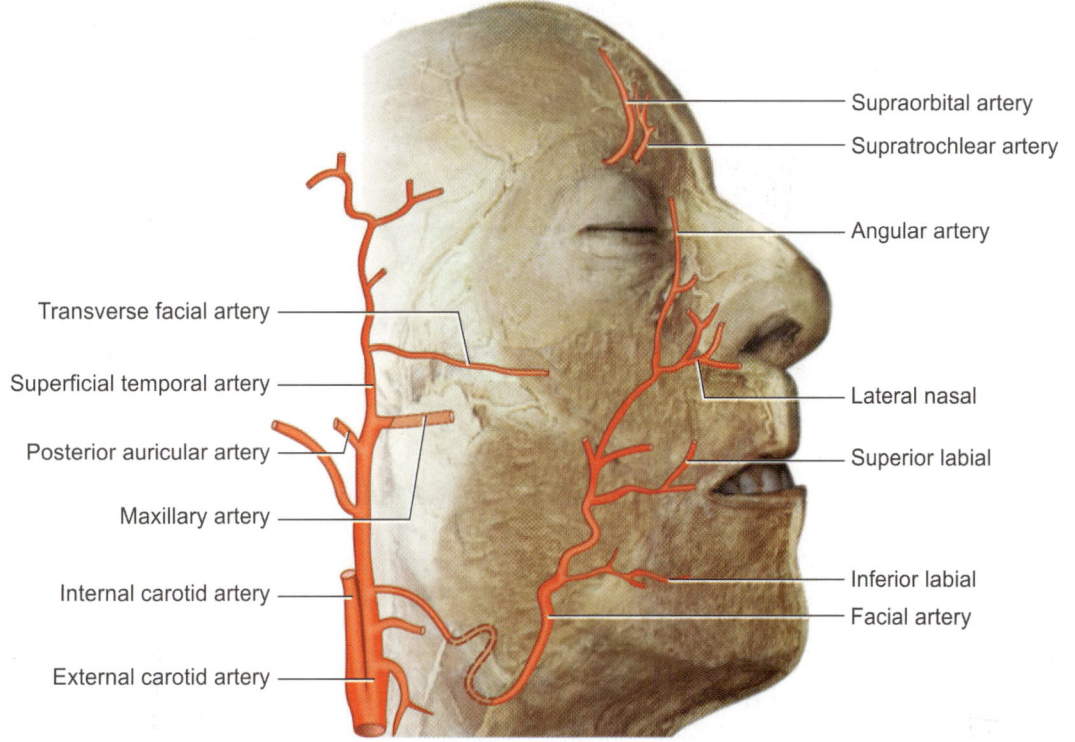

Supraorbital artery

Supratrochlear artery

Angular artery

Transverse facial artery

Superficial temporal artery

Lateral nasal

Posterior auricular artery

Superior labial

Maxillary artery

Internal carotid artery

Inferior labial

Facial artery

External carotid artery

Fig. 46.7b: Course of facial artery and its branches

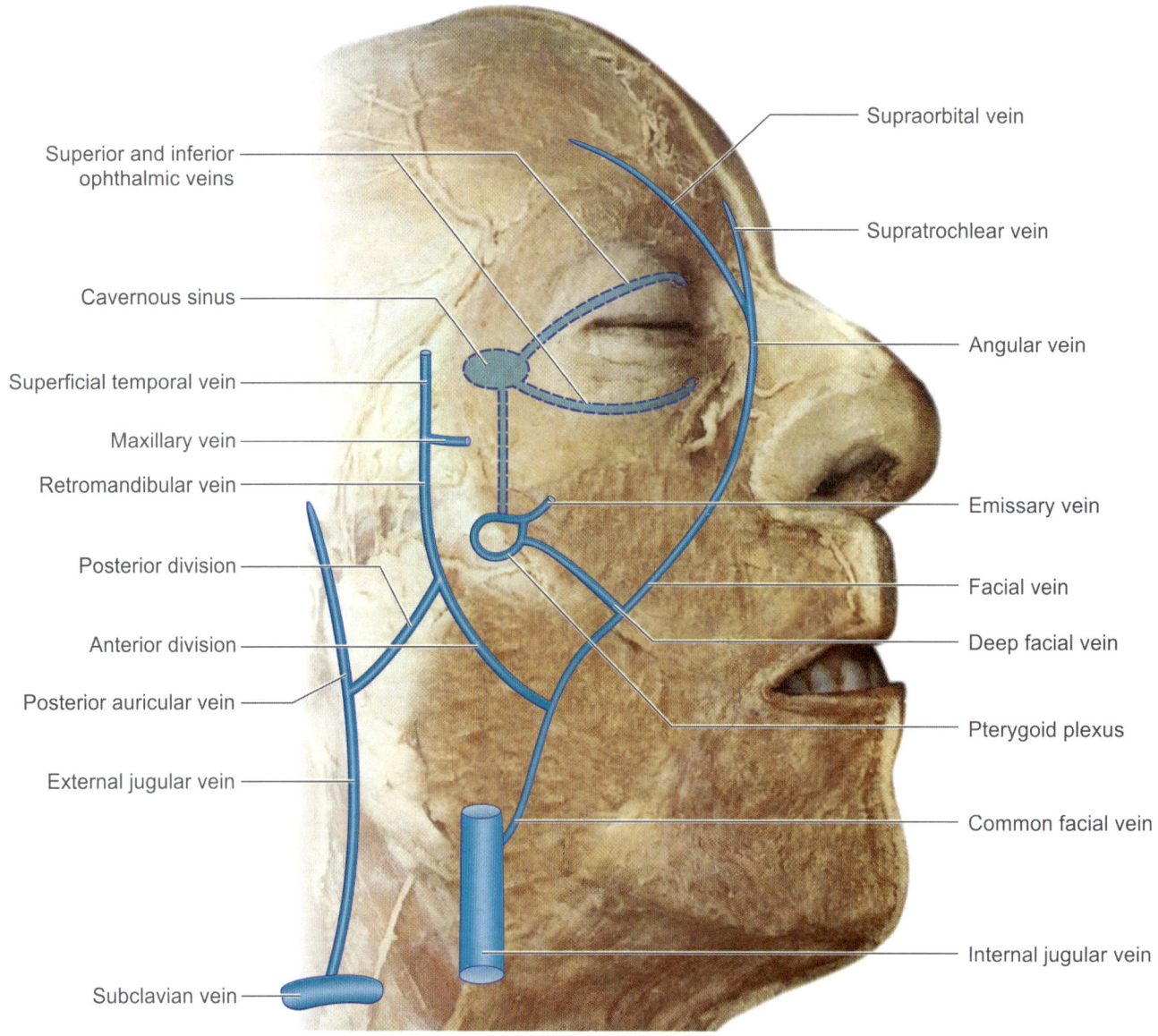

Fig. 46.8: Formation and course of facial and external jugular veins

bright light. They keep the cornea clean and moist. The upper eyelid is larger and more movable than the lower eyelid (Fig. 46.9).

- See that the skin is loose and identify the nerves and arteries as medial supratrochlear and lateral supraorbital.
- Identify the palpebral part of orbicularis oculi (sleeping muscle)
- Look for tarsal plate deep to the muscle.

- Identify levator palpebrae superioris getting inserted into upper margin and anterior surface of superior tarsal plate and also to the skin of upper eyelid including the superior conjunctival fornix.
- Appreciate that the lining of tarsal plate is the moist conjunctiva.
- Figure 46.9 shows some parts of lacrimal apparatus. These are lacrimal puncta and canaliculi, lacrimal sac and nasolacrimal duct.

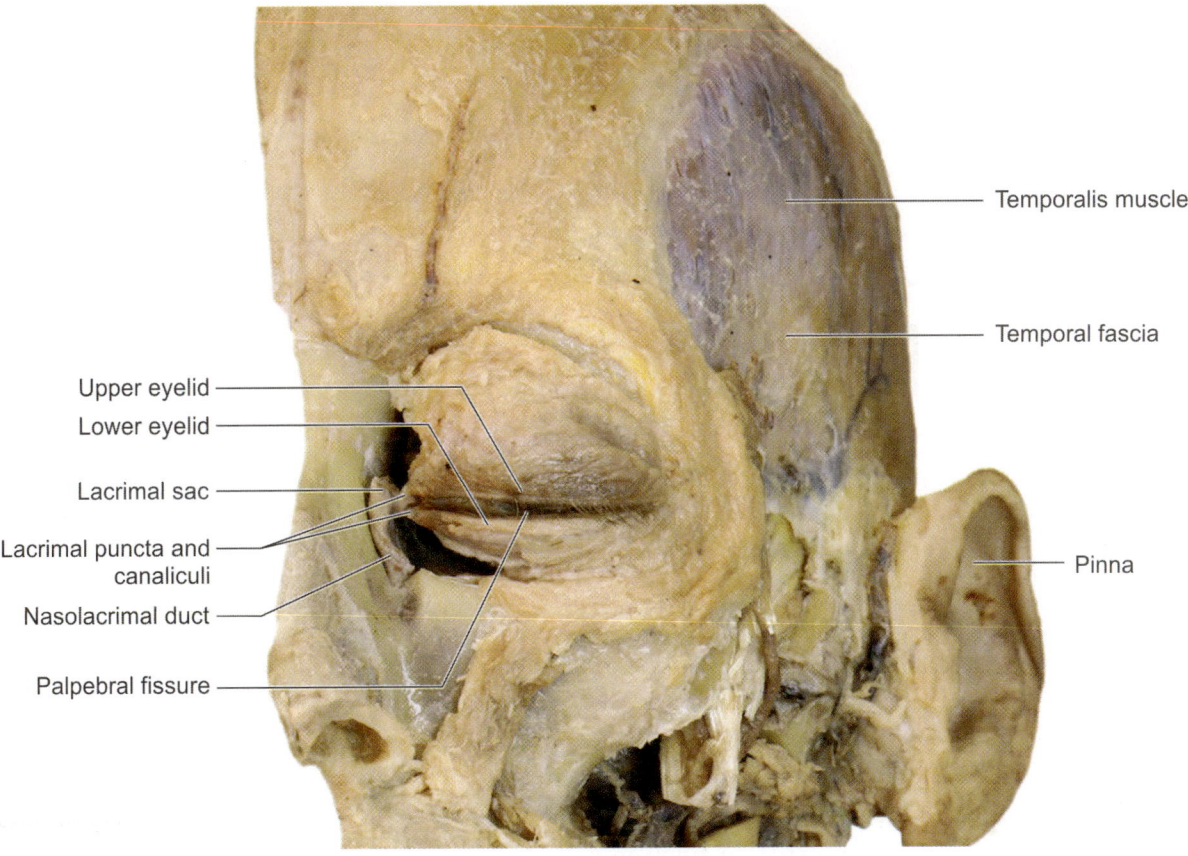

Fig. 46.9: Eyelids and parts of lacrimal apparatus

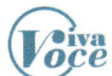 Viva Voce

- Name the sensory and motor nerves supplying the scalp.
- How is the external jugular vein formed?
- Name the parts of orbicularis oculi muscle.
- Name the muscles attached to the modiolus.
- Which is the dangerous area of face?
- Enumerate the parts of lacrimal apparatus.

- Why is buccinator muscle an accessory muscle of mastication?
- Name the layers of upper eyelid.
- What are the effects of left Bell's palsy on the face?
- Which arteries are called 'an anaesthetist's arteries' and why?

CHAPTER 47

Side of the Neck and Posterior Triangle

Learning Objectives

One should be able to

1. Enumerate branches of cervical plexus seen in superficial fascia of posterior triangle.
2. Name the boundaries and contents of posterior triangle.
3. Discuss origin insertion, important relations, nerve supply, actions and effects of paralysis of SCM muscle.

OVERVIEW

Most important landmark in the side of neck is sternocleidomastoid muscle (SCM).

Superficial fascia of neck contains some cutaneous nerves. These are great auricular, lesser occipital, transverse cutaneous nerve of neck and supraclavicular nerves. All these are branches of cervical plexus. In addition, the fascia contains external jugular vein which runs vertically over oblique SCM muscle to drain into subclavian vein. If this vein gets cut, there may be air embolism. Neck is invested by deep fascia known as cervical fascia. Cervical fascia has many divisions. These are investing layer, pretracheal layer, prevertebral layer, carotid sheath, buccopharyngeal and pharyngobasilar fasciae.

The posterior triangle is placed between SCM muscle, trapezius muscle and middle 1/3rd of clavicle. Its apex is above and base is below. Its roof is formed by investing layer of deep cervical fascia. Embedded in this roof lies the spinal root of accessory nerve. It leaves the SCM, runs in the roof of posterior triangle and ends by innervating the trapezius muscle. Close to this important nerve are the cutaneous branches

which have been seen in the superficial fascia. In the lower and medial part of triangle are 5 roots forming 3 trunks of the brachial plexus. This is the supraclavicular part of brachial plexus.

Close to lower trunk is the third part of subclavian artery. Other two arteries are branches of 1st part of subclavian artery.

Inferior belly of omohyoid is seen to divide the posterior triangle into an upper occipital part and lower supraclavicular or subclavian part.

Competency achievement: The student should be able to:

AN 29.1 Describe and demonstrate attachments, nerve supply, relations and actions of sternocleidomastoid.

STEPS OF DISSECTION

- Give a median incision from the chin downwards towards the suprasternal notch situated above the manubrium of sternum. Make one incision in the skin of base of mandible and continue it by oblique incision along posterior border of ramus of mandible up to the mastoid process and further along the superior nuchal line till the external occipital protuberance (Fig. 47.1).

312

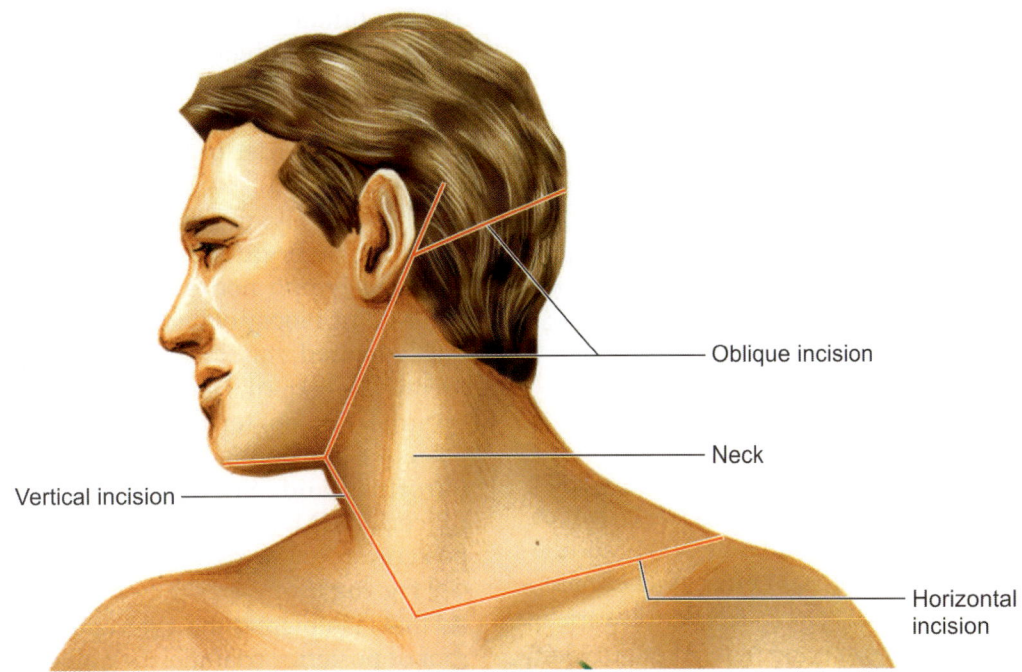

Fig. 47.1: Lines of incision

- One incision is given along the upper border of clavicle. Reflect only the skin up towards the anterior border of trapezius muscle.
- Identify the platysma muscle. Reflect it towards the mandible.
- Identify the anterior or transverse cutaneous nerve of neck in the upper part of superficial fascia.
- Look for external jugular vein running vertically away from the median plane.
- Remove the superficial fascia to be able to see the deep fascia.
- Identify the external jugular vein above the clavicle. See it piercing the deep fascia to drain into the subclavian vein.
- *To open up the suprasternal space:* Make a horizontal incision just above the sternum. Extend the incision along the anterior border of sternocleidomastoid muscle for 3–4 cm which reflects the superficial lamina to expose the suprasternal space and identify its contents.
- Identify the contents of suprasternal space. These are: Sternal heads of right and left SCM, jugular venous arch, a lymph node and interclavicular ligament.

Competency achievement: The student should be able to:

AN 35.1 Describe the parts, extent, attachments, modifications of deep cervical fascia.

- Identify the various layers of deep cervical fascia one by one. These are:
  - i. Investing layer
  - ii. Pretracheal layer
  - iii. Prevertebral layer
  - iv. Carotid sheath
  - v. Buccopharyngeal fascia
  - vi. Pharyngobasilar fascia

Learn the attachments of investing layer from BD Chaurasia's *Human Anatomy*.

- Identify that this fascia encloses:
  - i. 2 glands—parotid and submandibular
  - ii. 2 muscles—sternocleidomastoid and trapezius
  - iii. 2 spaces—supraclavicular and suprasternal
  - iv. 2 pulleys—for digastrics and omohyoids
  - v. Roof for 2 triangles—anterior and posterior triangles

Pretracheal layer encloses and supports the thyroid gland.

Prevertebral layer lies anterior to cervical vertebrae, forms the floor of posterior triangle and then continues as axillary sheath in the axilla.

Carotid sheath is formed by condensation of pretracheal and prevertebral fasciae. It encloses common carotid/internal carotid arteries, internal jugular vein and vagus nerve.

Two small fasciae are well seen in relation to superior constrictor muscle. Inner layer is pharyngobasilar fascia and outer layer is buccopharyngeal fascia.

POSTERIOR TRIANGLE

Steps of Dissection

- Try and dissect the cutaneous nerves which pierce the investing layer of cervical fascia at the middle of the posterior border of SCM muscle. These are:
  - i. Lesser occipital nerve going behind the auricle
  - ii. Great auricular nerve lying in front of auricle
  - iii. Transverse cutaneous nerve of neck
  - iv. Supraclavicular nerves with its three branches

The important motor nerve emerging in relation to this area is the spinal root of accessory nerve. It lies just deep to the fascial roof of the triangle, courses downwards and laterally across the triangle to enter the anterior border of trapezius which it supplies (Fig. 47.2a and b).

- Identify small lymph nodes around the spinal root of accessory nerve. The nerve may get entangled in enlarged lymph nodes. So one has to be careful while doing biopsy of lymph nodes. The nerve must not be injured.
- Identify the external jugular vein. See its formation by union of posterior auricular vein with the posterior division of retromandibular vein in the parotid gland. See it crossing the obliquely placed, SCM, running vertically across the posterior triangle to drain into the subclavian vein (*see* Fig 46.8).

As this vein pierces the anteroinferior angle of the roof of posterior triangle, its wall gets fused to the fascia. So the vein cannot retract leading to air embolism.

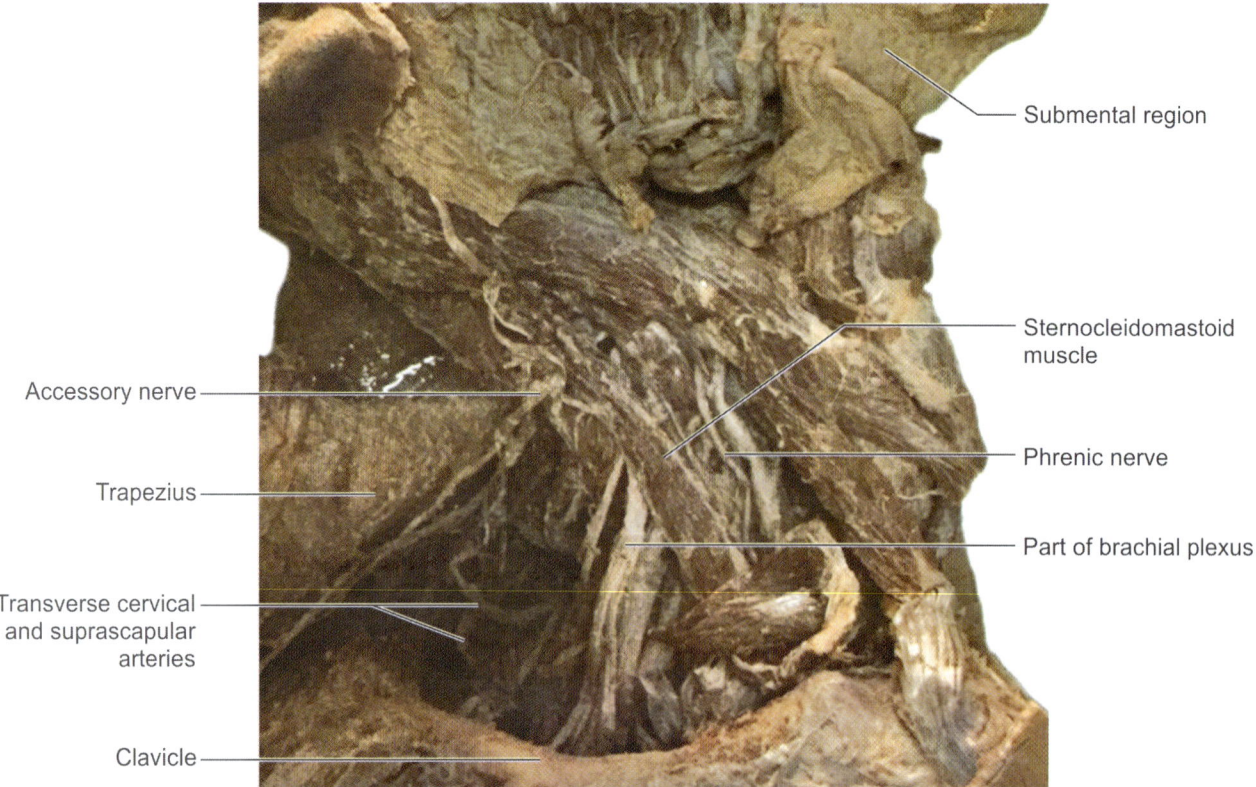

Fig. 47.2a: Some contents of posterior triangle of neck

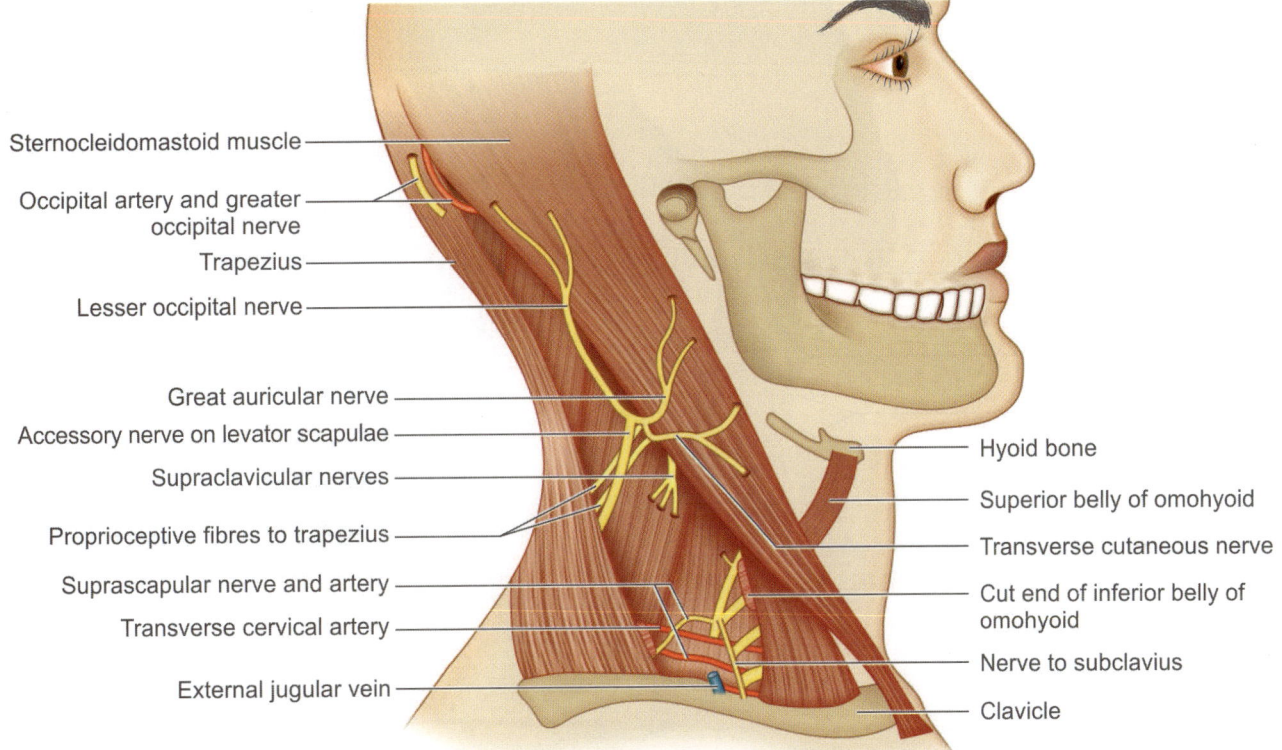

Sternocleidomastoid muscle

Occipital artery and greater occipital nerve

Trapezius

Lesser occipital nerve

Great auricular nerve

Accessory nerve on levator scapulae

Supraclavicular nerves

Proprioceptive fibres to trapezius

Suprascapular nerve and artery

Transverse cervical artery

External jugular vein

Hyoid bone

Superior belly of omohyoid

Transverse cutaneous nerve

Cut end of inferior belly of omohyoid

Nerve to subclavius

Clavicle

Fig. 47.2b: Boundaries and contents of posterior triangle

- Look for a thin muscle, the inferior belly of omohyoid coming from scapula (Fig. 47.2b). It courses upwards and medially to get inserted into a central tendon which lies on the internal jugular vein at the level of cricoid cartilage (under SCM). See that inferior belly divides the posterior triangle into an upper larger occipital triangle and a lower smaller subclavian or supraclavicular triangle.

- Identify transverse cervical artery along the upper border of inferior belly of omohyoid. Trace it both ways. See it arising in the anterior triangle from thyrocervical trunk and then passing in relation to muscles attached to scapula (Fig. 47.2b).

- Identify suprascapular artery running just above the clavicle (Fig. 47.2b). Both transverse cervical and suprascapular arteries take part in the anastomoses around the scapula along with circumflex scapular from subscapular artery, branch of 3rd part of axillary artery.

- The main contents of subclavian triangle are the upper, middle and lower trunks of the brachial plexus. Identify the three trunks (Figs 47.2b and 47.3).

Try to locate some of its branches, e.g. suprascapular and nerve to subclavius.

- Identify deeply placed long thoracic nerve arising from C5, C6 and C7 roots of brachial plexus and dorsal scapular from C5 segment. In the lowest part of subclavian triangle, the third part of subclavian artery and subclavian vein may be seen.

- Identify the contents of occipital triangle. These are accessory nerve and four cutaneous branches mentioned earlier (Fig. 47.2a).

- The branches from C3 and C4 for levator scapulae muscle and trapezius may be identified.

- Look for large occipital artery near apex of triangle (Fig. 47.2b). See its muscular branches especially to SCM muscle.

- A little away from occipital artery look for greater occipital nerve (dorsal ramus of C2 nerve).

- Lastly identify the muscles forming the floor of the triangle (Fig. 47.2b). These are:
    i. Scalenus medius in the lower part
   ii. Levator scapulae in middle part
  iii. Splenius capitis in upper part

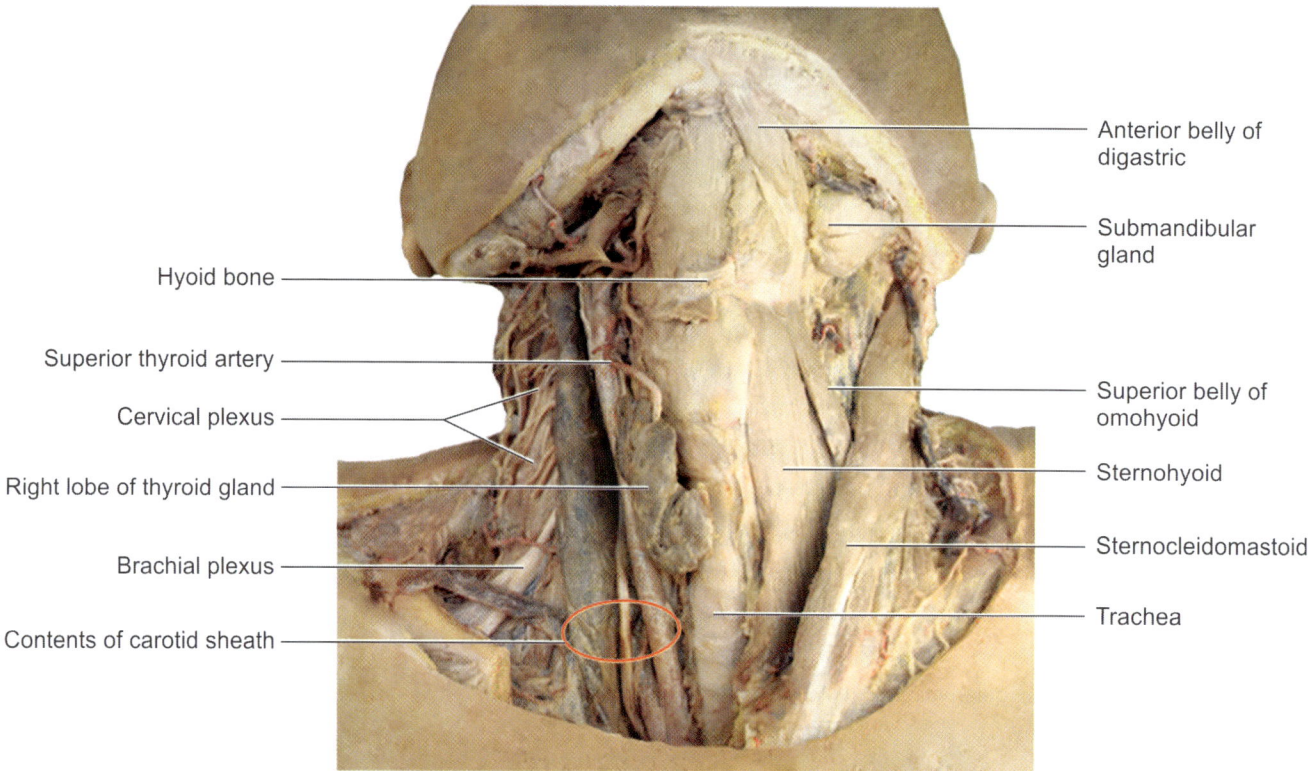

Hyoid bone

Superior thyroid artery

Cervical plexus

Right lobe of thyroid gland

Brachial plexus

Contents of carotid sheath

Anterior belly of digastric

Submandibular gland

Superior belly of omohyoid

Sternohyoid

Sternocleidomastoid

Trachea

Fig. 47.3: Parts of brachial plexus in posterior triangle. Structures in median region of neck also seen

- See that this muscular floor is covered by the prevertebral fascia which extends into the axilla to form the axillary sheath.
- Identify again the big muscle—the sternocleido-mastiod, arising from manubrium sterni and clavicle. See it extending upwards and laterally to the lateral surface of the mastoid process and lateral half of superior nuchal line (Fig. 47.3).
- Appreciate that SCM is a landmark in the neck and it divides the neck into an anterior and a posterior triangle.

- Identify:
  - i. Bones and joints, i.e. mastoid process and sternoclavicular joint
  - ii. Carotid sheath
  - iii. Many muscles, arteries, veins, nerves and lymph nodes beneath this important muscle.
- One important muscle is the serrated scalenus anterior muscle covered by prevertebral fascia. Locate the phrenic nerve between the scalenus anterior muscle and the fascia.

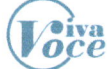

- Enumerate the contents of suprasternal space.
- What is the function of ligament of Berry.
- Name the contents of carotid sheath.
- Which layer of cervical fascia forms the axillary sheath?

- What are the boundaries of posterior triangle of neck?
- Which are the muscles supplied by spinal root of XI nerve?
- Name the arteries supplying the sternocleidomastoid muscle.

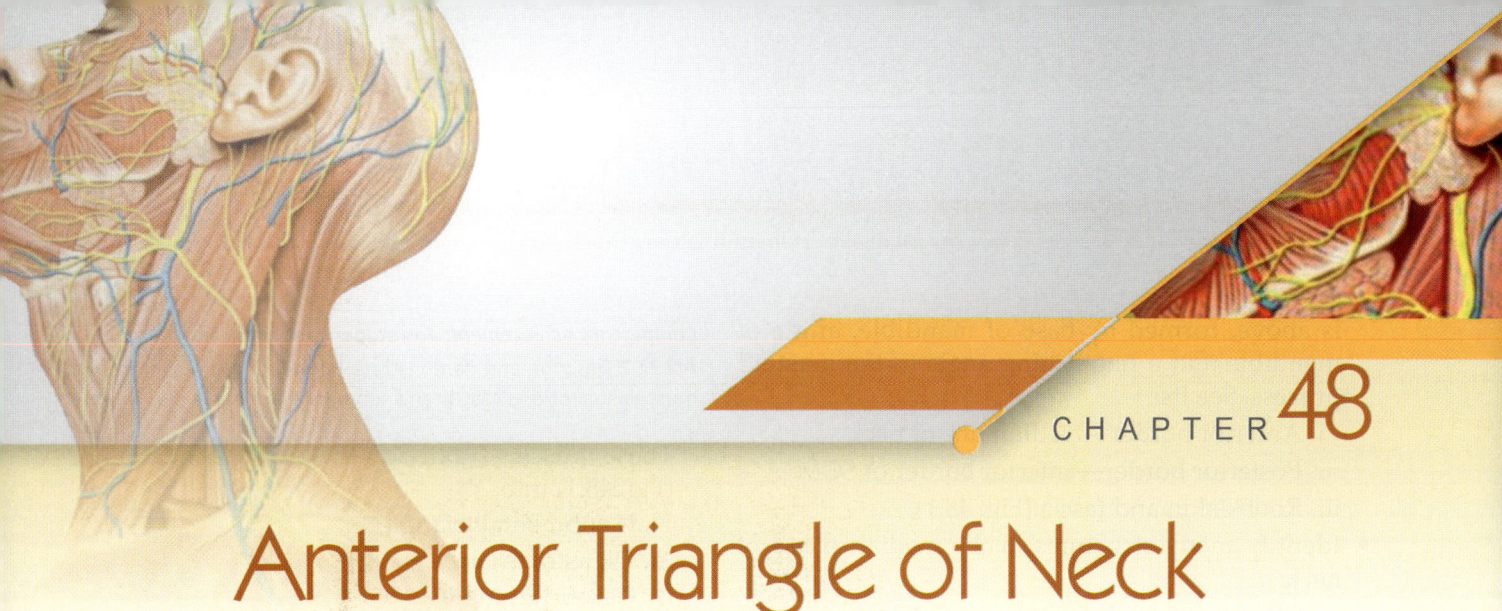

Anterior Triangle of Neck

OVERVIEW

Structures in the median line of neck: These are chin, raphe of mylohyoid muscle, hyoid bone, thyrohyoid membrane, cricothyroid membrane, rings of trachea and thyroid gland.

Boundaries of Anterior Triangle

Anteriorly by anterior median line and laterally by obliquely placed SCM muscle. Its apex is below. The upper border is formed by base of mandible and line joining the angle of mandible to the mastoid process.

Each of the anterior triangles is subdivided by the digastric muscles and superior belly of omohyoid into following smaller triangles. These are half submental triangle between anterior belly of digastric, median plane and the chin. Whole submental triangle is between both the anterior bellies of digastric muscles.

Digastric triangle lies between posterior and anterior bellies of digastric muscles.

Carotid triangle lies between anterior border of SCM, posterior belly of digastric and superior belly of omohyoid muscles.

Muscular triangle lies between anterior median line, anterior border of SCM and superior belly of omohyoid muscles.

Contents of the Triangles

Submental triangle contains submental lymph nodes.

Digastric triangle contains superficial part of submandibular gland. Carotid triangle contains common carotid, internal carotid and external carotid arteries with some of its branches; internal jugular vein, cranial nerves parts of IX, X, XI, XII, deep cervical lymph nodes.

Muscular triangle contains only muscles two superficial and two deep muscles.

Competency achievement: The student should be able to:

AN 32.1 Describe boundaries and subdivisions of anterior triangle.

ANTERIOR TRIANGLE

Steps of Dissection

• The anterior triangle of neck lies between median plane of neck and anterior border of SCM. Its base is above, formed by base of mandible, angle of mandible and a line joining angle to the mastoid process. See its:

   i. Anterior border—median line of neck
  ii. Posterior border—anterior border of SCM
 iii. Roof—skin and fascia (Fig. 48.1)

- Identify many structures in the median plane of neck:

   i. Chin/symphysis menti
  ii. Both mylohyoid muscles and the raphe of their insertion
 iii. Hyoid bone with many muscles attached to it (*see* Fig. 47.3)
 iv. Thyrohyoid membrane pierced by internal laryngeal nerve and superior laryngeal vessels
  v. Cricothyroid muscles
 vi. Cricotracheal membrane
 vii. Rings of trachea covered by thyroid gland

- In the anterior triangle there are anterior and posterior bellies of digastric muscles in upper part.
- Identify superior belly of omohyoid in lower part of triangle (*see* Fig. 47.3).

Competency achievement: The student should be able to:
AN 32.2 Describe and demonstrate boundaries and contents of muscular, carotid, digastric and submental triangles.

These muscles subdivide the big anterior triangle (Fig. 48.1) into:

   i. ½ submental triangle
  ii. Digastric triangle
 iii. Carotid triangle
 iv. Muscular triangle

- Look at the neck from front and see the boundaries of submental triangle. Appreciate that there is one submental triangle in the neck (half on each side). Dissect its boundaries and contents:

   i. Anterior bellies of digastric muscle
  ii. Body of hyoid bone (*see* Fig. 47.3)
 iii. Floor by mylohyoid muscles

- See the contents. These are a few submental lymph nodes and submental veins which join to form anterior jugular vein.
- Identify the digastric triangle (Fig. 48.2). This triangle is present on each side of the neck. Its boundaries are:

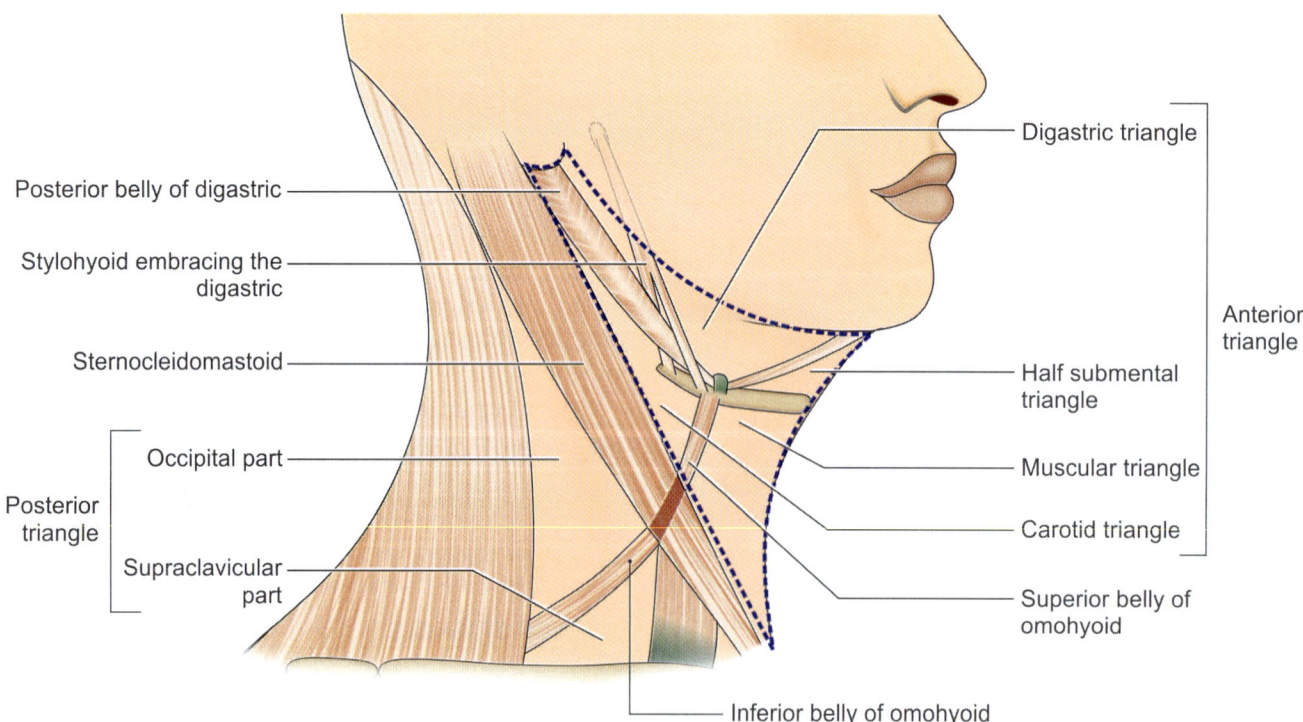

Fig. 48.1: Subdivisions of anterior and posterior triangles of neck

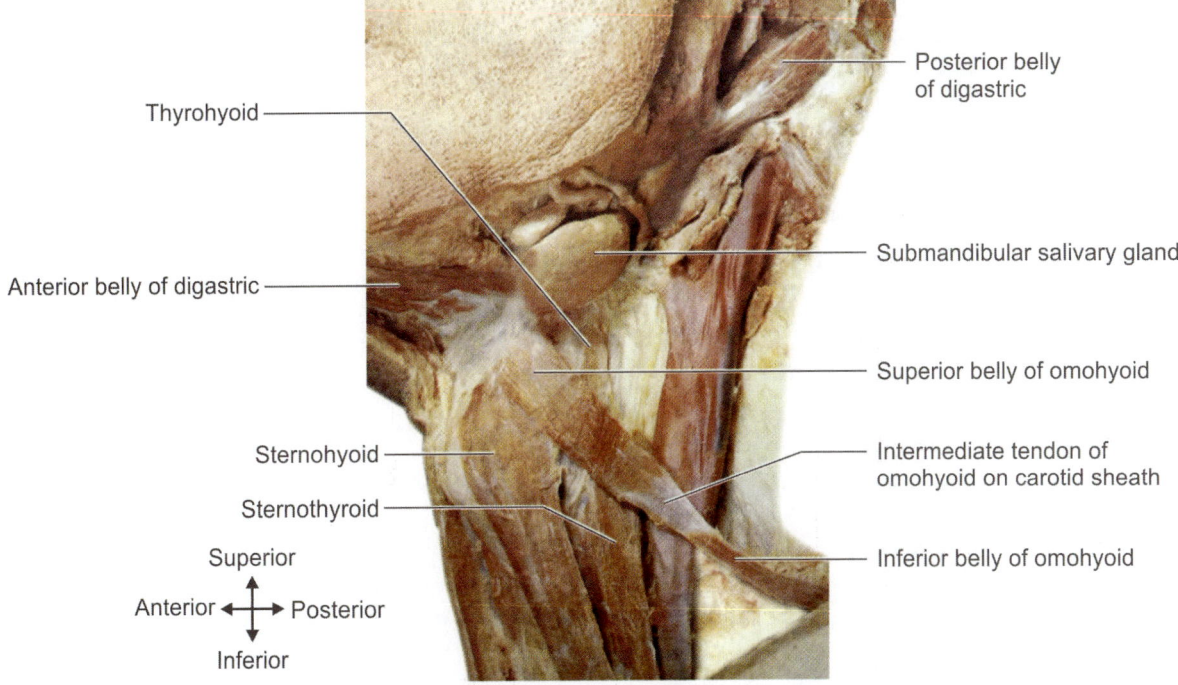

Thyrohyoid

Anterior belly of digastric

Posterior belly of digastric

Submandibular salivary gland

Superior belly of omohyoid

Intermediate tendon of omohyoid on carotid sheath

Sternohyoid

Sternothyroid

Inferior belly of omohyoid

Superior

Anterior ← → Posterior

Inferior

Fig. 48.2: Boundaries and contents of digastric and muscular triangles

i. Anterior belly of digastric muscle

ii. Posterior belly of digastric supplemented above by stylohyoid muscle

iii. Inferior border/base of mandible

- See that the two bellies are joined by an intermediate tendon attached to hyoid bone. This is the apex of the triangle. The base is the lower border of mandible and a line joining angle of mandible to mastoid process.

- The floor is formed by mylohyoid and hyoglossus muscles

- Identify some of the contents:

  i. Submandibular salivary gland (Fig. 48.2)

  ii. Submandibular lymph nodes

  iii. Nerve to mylohyoid

  iv. Submental artery

  v. Part of parotid gland

  vi. Distal part of external carotid artery before entering the parotid gland

  vii. IX cranial nerve

  viii. Pharyngeal branch of X cranial nerve

  ix. Styloid process with its attached structures

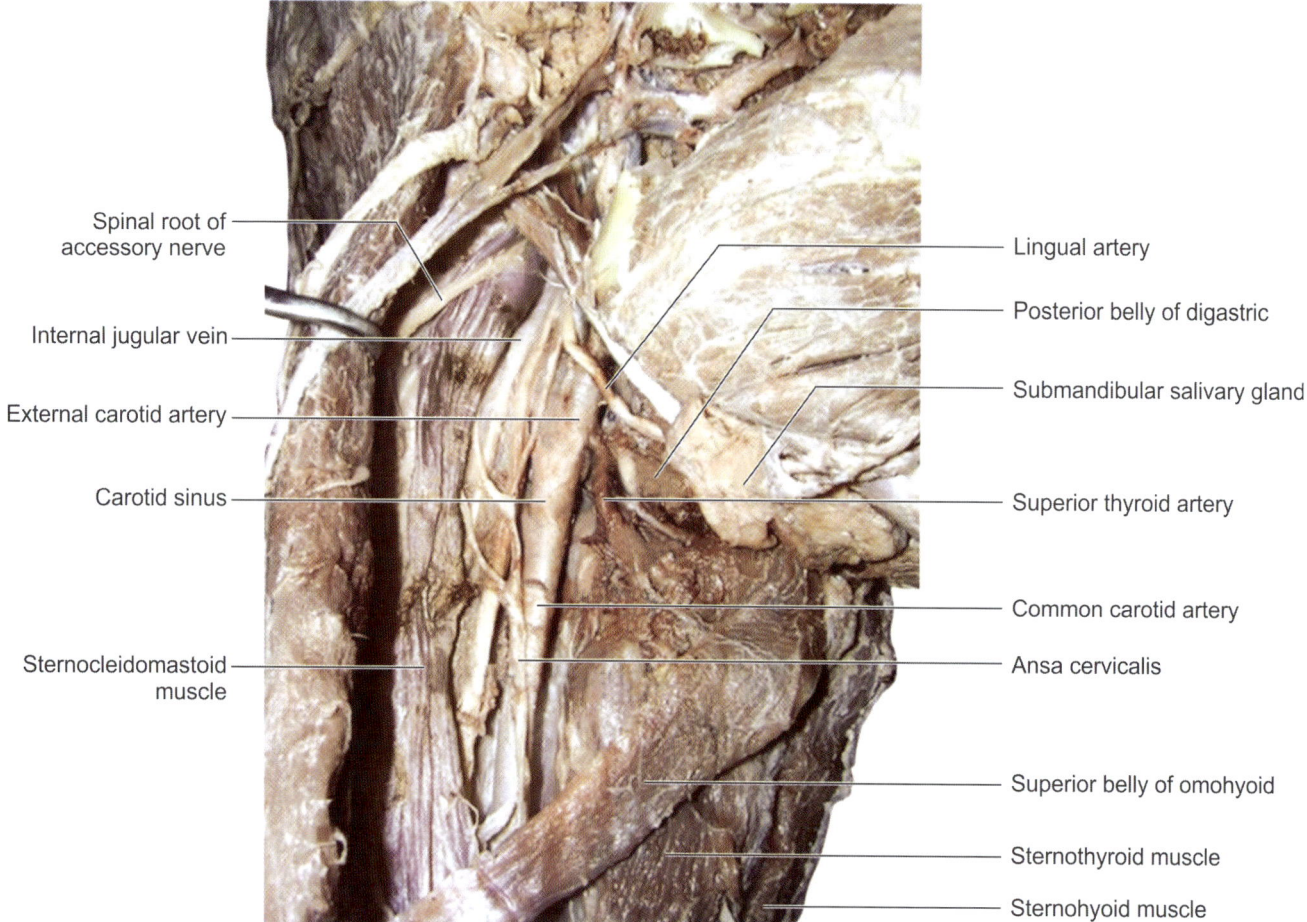

Spinal root of
accessory nerve

Internal jugular vein

External carotid artery

Carotid sinus

Sternocleidomastoid
muscle

Lingual artery

Posterior belly of digastric

Submandibular salivary gland

Superior thyroid artery

Common carotid artery

Ansa cervicalis

Superior belly of omohyoid

Sternothyroid muscle

Sternohyoid muscle

Fig. 48.3: Boundaries and some contents of carotid triangle

CAROTID TRIANGLE

• Clean the area between posterior belly of digastric muscle (bipennate); superior belly of omohyoid and anterior border of SCM muscle. This is carotid triangle (Fig. 48.3). Locate and identify three carotid arteries, i.e. common carotid and its two branches,

the internal carotid and external carotid, with laterally placed internal jugular vein (Fig. 48.4).

• Trace IX, X, XI and XII cranial nerves in relation internal carotid artery and internal jugular vein.

• IX nerve traverses between internal and external carotid arteries to reach submandibular region.

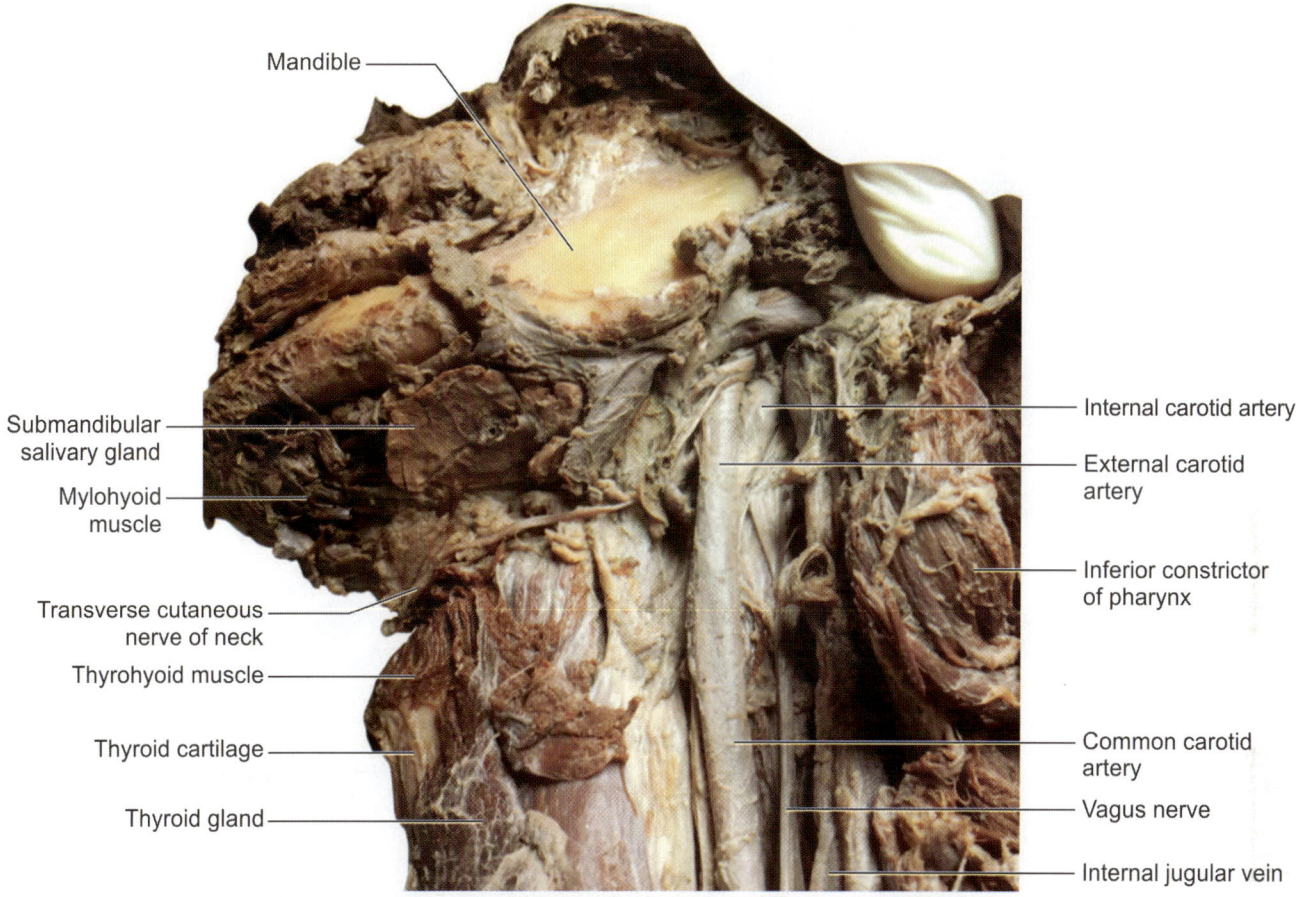

Mandible

Submandibular salivary gland

Mylohyoid muscle

Transverse cutaneous nerve of neck

Thyrohyoid muscle

Thyroid cartilage

Thyroid gland

Internal carotid artery

External carotid artery

Inferior constrictor of pharynx

Common carotid artery

Vagus nerve

Internal jugular vein

Fig. 48.4: Common carotid artery and its two branches

- X nerve courses between internal jugular vein and internal carotid artery (Fig. 48.5).
- Spinal root of XI crosses laterally over the internal jugular vein to reach SCM muscle (Fig. 48.3).
- XII nerve passes medially superficial to both internal and external carotid arteries (Fig. 48.3), then it crosses the loop of lingual artery to reach submandibular region for supplying 7/8 muscles of tongue.

- Identify branches of external carotid given off in the carotid triangle. Remember that internal carotid artery gives no branches in its cervical course.
- Clean the branches of external carotid artery. These are:
1. Superior thyroid for the thyroid gland (*see* Fig. 47.3). See this artery accompanying the external laryngeal branch of superior laryngeal of vagus till close to the apex of thyroid gland. At that point the nerve deviates medially to

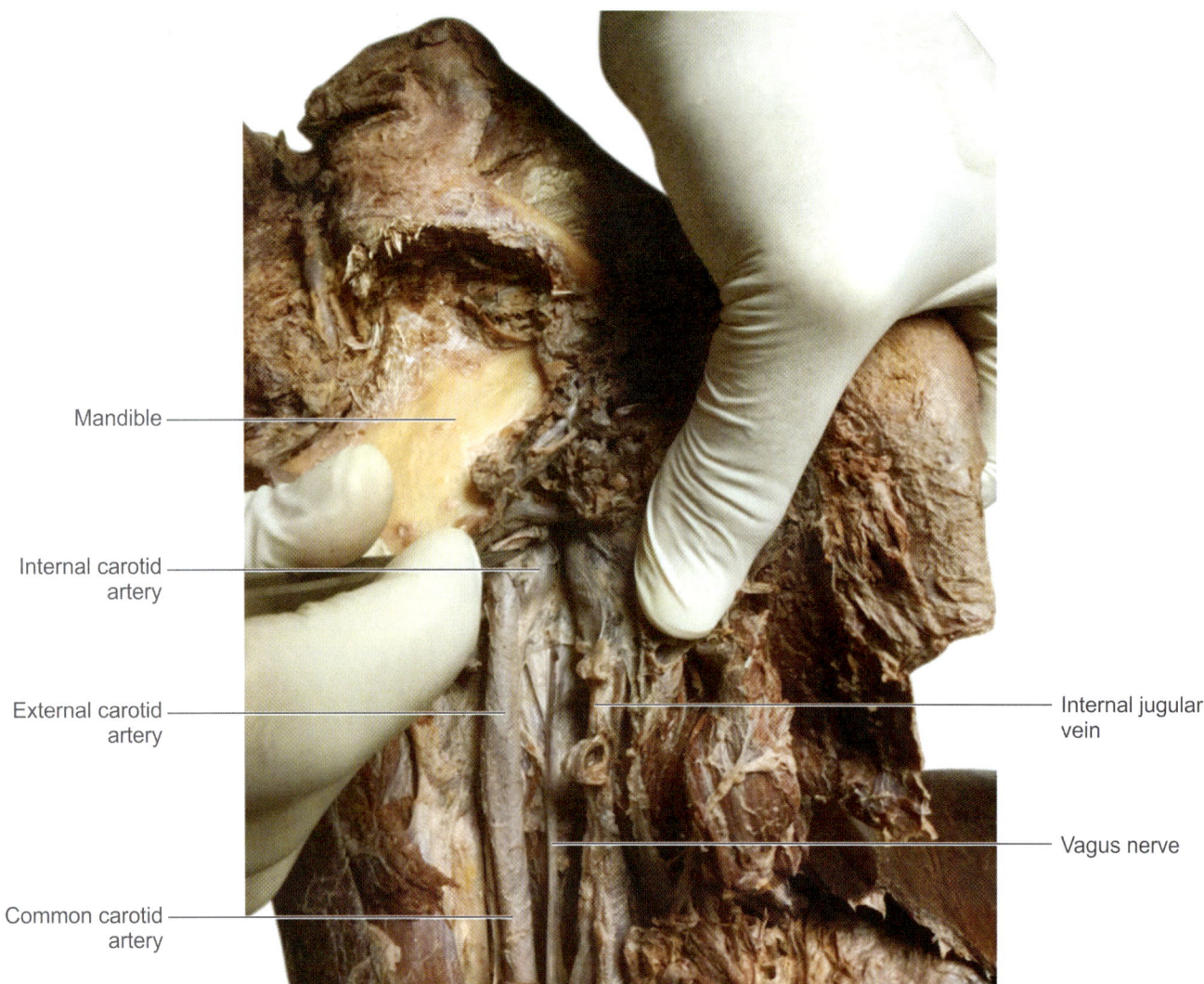

Mandible

Internal carotid artery

External carotid artery

Internal jugular vein

Vagus nerve

Common carotid artery

Fig. 48.5: Vagus nerve as a content of carotid triangle

innervate cricothyroid muscle and the artery reaches the thyroid gland.

2. Lingual is the next big tortuous branch (Fig. 48.6). It shows a loop at the beginning which is crossed by XII nerve. The artery reaches the sub-mandibular region and is the main supply of the muscles and mucous membrane of the tongue.

3. Third branch is again the tortuous facial artery (Fig. 48.7). It ascends along the pharynx in the cervical part to reach posterior end of submandibular salivary gland. It makes an 'S' shaped bend. Then it lies at the anteroinferior angle of masseter muscle to enter the face. It is palpable at this point.

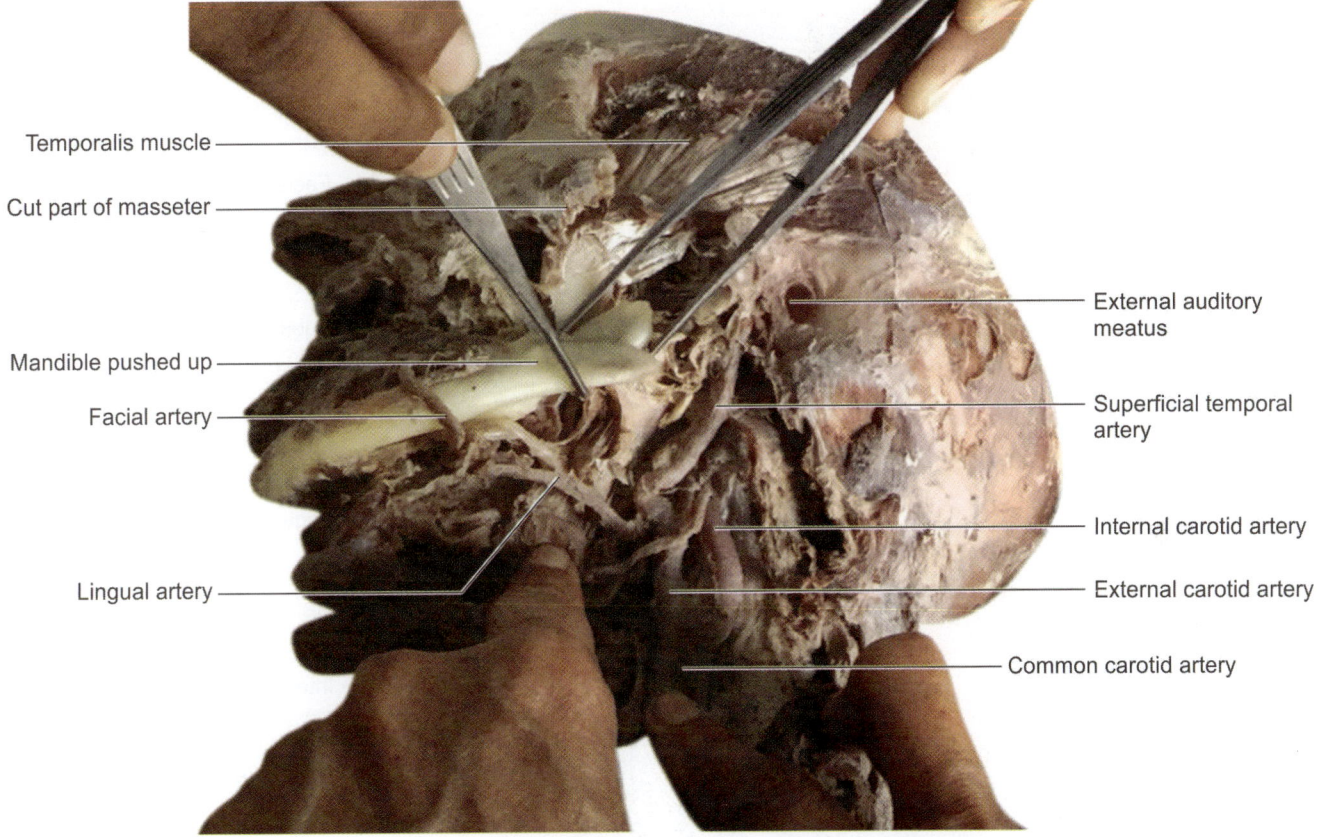

Temporalis muscle

Cut part of masseter

Mandible pushed up

Facial artery

Lingual artery

External auditory meatus

Superficial temporal artery

Internal carotid artery

External carotid artery

Common carotid artery

Fig. 48.6: Lingual branch of external carotid artery

4. Identify a small branch—ascending pharyngeal artery from medial aspect of external carotid artery. It gives branches to pharynx and palatine tonsil.

5. See its last branch given off in the carotid triangle. This is the occipital artery lying along lower border of bipennate posterior belly of digastric muscle (*see* Fig. 47.2b).

Veins accompanying most of these arteries end up in internal jugular vein (Figs 48.3 and 48.5).

- Identify a dilatation at terminal part of common carotid artery or beginning of internal carotid artery. This is the carotid sinus (Fig. 48.3). It acts as a baroreceptor for regulation of blood pressure.
- Locate a small brown body (2–5 mm) behind bifurcation of common carotid artery. This body is the carotid body. It acts as chemoreceptor for regulation of respiration.

- Identify the superior root of ansa (loop) cervicalis from C1 nerve joining inferior root of ansa cervicalis from C2 and C3 nerves to form a loop of ansa cervicalis (Fig. 48.3). Branches from these nerves supply the infrahyoid muscles of the muscular triangle.
- Posterior to carotid sheath identify the sympathetic trunk.

MUSCULAR TRIANGLE

- Cut through the origin of SCM muscle and reflect it upwards.
- Identify infrahyoid muscles. These are:
  i. Sternohyoid and superior belly of omohyoid forming the superficial layer (Fig. 48.2)
  ii. Sternothyroid and thyrohyoid forming the deep layer (Fig. 48.2).

These muscles are supplied by branches of superior root, inferior root of ansa cervicalis or by ansa itself.

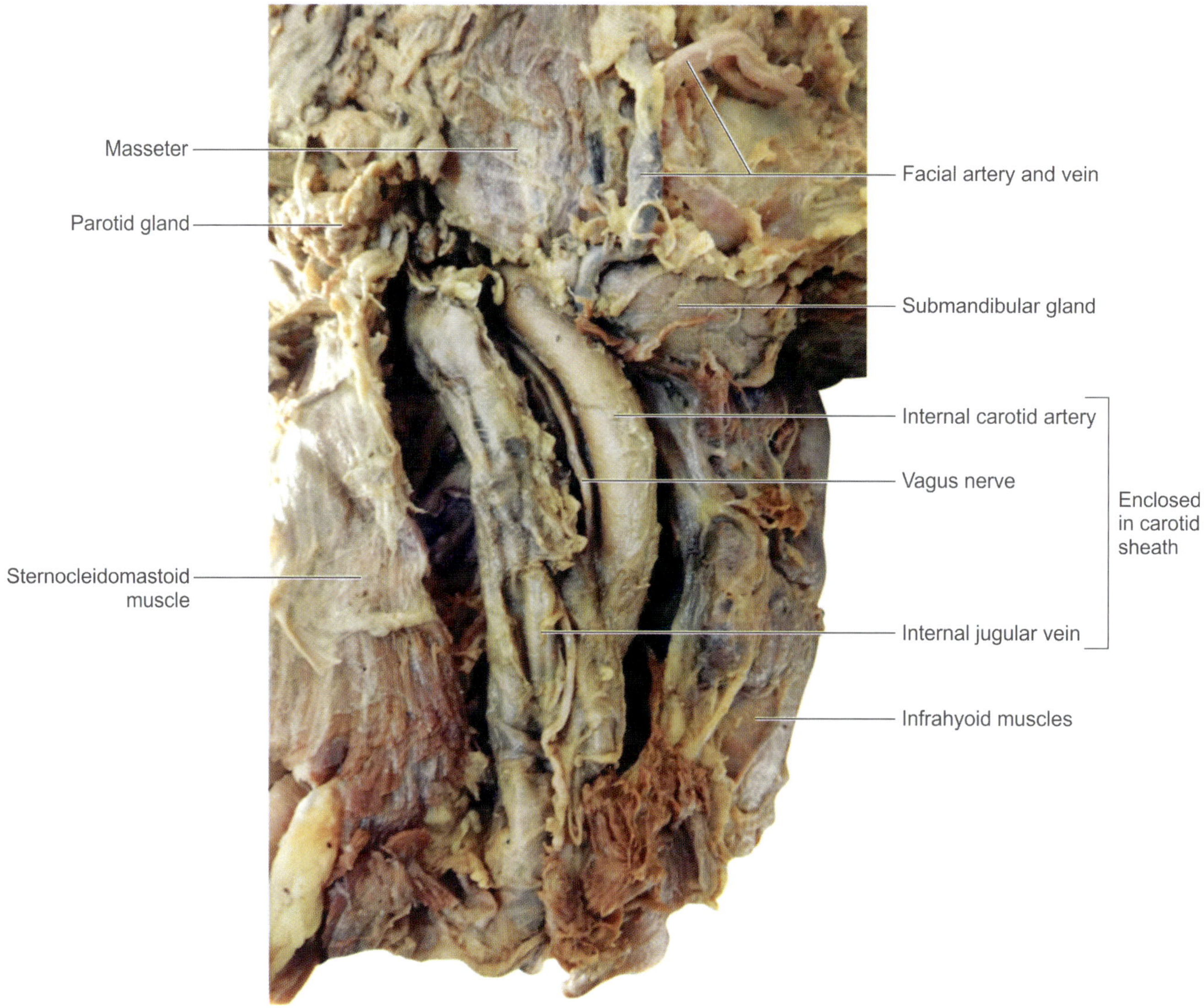

Masseter —

Parotid gland —

Facial artery and vein

Submandibular gland

Internal carotid artery

Vagus nerve

Enclosed in carotid sheath

Sternocleidomastoid muscle

Internal jugular vein

Infrahyoid muscles

Fig. 48.7: Carotid sheath as a content of carotid triangle

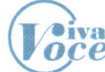

- Enumerate the boundaries of carotid triangle. Name the structures piercing the thyrohyoid membrane.
- Name the branches of external carotid artery given off in the carotid triangle.
- How is ansa cervicalis formed? What are its branches?
- Name the main contents of digastric triangle. How does hyoid bone develop?

Parotid Region

OVERVIEW

The parotid region contains the largest salivary gland, the parotid gland. It is enclosed by the investing layer of superficial fascia. Area of skin over parotid gland is supplied by ventral ramus of C2 nerve.

Parotid gland is comprised of base above, apex below, anterior and posterior borders and a medial border on its deeper surface. Many structures emerge from its borders and some are lying in its substance.

Secretomotor fibres reach from a branch of glossopharyngeal nerve. Parotid duct starts from its substance and leaves the gland at its anterior border. It passes forwards on the cheek and opens into vestibule of mouth opposite 2nd upper molar tooth.

Parotid gland is a purely serous gland with many small ducts and connective tissue.

> *Competency achievement:* The student should be able to:
> **AN 28.9** Describe and demonstrate the parts, borders, surfaces, contents, relations and nerve supply of parotid gland with course of its duct and surgical importance.

STEPS OF DISSECTION

- Remove the fascial covering of the parotid gland, formed by the cervical fascia. Remember that the skin overlying parotid gland is innervated by great auricular nerve (C2).

  The parotid gland comprises a concave base above, a narrow apex below and an anterior border with emerging parotid duct (Fig. 49.1).

- See that anteromedial surface is related to ramus of mandible with masseter and medial pterygoid muscles.

- Look that the posteromedial surface is related to mastoid process with SCM and posterior belly of digastric muscle and styloid process and structures attached to it.

  There are number of structures entering and leaving surfaces and borders of the gland. These will be dissected and identified.

- Identify the structures lying at the base of the gland. These are auriculotemporal nerve and superficial temporal vessels. This nerve carries secretomotor fibres from IX nerve to parotid gland.

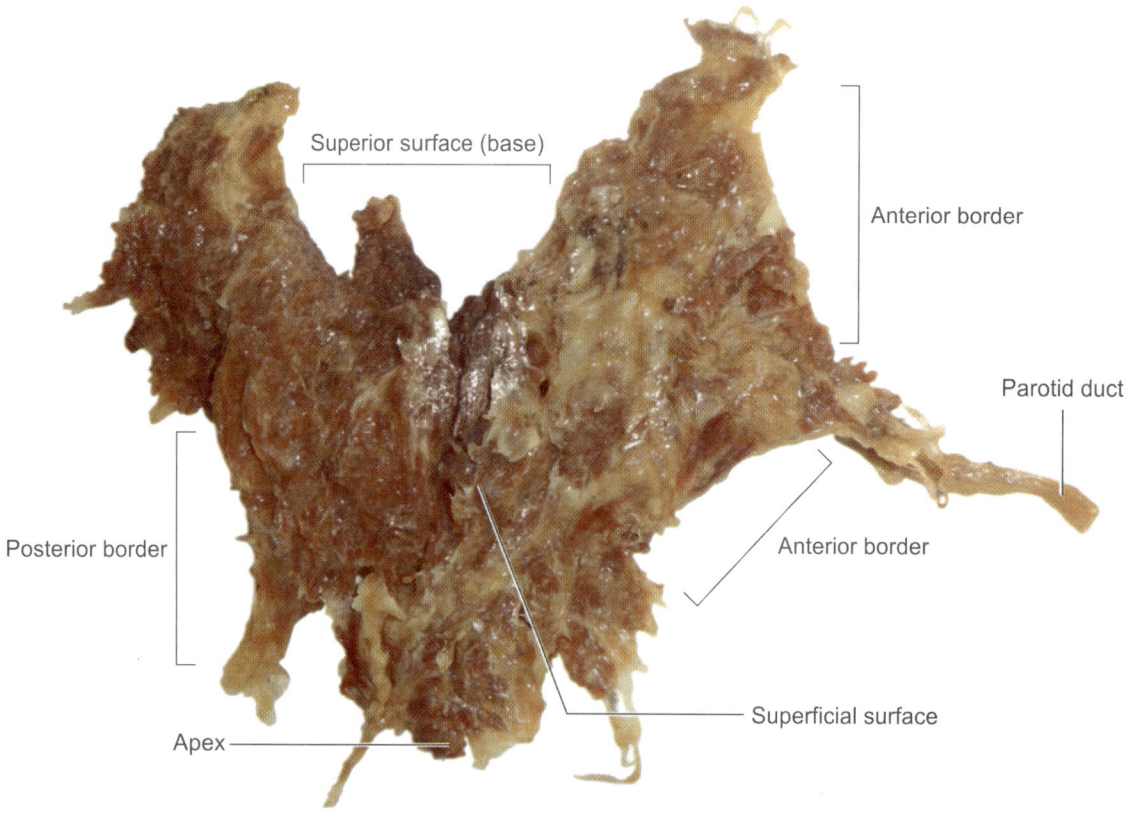

Fig. 49.1: Gross features of parotid gland with parotid duct emerging from its anterior border

- Clean the structures present at the anterior border. These are transverse facial artery and parotid duct and branches of facial nerve, i.e. temporal, zygomatic, buccal and marginal mandibular (Fig. 49.2a and b). See the lowest branch, the cervical branch, exists from the apex of the gland.
- In addition to cervical branch, the anterior and posterior divisions of retromandibular vein also exit from apical region of the gland.
- From its short posterior border identify posterior auricular nerve and posterior auricular vessels.
- Trace zygomatic branch of facial nerve inside the gland to reach the trunk of nerve. The trunk can be followed till the stylomastoid foramen. The trunk may be seen to divide into two branches, temporofacial and cervicofacial (Fig. 49.2b).
- Trace the course of retromandibular vein (*see* Fig. 46.8). See its formation by union of maxillary and superficial temporal veins. It runs downwards in the substance of parotid gland and divides into anterior and posterior divisions

- See the anterior division joining the facial vein to form common facial vein draining into internal jugular vein.
- Trace the posterior division of retromandibular vein joining posterior auricular vein to form external jugular vein.
- Follow the external carotid artery along the posterior border of ramus of mandible to enter parotid gland (Fig. 49.3). Here it is seen to divide into larger maxillary artery and palpable superficial temporal artery.
- Identify some of the parotid lymph nodes in the fascia and in the substance of the gland. These drain the middle ear, upper part of cheek, side of scalp, temple, etc.
- The parotid duct (Stenson's duct) leaves from the middle of anterior border of the gland (Fig. 49.1), runs forwards on the masseter muscle, pierces few structures. See its opening into vestibule of mouth opposite 2nd upper molar tooth.

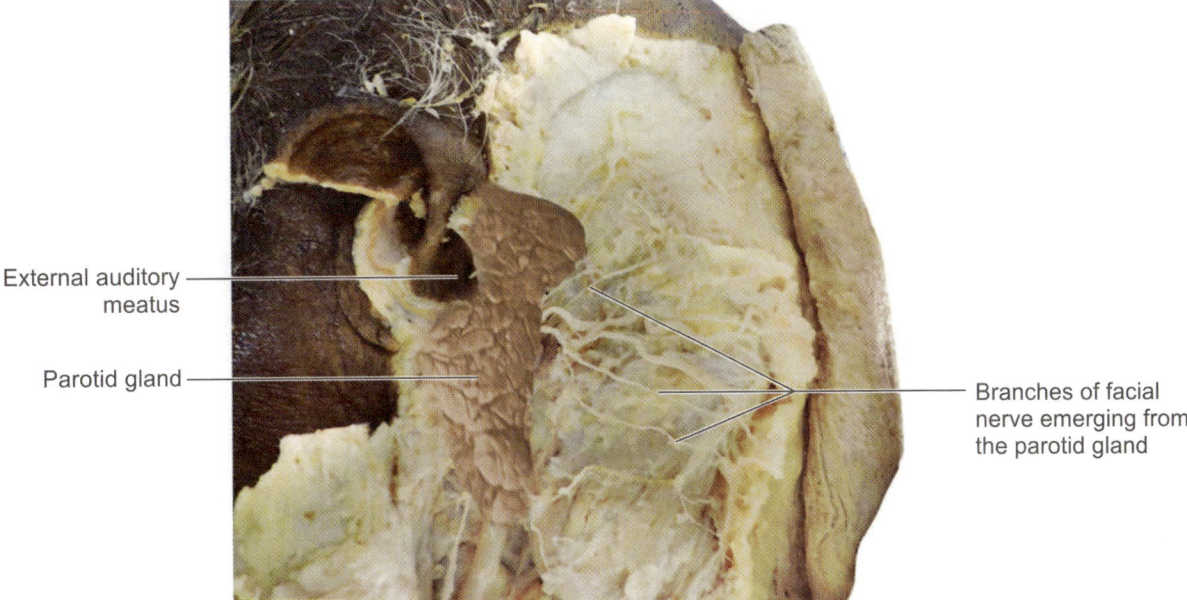

External auditory meatus

Parotid gland

Branches of facial nerve emerging from the parotid gland

Fig. 49.2a: Parotid gland with branches of facial nerve emerging from its anterior border

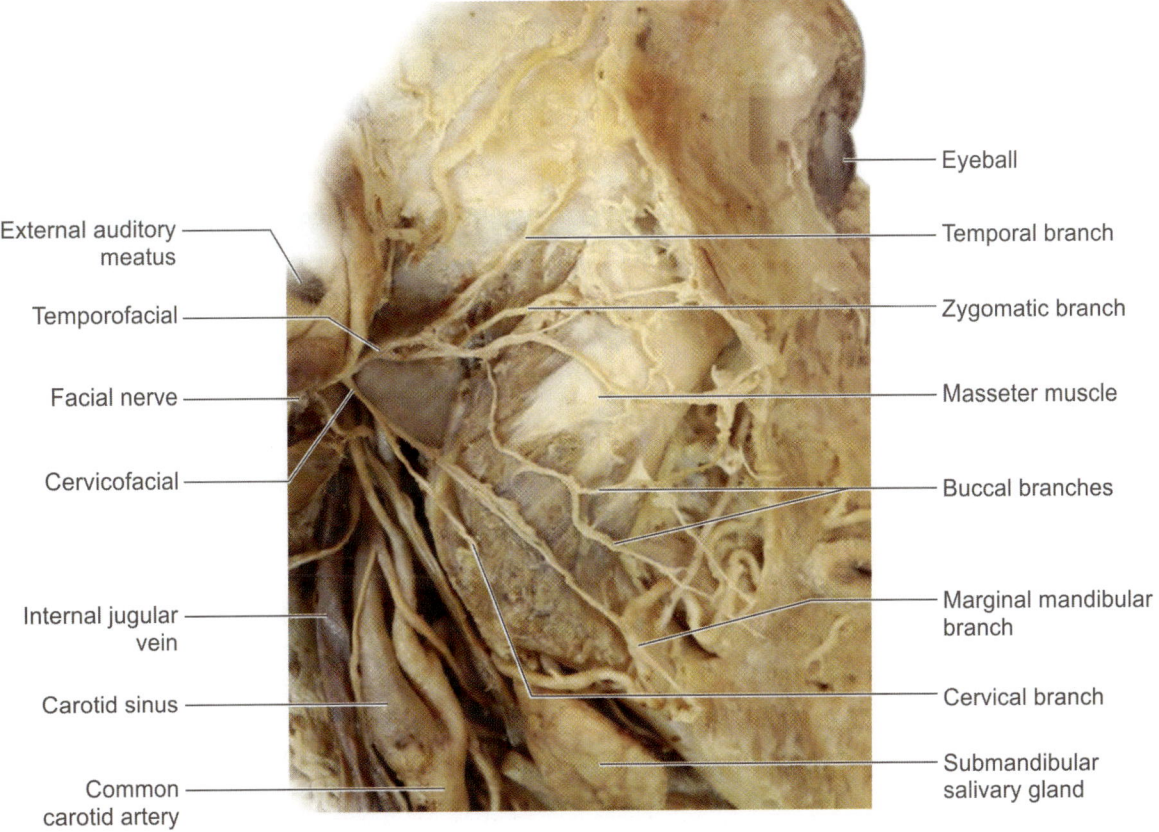

External auditory meatus

Temporofacial

Facial nerve

Cervicofacial

Internal jugular vein

Carotid sinus

Common carotid artery

Eyeball

Temporal branch

Zygomatic branch

Masseter muscle

Buccal branches

Marginal mandibular branch

Cervical branch

Submandibular salivary gland

Fig. 49.2b: Facial nerve dissected within parotid gland

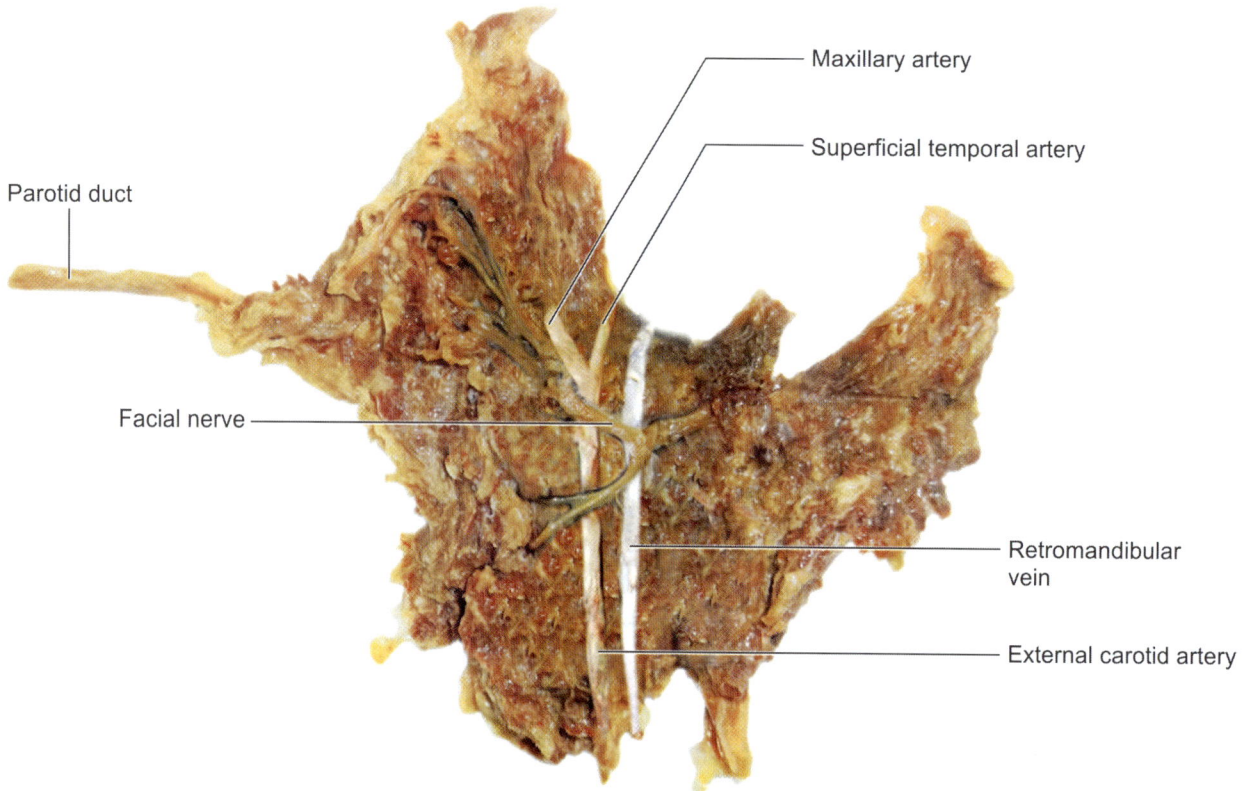

Parotid duct

Facial nerve

Maxillary artery

Superficial temporal artery

Retromandibular vein

External carotid artery

Fig. 49.3: Structures on the deep aspect of parotid gland

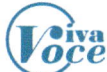

- Enumerate the structures emerging from the anterior border of parotid gland.
- What structures lie within the parotid gland?

- Trace the secretomotor nerve supply of the parotid gland.
- What is Hilton's method of drainage of parotid abscess?

CHAPTER 50

Temporal and Infratemporal Fossae

Learning Objectives

One should be able to

1. Revise the attachments and actions of muscles of mastication
2. Enumerate the branches of 3 parts of maxillary artery
3. Recapitulate relations of TMJ.
4. Enumerate roots and branches of otic ganglion

OVERVIEW

Temporal and infratemporal fossae contain the muscles of mastication, temporomandibular joint (TMJ), maxillary artery, and mandibular nerve with otic ganglion.

Muscles of mastication are temporalis, masseter, lateral pterygoid and medial pterygoid. These muscles cause various movements at TMJ and help in opening, closing, protraction, retraction and side to side movements of lower jaw. Lateral pterygoid is the only muscle out of these four muscles which lowers or depresses the jaw; other three are elevators of jaw and thus are antigravity muscles.

TMJ is a synovial joint of condylar variety. Movements at both TMJ mostly occur simultaneously. The articular ends are lined/covered by fibrocartilage. The interior of the joint contains an intra-articular disc which is also fibrocartilaginous in nature.

The disc divides the single joint cavity into two cavities so that diverse movements can take place in each of the two cavities. The joint permits elevation, depression, protraction, retraction and side to side movements. TMJ is closely related to branches of facial nerve and auriculotemporal nerve.

Maxillary artery is the larger terminal branch of external carotid artery. This artery gives branches which supply upper eight and lower eight teeth of one side of the face. Besides it gives branches which supply meninges, muscles of mastication, hard and soft palates, pharynx and septum of nose. Two of its branches are clinically important. These are middle meningeal artery, its rupture causes extradural hemorrhage and the other one is the terminal branch-sphenopalatine artery which is the artery of epistaxis (bleeding from nose).

Mandibular nerve is a mixed nerve. It is the largest branch of trigeminal nerve and is related to two parasympathetic ganglia, e.g. otic and submandibular ganglia. This nerve innervates four muscles of mastication and four other small muscles.

Its trunk leaves the skull through foramen ovale. There are two branches from trunk. The trunk divides into small anterior and large posterior divisions. Anterior division supplies three muscles of mastication and gives a sensory buccal branch.

Posterior division gives auriculotemporal nerve which arises by two roots. Then it divides into a lingual branch which proceeds towards the tongue and inferior alveolar for supplying lower eight teeth. The submandibular ganglion is suspended from the lingual nerve. This nerve gives a branch—the nerve to mylohyoid for innervating mylohyoid muscle and the anterior belly of digastric muscle.

Otic ganglion is related to nerve of medial pterygoid, a branch of trunk of V3 nerve. Topographically it is related to V3, but functionally it is related to IX nerve. Lesser petrosal nerve, branch of IX nerve, relays in otic ganglion. Postganglionic fibres reach auriculotemporal nerve which supplies parotid gland. Sympathetic fibres are from sympathetic plexus around middle meningeal artery. This ganglion has four roots and gives branches to two muscles and parotid gland.

> Competency achievement: The student should be able to:
> AN 33.1 Describe and demonstrate extent, boundaries and contents of temporal and infratemporal fossae.
> AN 33.2 Describe and demonstrate attachments, direction of fibres, nerve supply and actions of muscles of mastication.

Steps of Dissection

- Identify temporalis muscle on the lateral side of skull till coronoid process of mandible (Fig. 50.1).
- Identify masseter muscle extending from the zygomatic arch above to the ramus of mandible below (see Fig 46.7a). Cut the zygomatic arch in front of and behind the attachment of masseter muscle and reflect it downwards.
- Identify the nerve to masseter from anterior branch of mandibular nerve. Look for its arterial supply. Cut these structures. Clean the ramus of mandible by stripping off the masseter muscle from it.
- Give an oblique cut from the centre of mandibular notch to lower end of anterior border of ramus of mandible. Turn this part of the bone including insertion of temporalis upwards. Strip the muscle from the skull. Identify two deep temporal nerves arising from mandibular nerve and deep temporal artery arising from maxillary artery.
- Make one cut through the neck of mandible. Give another cut through the ramus at a distance of 4 cm from the neck.
- Remove the bone carefully in between these two cuts, avoiding injury to the underlying structures.
- The lateral pterygoid is exposed in the upper part while medial pterygoid is exposed in the lower part

of dissection (Fig. 50.2). Learn the attachments and actions of these muscles from BD Chaurasia's *Human Anatomy*.

- The lateral pterygoid muscle is the key of this region. Identify its relations:
  Superficial: Masseter, ramus of mandible, temporalis and 2nd part of maxillary artery.
  Deep: Mandibular nerve, middle meningeal artery and deep head of medial pterygoid
- Identify branches of mandibular nerve emerging at upper and lower borders of lateral pterygoid muscle.
- At upper border: Deep temporal nerves (Fig. 50.2) and masseteric nerve.
- At lower border: Lingual and inferior alveolar nerves.
- Coursing between the two heads of lateral pterygoid are the buccal branch of mandibular nerve and 3rd part of maxillary artery.

Maxillary Artery

- Identify external carotid artery that runs along the posterior border of ramus of mandible, then on the anteromedial surface of the parotid gland. There it divides into a smaller superficial temporal and a larger maxillary artery (Fig. 50.2).
- Trace the maxillary artery running along the inferior border of lower head of lateral pterygoid as its 1st part; then on the surface of its lower head as its 2nd part and finally between the two heads of this muscle as its 3rd part.
- Identify the important branches of its three parts:
  i. The middle meningeal artery coursing deep to the lateral pterygoid, then emerging at its upper border. It finally leaves the neck region by passing through foramen spinosum of middle cranial fossa.
  ii. Inferior alveolar artery runs medial to ramus of mandible to enter mandibular foramen and mandibular canal. Identify its mylohyoid branch as well as muscular branches. These are masseteric, anterior and posterior temporal arteries and pterygoid branches. Its last branch is buccal branch for the skin of cheek.
  iii. Posterior superior alveolar artery for molar teeth and maxillary air sinus.
  iv. Infraorbital artery for other five upper teeth, lacrimal sac, nose and upper lip.

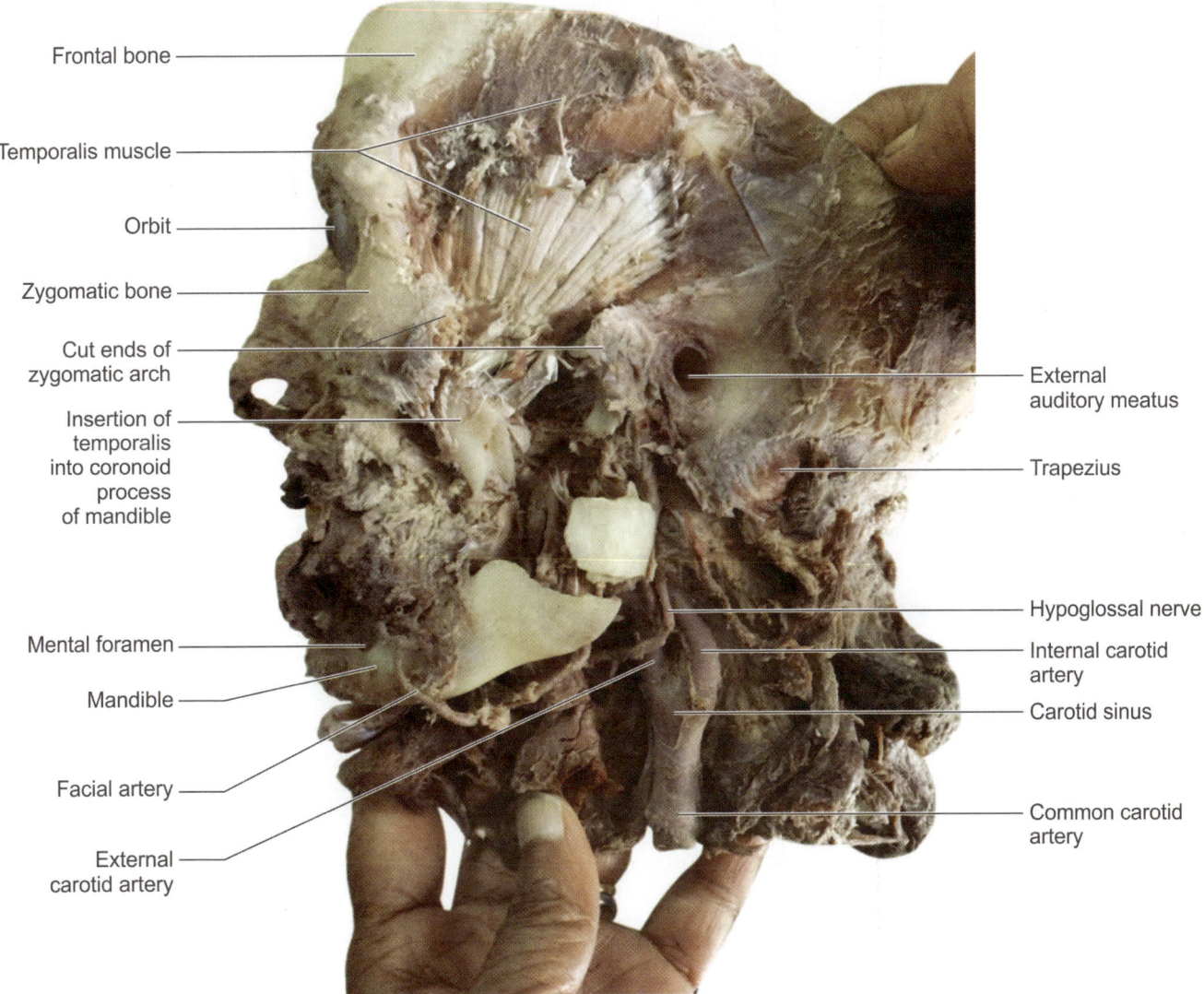

Fig. 50.1: Temporalis muscle

v. Other branches are greater palatine, lesser palatine, pharyngeal branch, artery to pterygoid canal.

vi. The terminal branch is sphenopalatine artery which lies in the nasal cavity. This artery will be seen in the chapter on nose and paranasal sinuses. It is clinically known as artery of "epistaxis".

Competency achievement: The student should be able to:

AN 33.4 Explain the clinical significance of pterygoid venous plexus.

Pterygoid Venous Plexus

The pterygoid venous plexus is around and within lateral pterygoid muscle. This plexus is drained by maxillary vein which unites with superficial temporal vein to form retromandibular vein. The plexus communicates with facial vein via deep facial vein and with cavernous sinus via an emissary vein. Infection from face can travel to cavernous sinus via this pathway.

Competency achievement: The student should be able to:

AN 33.3 Describe and demonstrate articulating surface, type and movements of temporomandibular joint.

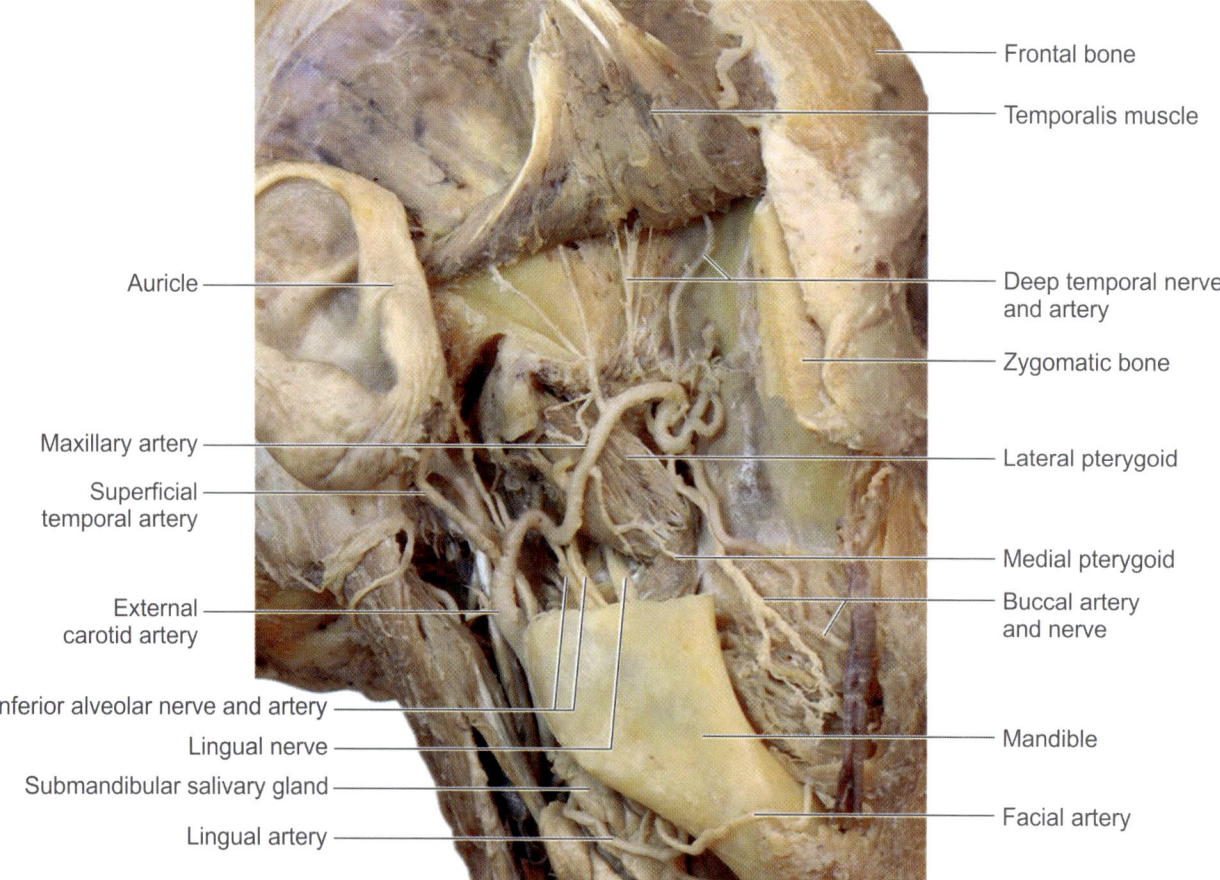

Auricle

Maxillary artery

Superficial
temporal artery

External
carotid artery

Inferior alveolar nerve and artery

Lingual nerve

Submandibular salivary gland

Lingual artery

Frontal bone

Temporalis muscle

Deep temporal nerve
and artery

Zygomatic bone

Lateral pterygoid

Medial pterygoid

Buccal artery
and nerve

Mandible

Facial artery

Fig. 50.2: Branches of maxillary artery with some branches of mandibular nerve

TEMPOROMANDIBULAR JOINT (TMJ)

Steps of Dissection

- Cut the lateral pterygoid close to its insertion into the neck of mandible (Fig. 50.3). This muscle is inserted into the neck of mandible. This muscle is also inserted into the articular disc of the joint and into the capsule of TMJ.
- Identify the loose capsule of the joint attached to articular tubercle and neck of mandible (Figs 50.3 and 50.4).
- Identify the lateral ligament, sphenomandibular ligament, stylomandibular ligament and pterygomandibular ligaments of TMJ (Fig. 50.4). Study their attachments from BD Chaurasia's *Human Anatomy*.
- Dislodge the head of mandible from the inferior aspect of the articular disc. Identify the fibro-

cartilages covering the head of mandible and concave mandibular fossa (Fig. 50.3a and b).
- Take out the articular disc and see its shape. It is concavoconvex on its superior aspects to fit against convex articular tubercle and concave mandibular fossa. The inferior aspect of the articular disc is only concave.
- See that the disc divides the joint cavity into upper or menisco-temporal compartment and a lower menisco-mandibular compartment. These would allow different varieties of movements in each of the two compartments.
- Study the movements of TMJ on dried bones. Upper compartment permits gliding movements while lower compartment permits rotational movements. Only the lateral pterygoid opens the jaw, i.e. it is depressor of TMJ. The other three muscles are all elevators of TMJ. These are antigravity muscles.

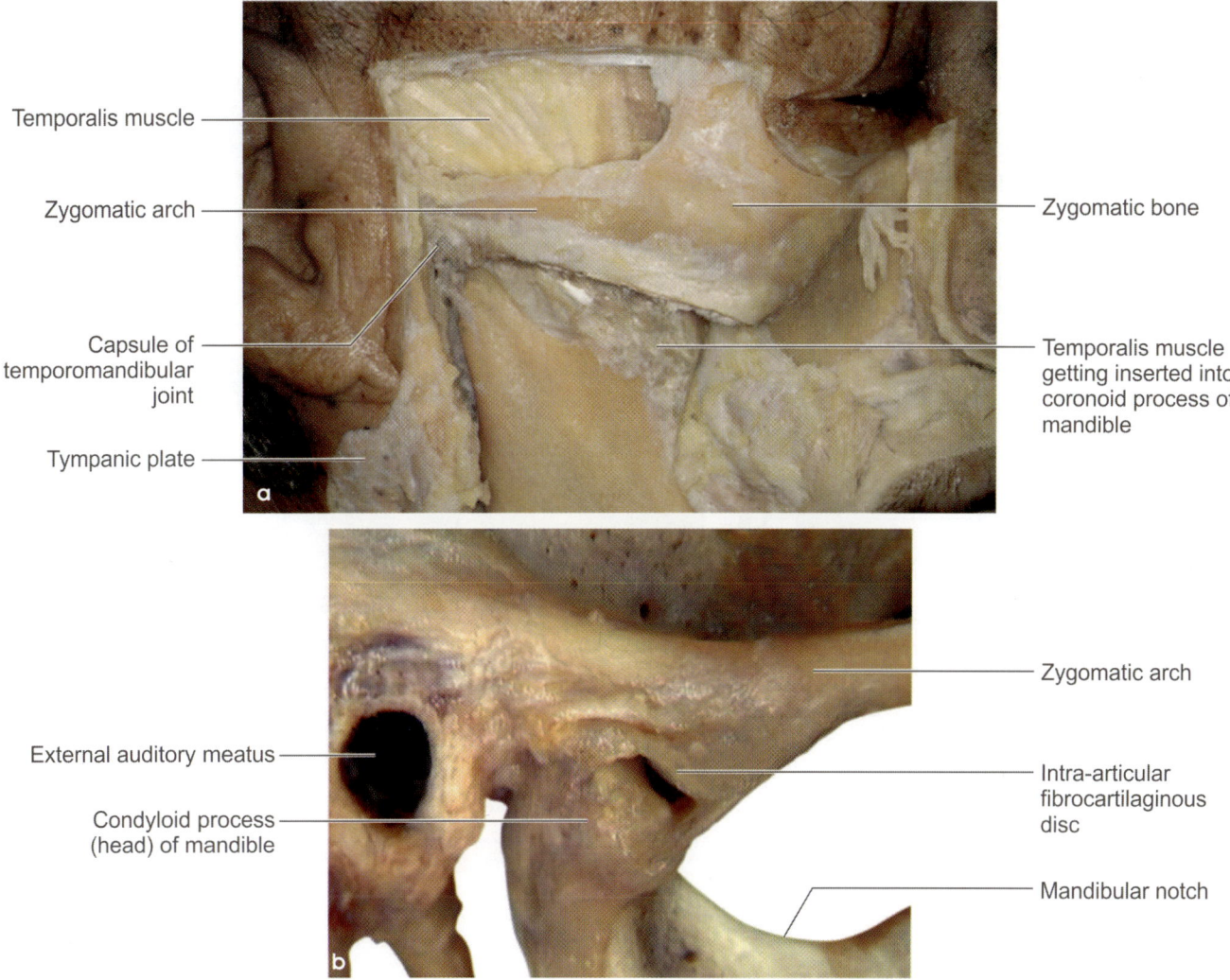

Temporalis muscle

Zygomatic arch

Capsule of temporomandibular joint

Tympanic plate

Zygomatic bone

Temporalis muscle getting inserted into coronoid process of mandible

External auditory meatus

Condyloid process (head) of mandible

Zygomatic arch

Intra-articular fibrocartilaginous disc

Mandibular notch

Fig. 50.3a and b: Temporomandibular joint

- The branches of auriculotemporal nerve and facial nerve are closely related to TMJ. One has to be careful during procedure on TMJ and protect the branches of these nerves.

Mandibular Nerve

- Middle meningeal artery has been identified as a branch of 1st part of maxillary artery. See that this artery is enclosed within two roots of the auriculotemporal nerve.
- Having identified auriculotemporal nerve, trace the two roots to the posterior division of mandibular nerve, and then to the trunk and anterior division of the largest mixed branch of the trigeminal nerve.

- Try to dissect branches of its trunk, anterior and posterior divisions separately (Fig. 50.5).
- Lift the trunk of mandibular nerve laterally to see the nerve to medial pterygoid and otic ganglion. Nerve to medial pterygoid innervates this muscle from its deep surface. This nerve gives a motor twig to otic ganglion which supplies tensor tympani of middle ear and tensor veli palatini of soft palate without relaying in the ganglion.
- See the branches for muscles of this region from its anterior branch. These go to temporalis, masseter and lateral pterygoid muscles. It continues as buccal nerve for the skin of cheek.

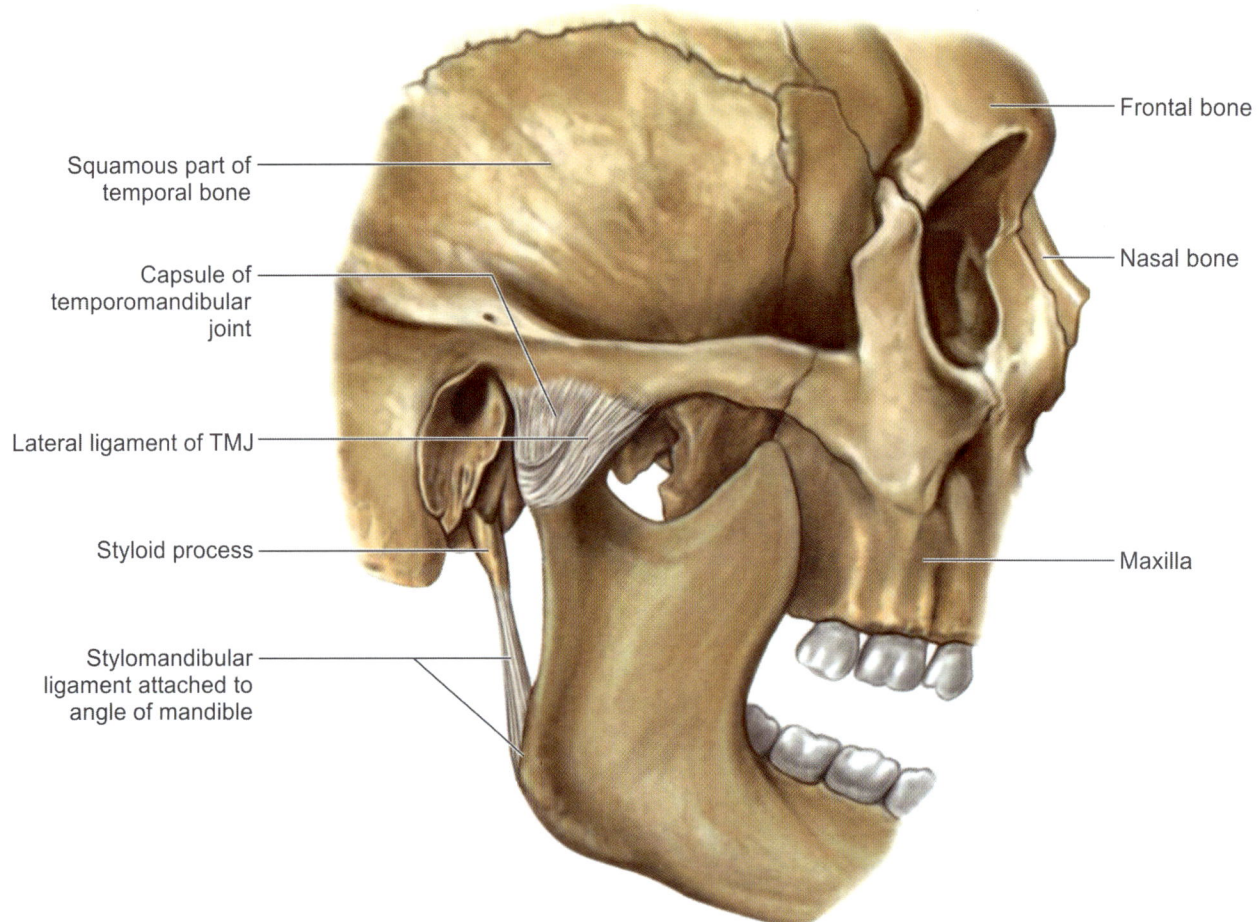

Squamous part of
temporal bone

Capsule of
temporomandibular
joint

Lateral ligament of TMJ

Styloid process

Stylomandibular
ligament attached to
angle of mandible

Frontal bone

Nasal bone

Maxilla

Fig. 50.4: Ligaments of temporomandibular joint

- Identify nerves from the thick posterior division. These are:
  - i. Two roots of auriculotemporal nerve join together and run with superficial temporal artery. It innervates the skin of pinna, temporal fossa, TMJ, and gives secretomotor fibres to the parotid gland.
  - ii. Lingual nerve given off 1 cm below the skull. Trace the chorda tympani (branch of facial nerve) emerging from petrotympanic fissure to join lingual nerve 2 cm below the skull.
  - iii. See important relation of lingual nerve to 3rd molar tooth. Then it reaches submandibular region.
  - iv. Identify inferior alveolar nerve running below and parallel to the lingual nerve towards the

mandibular foramen. Before it enters the foramen and the mandibular canal, see its branch—nerve to mylohyoid which also runs below the inferior alveolar nerve (in mylohyoid groove).
  - v. See the branches of nerve to mylohyoid being given to mylohyoid muscle and anterior belly of digastric muscle.

Otic Ganglion

- See the otic ganglion lying in relation to nerve to medial pterygoid (Fig. 50.5). See its position between the mandibular nerve and tensor tympani muscle.

Roots:
  - i. Sensory from auriculotemporal nerve.
  - ii. Sympathetic from plexus around middle meningeal artery.

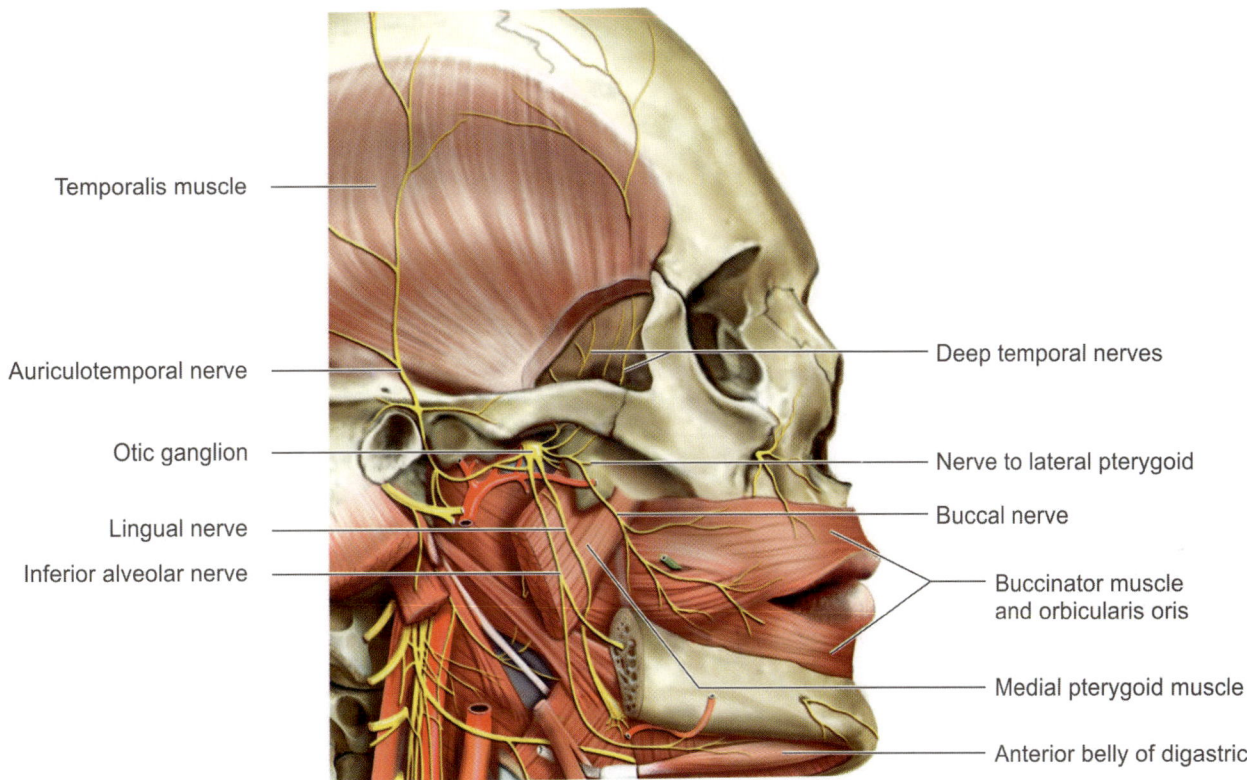

Temporalis muscle

Auriculotemporal nerve

Otic ganglion

Lingual nerve

Inferior alveolar nerve

Deep temporal nerves

Nerve to lateral pterygoid

Buccal nerve

Buccinator muscle and orbicularis oris

Medial pterygoid muscle

Anterior belly of digastric

Fig. 50.5: Branches of mandibular nerve including otic ganglion

iii. Secretomotor from lesser petrosal nerve, branch of IX

iv. Motor from nerve to medial pterygoid

Branches

i. Motor to tensor veli palatini and tensor tympani muscles.

ii. Secretomotor to parotid gland. These are fibres of IX nerve which relay in otic ganglion. The postganglionic fibres join the auriculotemporal nerve which gives branches to the largest salivary gland—the parotid gland.

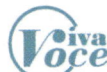

- Which parasympathetic ganglion has four roots? Name four roots and branches of the ganglion.
- Name the branches of all the parts of the maxillary artery.
- Which is the artery of epistaxis?
- Name the two compartments of temporomandibular joint. What movements occur in these compartments?
- What are the nerves related to the spine of sphenoid and what is their clinical importance?
- Which are the nerves related to TMJ?

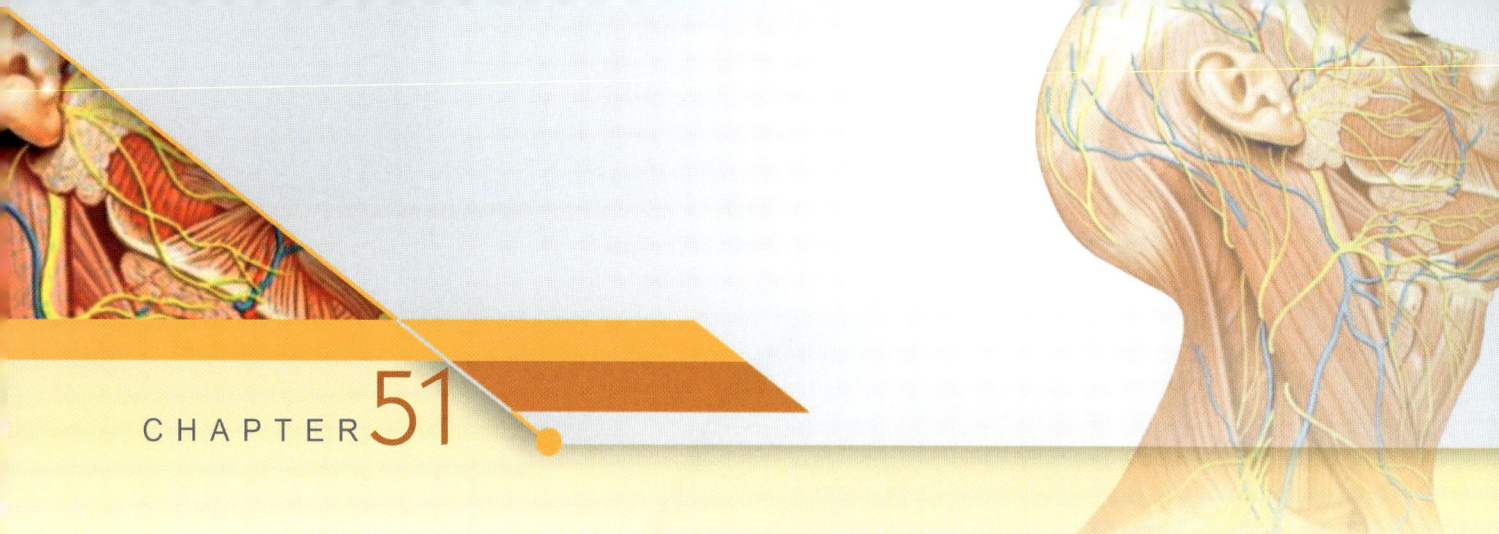

CHAPTER 51

Suprahyoid Muscles and Submandibular Gland

Learning Objectives

One should be able to

1. Recapitulate the nerve supply of suprahyoid muscles.
2. Learn the secretomotor nerve supply of submandibular salivary gland.

3. Position of four parts of lingual artery.
4. One should be able to recapitulate relations of superficial and deep parts of submandibular gland
5. Trace the roots and branches of submandibular ganglion

OVERVIEW

The suprahyoid muscles lie above the hyoid bone. Their attachment is to styloid process, mastoid process, tongue and mandible. These muscles are in four layers.

- 1st layer—anterior and posterior bellies of digastric and stylohyoid muscle supplementing the posterior belly (Fig. 51.1).
- 2nd layer—mylohyoid forming floor of mouth
- 3rd layer—hyoglossus and geniohyoid
- 4th layer—genioglossus

SUBMANDIBULAR REGION

The submandibular region lies between mandible above and hyoid below. Its sides are formed by the anterior and posterior bellies of digastric muscles.

Muscles in this region are present in following layers:

- 1st layer—digastric and stylohyoid
- 2nd layer—mylohyoid
- 3rd layer—geniohyoid and hyoglossus
- 4th layer—genioglossus

Most noticeable structure is the submandibular salivary gland including submandibular lymph nodes.

This gland is partly made of serous and partly of mucus acini. The gland comprises a large superficial and a small deep part. Facial artery is related to the posterior end of the superficial part. Then the artery makes a 'S' shaped bend and is seen at anteroinferior angle of the masseter muscle, where it enters the face. The lymph nodes on and inside the salivary gland drain medial part of forehead, face, upper lip and even the lateral and upper surface of the tongue. Thus cancer of tongue may spread to these lymph nodes.

The deep part of the gland lies on hyoglossus muscle, accompanied by lingual and hypoglossal nerves. Suspended from lingual nerve is submandibular parasympathetic ganglion. Chorda tympani, a branch of facial nerve, joins lingual nerve in infratemporal fossa, travels with lingual nerve to reach submandibular ganglion. This chorda tympani nerve forms secretomotor root to the ganglion. Its fibers relay and postganglionic fibres supply submandibular salivary gland and even sublingual salivary gland.

Competency achievement: The student should be able to:

AN 34.1 Describe and demonstrate the morphology, relations and nerve supply of submandibular salivary gland and submandibular ganglion.

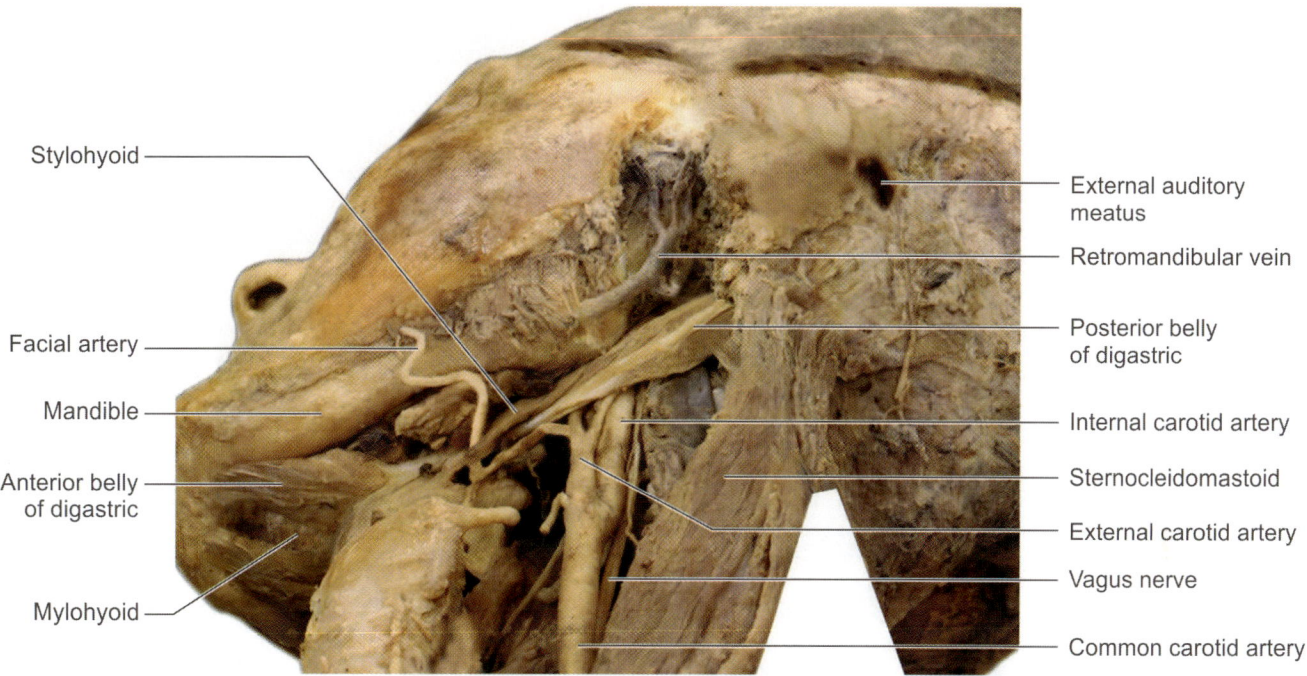

Stylohyoid

Facial artery

Mandible

Anterior belly
of digastric

Mylohyoid

External auditory
meatus

Retromandibular vein

Posterior belly
of digastric

Internal carotid artery

Sternocleidomastoid

External carotid artery

Vagus nerve

Common carotid artery

Fig. 51.1: Digastric triangle with tortuous facial artery and retromandibular vein

STEPS OF DISSECTION

- Cut the facial artery and vein present at the anteroinferior angle of masseter muscle (Fig. 51.1).
- Separate the origin of anterior belly of digastric from digastric fossa near symphysis menti.
- Cut mandible in median plane and carefully remove the base and remaining ramus of mandible. Push the mandible up.
- Trace the origin of posterior belly of digastric from mastoid notch (Fig. 51.1) and the origin of stylohyoid from the styloid process. Stylohyoid envelops the tendon of posterior belly of digastric muscle. Incise the pulley of digastric muscle and reflect digastric posteriorly.
- Identify mylohyoid arising from mylohyoid line of mandible. See the obliquity of these fibres. These form a median raphe attached to the chin above and to hyoid bone below (Fig. 51.1).
- See geniohyoid as a thin muscle arising from the lower genial tubercle of mandible to the hyoid bone.
- Identify quadrangular hyoglossus muscle arising from grater cornua of hyoid bone to the side of tongue.

- Identify the big fan shaped, bulky *lifesaving* genioglossus muscle. See it arising from the upper genial tubercle of mandible and going upwards to the tip, dorsum and base of tongue.
  Hyoglossus forms an important landmark in this region (Figs 51.2 and 51.3).
- See the structures on superficial surface of hyoglossus:
  i. Styloglossus lying on its upper border.
  ii. Identify lingual nerve (Fig. 51.2) with sub-mandibular ganglion suspended by its roots.
  iii. Below the ganglion is the deep part of sub-mandibular gland.
  iv. See the duct of gland emerging from its deep part and coursing towards the sublingual fold where it opens onto summit of sublingual fold.
  v. Identify the lingual nerve crossing over the submandibular duct (Fig. 51.3).
  vi. Lowest is most important hypoglossal nerve innervating 7/8 muscles of each half of the tongue (Fig. 51.3).
- Deep to the hyoglossus muscle are seen:
  i. Glossopharyngeal nerve innervating tongue with sensory and taste fibres.

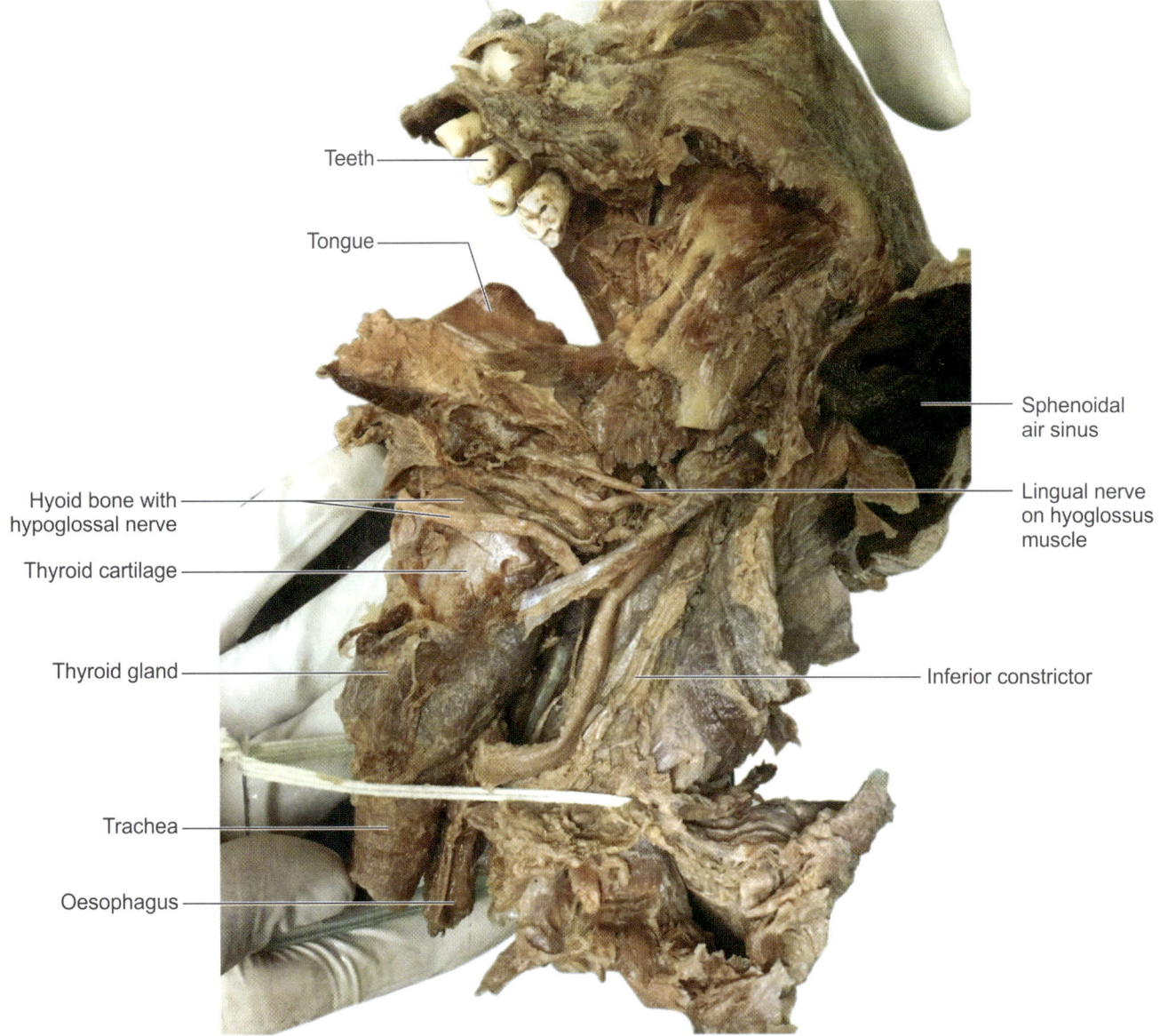

Teeth

Tongue

Hyoid bone with
hypoglossal nerve

Thyroid cartilage

Thyroid gland

Trachea

Oesophagus

Sphenoidal
air sinus

Lingual nerve
on hyoglossus
muscle

Inferior constrictor

Fig. 51.2: Relations of hyoglossus muscle

ii. The lingual artery arising from external carotid, passing deep to lower border of hyoglossus to enter the tongue as its deep branch.
• Carefully release hyoglossus from hyoid bone and reflect it towards the tongue.

Submandibular Salivary Gland

• See that the superficial large part of mixed salivary gland lies in the digastric triangle in between two bellies of digastric muscle (*see* Fig. 48.2), superficial to mylohyoid muscle. Push the superficial part posteriorly to see the whole of mylohyoid muscle.
• The deep smaller part of submandibular gland lies deep to the mylohyoid muscle (Fig. 51.3). Appreciate that mylohyoid indents this gland dividing it into a large superficial part and a small deep part.
• See the facial artery indenting the posterior end of the gland, and anteroinferior angle of masseter muscle at the base of mandible. Study the relations from BD Chaurasia's *Human Anatomy*.

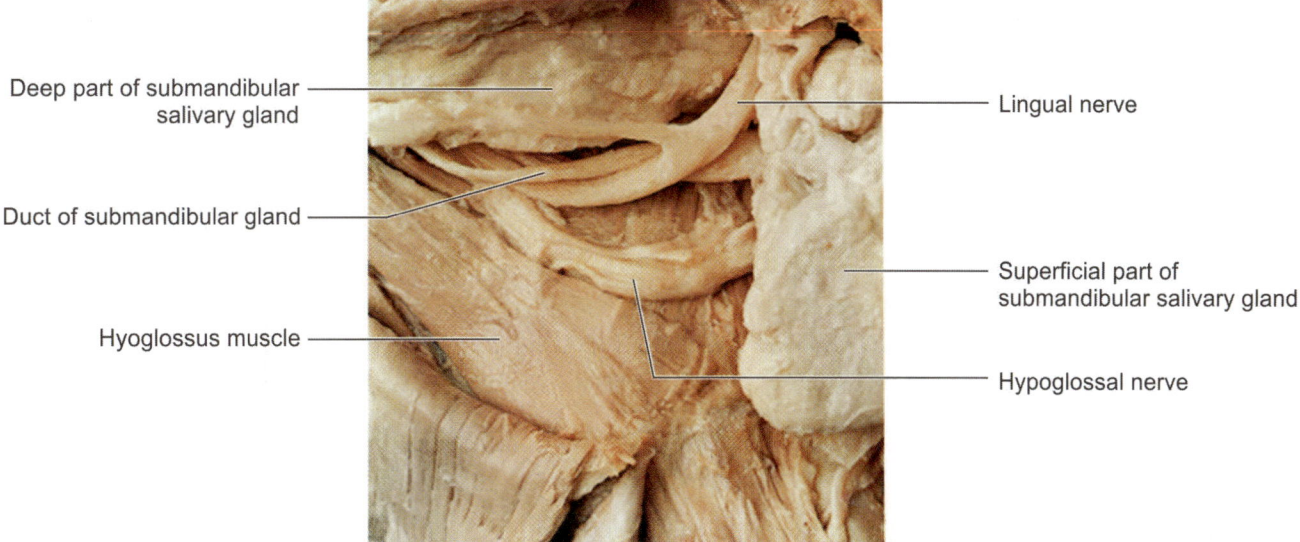

Deep part of submandibular salivary gland

Duct of submandibular gland

Hyoglossus muscle

Lingual nerve

Superficial part of submandibular salivary gland

Hypoglossal nerve

Fig. 51.3: Relation of lingual artery to duct of submandibular gland

Sublingual Salivary Gland

The smallest mucous salivary gland is present below the mucous membrane, close to the median plane. It rests on the mylohyoid muscle in the sublingual fossa of the mandible. The two glands almost meet in the median plane. Its nerve supply and blood supply is same as the submandibular gland. Both are supplied by branches of submandibular ganglion and facial artery.

Submandibular Ganglion

- Identify the submandibular parasympathetic ganglion. See its situation on the surface of hyoglossus muscle between lingual nerve above and hypoglossal nerve below (Fig. 51.2).

- See its roots:
  i. Sensory—2 branches of lingual nerve

ii. Sympathetic—sympathetic plexus around facial artery

iii. Secretomotor—chorda tympani, branch of facial nerve as it exits from petrotympanic fissure to join lingual nerve at an acute angle in the infratemporal fossa. These fibres only relay in the ganglion. Postganglionic fibres are given to the submandibular gland. Some fibres pass back to the lingual nerve and get distributed to sublingual salivary gland and glands in the anterior part of oral cavity.

As secretion of the gland is viscous, it is vulnerable to formation of calculi.

Submandibular lymph nodes are present within and on the submandibular salivary gland. These nodes drain tongue, side of cheek, part of forehead, etc. Cancer cells from tongue may reach these lymph nodes and even spread into the mandible.

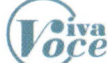

- Name the layers of suprahyoid muscles. Which nerves supply these muscles?
- Which muscle divides the submandibular gland into a superficial and deep part?

- Name the roots of the submandibular ganglion. What are its branches?
- Why are facial and lingual arteries tortuous?

CHAPTER **52**

Structures in the Neck

Learning Objectives

One should be able to

1. Discuss blood supply of thyroid gland and its clinical anatomy
2. Give functional importance of parathyroid glands
3. Enumerate the branches of subclavian and external carotid arteries.

4. Name the lymph nodes in the neck.
5. Name the muscles attached to styloid process with their nerve supply.
6. Enumerate the muscular branches of IX, X, XI and XII cranial nerves.

OVERVIEW

Deep Structures in the Neck

The structures are:

- Thyroid gland, parathyroid glands
- Blood vessels of neck
- Lymph nodes
- Styloid apparatus

Thyroid gland is an endocrine gland in front of upper part of trachea. It comprises two lobes and an isthmus. Each lobe has an apex, base, lateral, medial and posterior surfaces and anterior and posterior borders. The gland is richly supplied by a pair of superior and inferior thyroid arteries. There are two pairs of parathyroid glands on its posterior surface.

Thyroid gland moves with deglutition. It is palpated from the back.

Parathyroid glands lie along the posterior border of the thyroid gland. Superior parathyroids (parathyroid IV) lie near the middle of the gland while inferior parathyroids (parathyroid III) lie near lower pole of thyroid gland.

Thymus is a lymphoid organ which is big during childhood and gets involuted at the age of puberty. It

develops from endoderm of third pharyngeal pouch in conjunction with inferior parathyroid. Thymus controls lymphopoiesis as well as development of peripheral lymphoid tissues of the body during neonatal period.

Blood Vessels

Large arteries in neck are subclavian and common carotid arteries. Subclavian gives vertebral artery as its first branch which travels up to the cranial cavity to supply the brain. Other branch is thyrocervical trunk which gives branches to supply neck muscles and important thyroid gland. Common carotid divides into external carotid for supplying face, neck tongue, etc. and an internal carotid which also reaches up the cranial cavity to supply the brain. Main vein in the region is internal jugular vein, the continuation downwards of the sigmoid sinus.

Lymph Nodes

The lymph nodes are arranged in a superficial circle, deep circle and innermost circle known as Waldeyer's ring. Lymph from head and neck drains into jugular lymph trunk. This trunk drains into thoracic duct on the left side and right lymphatic duct on the right side. These ducts drain into respective brachiocephalic veins.

Styloid process is a needle like process. Its base is related to facial nerve and apex to external carotid artery. Three muscles and two ligaments are attached to it.

LAST FOUR CRANIAL NERVES

Cranial nerve IX, the glossopharyngeal nerve supplies only one muscle—the stylopharyngeus. It carries secretomotor fibres to the parotid gland and carries taste from posterior 1/3rd of tongue including the circumvallate papillae.

Cranial nerve X, the vagus carries the parasympathetic component of autonomic nervous system to the thoracic and abdominal viscera. It is joined by cranial root of XI, the accessory nerve which innervates 4/5 muscles of soft palate, 5/6 muscles of pharynx and all the muscles of larynx.

Cranial nerve XI, the accessory has two roots, the cranial and spinal roots. Cranial root joins vagus and gets distributed with it. The spinal root innervates the sternocleiodmastoid muscle (landmark muscle), runs through roof of posterior triangle and ends in the trapezius muscle.

Cranial nerve XII, the hypoglossal leaves the skull through hypoglossal canal, runs downwards, crosses the loop of lingual artery and supplies 7/8 muscles of the mobile tongue.

> **Competency achievement:** The student should be able to:
>
> **AN 35.2** Describe and demonstrate location, parts, borders, surfaces, relations and blood supply of thyroid gland.

Steps of Dissection

- Sternocleidomastiod muscles have been reflected upwards. Cut the sternothyroid muscles and intermediate tendon of omohyoid and reflect them upwards.
- Clean the surface of trachea and identify inferior thyroid veins draining into left brachiocephalic vein.
- Try to see some remnants of thymus gland close to inferior thyroid vein.
- Remove the pretracheal fascia enclosing thyroid gland.

- Identify the isthmus of thyroid gland overlapping 2nd–4th rings of trachea (Fig. 52.1). See if pyramidal lobe is present projecting from the upper border of the isthmus (Fig. 52.2).
- Look for gross anatomy of thyroid gland, these being apex, base; superficial, medial and postero-lateral surfaces; anterior and posterior borders (Fig. 52.2).
- Identify borders and surfaces of isthmus of thyroid gland. These are upper and lower borders and superficial and deep surfaces.
- Study the relations of the lobes and isthmus from BD Chaurasia's *Human Anatomy*.
- Identify the arteries supplying the gland. These are superior thyroid and inferior thyroid (Fig. 52.3).
- Recollect that superior thyroid artery is the first branch of external carotid artery (Fig. 52.4, *see* Fig 47.3). It descends down with superior laryngeal nerve, (branch of vagus) and then with external laryngeal nerve. See the latter nerve diverging medially near the apex of the lobe to reach the cricothyroid muscle. So the superior thyroid artery must be ligated close to the apex avoiding injury to the external laryngeal nerve.
- See that the inferior thyroid artery is a branch of thyrocervical trunk of 1st part of subclavian artery (Fig. 52.4). Trace the inferior thyroid artery upwards, backwards and medially to reach tracheo-oesophageal groove and thyroid gland where it lies in close contact with recurrent laryngeal nerve. If required some branches of inferior thyroid artery should be ligated so that blood supply to the parthyroid glands is maintained.
- Veins accompany the two thyroid arteries drain into internal jugular vein.
- In addition notice a middle thyroid vein unaccompanied by any artery which also drains into internal jugular vein.

Parathyroid Glands

- Identify the two parathyroid glands on each side between the true and false capsules of the gland.
- Trace their blood supply through an anastomotic branch between superior thyroid artery and inferior thyroid artery.

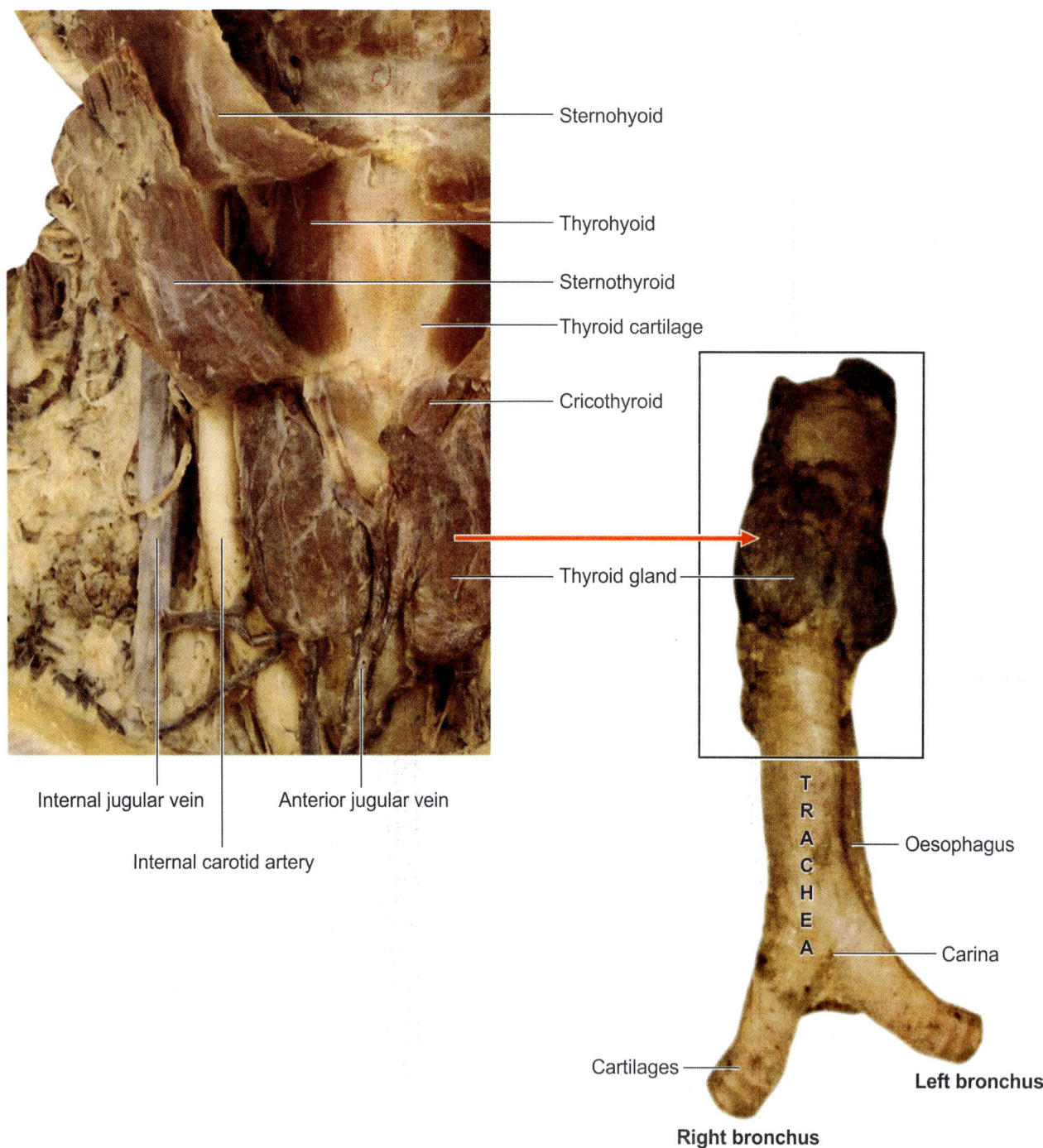

Fig. 52.1: Thyroid gland and related vessels

Thymus Gland

Try to identify remnants of thymus gland in the lower part of neck. It is darker in colour than fat. The gland produces T lymphocytes which are important for body's immunity.

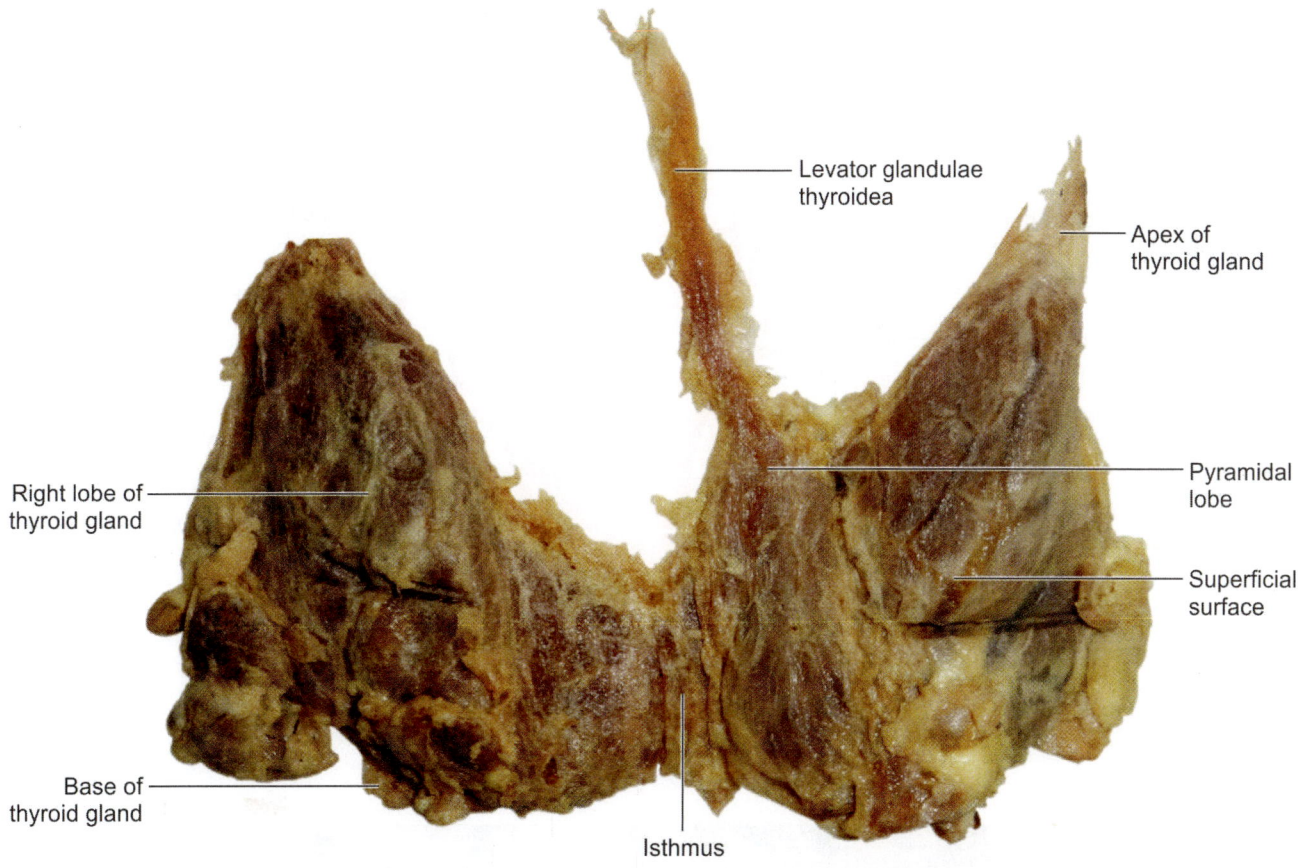

Levator glandulae thyroidea

Apex of thyroid gland

Pyramidal lobe

Superficial surface

Right lobe of thyroid gland

Base of thyroid gland

Isthmus

Fig. 52.2: Gross anatomy of thyroid gland. Pyramidal lobe also seen

Blood Vessels

- Identify scalenus anterior muscle in the antero-inferior part of the neck, partly under the sterno-cleidomastiod muscle.
- Look for subclavian artery which gets divided into three parts from medial to lateral side by the scalenus anterior muscle.
- Trace the branches of 1st part of subclavian artery. These are vertebral artery going above, internal thoracic passing below and thyrocervical trunk whose branches course laterally and above.
- Only one branch, i.e. costocervical trunk arises from 2nd part of subclavian on the right side only. The

left costocervical trunk arises from 1st part itself. 3rd part mostly gives no branch. Learn the course of these arteries from BD Chaurasia's *Human Anatomy*.

Common Carotid Artery (CCA)

- Common carotid artery has been exposed in the carotid triangle (*see* Fig. 48.3). Clean its entire course.
- Common carotid artery ends by dividing into internal and external carotid arteries.
- Identify the internal carotid artery (ICA) and trace it upwards till it leaves the neck (*see* Fig. 51.1).
- Try to look for carotid body behind bifurcation of common carotid artery, this body is 2–5 mm in size and acts as a chemoreceptor for controlling the respiration.
- Also identify the carotid sinus (*see* Figs 48.3 and 50.1), a little dilatation at beginning of internal

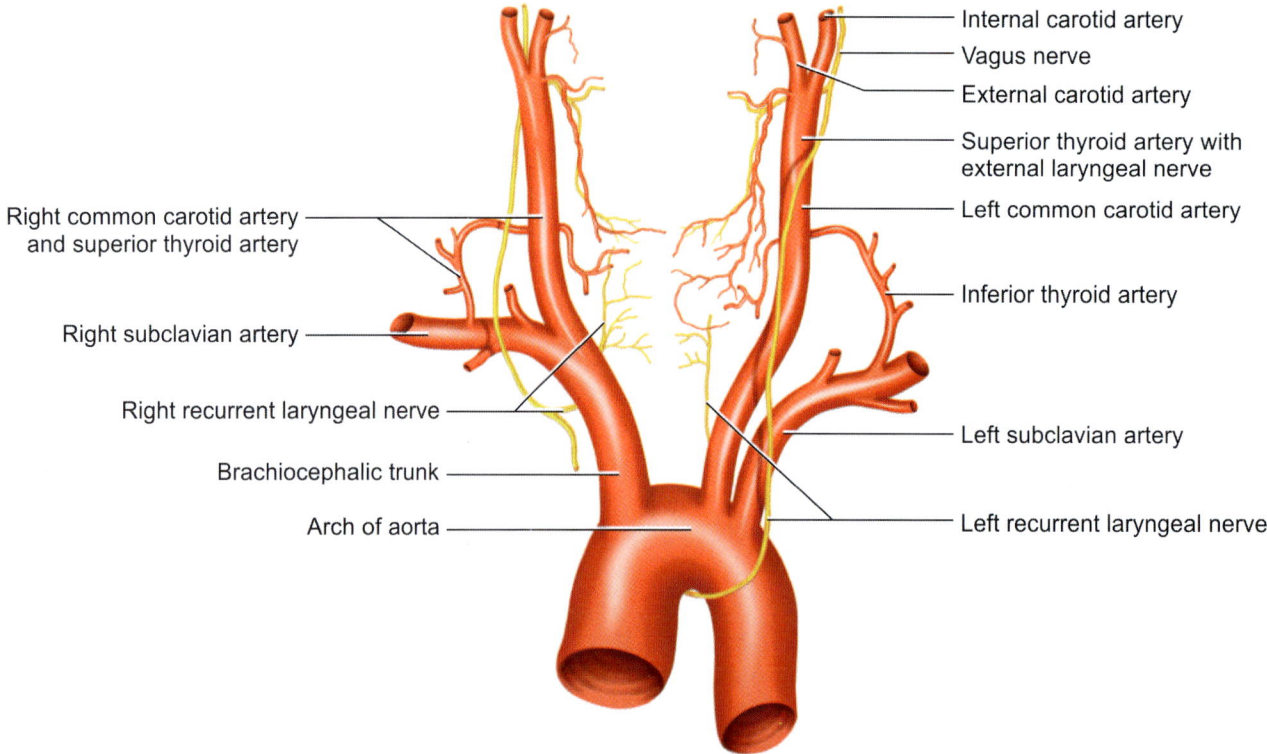

Internal carotid artery
Vagus nerve
External carotid artery
Superior thyroid artery with external laryngeal nerve
Left common carotid artery
Inferior thyroid artery
Left subclavian artery
Left recurrent laryngeal nerve

Right common carotid artery and superior thyroid artery
Right subclavian artery
Right recurrent laryngeal nerve
Brachiocephalic trunk
Arch of aorta

Fig. 52.3: Arteries of thyroid gland

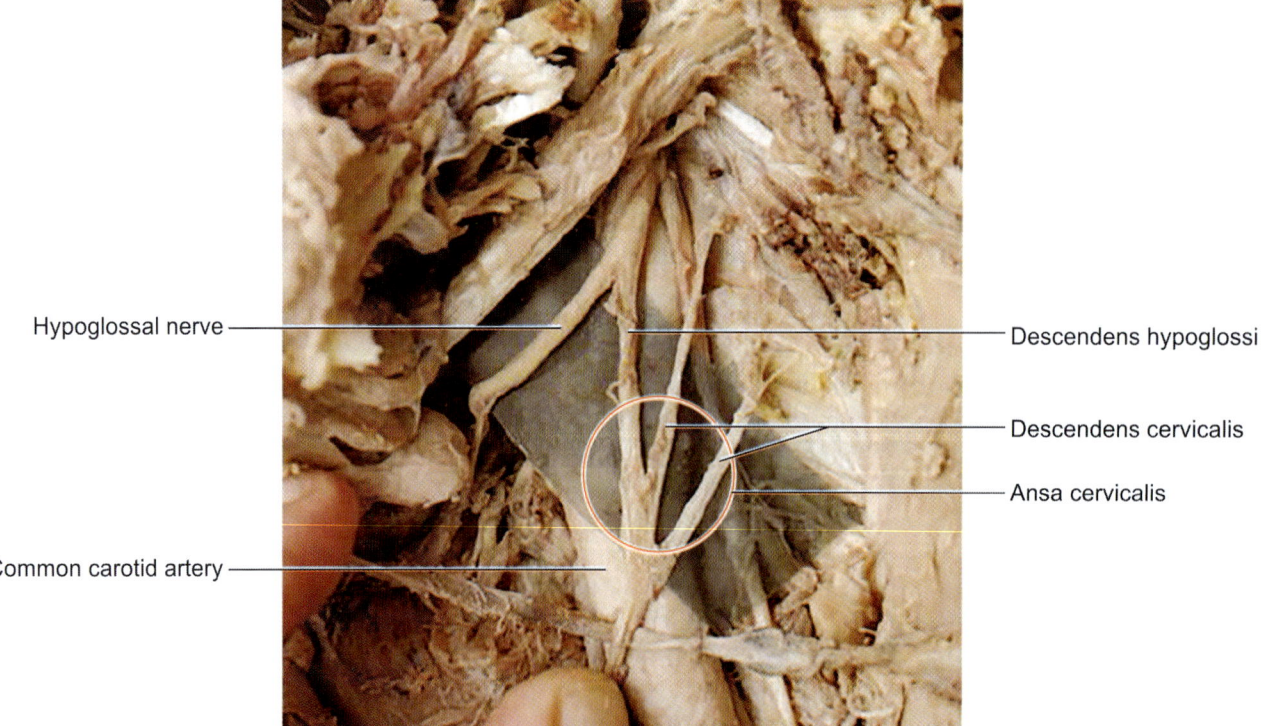

Hypoglossal nerve
Common carotid artery

Descendens hypoglossi
Descendens cervicalis
Ansa cervicalis

Fig. 52.4: Descendens hypoglossi, descendens cervicalis and the ansa cervicalis

carotid artery or termination of CCA. It acts as a baroreceptor to control blood pressure.

- Both carotid body and carotid sinus are innervated by IX, X and sympathetic nerves.

> *Competency achievement:* The student should be able to:
> **AN 35.4** Describe and demonstrate origin, course, relations, tributaries and termination of internal jugular and brachiocephalic veins.

Veins

- Identify the internal jugular vein (IJV) (Fig. 52.3, *see* Figs 48.3, 48.7) and subclavian veins on both sides of neck. These two veins join to form brachiocephalic vein on both the sides.
- See that the left brachiocephalic vein is longer and it joins short right brachiocephalic vein to form the superior vena cava.

The internal jugular vein is accessible deep in the lesser supraclavicular fossa present between the sternal and clavicular heads of SCM muscle.

Pulsations of CCA and ICA can be felt at the anterior border of SCM. These are also called anaesthetist's arteries.

> *Competency achievement:* The student should be able to:
> **AN 35.7** Describe the course and branches of IX, X, XI and XII nerve in the neck.

Glossopharyngeal (IX) Nerve

- The rootlets are attached between olive and inferior cerebellar peduncle of medulla oblongata above those of X and XI nerves (*see* Fig. 67.4).
- See the nerve exit from anterior most part of jugular foramen.
- See the nerve descending between internal jugular vein and ICA deep to the muscles attached to the styloid process.
- Trace it passing forwards between ICA and ECA to reach side of pharynx. Then it enters submandibular region by passing deep to hyoglossus muscle, where it ends by dividing into tonsillar and lingual branches.
- Trace the branches:
  - i. Tympanic branch forms tympanic plexus which gives lesser petrosal nerve. This nerve supplies parotid gland after relaying in the otic ganglion (general visceral efferent—GVE)
  - ii. Carotid branch to carotid sinus and carotid body
  - iii. Pharyngeal branch for mucous membrane of palate, pharynx and tonsils—General visceral afferent (GVA)
  - iv. Muscular branch for stylopharyngeus muscle—special visceral efferent (Sp VE)
  - v. Lingual branches for general sensation from posterior 1/3rd of tongue including taste sensations from circumvallate papillae. General visceral afferent (GVA) and special visceral afferent (Sp VA)

Vagus (X) Nerve

Vagus nerve has an extensive course through head and neck, thorax and abdomen. Fibres of cranial root of XI are also distributed through vagus nerve.

Vagus nerve carries parasympathetic fibres for the glands of respiratory tract and gastrointestinal tract.

Functional components

Nucleus ambiguus for muscles—speical visceral efferent (SVE)

Dorsal nucleus of vagus—general visceral efferent and general visceral afferent (GVE and GVA)

Nucleus of tractus solitarius—special visceral afferent (SVA)

Nucleus of spinal tract of V—general somatic efferent (GSA)

Course

- The rootlets lie in the groove between olive and inferior cerebellar peduncle behind IX nerve
- The nerve exists from jugular foramen and lies in the carotid sheath on a posterior plane between internal jugular vein and internal carotid artery or common carotid artery (*see* Figs 48.4, 48.7 and 51.1).
- At the root of neck the right vagus crosses 1st part of the subclavian artery inclining medially behind brachiocephalic vessels to reach right side of trachea.
- At the root of neck the left vagus lies between left CCA and left subclavian arteries, then behind left internal jugular vein and brachiocephalic vein to reach the thorax.
- Trace its branches in head and neck:
  - i. Meningeal—for meninges of posterior cranial fossa

ii. Auricular—for pinna and external auditory meatus

iii. Pharyngeal—for muscles of palate and pharynx

iv. Carotid—for carotid body and sinus

v. Superior laryngeal—for cricothyroid muscle and part of mucous membrane of larynx

vi. Recurrent laryngeal—for all muscles of larynx and mucous membrane of part of larynx

vii. Cardiac—for heart

Accessory (XI) Nerve

Accessory nerve comprises 2 roots:

i. Cranial root arising from a nucleus in medulla oblongata (see Fig. 67.4)

ii. Spinal root arising from C1–C5 segments of spinal cord

Functional components

Cranial root—special visceral efferent (SVE) fibres of cranial root of XI get distributed via X nerve to muscles of soft palate, pharynx and larynx

Spinal root—also special visceral efferent fibres. Its fibres supply SCM and trapezius muscles.

Nuclei—lowest part of nucleus ambiguus and spinal nucleus of XI.

Course

The cranial root is attached to the groove between olive and inferior cerebellar peduncle of medulla oblongata below IX and X cranial nerves. As it exits from cranial cavity through jugular foramen it joins spinal root of XI for a short distance. But the two roots again separate and cranial root finally joins X nerve and gets distributed through X to supply muscles of soft palate, pharynx and larynx.

Spinal Root of XI

After its origin from C1–C5 segments, the spinal root ascends up to the cranial cavity through foramen magnum. There it runs laterally and fuses for a short distance with cranial root. As it passes out of the jugular foramen it separates from the cranial root.

The spinal root descends between IJV and ICA deep to styloid process. Nearly 3 cm below the base it runs backwards over IJV in the anterior triangle of neck (see Fig. 48.3).

The nerve pierces anterior border of SCM at junction of upper 1/4th and lower 3/4th. It supplies SCM and exits from here at its posterior border a little above its middle (see Fig. 47.2b).

Thus it reaches posterior triangle of neck. It runs across the posterior triangle, embedded in its roof lying over the levator scapulae muscle (see Fig. 47.2b).

The nerve leaves posterior triangle as it passes deep to anterior border of trapezius 5 cm above the clavicle.

The nerve supplies both the boundary muscles of posterior triangle of neck. It is accompanied by number of lymph nodes in its course in posterior triangle.

While taking biopsy of lymph nodes of posterior triangle, one must be careful of not injuring the spinal root of XI nerve.

Hypoglossal (XII) Nerve

Hypoglossal nerve is meant for supplying muscle of the tongue. Seven out of eight muscles of each side of tongue are innervated by XII nerve.

Functional components

General somatic efferent (GSE) column gives fibres for supply to muscles of tongue.

Nucleus lies in floor of IV ventricle. Nucleus for genioglossus receives only contralateral fibres. Rest of the muscles receive both ipsilateral and contralateral fibres.

Course

The rootlets of XII nerve are attached in a groove between pyramid and olive. The nerve leaves the skull through hypoglossal/anterior condylar canal.

In the neck the nerve lies deep to IJV and ICA, then crosses vagus (X) and reaches anterior to vagus nerve.

At lower border of posterior belly of digastric muscle it crosses both ICA and ECA and the loop of lingual artery to enter submandibular region (see Figs 48.3 and 50.1).

Then the nerve runs on hyoglossus muscle to reach substance of tongue (Fig. 52.5, see Fig 51.3).

It gives branches to all four intrinsic muscles of tongue and innervates 3 out of 4 extrinsic muscles of tongue.

If XII nerve of right side is paralysed, the tongue on protrusion deviates to the right side.

Sympathetic Trunk

The sympathetic trunk was seen to lie posterior to the carotid sheath in carotid triangle. Now trace the trunk upwards and downwards to locate three cervical ganglia. These are superior, middle and inferior cervical ganglia. Details to be studied from BD Chaurasia's *Human Anatomy.*

Cervical Plexus

- Dissect and clean cervical plexus (ventral rami of C1–C4 nerves).
- Descendens hypoglossi from C1 and descendens cervicalis from C2, C3 join to form ansa cervicalis (Fig. 52.5). It lies anterior to carotid sheath in the carotid triangle of neck.
- Branches from both descendens nerves and from the loop innervate the infrahyoid muscles

  Other branches of the cervical plexus are four cutaneous nerves already seen in the posterior triangle of neck. The muscular branches from C1–C4 roots supply the prevertebral muscles.

- Identify one important branch of the plexus, i.e. the phrenic nerve. This is the sole motor supply of respective dome of the diaphragm.
- Trace this nerve lying on the surface of scalenus anterior muscle deep to the prevertebral fascia (*see* Fig. 47.2a).
- Follow it into the thorax where it lies on the fibrous pericardium, accompanied by pericardiacophrenic artery (branch of internal thoracic artery).
- It passes through diaphragm and supplies its musculature from the abdominal aspect. Sensory branches of phrenic nerve innervate fibrous and parietal layer of pericardium, parietal layer of pleura and parietal layer of peritoneum.

Lymph Nodes

See the various groups of lymph nodes in the neck (Fig. 52.6). These are the following groups:

A. *Superficial group:*

   1. Identify buccal nodes lying on buccinator

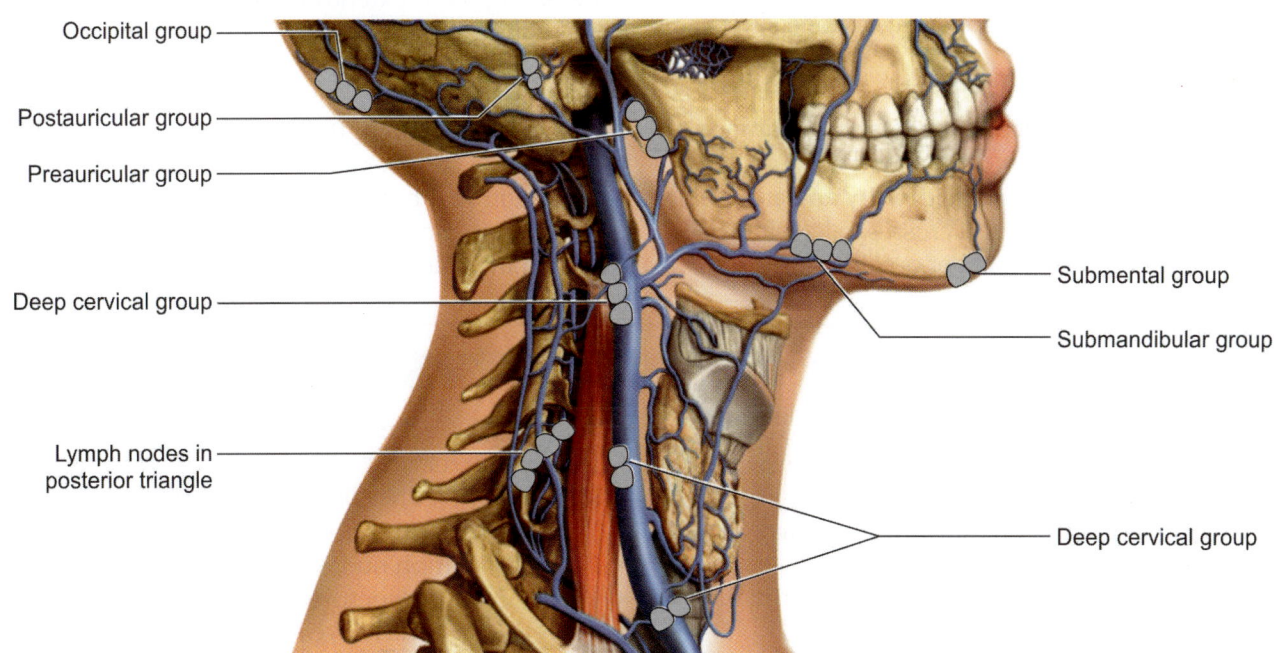

Fig. 52.5: Various groups of lymph nodes

2. Preauricular in front of ear
3. Posterior auricular behind the ear
4. Occipital near apex of posterior triangle
5. Anterior cervical along anterior jugular vein
6. Lateral cervical along external jugular vein

All these drain structures close to the respective lymph nodes.

B. *Deep group:*

Identify

1. Submental and submandibular nodes
2. Upper lateral group or jugulodigastric nodes where posterior belly of digastric crosses internal jugular vein IJV
3. Middle lateral group around IJV
4. Lower lateral group or jugulo-omohyoid nodes
5. Lymph nodes in posterior triangle around spinal root of XI nerve

Efferent of deep cervical lymph nodes form right jugular lymph trunks.

C. *Deepest lymph nodes*

1. Prelaryngeal/pretracheal
2. Paratracheal
3. Retropharyngeal
4. Waldeyer's ring/submucosal lymph nodes—these comprise lingual tonsil, palatine tonsil, tubal tonsil and nasopharyngeal tonsil.

Thoracic Duct

- Identify thoracic duct which starts in abdomen as continuation of cisterna chyli (*see* Fig. 14.2).
- Trace it entering the thoracic cavity and ascending up to T5 vertebra where it crosses to left side. See it ascending on the left side of oesophagus.

- See the thoracic duct terminating on the left side of the root of neck by opening at the angle of junction between left IJV and left subclavian veins. The thoracic duct drains:
  - Both lower limbs
  - Abdomen
  - Left side of head and neck
  - Left upper limb
  - Left side of thorax
- Identify one more lymphatic duct—right lymphatic duct draining right side of head and neck, right upper limb and right half of thorax.
- See this duct opening in the same angle of 2 veins on the right side.

Styloid Apparatus

- Identify the styloid process as a needle like process anteromedial to the mastoid process.
- See three muscles attached to it. These are:
  i. Stylopharyngeus muscle getting inserted into the posterior border of thyroid cartilage. This is the only muscle innervated by IX nerve.
  ii. Stylohyoid lies between styloid process and hyoid bone (*see* Fig. 51.1). See the two slips of this muscle envelope the intermediate tendon of digastric muscle. It is supplied by VII nerve.
  iii. Styloglossus extending between styloid process to the lateral margin of tongue and is supplied by XII nerve.
  iv. Stylohyoid ligament is a remnant of 2nd pharyngeal arch. It extends from tip of styloid process to lesser cornua of hyoid bone.
  v. Stylomandibular ligament attached to styloid process above and angle of mandible below. It is a modification of cervical fascia.

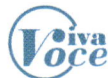

- What does the word 'thyroid' mean?
- Where does the thyroid venous plexus lie in relation to its capsules?
- Where is superior thyroid artery ligated during thyroidectomy and why?
- Which artery is the guide to location of the parathyroid glands?
- Why is "parathyroid III" called the inferior parathyroid gland?

- Name the branches of 1st part of subclavian artery.
- How many cervical sympathetic ganglia are there? Name the branches of superior cervical ganglion.
- What are the features of Horner's syndrome?
- Name the lymph nodes forming Waldeyer's ring.
- What are the structures attached to the styloid process? Give the nerve supply of these muscles.
- Enumerate the muscles supplied by ansa cervicalis and its roots.

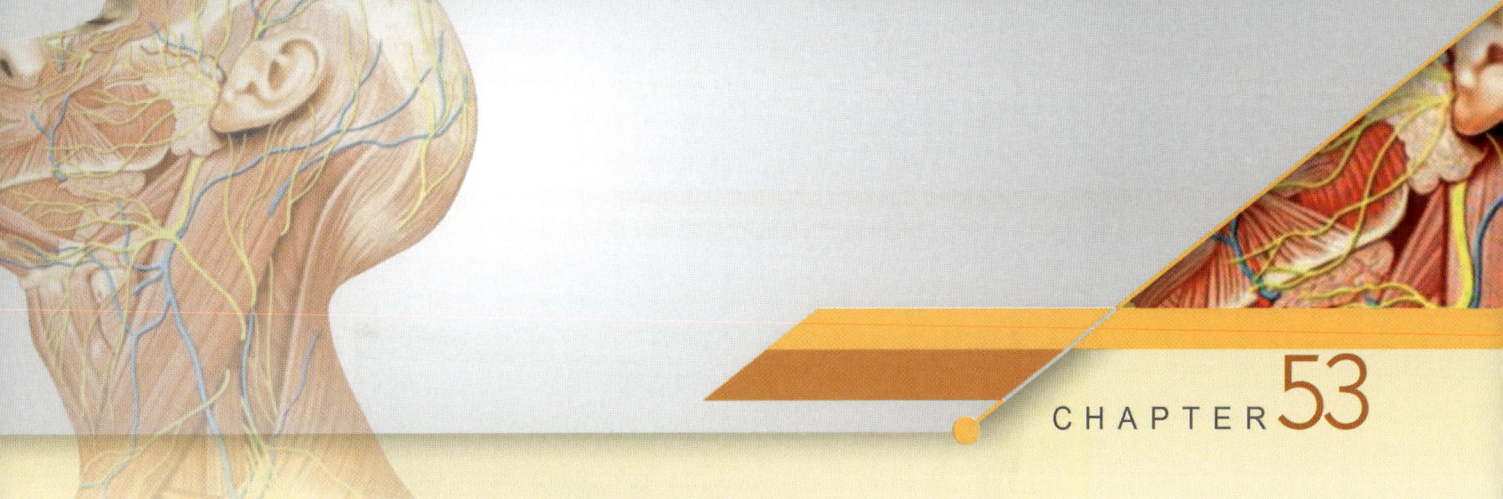

Prevertebral and Paravertebral Regions

OVERVIEW

Prevertebral region lies anterior to the cervical vertebrae, contains few muscles including the important vertebral artery. Paravertebral region contains the three pairs of scalene muscles.

This region also contains atlantooccipital, atlantoaxial and other cervical joints. The atlantooccipital joint is an ellipsoid variety of synovial joint permitting movements of "Yes" (nodding).

Median atlantoaxial joint is a pivot variety of synovial joint permitting rotation of the head, as in saying "No".

Ligaments connecting axis and occipital bone:
 i. Membrana tectoria, the continuation upwards of the posterior longitudinal ligament
 ii. Cruciate ligament comprised of transverse ligament and upper and lower vertical bands.
 iii. Apical ligament of dens, remnant of notochord
 iv. Alar ligament.

Vertebral Artery

The vertebral artery arising from the 1st part of subclavian artery has already been seen. It comprises 4 parts:

1st part lies in the scaleno-vertebral triangle.
• Identify the boundaries and contents of scaleno-vertebral triangle as:
  – Lateral—scalenus anterior
  – Medial—lower oblique part of longus colli
  – Apex—transverse process of C6 vertebra
  – Base—1st part of subclavian artery
  – Posterior wall—transverse process of C7, ventral ramus of C8 nerve, neck of 1st rib
  – Contents—1st part of vertebral artery, cervical part of sympathetic trunk

2nd part of the vertebral artery lies in the foramen transverseria of C6–C1 vertebrae (Fig. 53.1).
• To see this part, remove scalenus anterior muscle (if not already removed).
• Then identify deeply placed anterior and posterior intertransverse muscles to expose the 2nd part of vertebral artery.

The 3rd part will be seen in the suboccipital triangle (Fig. 53.1).

The vertebral artery is accompanied by venous plexus and a branch from stellate ganglion.

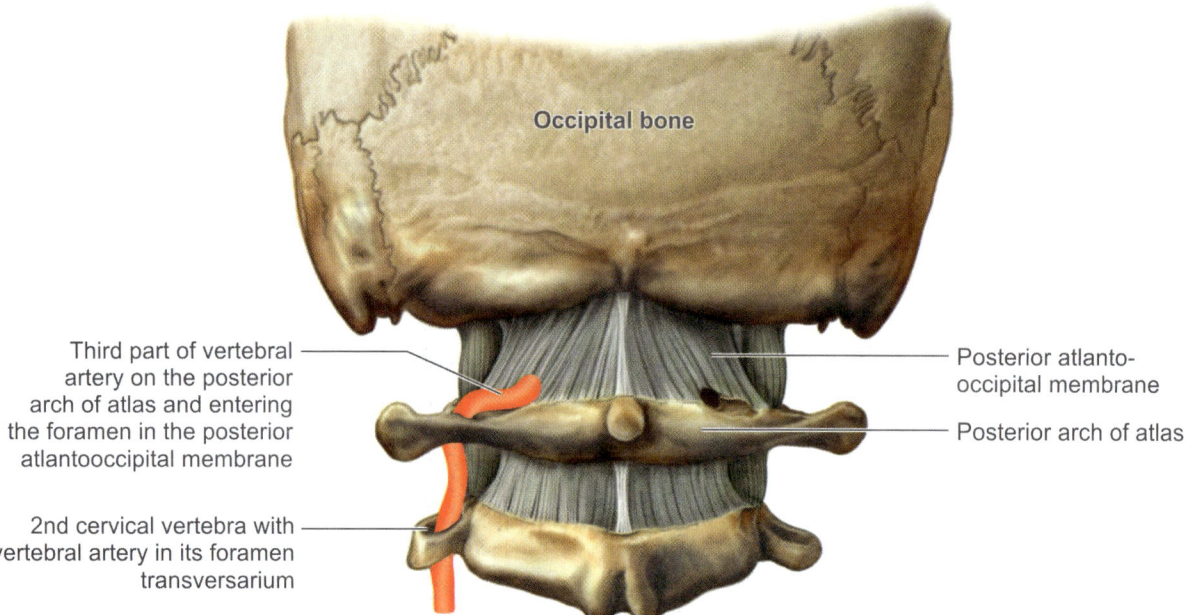

Fig. 53.1: Part of the course of vertebral artery

- See that the ventral rami of cervical nerves lie posterior to the artery.

4th part enters the cranial cavity through foramen magnum.

- See that the vertebral artery does not traverse foramen transversarium of C7 vertebra. This foramen only contains the vertebral vein.
- Identify rectus capitis lateralis and rectus capitis anterior as two muscles lying between the occiput and the atlas.
- Look for anterior primary ramus of C1 nerve emerging between these two muscles.

  Scalenus anterior muscle was seen earlier lying deep to lower part of SCM. It also divides the subclavian artery into 1st, 2nd and 3rd parts. Phrenic nerve also lies between this muscle and prevertebral fascia overlying this muscle.

- Identify scalenus medius forming the lower part of floor of posterior triangle of neck (*see* Fig. 47.2b). Scalenus posterior lies deep to scalenus medius muscle.
- Clean the anterior surfaces of cervical parts of trachea and oesophagus (Fig. 53.2).
- Identify cervical pleura at the root of neck. Look for the posterior relations of cervical pleura. These are: sympathetic trunk, first posterior intercostal

vein, superior intercostal artery and 1st thoracic nerve. Recapitulate these 4 structures are lying at the neck of 1st rib.

- Anteriorly cervical pleura is related to branches of 1st part of subclavian artery eg vertebral, anterior thoracic and 3 branches of thyrocervical trunk.
- Laterally the roots and trunks of brachial plexus are related to cervical pleura. Part of the pleura lies between scalenus anterior and scalenus medius muscles.
- See that the trachea begins as continuation of larynx at level of C6 vertebra. It has a small part in neck as it descends into superior mediastinum of thorax. Clean the isthmus of thyroid gland as it covers 2nd and 3rd tracheal rings (*see* Fig. 52.1 inset). Identify sternohyoid and sternothyroid muscles.
- Deep to trachea identify collapsible oesophagus (Fig. 53.2). Oesophagus also starts at the level of C6 vertebra. After a brief course it descends in the superior mediastinum of thorax.
- Identify right and left recurrent laryngeal nerves lying between trachea and oesophagus. The lobes of thyroid gland on each side are also related to both trachea and oesophagus. These nerves are related to arteries of neck and thorax (*see* Fig. 52.3)

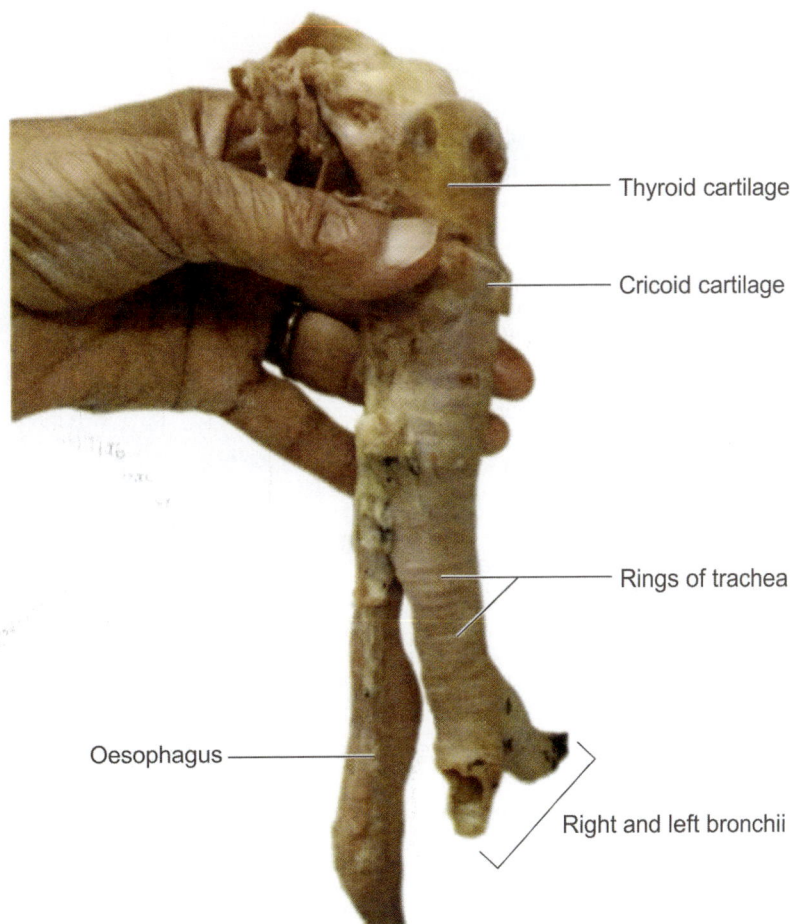

Thyroid cartilage

Cricoid cartilage

Rings of trachea

Oesophagus

Right and left bronchii

Fig. 53.2: Laryngeal cartilages with trachea and oesophagus

- On the left side of oesophagus, try to identify the beaded thoracic duct as it ascends up to root of neck to open at the angle present at junction of left subclavian and left internal jugular veins. Note the natural constrictions of the oesophagus at the level of C6 in the region of neck. Others are at level of T5, and T10 vertebra.

Joints of the Skull and Prevertebral Region

The various bones in the skull are mostly united by sutures.

Joints between teeth and their sockets are gomphosis.

Temporomandibular joints and joints between the ossicles of middle ear are synovial joints.

Joint between basisphenoid and basiocciput is primary cartilaginous joint.

- Observe that the anterior aspect of vertebral bodies are united by anterior longitudinal ligament (Fig. 53.3 inset).
- Notice that the adjacent surfaces of vertebral bodies are covered by hyaline cartilages and in between hyaline cartilages is the intervertebral disc (Fig. 53.3). This is the secondary cartilaginous joint.
- The intervertebral disc comprises:
  1. Central nucleus pulposus
  2. Peripheral annulus fibrosis
- Observe the lateral margins of the vertebral bodies. Both on upper surface and lower surface their margins/lips are raised (say C5 vertebra). These are lateral joints between the lower lip of vertebra C4 with upper lip of C5. Similarly there are joints between lower lip of C5 and upper lip of C6.

Thus there are four lateral joints and two central joints between three adjacent vertebrae (C4–C6). These

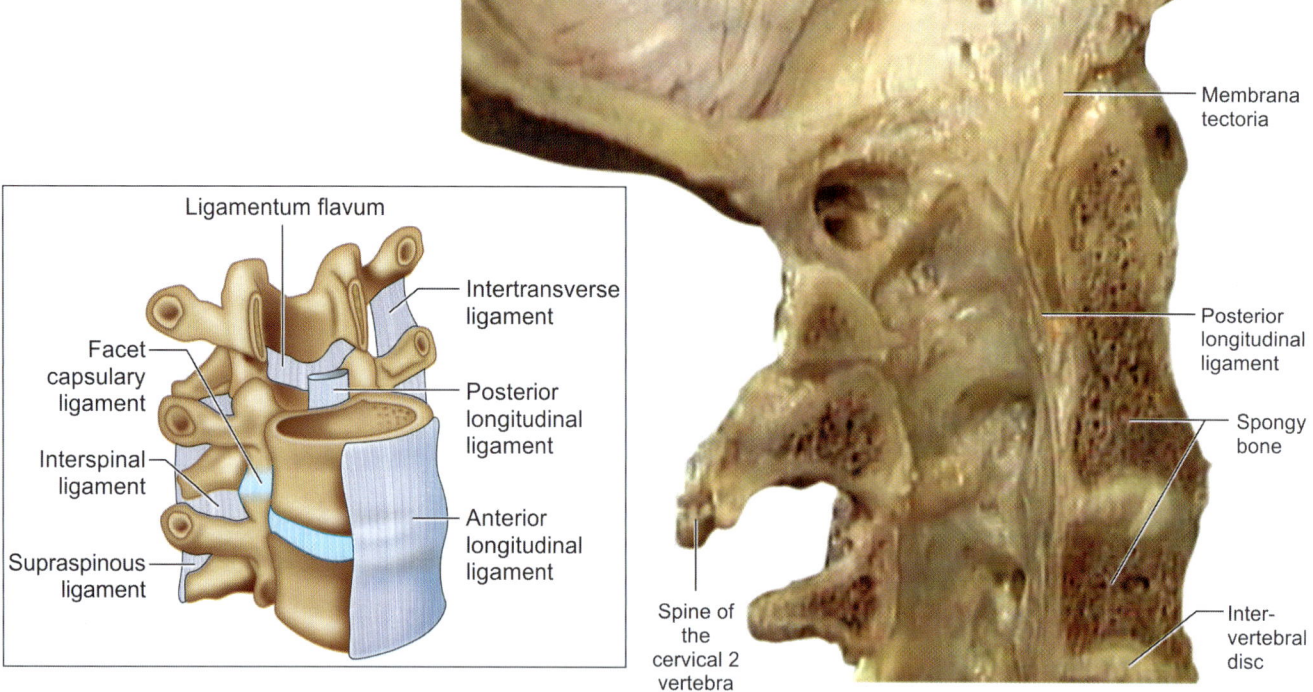

Fig. 53.3: Joints and ligaments of lower cervical vertebrae

are uncovertebral/Luschka joints. Study these joints on disarticulated bones.

- See the presence of synovial joints between articular processes of adjacent vertebrae (facet joints).

Competency achievement: The student should be able to:

AN 43.1 Describe and demonstrate the movements with muscles producing the movements of atlantooccipital joint and atlantoaxial joint.

- Identify the joints between occipital bone, atlas and axis vertebrae (Fig. 53.4). Atlantooccipital joints permit nodding/'yes' movements.
- There are three atlantoaxial joints, one median (Fig. 53.4) and two lateral. The median joint permits rotational movement/'no'.
- See the position of posterior atlantooccipital membrane stretching between posterior arch of atlas and posterior margin of foramen magnum.
- Identify and remove posterior arch of atlas and spine and lamina of axis vertebra.
- Now identify ligaments in relation to odontoid process. These are membrana tectoria, continuation upwards of posterior longitudinal ligament (Fig. 53.3). It lies between body of axis and anterior

margin of foramen magnum above. Remove this ligament.

- Now note the cruciate ligament (Fig. 53.4). It comprises:
  i. One very strong transverse ligament extending between two lateral masses of atlas, passing behind dens of axis.
  ii. Two vertical bands, one above to anterior margin of foramen magnum and one below to body of axis vertebra.
  iii. The alar ligaments extending from sides of odontoid process to medial side of occipital condyles.
- The apical ligament from the tip of odontoid process to anterior margin of foramen magnum. Note that the three structures are attached to basisphenoid beyond the anterior margin of foramen magnum.

These are from before backwards:
  i. The membrana tectoria
  ii. Upper vertical band of cruciate ligament
  iii. Apical ligament

- Identify accessory atlantoaxial ligaments present between posterior surface of body of dens and lateral masses of atlas vertebra (Fig. 53.4 inset).

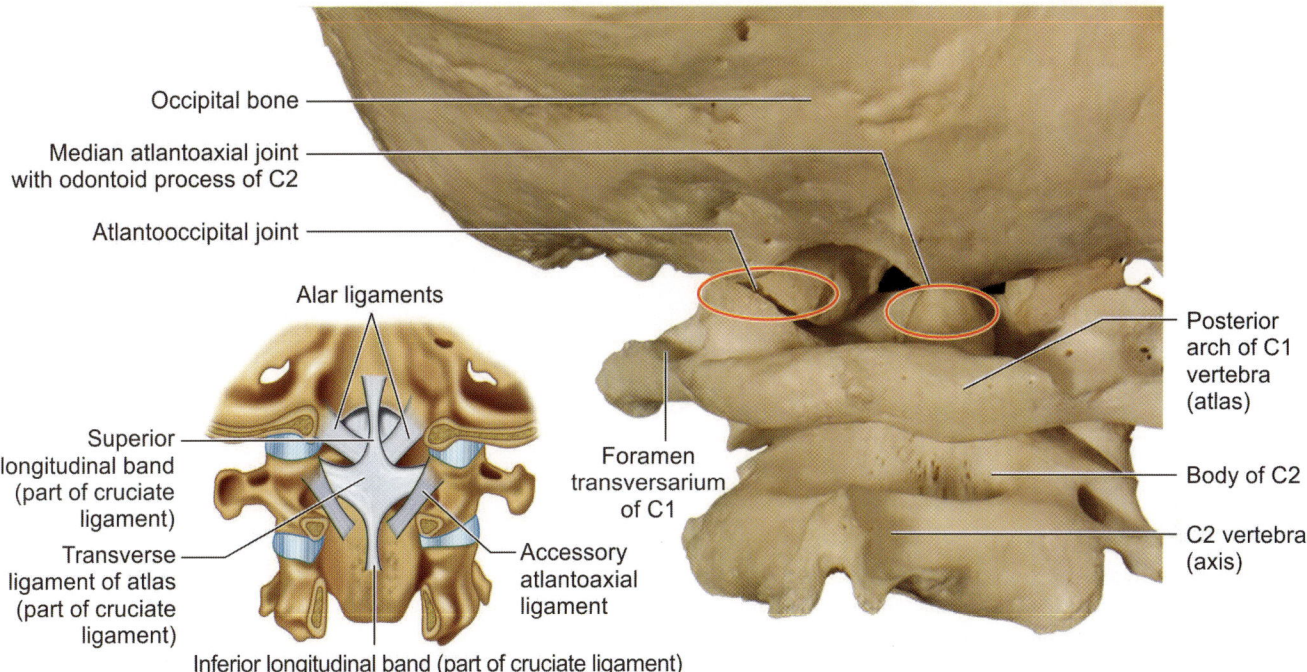

Fig. 53.4: Joints and ligaments between occipital bone, atlas and axis vertebrae

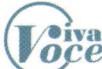

- Where are the various parts of vertebral artery placed?
- What is the relation of scalenus anterior muscle to the subclavian artery?
- What is tracheostomy and where is it performed?
- Name the ligaments between occipital bone and axis vertebra.

- Give the attachments of cruciate ligament of the atlas vertebra.
- What type of joint is median atlantoaxial joint?
- What type of joint is atlantooccipital joint?

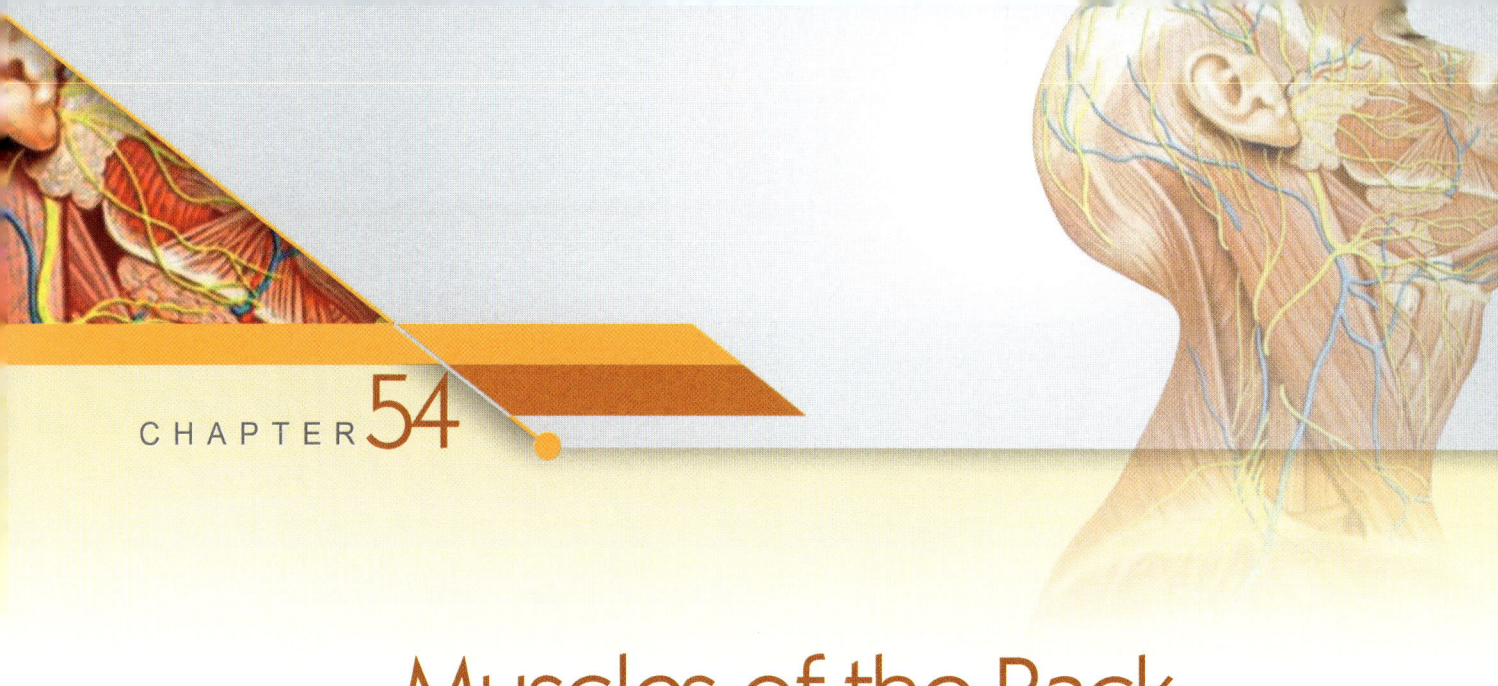

CHAPTER 54

Muscles of the Back

Learning Objectives

One should be able to

1. Name the three parts of sacrospinalis/erector spinae muscle with their attachments.
2. Name the parts of vertebral artery and their location.

OVERVIEW

Muscles of the back are disposed in 4 layers. Muscles of 1st and 2nd layers belong to upper limb and get innervated from brachial plexus. Only splenius of second layer is a true muscle of the back.

Muscles of 3rd and 4th layers are true muscles of the back. These are supplied by the dorsal rami of spinal nerves. These muscles are extensors of back.

In the uppermost part of back is a small triangle known as suboccipital triangle. It is bounded by 3 muscles. Most important content is the third part of vertebral artery and dorsal ramus of C1 nerve. This third part of the vertebral artery enters foramen magnum of occipital bone as the fourth part and unites with opposite artery to form a single median basilar artery.

STEPS OF DISSECTION

- The skin of back of neck has already been removed while the back of upper limb was dissected. If not, see the lines of incision on the "back" of upper limb (Fig. 54.1).
- Reflect the thick skin and fascia. The skin of back is innervated by dorsal rami of cervical nerves.

- Muscles of the back are disposed in four layers:
  1. Trapezius and latissimus dorsi (Fig. 54.2)
  2. a. Levator scapulae, rhomboids (Fig. 54.2)
     b. Serratus posterior superior and inferior
     c. Splenius cervicis and splenius capitis
  3. Erector spinae/sacrospinalis and semispinalis (Fig. 54.3)
  4. Multifidus, rotatoers, interspinales, intertransversarii and suboccipital muscles.

Competency achievement: The student should be able to:
AN 42.3 Describe the position, direction of fibres, relations, nerve supply, actions of semispinalis capitis and splenius capitis.

Their features are:

1. These form vertical bulges on either side of midline. These are innervated segmentally by dorsal primary rami of cervical, thoracic, lumbar and sacral nerves.
2. The erector spinae is arranged into three groups—medial, intermediate and lateral.

Medial group/spinal group consists of spinalis thoracis, spinalis cervicis and spinalis capitis.

Intermediate group/longissimus group consists of longissimus thoracis, longissimus cervicis and longissimus capitis.

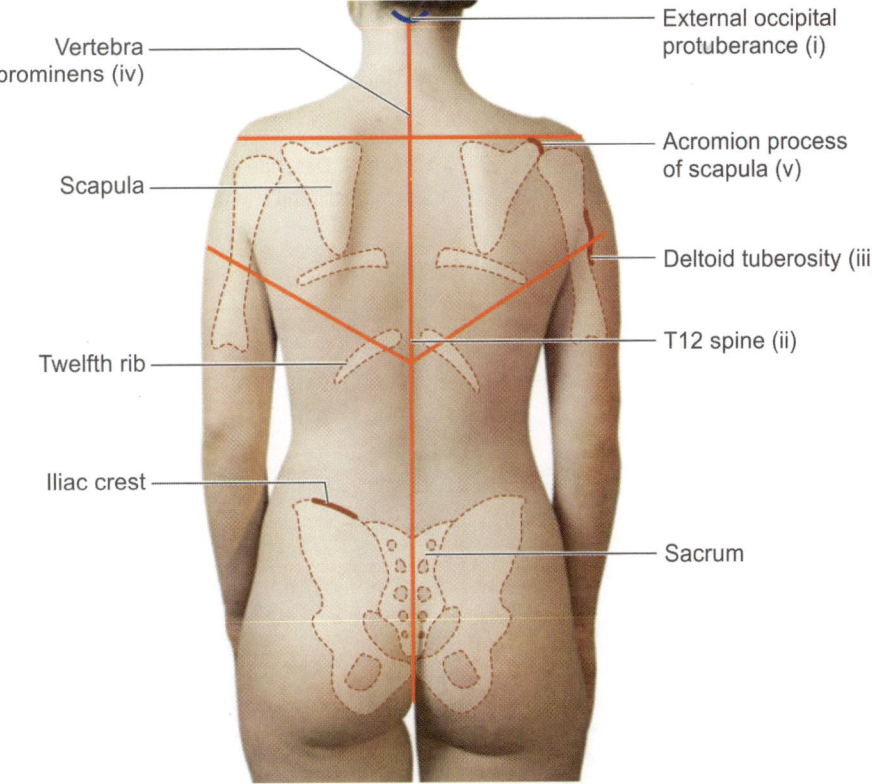

Vertebra prominens (iv)

External occipital protuberance (i)

Scapula

Acromion process of scapula (v)

Deltoid tuberosity (iii)

T12 spine (ii)

Twelfth rib

Iliac crest

Sacrum

Fig. 54.1: Lines of incision

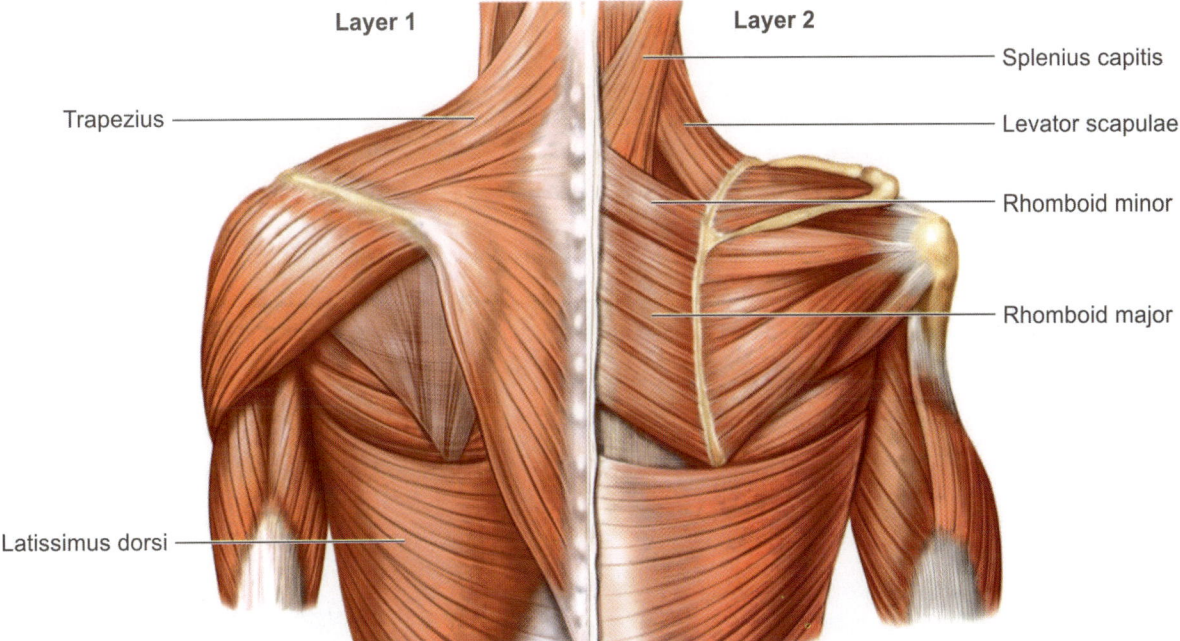

Layer 1

Layer 2

Splenius capitis

Trapezius

Levator scapulae

Rhomboid minor

Rhomboid major

Latissimus dorsi

Fig. 54.2: Muscles of 1st and 2nd layers of the back

The lateral group/iliocostocervical portion is composed of iliocostalis, costocostalis and costo-cervicalis.

The semispinalis portion of third layer consists of semispinalis thoracis, semispinalis cervicis and semispinalis capitis.

Multifidus, interspinales between the spines, intertransversarii between the transverse processes of adjacent vertebrae.

Competency achievement: The student should be able to:

AN 42.2 Describe and demonstrate the boundaries and contents of suboccipital triangle.

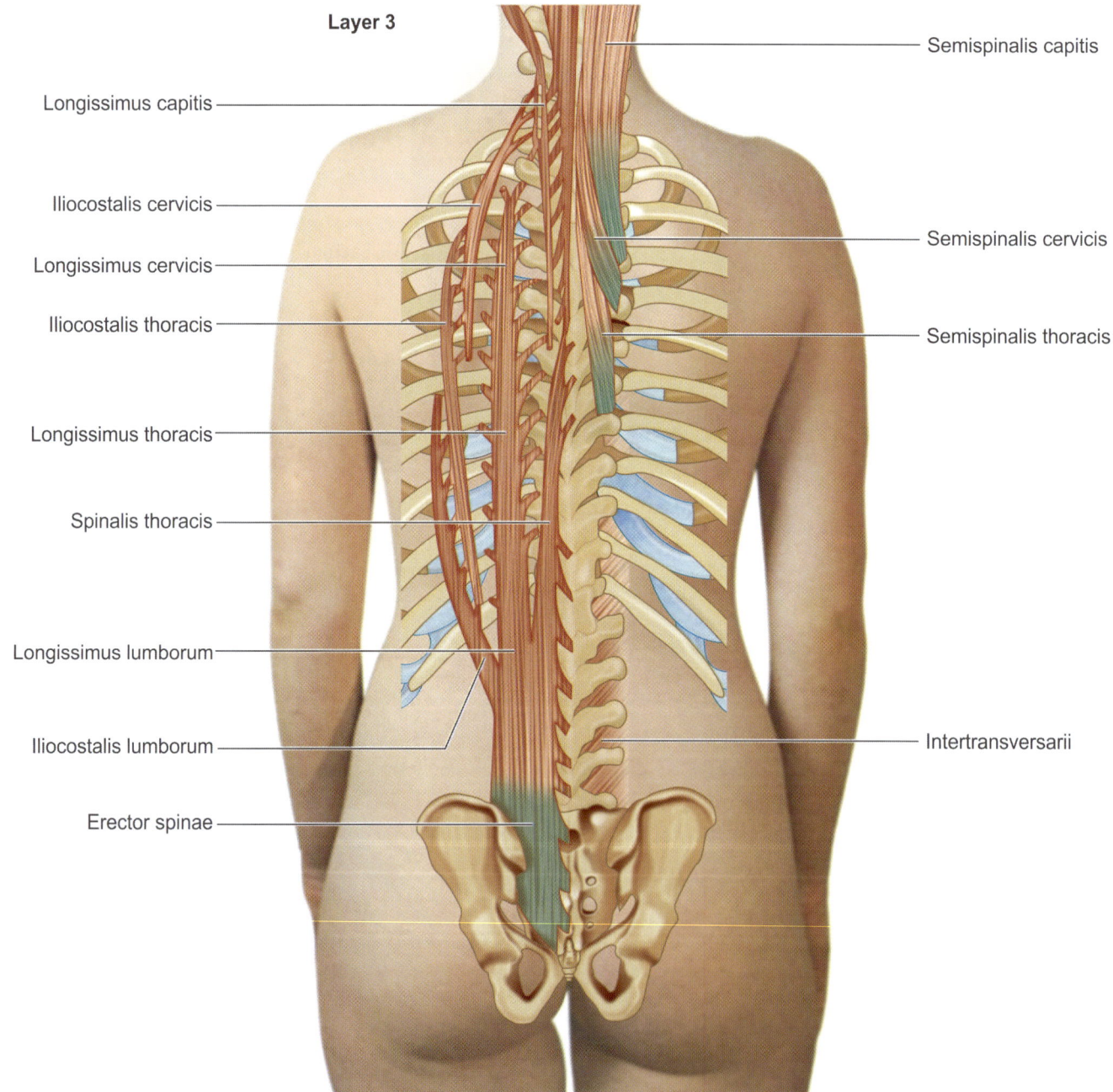

Fig. 54.3: Muscles of 3rd layer of the back

Suboccipital Triangle

- Dissect and clean the occipital artery as it emerges from under cover of the mastoid process and the muscles attached to it.
- Detach the trapezius muscle arising from the superior nuchal line and ligamentum nuchae.
- Identify splenius capitis extending between upper thoracic spines, lower ½ of ligamentum nuchae and transverse processes of C1 and C2 vertebrae and mastoid process. Separate the muscle from its origin and reflect it downwards.
- Identify semispinalis capitis attached to transverse processes of C1–C4 vertebrae and to medial ½ of area between superior and inferior nuchal lines (Fig. 54.4). Clean the thick great occipital nerve piercing this muscle.

- Detach the semispinalis capitis from its insertion and reflect it downwards. Identify great occipital nerve again and see its communication with a branch of dorsal ramus of C1 nerve (suboccipital nerve). Now trace the other branches of C1.
- Now identify the muscles forming the boundaries of suboccipital triangle. These are rectus capitis posterior major, obliquus capitis superior and obliquus capitis inferior (Fig. 54.4).
- The suboccipital nerve supplies all muscles forming boundaries of suboccipital triangle. Identify this nerve as it lies between 3rd part of vertebral artery and posterior arch of atlas. This nerve does not give any cutaneous branch.
- Trace the 3rd part of vertebral artery under the free margin of posterior atlantooccipital membrane (*see* Fig. 53.1). Clean and remove the suboccipital plexus of veins.

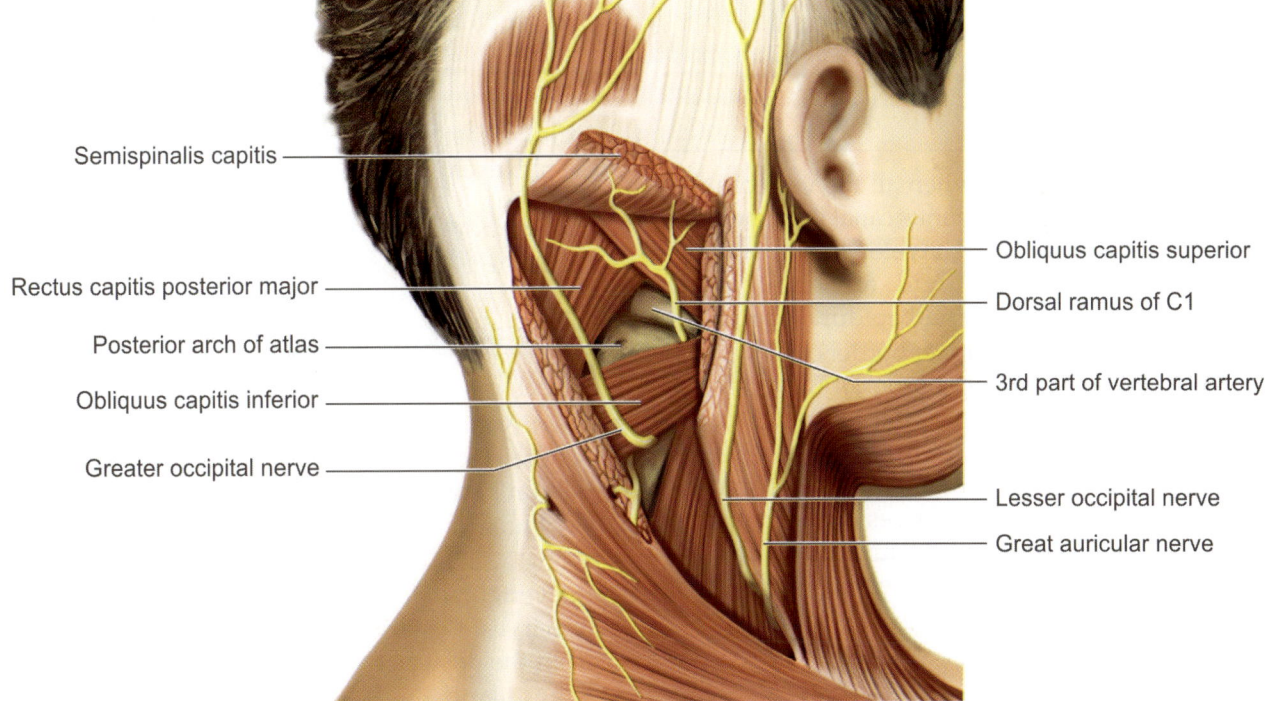

Fig. 54.4: Suboccipital triangle: Boundaries and contents

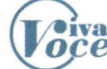

- Name the muscles in all 4 layers of the back.
- What are the boundaries of suboccipital triangle and name its contents?
- What are the parts of erector spinae muscle?
- Name the thickest cutaneous nerve of the body.

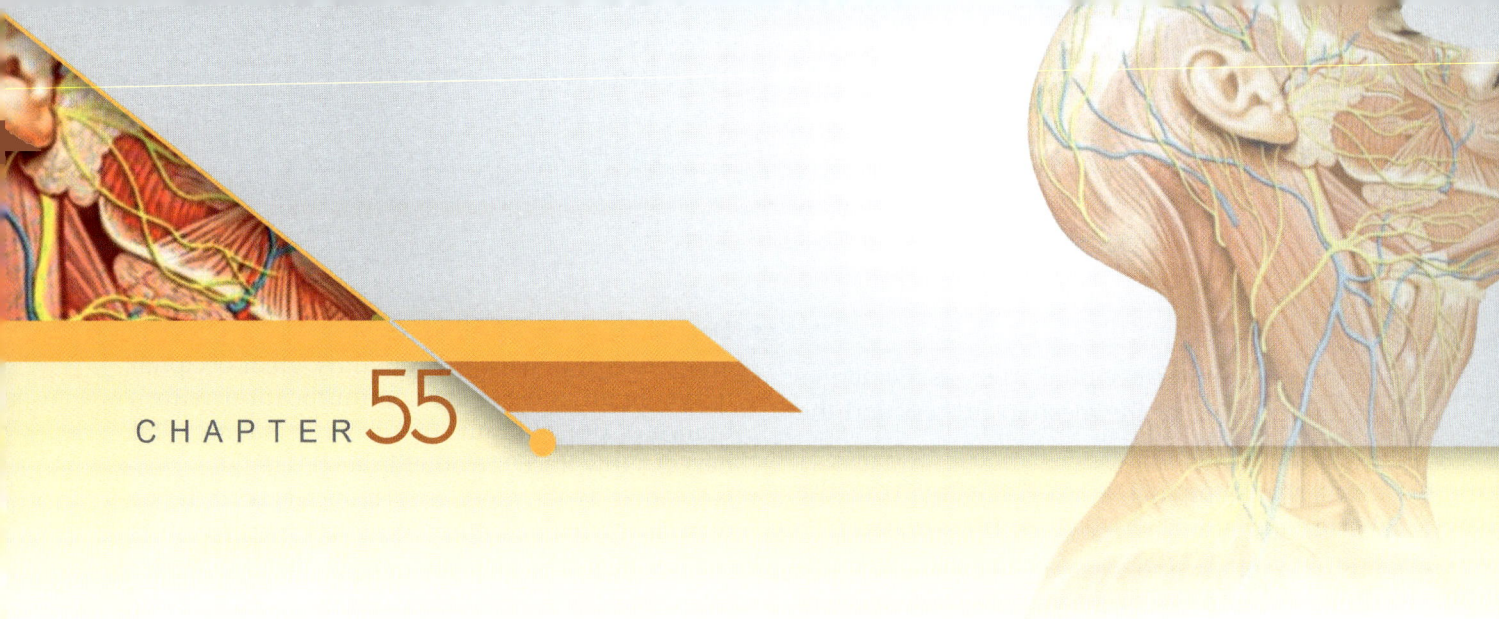

CHAPTER 55

Vertebral Canal

Learning Objectives

One should be able to

1. Comment on the formation and function of ligamentum denticulata?
2. Explain the procedure of lumbar puncture.

OVERVIEW

Vertebral canal is formed when all the vertebrae are put in sequence and a continuous canal is formed. The canal lodges the spinal cord enveloped by pia mater, subarachnoid space with fluid, arachnoid mater, subdural space, dura mater and epidural space.

Spinal cord starts at the upper border of C1 vertebra (Fig. 55.1) and ends at lower border of L1 vertebra in an adult. In a child it extends till L3 vertebra. The spinal cord gives rise to 31 pairs of spinal nerves. These are 8 cervical, 12 thoracic, 5 lumbar, 5 sacral and one coccygeal nerves. Cervical nerves lie horizontally, thoracic nerves obliquely and lumbar, sacral and coccygeal nerves vertically. The vertical nerve roots form the cauda equina.

Intervertebral foramen contains:

- Ends of dorsal and ventral nerve roots
- Dorsal root ganglion
- Nerve trunk
- Beginning of dorsal and ventral rami
- Spinal artery and vein

Vertebral venous plexus comprises external vertebral venous plexus, plexus within vertebral bodies and epidural plexus. Cancer cells from prostate, thyroid, breast, etc. can spread to cranial cavity via these plexuses.

Competency achievement: The student should be able to:

AN 42.1 Describe the contents of the vertebral canal.

STEPS OF DISSECTION

- Detach muscles on the back of vertebral column.
- Identify supraspinous and interspinous ligaments between the spines of vertebrae. Identify ligamentum flavum between the laminae of adjacent vertebrae (*see* Fig. 53.3 inset).
- Using a saw remove the spines and laminae of all the vertebrae. Identify the posterior primary rami of nerves. Posterior rami of sacral nerves emerge from the posterior sacral foramina.
- Now identify the space between vertebrae and dura mater—epidural space containing vertebral venous plexus.
- The dura mater extends from foramen magnum to S2 vertebra where it ends in a blind sac.
- Cut open the dura mater to see underlying delicate arachnoid mater. The subdural space between dura and arachnoid contains lymph for easy movements.

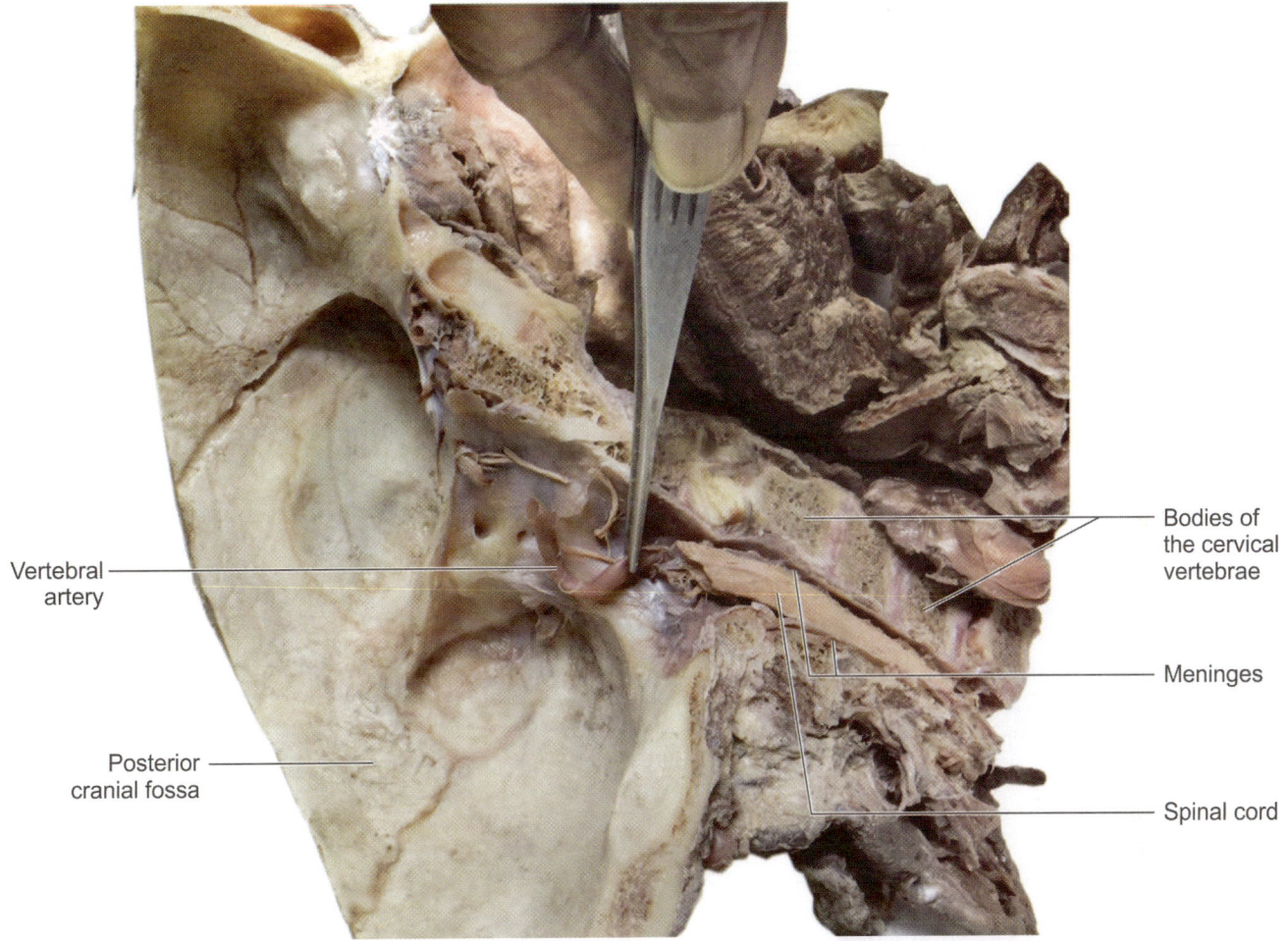

Fig. 55.1: Spinal cord in vertebral canal

Labels on figure:
Vertebral artery
Posterior cranial fossa
Bodies of the cervical vertebrae
Meninges
Spinal cord

Arachnoid mater continues with the arachnoid mater of cranial cavity and ends below at S2 level.

- The space deep to arachnoid mater is subarachnoid space. It is wide and contains cerebrospinal fluid (CSF) (Fig. 55.2).

- Remove a part of arachnoid mater to see firm pia mater. Trace pia mater beyond spinal cord as filum terminale till the back of coccyx.

- See the extensions of pia mater between dorsal and ventral primary rami as ligamentum denticulatum, which acts as a support to the spinal cord. Locate the lower end of spinal cord as conus medullaris around the lower border of L1 vertebra.

- Identify 31 pairs of spinal nerves arising from dorsal and ventral nerve roots. See that the upper nerves are horizontal, middle ones oblique and lower vertical ones are known as cauda equina (Fig. 55.3).

- Dorsal root of each spinal nerve is characterised by dorsal root ganglion. All these ganglia lie in the intervertebral foramina except C1 and C2 (placed on posterior arch of atlas and vertebral arch of axis) and sacral and coccygeal ganglia which lie in the sacral canal.

- See the arteries and veins of spinal cord.

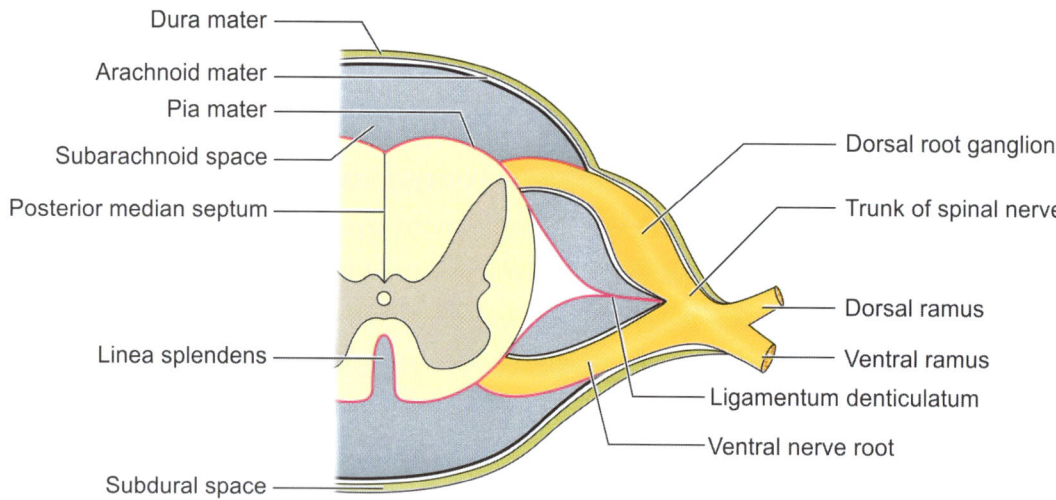

Fig. 55.2: Meninges around the spinal cord. Subarachnoid space filled with cerebrospinal fluid

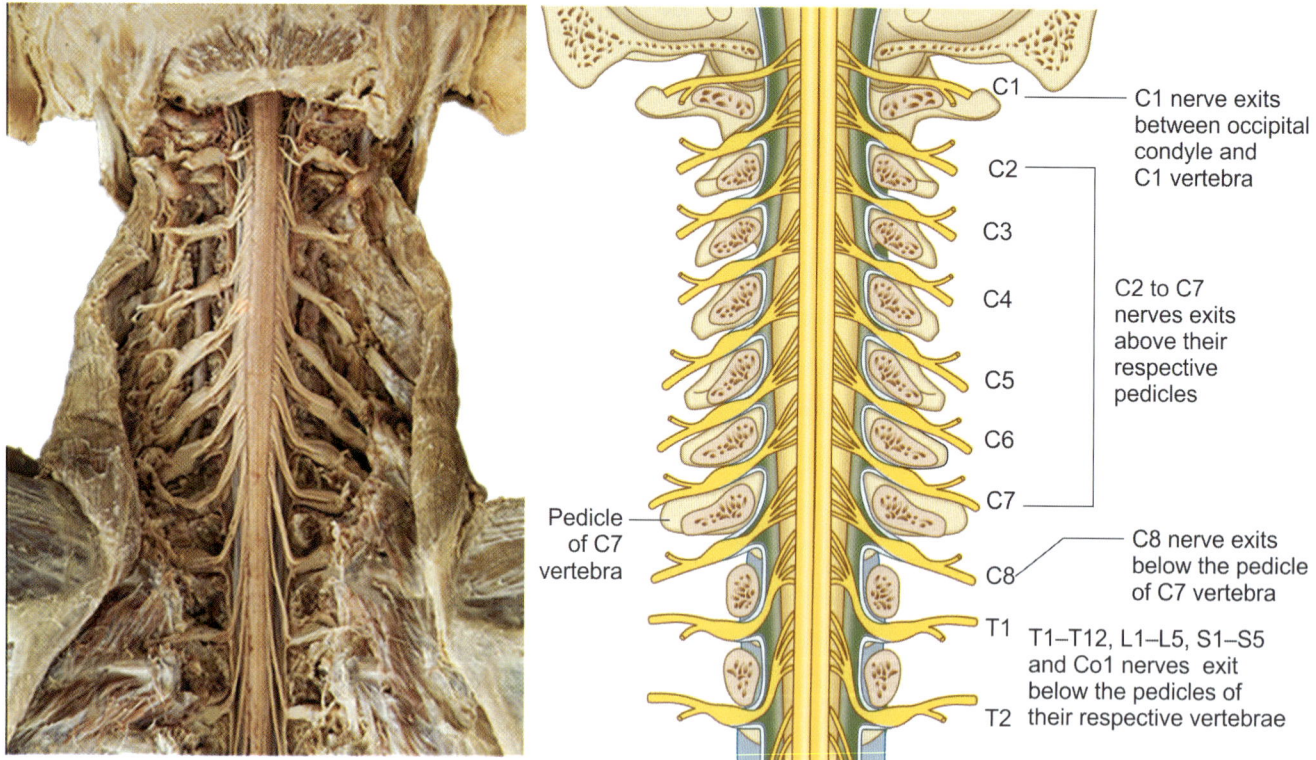

Fig. 55.3: Upper, middle and lower spinal nerves

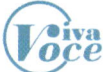

- Name the supports of the spinal cord.
- What is ligamentum denticulatum?
- Name the contents of an intervertebral foramen.
- What are the symptoms of 'cauda equina syndrome'?
- Name the parts of vertebral venous plexus.

Cranial Cavity

OVERVIEW

Cranial cavity is a space within the calvaria/brain box which is highest placed cavity in the body and houses the vital brain, meninges, venous sinuses, endocrine glands, etc. The cranial cavity contains numerous foramina for passage of nerves, veins, arteries and lowest part of medulla oblongata.

STEPS OF DISSECTION

- Detach the epicranial aponeurosis, if not already done, laterally till the inferior temporal line in the region of temple. Detach the temporalis muscle with its covering fascia and reflect these downwards over the pinna.
- Mark 2 points: 1st point—2 cm above supraorbital margin and 2nd point—1 cm above the inion/external occipital protruberance. Connect these two points by a line passing around the skull on each side (Fig. 56.1).
- Saw through the outer table of skull and observe the diploe (Fig. 56.2a).
- Gently break the inner table with a hammer and chisel. See that the brain is not damaged.

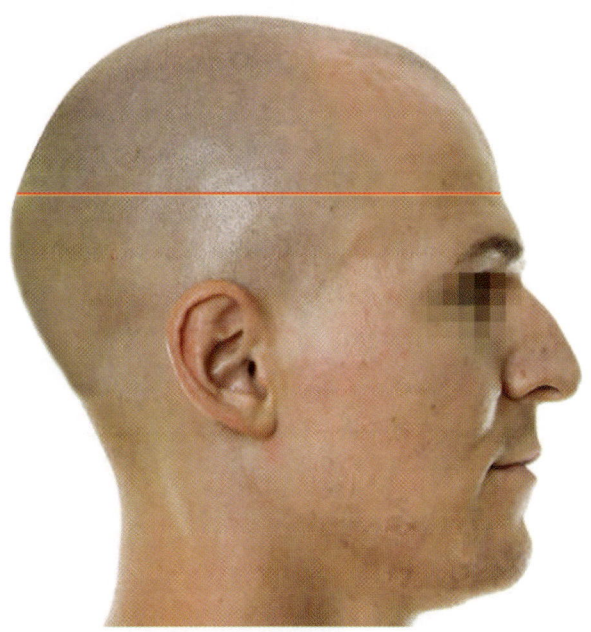

Fig. 56.1: Line of incision

- Examine the endosteal layer of dura mater—see this layer fusing with meningeal layer, except at the site of venous sinuses (Fig. 56.2a).

- Identify the veins and arteries on the dura mater (Fig. 56.2a and b). The veins are superficial as compared to the arteries and produce the grooves on the inner aspect of skull.

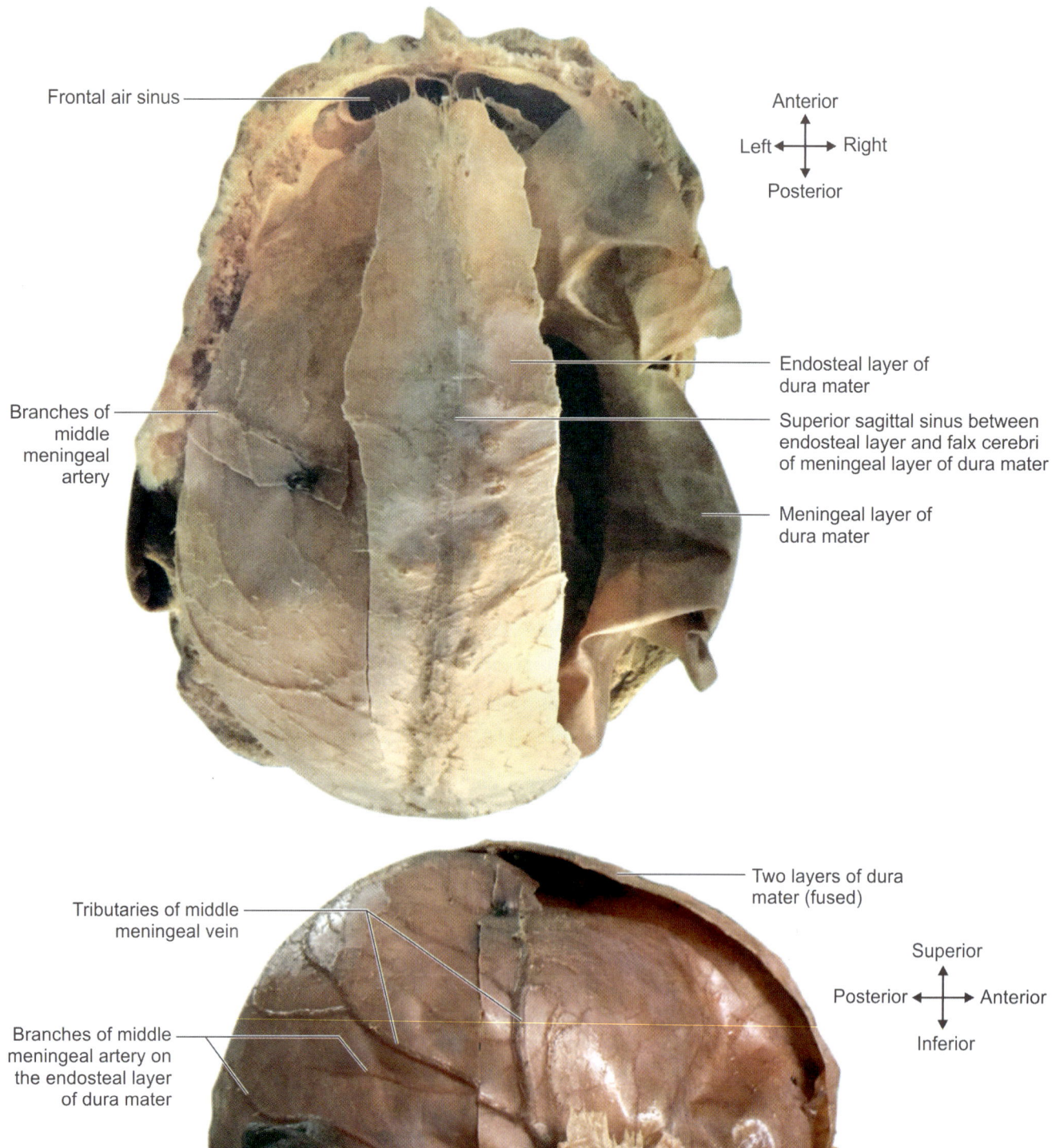

Frontal air sinus

Branches of middle meningeal artery

Anterior
Left ← → Right
Posterior

Endosteal layer of dura mater

Superior sagittal sinus between endosteal layer and falx cerebri of meningeal layer of dura mater

Meningeal layer of dura mater

Tributaries of middle meningeal vein

Branches of middle meningeal artery on the endosteal layer of dura mater

Two layers of dura mater (fused)

Superior
Posterior ← → Anterior
Inferior

Fig. 56.2: Meningeal vessels in the endosteal layer of dura mater

- Slit the outer layer of dura mater in the sagittal plane and see the superior sagittal sinus.
- Clean the sinus and identify the arachnoid villi/granulations projection into the sinus. Trace some cerebral veins draining into the sinus.

Competency achievement: The student should be able to:

AN 30.3 Describe and identify dural folds and dural venous sinuses.

- Give an incision on both side of superior sagittal sinus and a cut close to crista galli. Then try to pull out a fold of meningeal layer of dura mater—the falx cerebri between two cerebral hemispheres (Figs 56.3 and 56.4a). This fold can be pulled till the occipital lobes.
- See that falx cerebri is sickle shaped (Fig. 56.3). At its inferior border identify a thin inferior sagittal sinus (Fig. 56.3).
- Pull backwards a similar fold of dura mater between two lobes of cerebellum—the falx cerebelli.
- Identify the attachments of tentorium cerebelli (Figs 56.4a and b). Its attached border is attached to lips of groove for the transverse sinus, superior border of petrous temporal bone and posterior clinoid process. Its free border is attached to anterior clinoid processes.
- Try to look for diaphragma sellae over the hypophyseal fossa.

Competency achievement: The student should be able to:

AN 30.1 Describe the cranial fossae and identify related structures.

Anterior Cranial Fossa

- Put 2–3 blocks under the shoulder so that head falls backwards. Lift the frontal lobes of the brain. This will expose the olfactory bulbs. Look for olfactory rootlets emerging from cribriform plate of ethmoid joining the olfactory bulb.
- Identify optic nerve, ophthalmic artery, branch of internal carotid artery entering the optic canal.
- The lesser wing of sphenoid forms posterior boundary of anterior cranial fossa (Fig. 56.5). Identify a venous sinus—sphenoparietal sinus lying along free border of lesser wing. Incise the dura here.
- Identify anterior clinoid process to which free border of tentorium cerebelli is attached (Fig. 56.5).

Middle Cranial Fossa

Middle cranial fossa lies between anterior and posterior fossa (Fig. 56.5). Its boundary is formed by superior border of petrous temporal bone laterally and dorsum sellae in the midline.

- Identify concave depression in the body of sphenoid called the sella turcica. A fold of dura mater is placed horizontally over this sella/

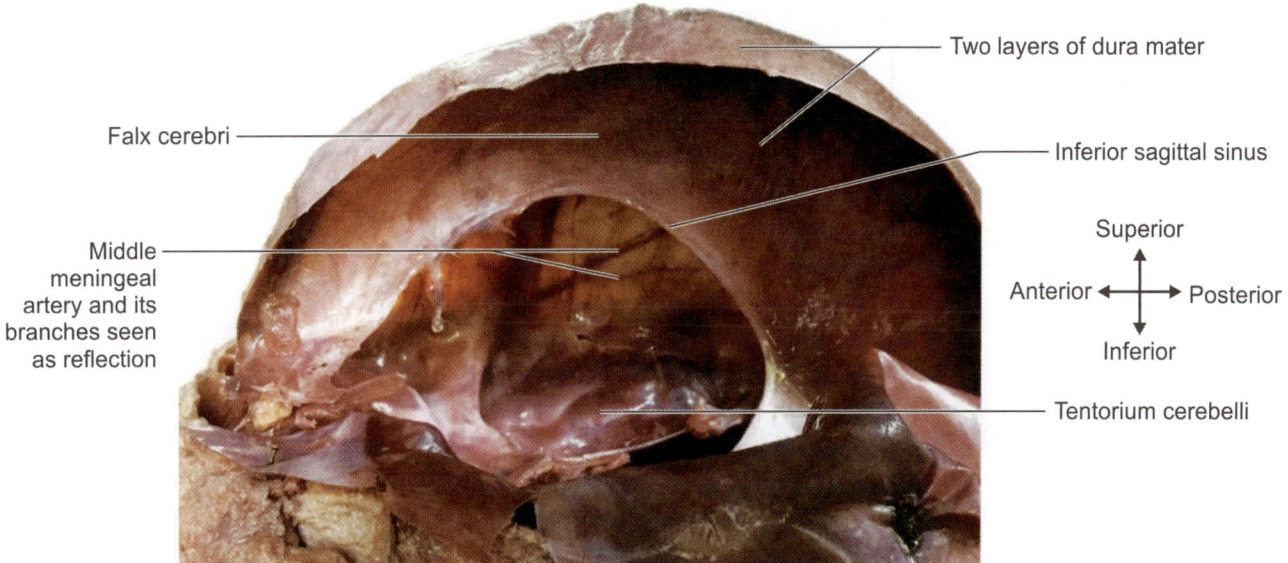

Fig. 56.3: Falx cerebri with venous sinuses

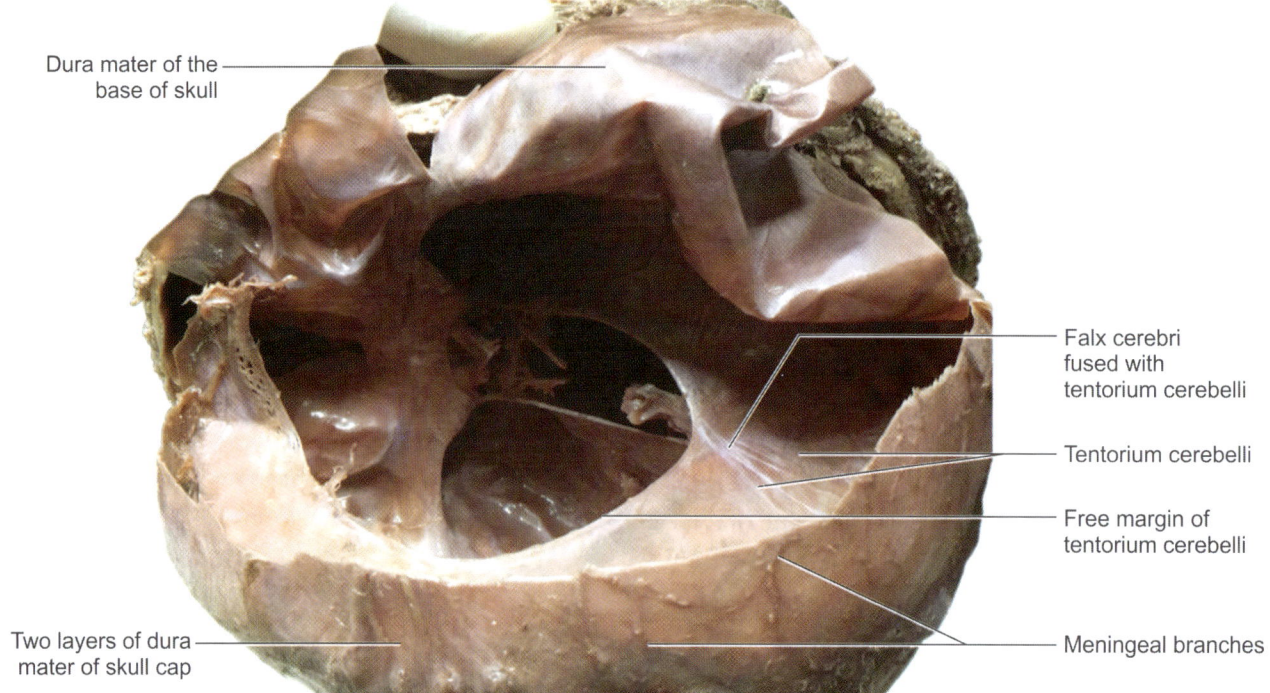

Dura mater of the base of skull

Falx cerebri fused with tentorium cerebelli

Tentorium cerebelli

Free margin of tentorium cerebelli

Two layers of dura mater of skull cap

Meningeal branches

Fig. 56.4a: Tentorium cerebelli(upside down)

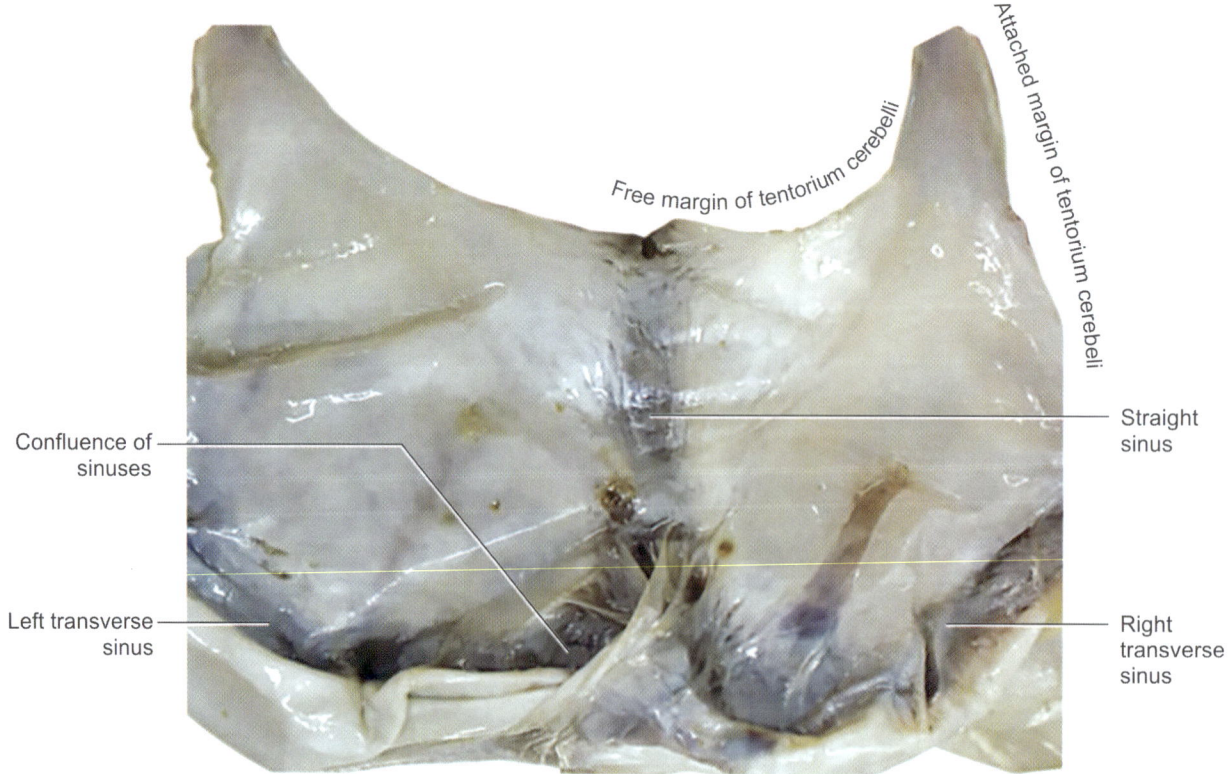

Free margin of tentorium cerebelli

Attached margin of tentorium cerebeli

Confluence of sinuses

Straight sinus

Left transverse sinus

Right transverse sinus

Fig. 56.4b: Tentorium cerebelli with related venous sinuses

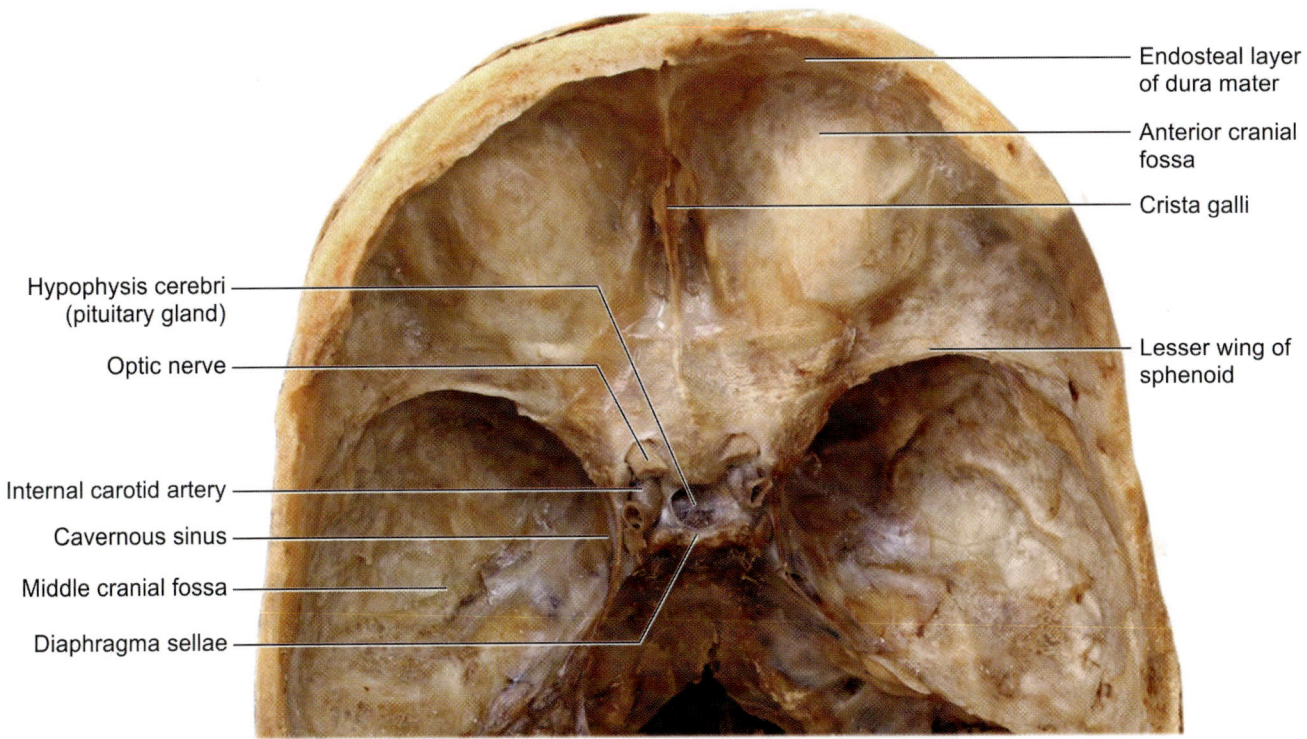

Hypophysis cerebri
(pituitary gland)

Optic nerve

Internal carotid artery

Cavernous sinus

Middle cranial fossa

Diaphragma sellae

Endosteal layer
of dura mater

Anterior cranial
fossa

Crista galli

Lesser wing of
sphenoid

Fig. 56.5: Structures in anterior and middle cranial fossae

hypophyseal fossa. The fold is diaphragma sellae (Fig. 56.5). It protects the hypophysis cerebri from being pressed by the cerebrum.

- Look for cavernous sinus present on either side of body of sphenoid (Fig. 56.6). Cut through it between the anterior and posterior ends and locate its contents (Fig. 56.6). Define its connections with other venous sinuses.

- Identify oculomotor nerve piercing the dura mater between free and attached margins of tentorium cerebelli to enter cavernous sinus.

- See trochlear nerve below oculomotor nerve.

- Below trochlear nerve is ophthalmic division (V_1) of trigeminal (V) nerve, and below ophthalmic is maxillary division (V_2) of V nerve.

- Trace both V_1 and V_2 divisions backwards till the trigeminal ganglion lying at the anterior face of petrous temporal bone.

- Identify the dural fold, cavum trigeminale and incise it to see ganglion of V nerve. Trace the motor root of V nerve under the V ganglion. It joins V_3 nerve.

- The mandibular division (V_3) of V nerve arises from lateral side of ganglion and exits from the cranial cavity via the foramen ovale. Remove the dura mater forming the lateral wall of cavernous sinus and identify internal carotid artery and abducent (VI) nerve.

- Try to remove the dura mater from anterior surface of petrous temporal bone and look for greater petrosal nerve which joins with deep petrosal (sympathetic) to form nerve of pterygoid canal.

- Below greater petrosal, look for a slender lesser petrosal nerve which exits skull through foramen ovale.

- See the middle meningeal artery entering the skull through foramen spinosum. After a short course, it divides into a larger anterior branch and a smaller posterior branch. The anterior branch runs till inner aspect of pterion and then upwards and medially almost parallel to precentral sulcus (Fig. 56.7). The posterior branch runs up to the lambda.

- Identify the temporal lobe in the lateral part of middle cranial fossa. In its central part lies the diencephalon.

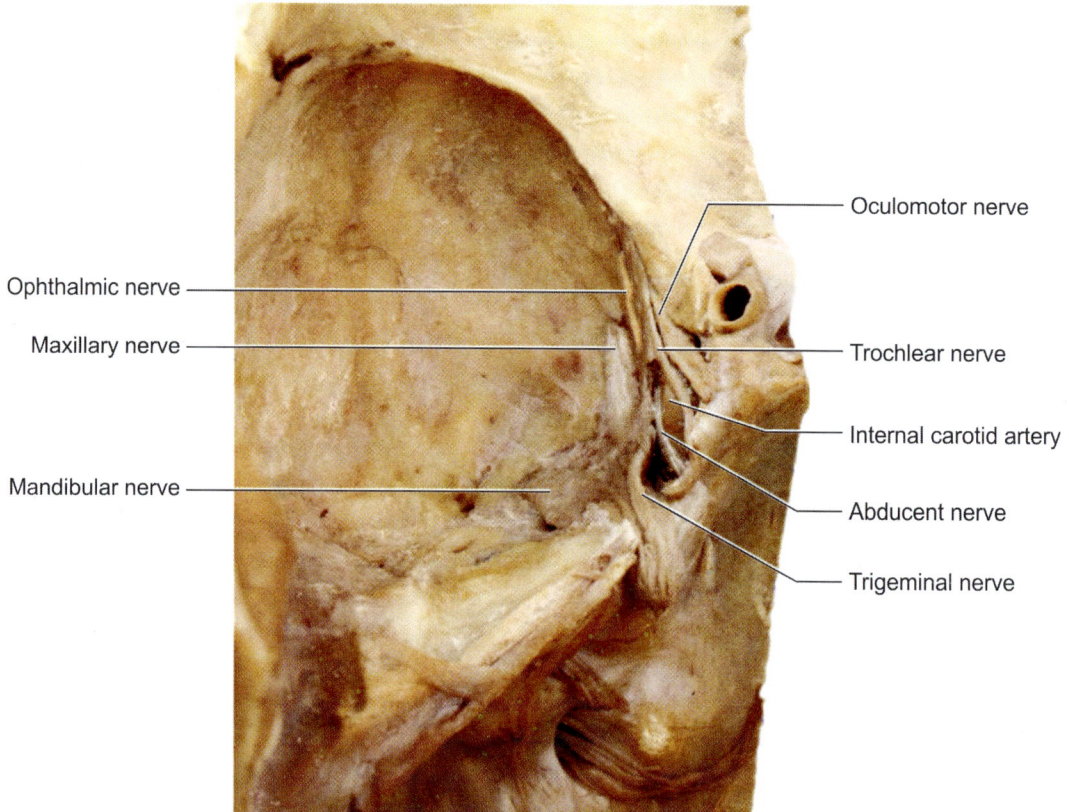

Ophthalmic nerve

Maxillary nerve

Mandibular nerve

Oculomotor nerve

Trochlear nerve

Internal carotid artery

Abducent nerve

Trigeminal nerve

Fig. 56.6: Contents of cavernous venous sinus

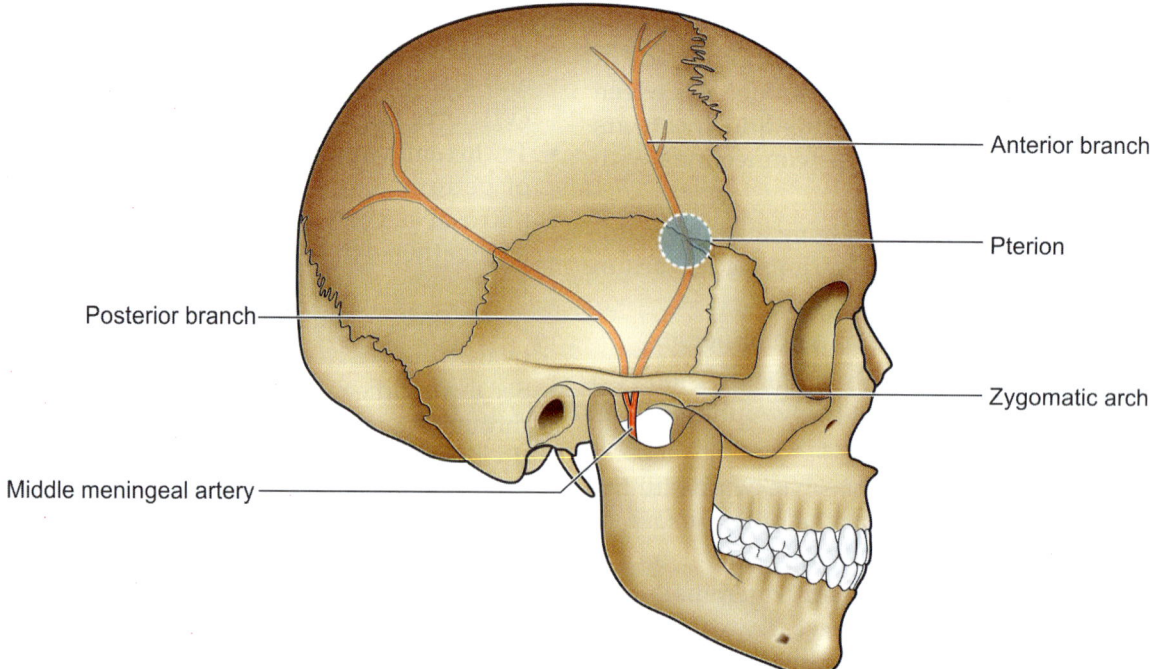

Posterior branch

Middle meningeal artery

Anterior branch

Pterion

Zygomatic arch

Fig. 56.7: Course of middle meningeal artery

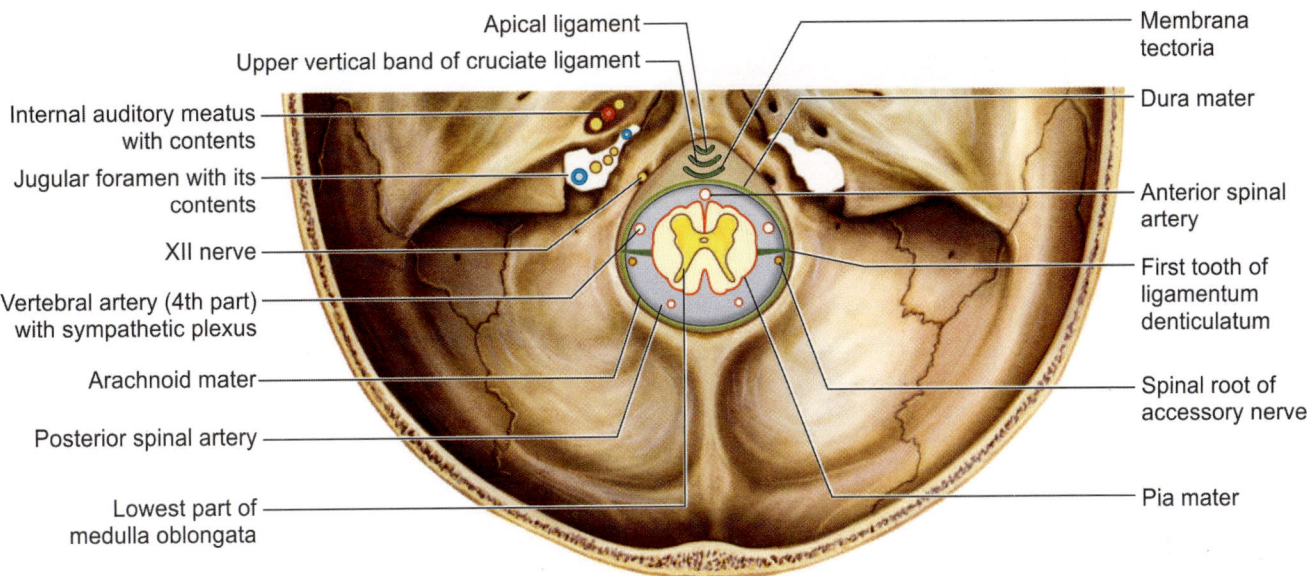

Apical ligament
Upper vertical band of cruciate ligament
Membrana tectoria
Internal auditory meatus with contents
Dura mater
Jugular foramen with its contents
XII nerve
Anterior spinal artery
Vertebral artery (4th part) with sympathetic plexus
First tooth of ligamentum denticulatum
Arachnoid mater
Spinal root of accessory nerve
Posterior spinal artery
Lowest part of medulla oblongata
Pia mater

Fig. 56.8: *Structures in posterior cranial fossa*

Posterior Cranial Fossa

Posterior cranial fossa is the deepest fossa. The 2 lobes of cerebellum (below) and 2 occipital lobes of cerebrum (above) are situated in this fossa. It also has the largest foramen—foramen magnum through which medulla oblongata continues as the spinal cord.

Identify VI nerve—the abducent nerve piercing dura mater over the clivus.

Identify VII nerve—the facial nerve with VIII-vestibulocochlear nerve and labyrinthine vessels entering internal acoustic meatus (Fig. 56.8).

Look for IX, X, XI nerves leaving through the middle part of jugular foramen (Fig. 56.8). Its anterior part gives passage to inferior petrosal sinus, while its posterior part gives exit to sigmoid sinus which continues as internal jugular vein.

XII nerve—the hypoglossal nerve exits through anterior condylar canal/hypoglossal canal (Fig. 56.8).

Through the foramen magnum identify the beginning of spinal cord, three meninges, anterior and posterior spinal arteries, vertebral arteries, spinal root of XI nerve. Three ligaments—apical ligament, upper band of cruciate ligament and membrana tectoria pass through anterior most part.

Note the following venous sinuses:

1. Superior sagittal sinus (Fig. 56.2)
2. Inferior sagittal sinus (Fig. 56.3)
3. Superior petrosal sinus
4. Inferior petrosal sinus
5. Transverse sinus (Fig. 56.4b)
6. Straight sinus (Fig. 56.4b)
7. Sigmoid sinus
8. Occipital sinus

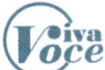

Viva Voce

- Where do superior sagittal and inferior sagittal venous sinuses lie?
- How many roots are there in trigeminal ganglion? Name its branches.
- Name the structures present in the lateral wall of cavernous sinus.
- Name the cranial nerves in order.
- Name the four parts of internal carotid artery.
- Which artery lies on the inner aspect of the pterion?

Orbit

OVERVIEW

The orbit is a big hollow cavity in the upper part of skull on each side. It is a deep socket, bounded by frontal bone superiorly, zygomatic bone laterally, nose medially and maxilla bone inferiorly (Fig. 57.1). All these structures provide support and protection to the contents of orbital cavity. It gives accommodation to the eyeball, extraocular muscles, nerves, blood vessels, ligaments and the lacrimal apparatus.

The seven voluntary muscles are superior, inferior, medial and lateral recti, superior and inferior obliques and levator palpebrae superioris. Involuntary muscles are superior and inferior tarsal muscles. Nerves for the extraocular muscles are III, IV and VI cranial nerves. Involuntary muscles are innervated by sympathetic fibres. Ophthalmic artery is the artery of the orbit. Its most important branch is the central artery of retina which is an end artery. The sensory nerves for the orbit are from branches of ophthalmic division of trigeminal nerve.

Competency achievement: The student should be able to:

AN 31.1 Describe and identify extraocular muscles of eyeball.

STEPS OF DISSECTION

- Strip the endosteum from the floor of the anterior cranial fossa. Gently break the orbital plate of frontal bone forming the roof of the orbit and remove it in pieces so that orbital periosteum is clearly visible.
- On the medial aspect of orbit, identify ethmoidal nerves and vessels.
- Posteriorly identify optic canal and superior orbital fissure. Identify the optic nerve and ophthalmic artery passing through optic canal.
- Identify and trace chiefly the nerves traversing the superior orbital fissure. From lateral to medial side these are:
  i. Lacrimal, frontal and trochlear nerves
  ii. Upper division of oculomotor
  iii. Nasociliary
  iv. Lower division of oculomotor
  v. Abducent nerve most laterally.
- Ophthalmic veins also traverse this fissure, superior ophthalmic vein in upper part and inferior ophthalmic vein in lower part of superior orbital fissure. Revise these structures on dried skull.

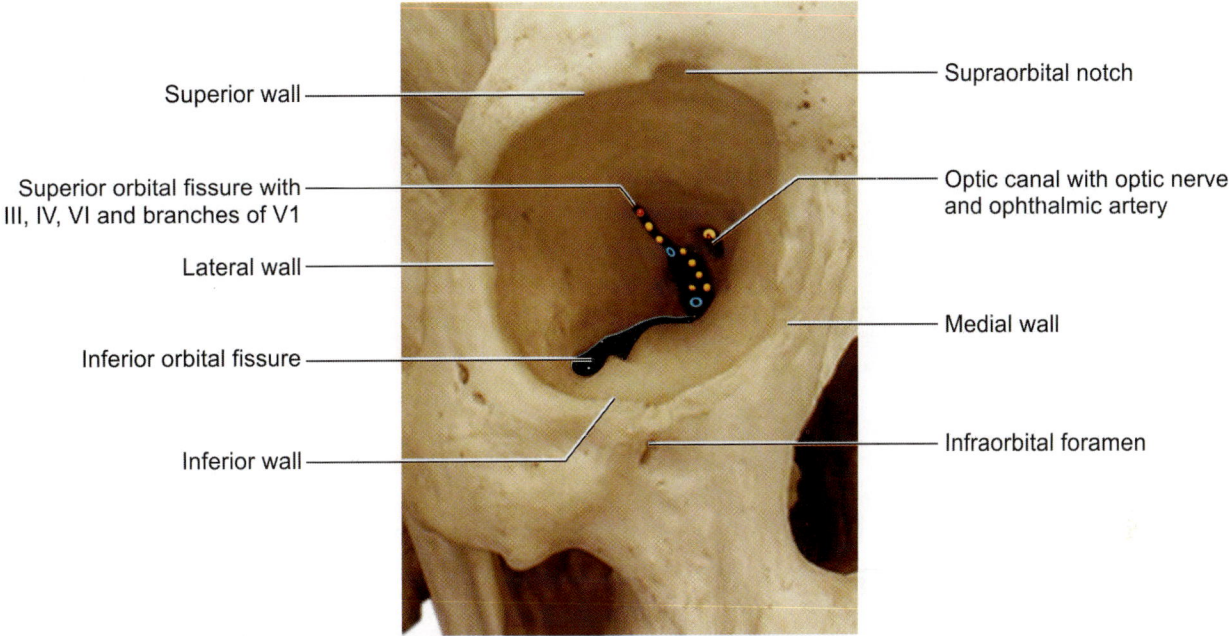

Superior wall

Superior orbital fissure with III, IV, VI and branches of V1

Lateral wall

Inferior orbital fissure

Inferior wall

Supraorbital notch

Optic canal with optic nerve and ophthalmic artery

Medial wall

Infraorbital foramen

Fig. 57.1: Bony boundaries of the orbit

- Define the orbital fascia and fascial sheath of the eyeball.
- Divide the orbital periosteum along the middle of the orbit anteroposteriorly. Cut through it horizontally close to the anterior margin of orbit.
- Now the superficial structures in the orbit are visible.
- Identify superior oblique muscle placed in a sagittal plane along the medial wall of orbit (Fig. 57.2).
- Identify and preserve trochlear nerve entering the superior oblique muscle in the superomedial angle of the orbit (Fig. 57.2).
- Find the frontal nerve lying in the midline on levator palpebrae superioris muscle. See it dividing into its two terminal divisions in the anterior part of orbit (Fig. 57.2).
- Identify superior rectus beneath the levator palpebrae superioris muscle (Fig. 57.3).
- Trace the upper division of oculomotor nerve lying between these two muscles and innervating both of them.
- Identify the lacrimal nerve and artery running along the lateral wall of the orbit. These reach the superolateral corner of the orbit. Lacrimal nerve carries secretomotor fibres from pterygopalatine ganglion to the lacrimal gland.

- Follow the tendon of superior oblique muscle passing superolaterally beneath the superior rectus to be inserted into the sclera behind its equator. It is inserted just above the insertion of inferior oblique muscle.
- Now divide frontal nerve, levator palpebrae superioris and superior rectus in their middle and reflect them apart.
- Now identify deeper structures in the orbit (Fig. 57.4).
- Locate the optic nerve coursing laterally from the optic foramen/canal. This is a thick nerve easily identifiable (Fig. 57.4).
- Identify the structures crossing optic nerve superficially from lateral to medial side. These are nasociliary nerve (Fig. 57.4), ophthalmic artery and superior ophthalmic vein.
- See the branches of nasociliary nerve:
  i. Communicating branch to ciliary ganglion
  ii. 2–3 long ciliary nerves (Fig. 57.4)
  iii. Posterior ethmoidal nerve
  iv. Infratrochlear nerve
  v. Anterior ethmoidal nerve
- Locate the branches of ophthalmic artery:
  i. Central artery of retina—most important branch as it is an end artery.

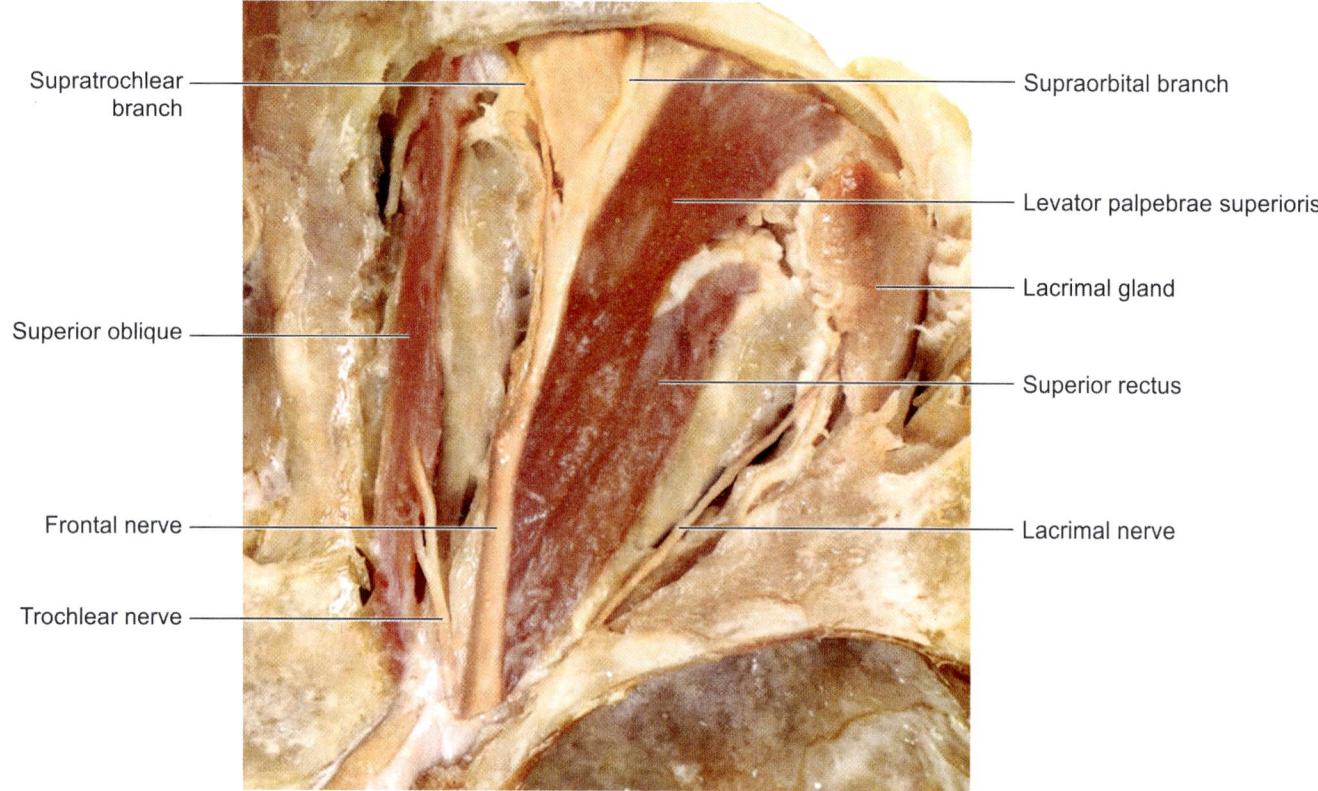

Supratrochlear branch

Superior oblique

Frontal nerve

Trochlear nerve

Supraorbital branch

Levator palpebrae superioris

Lacrimal gland

Superior rectus

Lacrimal nerve

Fig. 57.2: Superficial dissection of the orbit

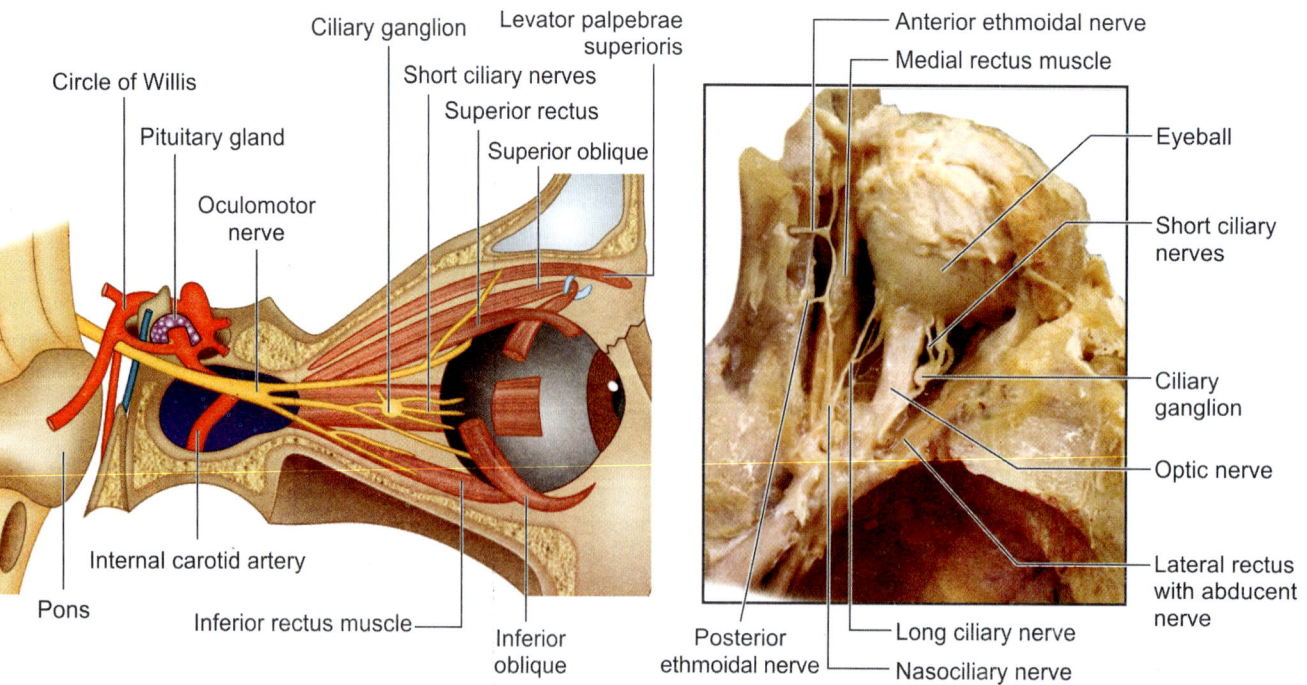

Ciliary ganglion

Levator palpebrae superioris

Short ciliary nerves

Superior rectus

Superior oblique

Circle of Willis

Pituitary gland

Oculomotor nerve

Internal carotid artery

Pons

Inferior rectus muscle

Inferior oblique

Fig. 57.3: Oculomotor nerve and related muscles

Anterior ethmoidal nerve

Medial rectus muscle

Eyeball

Short ciliary nerves

Ciliary ganglion

Optic nerve

Lateral rectus with abducent nerve

Posterior ethmoidal nerve

Long ciliary nerve

Nasociliary nerve

Fig. 57.4: Deep structures in the orbit

ii. Lacrimal artery giving branches to lacrimal gland

iii. Zygomatic branches

iv. Lateral palpebral

v. Muscular branches.

vi. Long and short posterior ciliary arteries

vii. Supraorbital and supratrochlear branches

viii. Anterior and posterior ethmoidal branches, medial palpebral and dorsal nasal branches.

- Look for two long ciliary nerves and 12–20 short ciliary nerves (Fig. 57.4).
- Remove the orbital fat. Look carefully in the posterior part of the interval between optic nerve and lateral rectus muscle along the lateral wall of the orbit to locate and identify pin head sized ciliary ganglion (Fig. 57.3).
- Trace the roots connecting the ganglion to the nasociliary nerve (sensory root), nerve to inferior oblique (parasympathetic root) and nerve fibres from long ciliary artery (sympathetic root).

- Now identify the abducent nerve closely adherent to the medial surface of lateral rectus muscle (Fig. 57.3).
- Incise the inferior fornix of conjunctiva and palpebral fascia. Elevate the eyeball and remove fat and fascia to identify the origin of inferior oblique muscle from the floor of orbit anteriorly.
- Identify levator palpebrae superioris and superior rectus above the eyeball; superior oblique superomedially; medial rectus medially; lateral rectus laterally and inferior rectus inferiorly (Figs 57.2 and 57.3).
- These seven extraocular muscles are seen as miniature ribbon muscles having short tendon of origin and long tendons of insertion.
- See that four recti muscles are inserted anterior to the equator; two obliques are inserted behind the equator and levator palpabrae superioris gets inserted into upper tarsal plate, skin of upper eyelid and into superior conjunctival fornix.

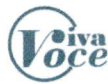 **Viva Voce**

- Name the extraocular muscles with their nerve supply.
- What nerves course through superior orbital fissure?
- What type of artery is 'central artery of retina' and why?

- Name the roots and branches of the ciliary ganglion.
- What are the nerve supply and insertions of levator palpebrae superioris muscle?
- Which are the muscles innervated by fibres of Edinger-Westphal nucleus?

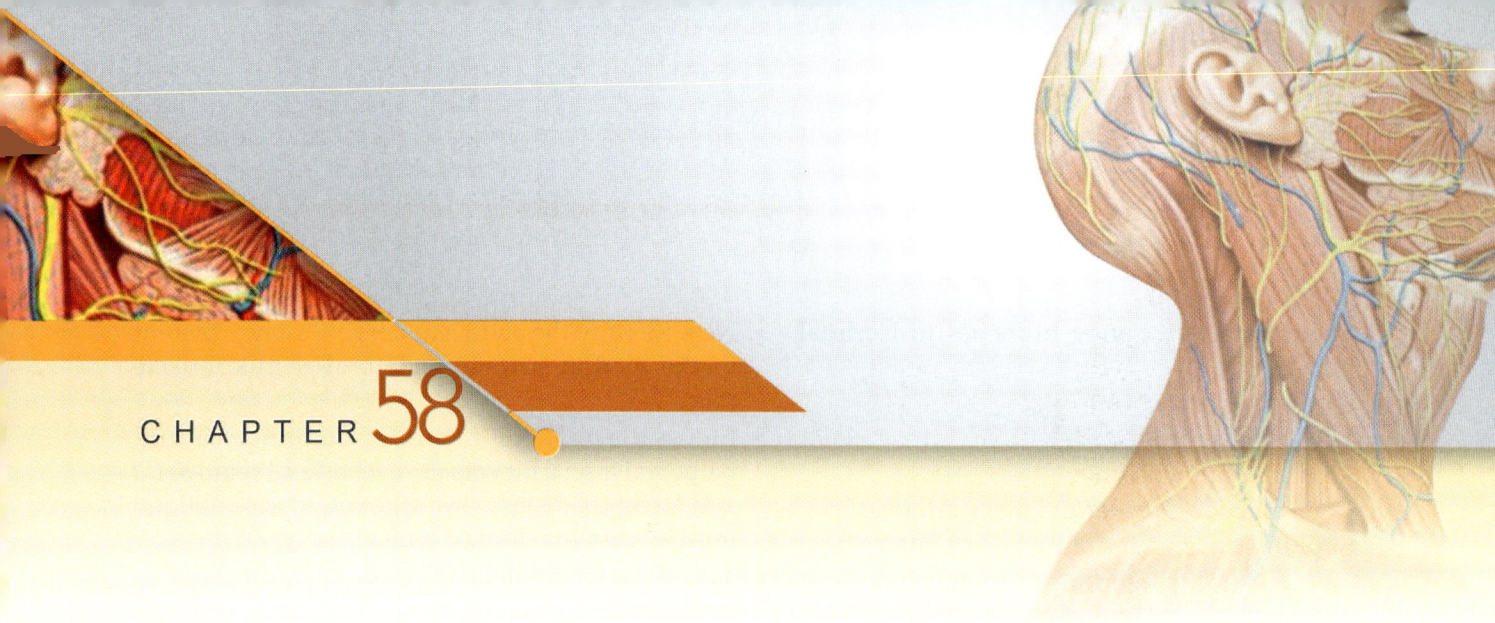

CHAPTER 58

Mouth and Pharynx

Learning Objectives

One should be able to

1. Identify the opening of parotid duct in the vestibule of mouth.
2. Learn nerve supply and blood supply of upper and lower teeth.
3. Name the arteries supplying the palatine tonsil.

OVERVIEW

Mouth hardly needs dissection. The structures in the mouth are seen in each other's mouth. These can also be seen in self with the help of a hand mirror.

Look at the lips, cheeks, oral cavity proper and vestibule on each side of oral cavity.

Oral cavity proper is the cavity bounded by all the upper and lower teeth. Tongue is the biggest content of this cavity.

On each side of oral cavity proper between the teeth and cheek is a space called vestibule. In the vestibule is the opening of the parotid duct opposite the crown of 2nd upper molar tooth.

The vestibule opens into the mouth cavity proper behind the 3rd molar.

The two lips form the upper and lower boundaries of the oral fissure. Lips are lined by skin on the outside and by mucous membrane on the inner aspect and muscles (orbicularis oris) in between.

The cheeks form a large part of the face. Nasolabial folds indicate the junction of lips and cheeks.

Oral Cavity Proper

Identify the following structures—teeth, gums, alveolar arches of the jaws. Sublingual region shows sublingual fold with a papilla medially for the opening of the duct of the submandibular gland and 8–10 ducts of sublingual gland.

The tongue occupies most of this cavity. Roof is seen to be formed by hard palate and soft palate.

Oral cavity continues with oropharynx posteriorly. The junction is called oropharyngeal isthmus.

STEPS OF DISSECTION

- Make a soft sagittal section of head and neck.
- Cut through the centre of the frontal bone, internasal suture, intermaxillary suture, chin, hyoid bone, thyroid, cricoid and tracheal cartilages. Carry the incision through the septum of the nose, nasopharynx, tongue and both the hard and soft palates.
- Cut through the centre of remaining occipital bone and cervical vertebrae. This will complete the sagittal section of head and neck (Fig. 58.1).

Hard Palate

- See the hard palate on a dried skull. Identify the various foramina and revise the structures passing through these foramina. Strip the mucoperiosteum of hard palate. The mucous membrane and the overlying periosteum are intimately fused to each other. The two together are called mucoperiosteum. See that the hard palate separates the nasal cavity above from the oral cavity below (Fig. 58.1). Identify the greater palatine artery entering the region of hard palate. It is a branch of 3rd part of maxillary artery.
- Look for nasopalatine and anterior palatine nerves, branches of pterygopalatine ganglion.

Competency achievement: The student should be able to:

AN 36.1 Describe the: (1) morphology, relations, blood supply and applied anatomy of palatine tonsil, (2) composition of soft palate.

Soft Palate

- Identify the half of the soft palate in the sagittal section of head and neck (Fig. 58.1).
- *Identify its:*
    i. 2 surfaces—anterior concave surface and posterior convex surface.
    ii. 2 borders—attached superior border and free inferior border

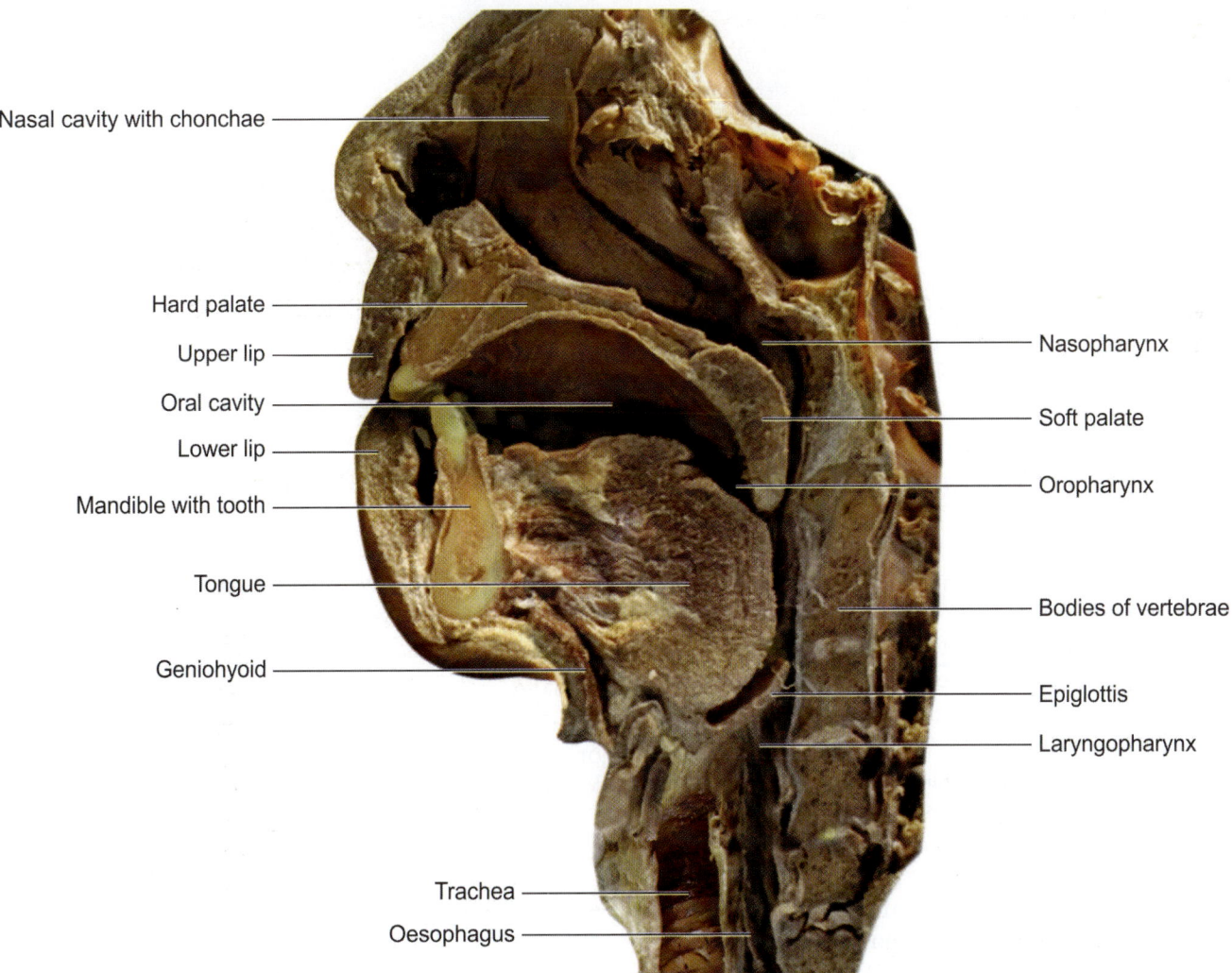

Fig. 58.1: Sagittal section of head and neck

Labels: Nasal cavity with chonchae, Hard palate, Upper lip, Oral cavity, Lower lip, Mandible with tooth, Tongue, Geniohyoid, Trachea, Oesophagus, Nasopharynx, Soft palate, Oropharynx, Bodies of vertebrae, Epiglottis, Laryngopharynx

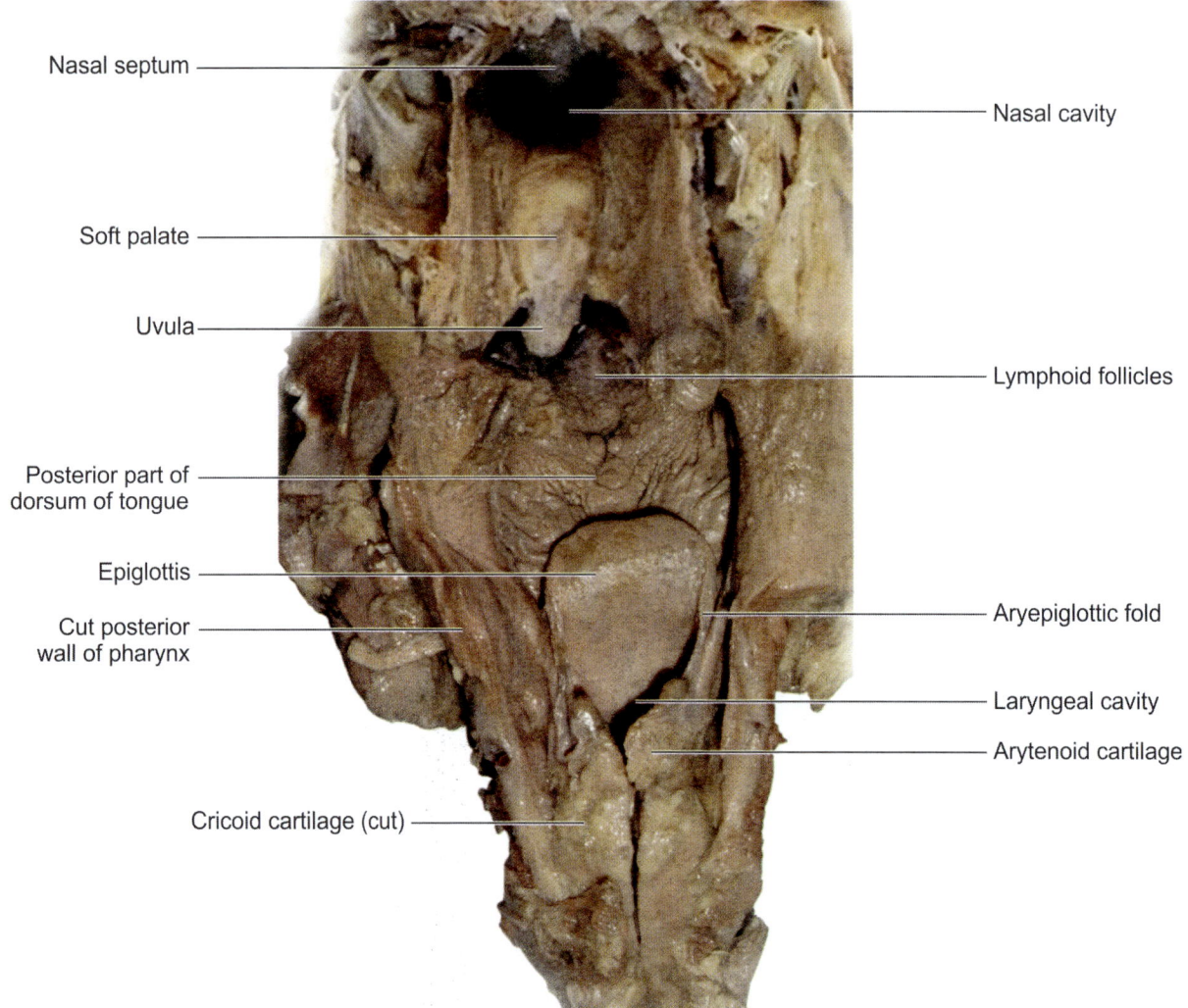

Nasal septum

Nasal cavity

Soft palate

Uvula

Lymphoid follicles

Posterior part of
dorsum of tongue

Epiglottis

Aryepiglottic fold

Cut posterior
wall of pharynx

Laryngeal cavity

Arytenoid cartilage

Cricoid cartilage (cut)

Fig. 58.2: Parts of pharynx

iii. A conical projection from the free border known as uvula (Fig. 58.2)

- Soft palate can easily be visualised through a mirror. Identify the muscles of soft palate.
  1. Tensor veli palatini forms the palatine aponeurosis
  2. Levator veli palatini is attached to upper surface of palatine aponeurosis.
  3. Palatoglossus is attached to upper surface of palatine aponeurosis
  4. Palatopharyngeus is mainly attached to lower surface of palatine aponeurosis
  5. Musculus uvulae is a small muscle inserted into the uvula of the soft palate.

Four out of the five muscles (except palatoglossus) are innervated by vagoaccesory complex.

Pharynx

Pharynx is a muscular tube behind the nasal cavity, oral cavity and the larynx. It is approximately 12 cm long.

It comprises 3 parts (Figs 58.1 and 58.2):
1. Nasopharynx—behind the nasal cavity
2. Oropharynx—behind oral cavity
3. Laryngopharynx—behind the larynx

It ends at the level of C6 vertebra and continues as oesophagus.

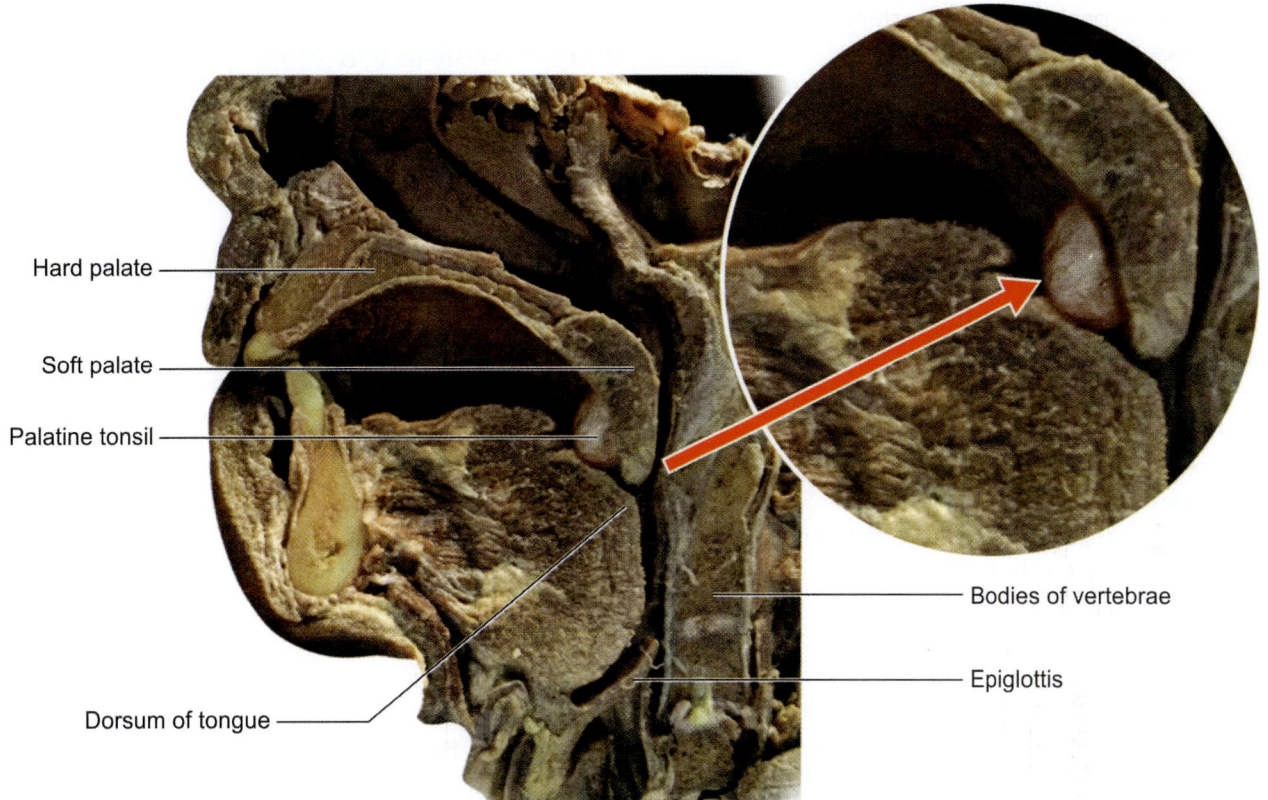

Fig. 58.3: Oropharynx with palatine tonsil

Labels: Hard palate, Soft palate, Palatine tonsil, Dorsum of tongue, Bodies of vertebrae, Epiglottis

The nasopharynx extends from base of skull (basisphenoid, basiocciput) till the soft palate.

The oropharynx extends from soft palate to upper border of epiglottis.

Laryngopharynx extends from upper border of epiglottis to lower border of cricoid cartilage.

Figure 58.2 shows the posterior parts of nasopharynx, oropharynx and laryngopharynx after reflecting the posterior wall of pharynx.

Learn the components of all three parts from BD Chaurasia's *Human Anatomy*.

See the components of Waldeyer's ring at the nasooro-pharyngeal isthmus. The components of the ring are:
1. Nasopharyngeal tonsil in the roof of nasopharynx
2. On each side are the tubal tonsils lying above the opening of the pharyngotympanic tube
3. On each side palatine tonsils are seen lying in the tonsillar fossa between palatoglossal arch anteriorly and palatopharyngeal arch posteriorly.
4. Lingual tonsils present in the posterior 1/3rd of the tongue.

Competency achievement: The student should be able to:

AN 36.1 Describe the: (1) morphology, relations, blood supply and applied anatomy of palatine tonsil, (2) composition of soft palate.

Palatine Tonsil

Try to see the palatine tonsils in children where these are easily seen (Fig. 58.3). After puberty all tonsillar tissues usually retrogress.

See the tonsillar fossa in yourself using a mirror. Its medial surface is seen projecting into the oral cavity.

The lateral surface of palatine tonsil is covered by the capsule, i.e. there is a hemicapsule.
- Identify the superior constrictor muscle forming the tonsillar bed.
- Identify the pharyngobasilar fascia on the inner aspect of the superior constrictor also forming the tonsillar bed.
- See that upper pole of tonsil reaches the soft palate, lower pole is related to the tongue (Fig. 58.3).
- Note the site of origin of facial artery as the 2nd anterior branch from external carotid artery. During

its cervical part, the facial artery gives tonsillar branches to the palatine tonsil.

- Identify few other arteries supplying the tonsil from greater palatine, ascending pharyngeal and lingual arteries.
- The palatine vein drains into facial vein. This vein is likely to be injured during tonsillectomy.

Muscles of Pharynx

- Identify the following structures:
  – Pharyngeal tubercle
  – Pterygoid hamulus
  – Pterygomandibular raphe
  – Posterior end of mylohyoid line
  – Posterior part of side of tongue
  – Lesser cornua and greater cornua of hyoid bone
  – Oblique line of thyroid cartilage
  – Cricoid cartilage
  – Styloid process of temporal bone
  – Soft palate
  – Pharyngeal end of pharyngotympanic tube
- Now identify the muscles of pharynx.

The 3 outer circular muscles are:
1. Superior constrictor
2. Middle constrictor
3. Inferior constrictor

All the three muscles are inserted into the pharyngeal raphae, which extends from pharyngeal tubercle on the base of skull to the posterior surface of cricoid cartilage (Fig. 58.4).

The 3 inner longitudinal muscles are:
1. Palatopharyngeus
2. Stylopharyngeus
3. Salpingopharyngeus
- See the pharyngobasilar fascia beneath the longitudinal muscle layer. It is thick and well developed from the base of skull till the upper end of superior constrictor muscle.
- Inner layers are submucosal and mucosa.
- Outside the outer circular layer is the bucco-pharyngeal fascia.

Thus the layers of pharynx from outside to inside are:
  i. Buccopharyngeal fascia
  ii. 3 constrictor muscles
 iii. 3 longitudinal muscles
 iv. Pharyngobasilar fascia
  v. Submucosa
 vi. Mucosa

Structures in between Pharyngeal Muscles

- Identify the structures above superior constrictor muscle. These are:
    i. Thickened pharyngobasilar fascia
    ii. Pharyngotympanic/auditory tube
   iii. Levator veli palatini muscle
   iv. Ascending palatine artery

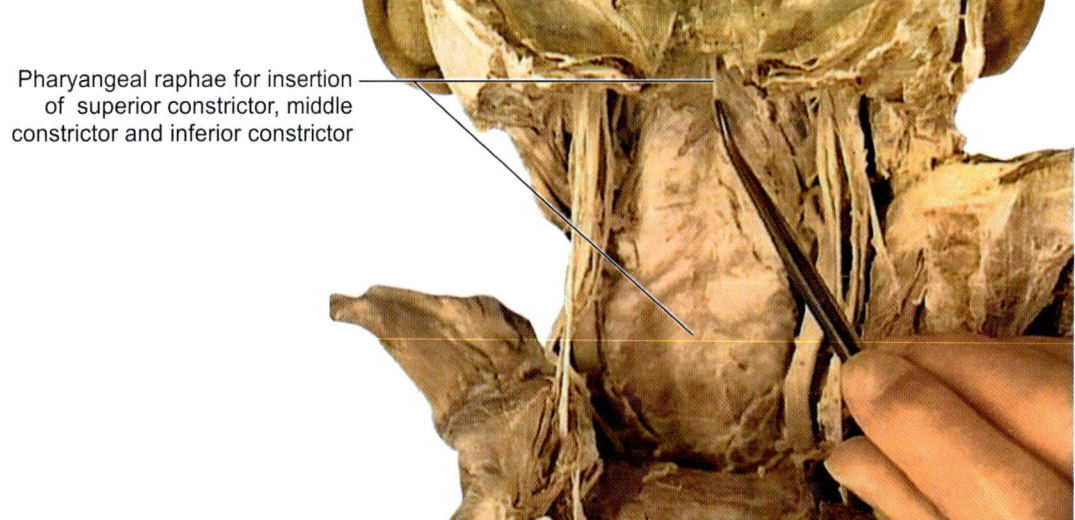

Pharyangeal raphae for insertion of superior constrictor, middle constrictor and inferior constrictor

Fig. 58.4: Pharyngeal raphe

- Define the attachments of superior, middle and inferior constrictors of pharynx by separating them from each other.
- Identify the structures traversing through the gaps between the three constrictor muscles (Fig. 58.5).
  - i. The structures traversing the gap between superior and middle constrictor muscles are the stylopharyngeus muscle and glossopharyngeal nerve.
  - ii. The structures between middle and inferior constrictor are internal laryngeal nerve, branch of X, and superior laryngeal branch of superior thyroid artery.
  - iii. Identify structures below inferior constrictor muscle. They are the recurrent laryngeal branch of X and inferior laryngeal artery, a branch of inferior thyroid artery.
- Cut through the tensor veli palatini and reflect it downwards. Remove the fascia and identify the mandibular nerve again with otic ganglion medial to it.
- Locate the middle meningeal artery at the foramen spinosum as it lies just posterior to mandibular nerve. See the course of this artery in the middle cranial fossa. It runs forwards and laterally grooving the squamous temporal bone before dividing into anterior and posterior branches. The anterior branch runs on the inner aspect of pterion. Then it runs upwards and backwards almost parallel to precentral sulcus (*see* Fig. 56.7).
- The posterior branch runs backwards about 4 cm above the zygomatic arch.

Auditory Tube

It is also called Eustachian tube. Correctly it should be named pharyngotympanic tube as it lies between the anterior wall of middle ear and the lateral wall of nasopharynx.

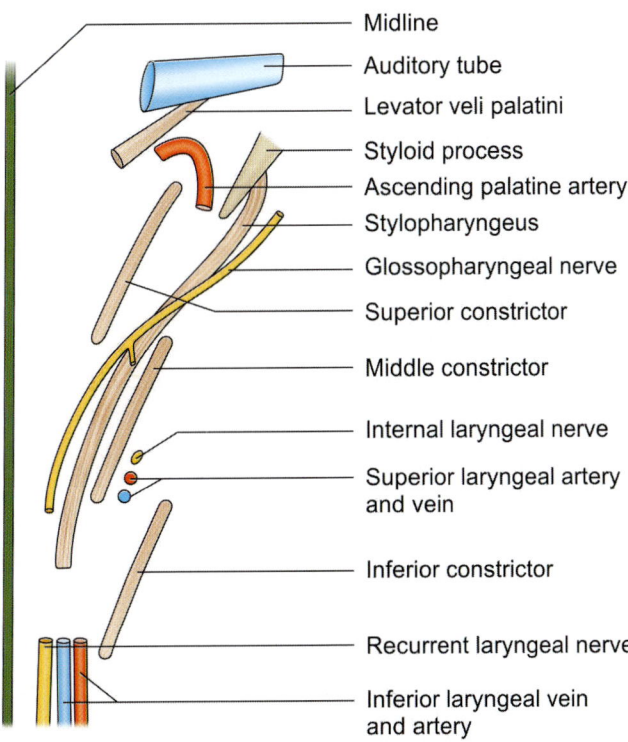

Fig. 58.4: Structures in the gaps between the constrictor muscles

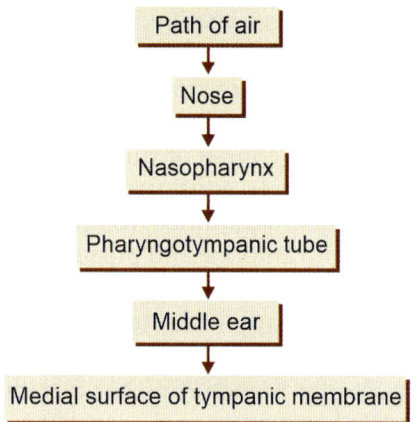

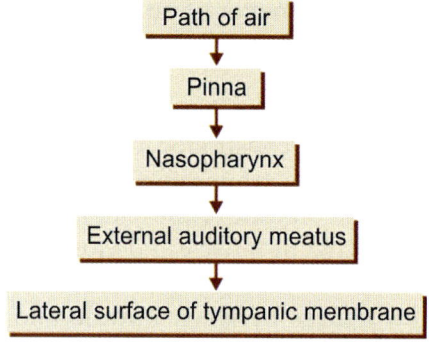

If pressure on both sides of tympanic membrane is equal, vibrations of tympanic membrane are harmonious. If pressure is less on medial side, vibrations are not proper and there is difficulty in hearing.

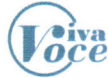 **Viva Voce**

- What are the parts of the patate?
- Name the muscles of the soft palate and give their nerve supply.
- Name the longitudinal and circular muscles of the pharynx with their nerve supply.

- Which all arteries supply the palatine tonsil.
- What is the function of auditory/pharyngo-tympanic tube? Name its parts and their length.

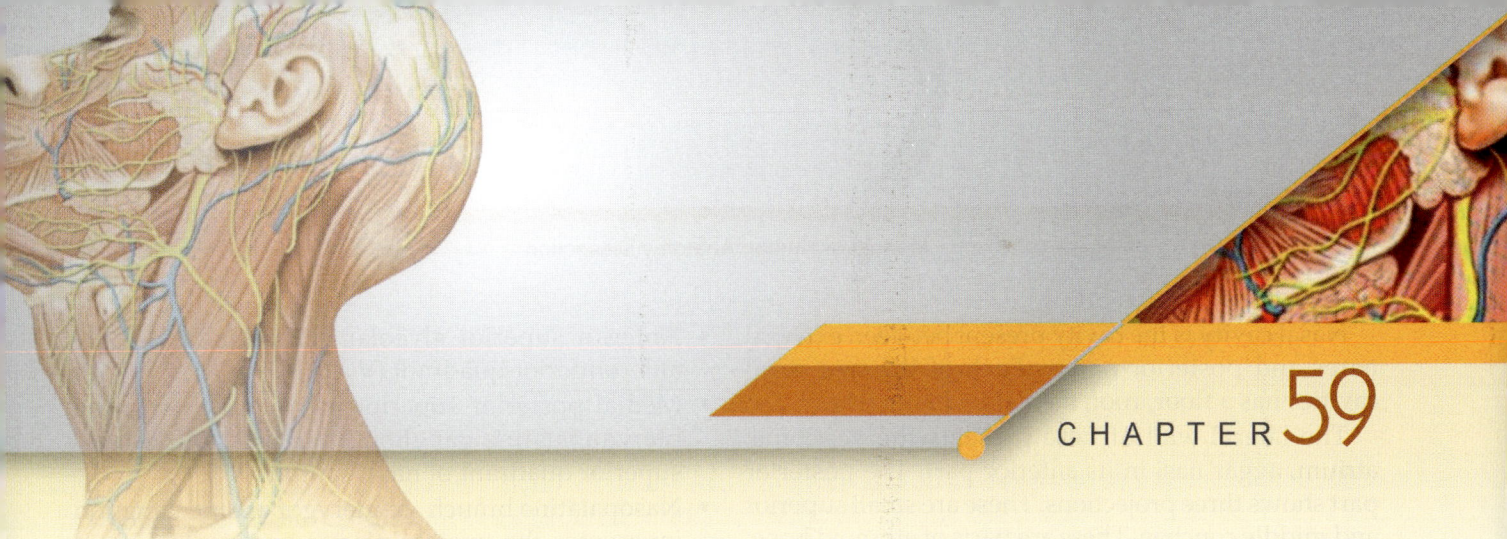

CHAPTER 59

Nose and Paranasal Sinuses

Learning Objectives

One should be able to
1. Learn the arteries and nerves supplying lateral wall of nose.
2. Course of the artery of epistaxis.
3. Openings of all the paranasal sinuses in the lateral wall of nose.
4. Roots and branches of pterygopalatine ganglion.

OVERVIEW OF NOSE

Nose is the most prominent part of the face. Its chief functions are olfaction (sense of smell) and respiration.

External nose comprises root, dorsum, tip, anterior nares and nasal septum.

The skeletal framework of nose is partly bony, partly cartilaginous and cuticular (Fig. 59.1).

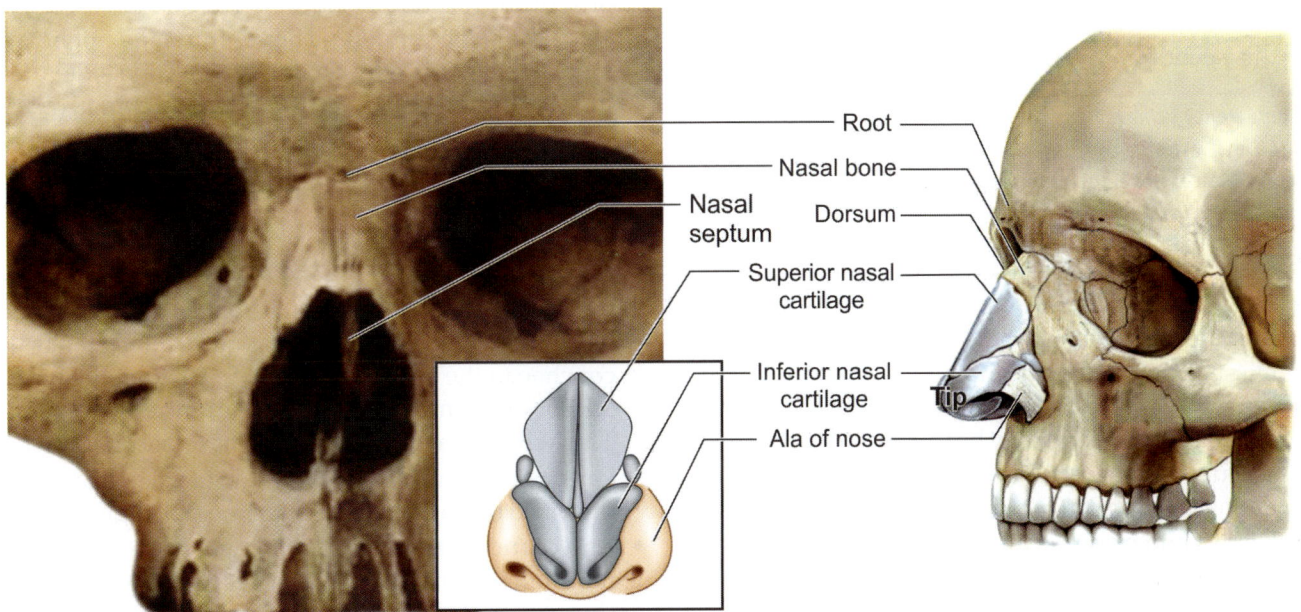

Root
Nasal bone
Nasal septum
Dorsum
Superior nasal cartilage
Inferior nasal cartilage
Ala of nose
Tip

Fig. 59.1: Skeletal framework of external nose

379

Nasal cavity is the cavity present between external nares and posterior nares. Each of the two nasal cavities has a floor, roof, medial and lateral walls.

The lateral wall of nose presents the vestibule, atrium, aggar nasi in its anterior part. The posterior part shows three projections. These are small superior and middle conchae. These are parts of ethmoid bone. The inferior concha is lowest and is an independent bone.

Below each concha is the respective meatus. So we see superior meatus below the superior concha; middle meatus below the middle concha and inferior meatus below the inferior concha.

Sphenoethmoidal recess is a small space between the roof of the nose and the superior concha.

OVERVIEW OF PNS

There are some bones around the nose that contain air filled spaces within them. The bones having air sinuses are called pneumatic bones. These bones are ethmoid, frontal, sphenoid and maxilla.

There are six pairs of air sinuses. These air sinuses are lined by secretory epithelium and secrete thin serous fluid which humidifies the air and warms up/cools down the inspired air.

NASAL SEPTUM

Get a sagittal section of dried skull. Identify the bones in this section.

Competency achievement: The student should be able to:

AN 37.1 Describe and demonstrate features of nasal septum, lateral wall of nose, their blood supply and nerve supply.

Steps of Dissection

- Take the soft sagittal section of head and neck prepared in Chapter 58.
- Dissect and remove mucous membrane of the septum of nose in small pieces. See the mucous membrane is covering both the surfaces of the septum of the nose. Identify the structures forming the nasal septum (Fig. 59.2).
- Dissect and preserve the nerves lying in the mucous membrane.
- Identify the anterior and posterior ethmoidal nerves (V$_1$) present in the anterosuperior quadrant.

- Anterior superior alveolar nerve innervates the anteroinferior quadrant (V$_2$).
- Medial posterior superior nasal branches of the pterygopalatine ganglion innervate the postero-superior quadrant of nasal septum (V$_2$).
- Nasopalatine branch of pterygopalatine ganglion innervates the posteroinferior quadrant of nasal septum(V$_2$).
- The special sensory nerves/olfactory nerves (I) remain confined to the uppermost part of nasal septum.
- Identify the arteries supplying nasal septum. These are:
  i. Anterior and posterior ethmoidal
  ii. Superior labial
  iii. Sphenopalatine. It contributes major part of arterial supply to the septum.

These arteries anastomose in the anteroinferior part of septum. Their capillaries may rupture in hot weather and cause bleeding from the nose—epistaxis. Thus sphenopalatine artery is called the *artery of epistaxis.*

- After removing all the mucous membrane, see the bones, cartilages and cuticular parts forming the nasal septum.
- Identify bones as perpendicular plate of ethmoid, vomer, cartilage as septal cartilage. The lowest part of septum formed by fibrofatty tissue covered by skin is called columella. The septum may not be in median plane. It may be deviated to one side and the condition is called *Deviated Nasal Septum.*
- Remove the structures forming the septum, see lateral wall of nose.

LATERAL WALL OF NOSE

Steps of Dissection

- Observe the superior, middle and inferior nasal conchae in the lateral wall (Fig. 59.3). Remove with scissors the anterior part of inferior nasal concha. This will reveal the opening of nasolacrimal duct.
- Pass a probe upwards through the nasolacrimal duct into the lacrimal sac at the medial angle of eye.
- Look under the nasal conchae to expose the meatuses lying below the respective conchae (Fig. 59.4). This will expose the openings of the sinuses present there:

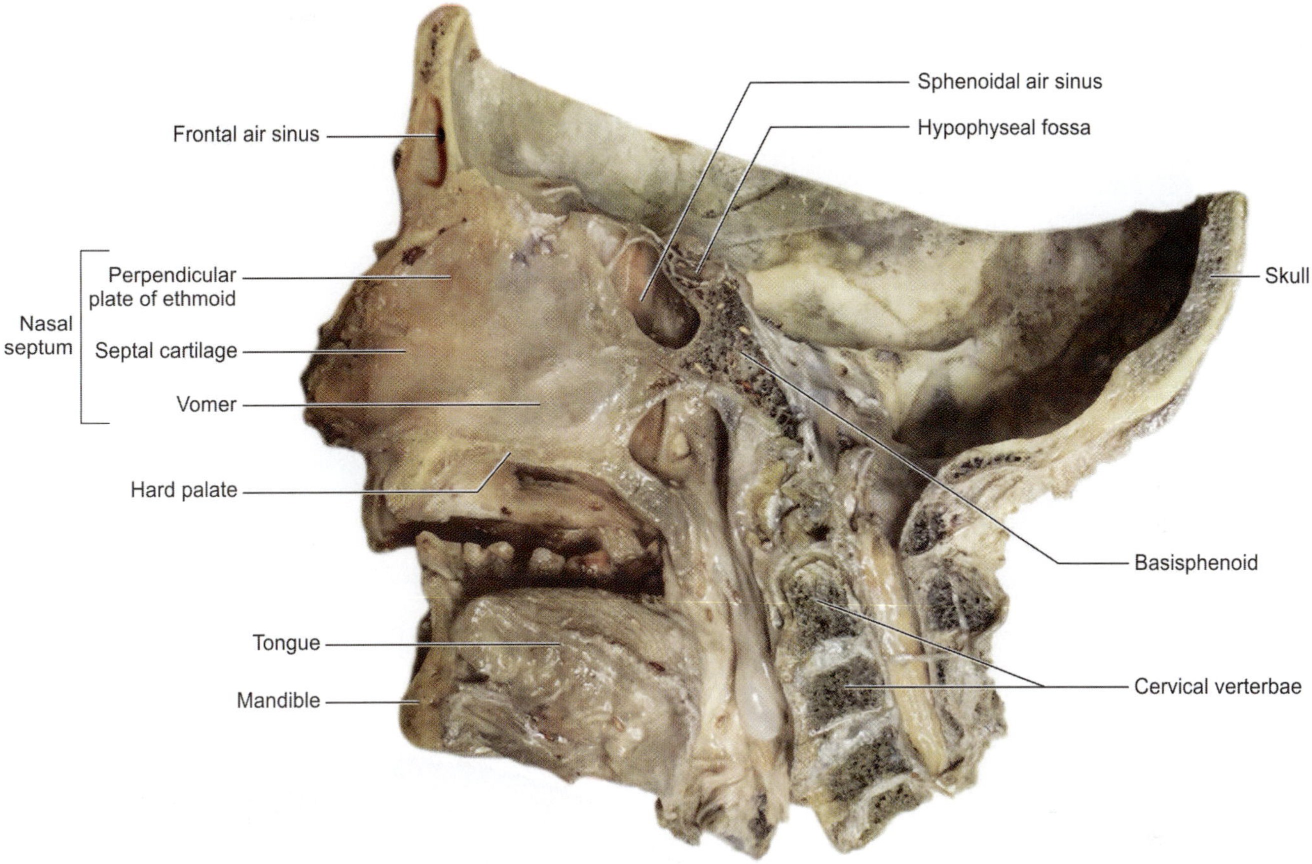

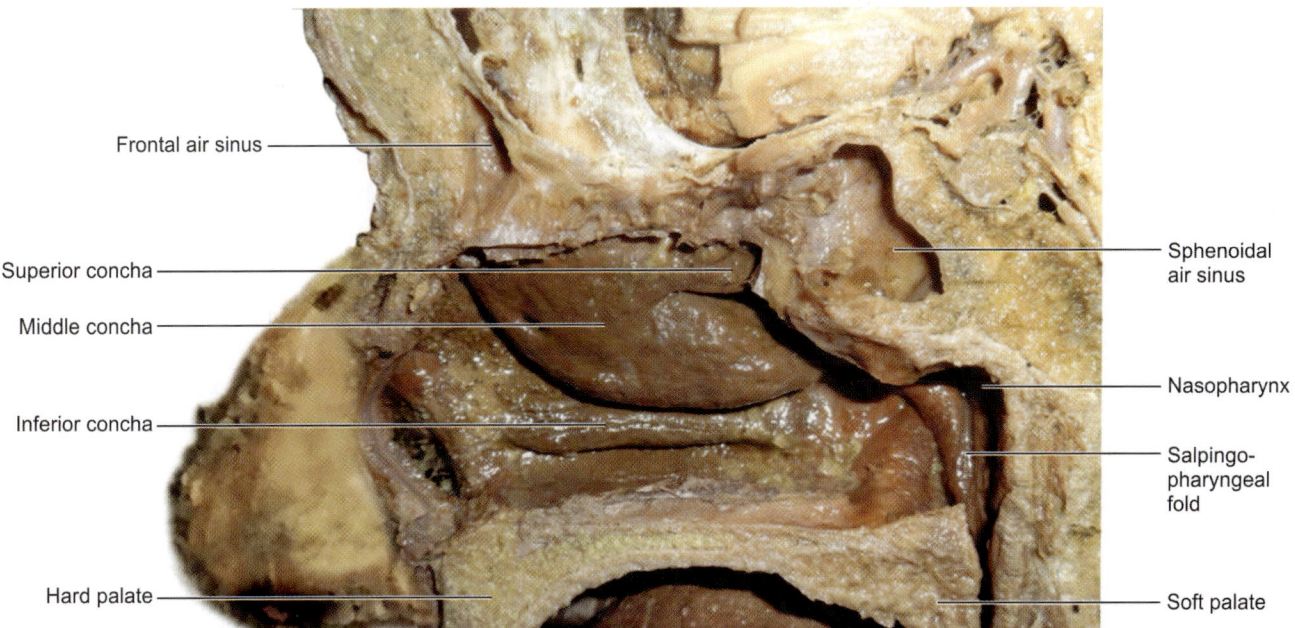

Fig. 59.2: Nasal septum

Sphenoidal air sinus

Hypophyseal fossa

Frontal air sinus

Skull

Perpendicular plate of ethmoid

Nasal septum

Septal cartilage

Vomer

Hard palate

Basisphenoid

Tongue

Mandible

Cervical verterbae

Frontal air sinus

Superior concha

Middle concha

Inferior concha

Hard palate

Sphenoidal air sinus

Nasopharynx

Salpingo-pharyngeal fold

Soft palate

Fig. 59.3: Lateral wall of nasal cavity with conchae

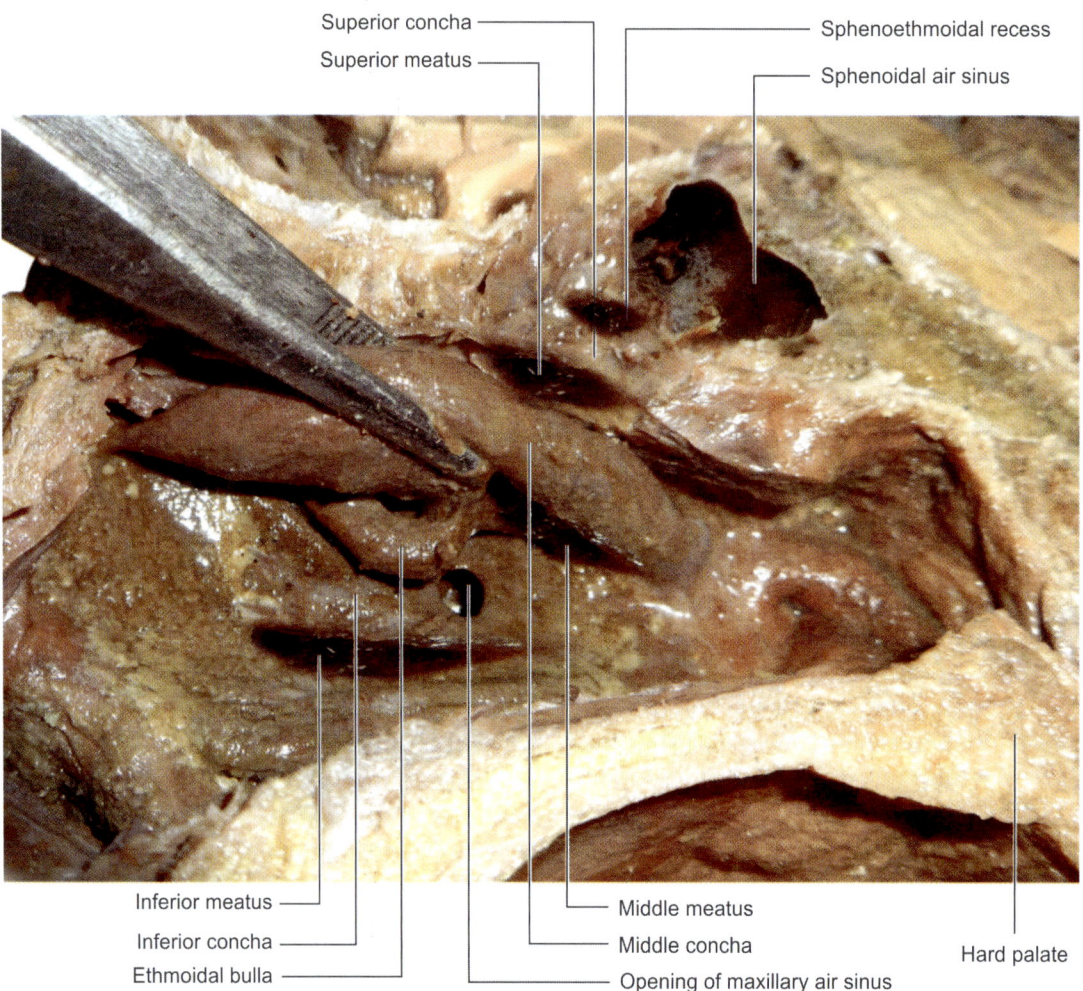

Superior concha — | Sphenoethmoidal recess
Superior meatus — | Sphenoidal air sinus

Inferior meatus — | Middle meatus
Inferior concha — | Middle concha
Ethmoidal bulla — | Opening of maxillary air sinus
Hard palate

Fig. 59.4: Meatuses in the lateral wall of nasal cavity

i. The sphenoethmoidal air sinus opens into sphenoethmoidal recess.

ii. Posterior ethmoidal air sinuses drain into superior meatus.

iii. Middle ethmoidal air sinuses open into ethmoidal bulla of middle meatus. Frontal air sinus, anterior ethmoidal air sinuses and maxillary air sinus open into hiatus semilunaris of middle meatus.

iv. Nasolacrimal duct opens into the inferior meatus of nose.

Arteries and Nerves

The arteries supplying the lateral wall of nose are:

i. Anterior and posterior ethmoidal arteries

ii. Branches of facial artery

iii. Branches from sphenopalatine artery

iv. Greater palatine is the main artery of the lateral wall of nose.

Sensory nerve supply is by the following nerves:

i. Anterior ethmoidal nerve (V_1) (Fig. 59.5)

ii. Anterior superior alveolar nerve(V_2)

iii. Lateral posterior superior nasal branches

iv. Branches of anterior/greater palatine nerves

Special sensory nerve is olfactory (I) in the uppermost part of the lateral wall of nose.

Competency achievement: The student should be able to:

AN 37.2 Describe location and functional anatomy of paranasal sinuses.

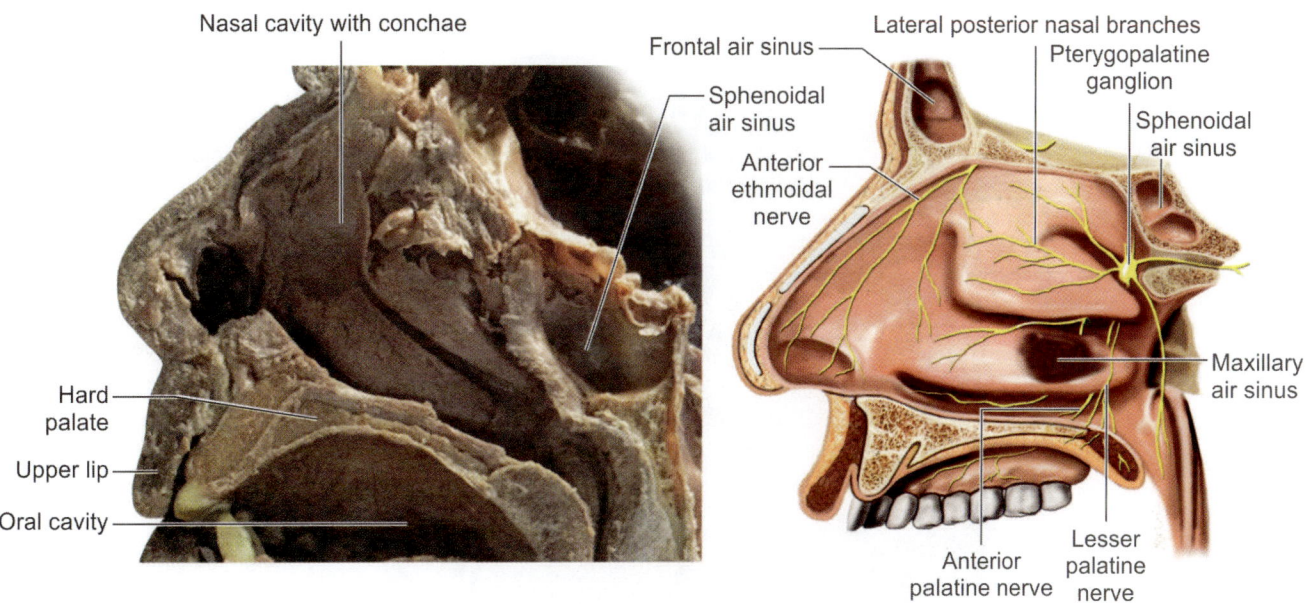

Fig. 59.5: Lateral wall of nasal cavity with its nerve supply. Some paranasal sinuses also seen

PARANASAL AIR SINUSES

There are six pairs of air sinuses. These are:
1. Sphenoidal air sinus ((Figs 59.2 to 59.6)
2. Frontal air sinus (Figs 59.2 and 59.3)
3. Anterior ethmoidal air sinus (8–10) (Fig. 59.6)
4. Middle ethmoidal air sinus (4–6)
5. Posterior ethmoidal air sinus (2–4)
6. Maxillary air sinus (Fig. 59.5)

Steps of Dissection

- Remove the thin walls of ethmoidal air sinuses cells and look for the continuity with the mucous membrane of the nose.
- Remove the medial wall of maxillary air sinus extending anteriorly from the opening of nasolacrimal duct till the greater palatine canal posteriorly. Now maxillary air sinus can be seen.

Pterygopalatine Ganglion

- Trace the connections and branches of pterygopalatine ganglion. It is responsible for supplying secretomotor fibres to the glands of the nasal cavity, palate, pharynx, lacrimal gland and paranasal sinuses. It is also called "ganglion of hay fever" as inflammation of the ganglion causes allergic sinusitis.
- Remove part of the roof of maxillary air sinus so that the maxillary nerve and pterygopalatine ganglion are identifiable in the pterygopalatine fossa (Fig. 59.5).
- Trace the infraorbital nerve in the infraorbital canal in the floor of the orbit. Try to locate he sinuous course of anterior superior alveolar nerve into upper incisor teeth.

Pterygopalatine ganglion is the largest para-sympathetic ganglion associated with facial (VII) nerve. Its roots are:

 i. Secretomotor is greater petrosal nerve arising from geniculate ganglion
 ii. The deep petrosal nerve arising from post-ganglionic fibres around internal carotid artery
iii. Sensory roots are the branches of maxillary nerve.

The greater petrosal and deep petrosal nerves unite to form "nerve of pterygoid canal". It reaches pterygo-palatine ganglion where only the fibres of greater petrosal nerve relay. These postganglionic secretomotor fibres reach the lacrimal, nasal, palatal, pharyngeal glands and paranasal sinuses.

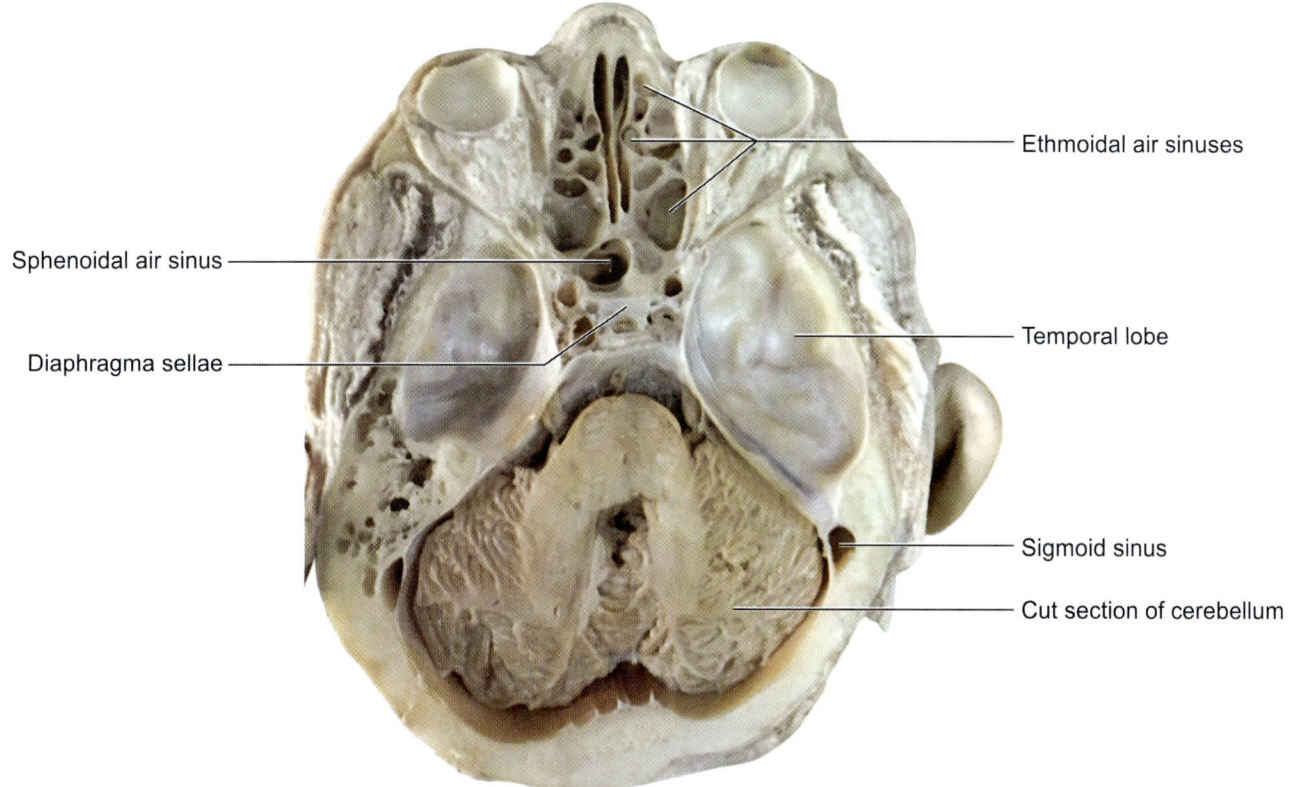

Fig. 59.6: Some paranasal sinuses

Labels on figure:
- Ethmoidal air sinuses
- Sphenoidal air sinus
- Diaphragma sellae
- Temporal lobe
- Sigmoid sinus
- Cut section of cerebellum

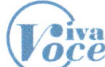

Viva Voce

- Name the structures forming the nasal septum.
- Which nerves supply the nasal septum?
- What is Little's area? Which arteries anastomose in this area?
- Name the openings in the middle meatus of nose.

- What are the roots of pterygopalatine ganglion? Name the branches of the pterygopalatine ganglion.
- How much of nasal cavity is lined by olfactory epithelium?

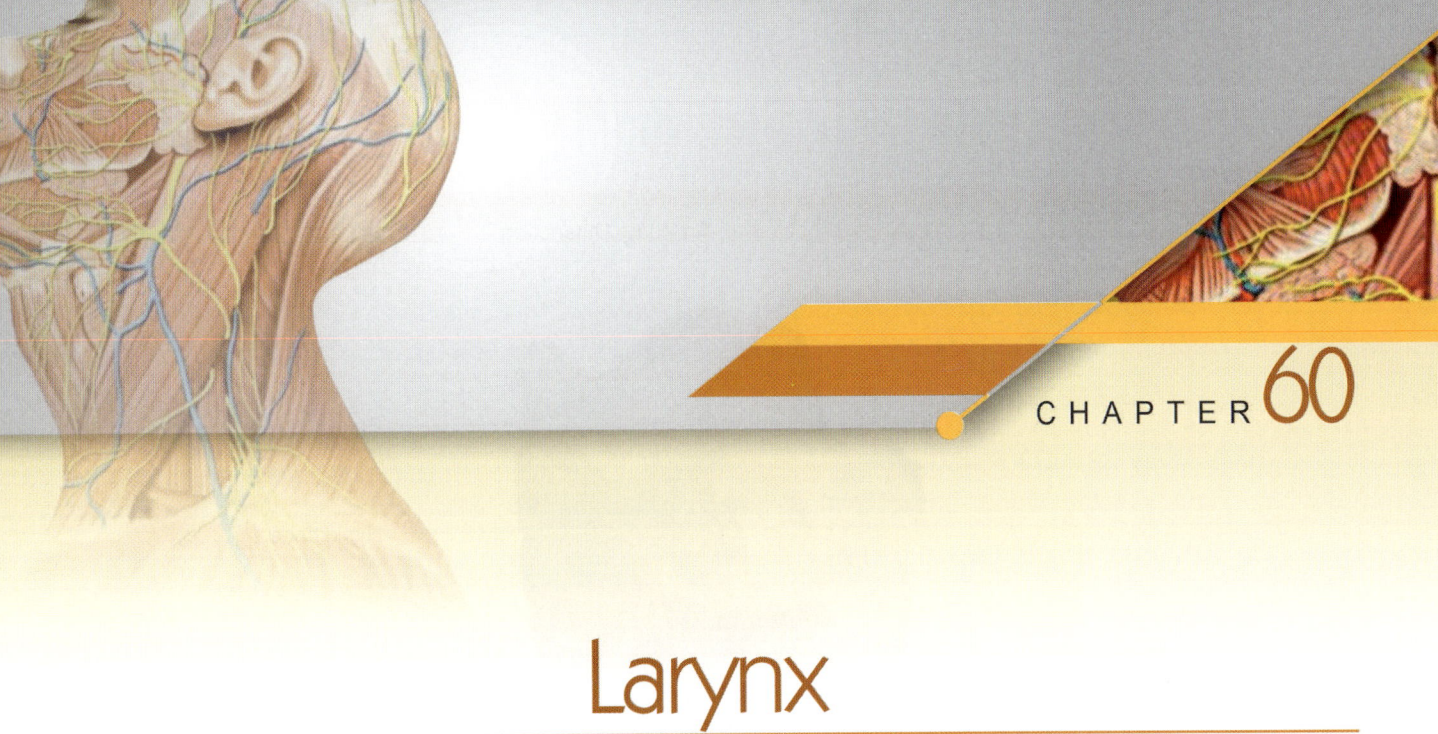

CHAPTER 60

Larynx

Learning Objectives

One should be able to
1. Explain action of abduction and adduction of vocal cords.
2. Explain action of opening and closing inlet of larynx.
3. Discuss the formation of teacher's/singer's nodules.

OVERVIEW

Larynx is the voice box and a respiratory organ. It only permits air into the lower respiratory passages and prevents entry of any food/fluid, etc. Larynx is comprised of cartilages and membranes and lies opposite 3rd–6th cervical vertebrae.

The unpaired cartilages are thyroid, cricoid and epiglottis while the paired cartilages are aryternoid, corniculate and cuneiform (Figs 60.1 and 60.2).

Thyroid cartilage is 'V' shaped cartilage made of right and left laminae. Muscles attached to its outer surface are cricothyroid, sternothyroid, thyrohyoid and inferior constrictor of pharynx. Muscles on its inner aspect are thyroarytenoid, thyroepiglottic. In addition vestibular and vocal folds of mucous membrane including thyroepiglottic ligament are attached.

Cricoid is a ring like cartilage. It gives attachment to cricothyroid, lateral cricoarytenoid and posterior cricoarytenoid muscles. Also provides attachment to cricothyroid and cricovocal membranes.

Epiglottis is a leaf like cartilage which is elastic in nature. It never gets calcified. Thyroepiglottic muscle opens the inlet of larynx; aryepiglottic muscle closes

the inlet of larynx. Epiglottis is attached to thyroid cartilage and is related to tongue and hyoid bone.

Arytenoid cartilages are paired in position. Its vocal process gives attachment to vocal ligament. Muscular process gives attachment to lateral cricoarytenoid muscles anteriorly and to posterior cricoarytenoid posteriorly. In addition it also provides attachment to transverse arytenoid and oblique arytenoid muscles.

Extrinsic membranes of larynx are thyrohyoid, hyoepiglottic and cricotracheal membranes. Intrinsic membranes are quadrate membrane between arytenoid and epiglottic cartilages. Its free border forms vestibular fold.

Other membrane is cricovocal membrane extending from cricoid cartilage and its upper free border forms the vocal fold.

Muscles are named according to their attachments. Cricothyroid is tensor of vocal cords (external laryngeal nerve). Thyroarytenoid is relaxer of vocal cords (recurrent laryngeal nerve). Posterior cricoarytenoid is the only abductor of vocal cords (recurrent laryngeal nerve). Lateral cricoarytenoid, transverse arytenoid and oblique arytenoid are

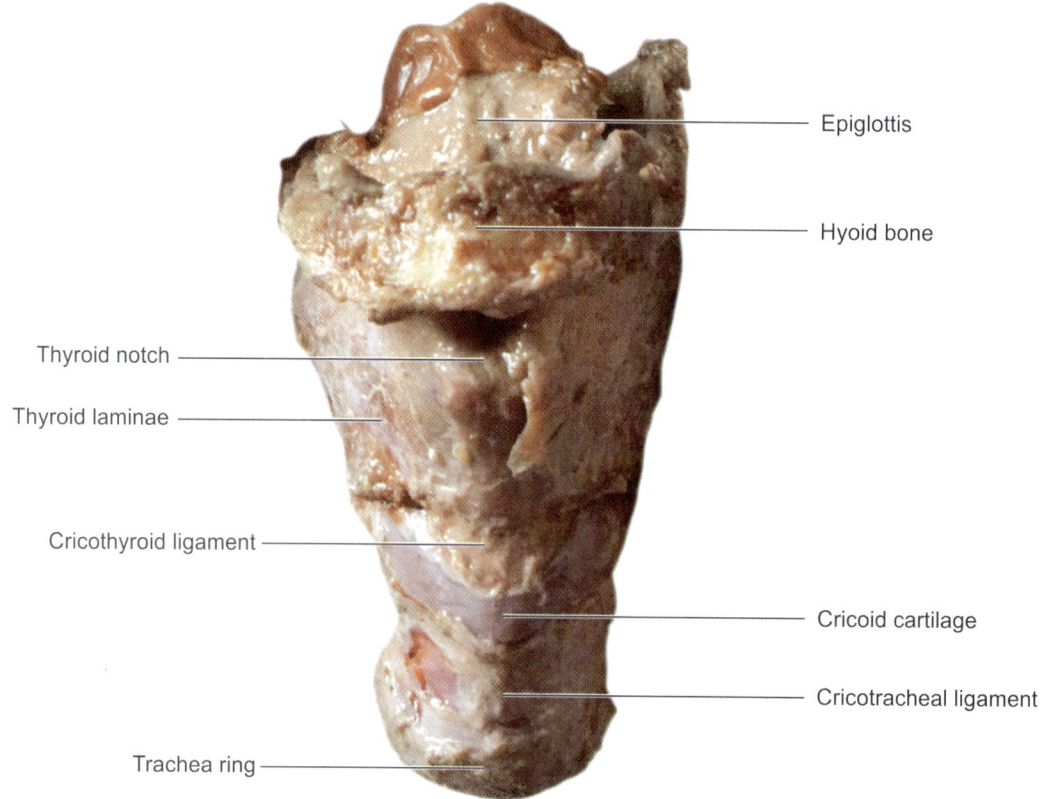

Epiglottis

Hyoid bone

Thyroid notch

Thyroid laminae

Cricothyroid ligament

Cricoid cartilage

Cricotracheal ligament

Trachea ring

Fig. 60.1: Cartilages of larynx (anterior view)

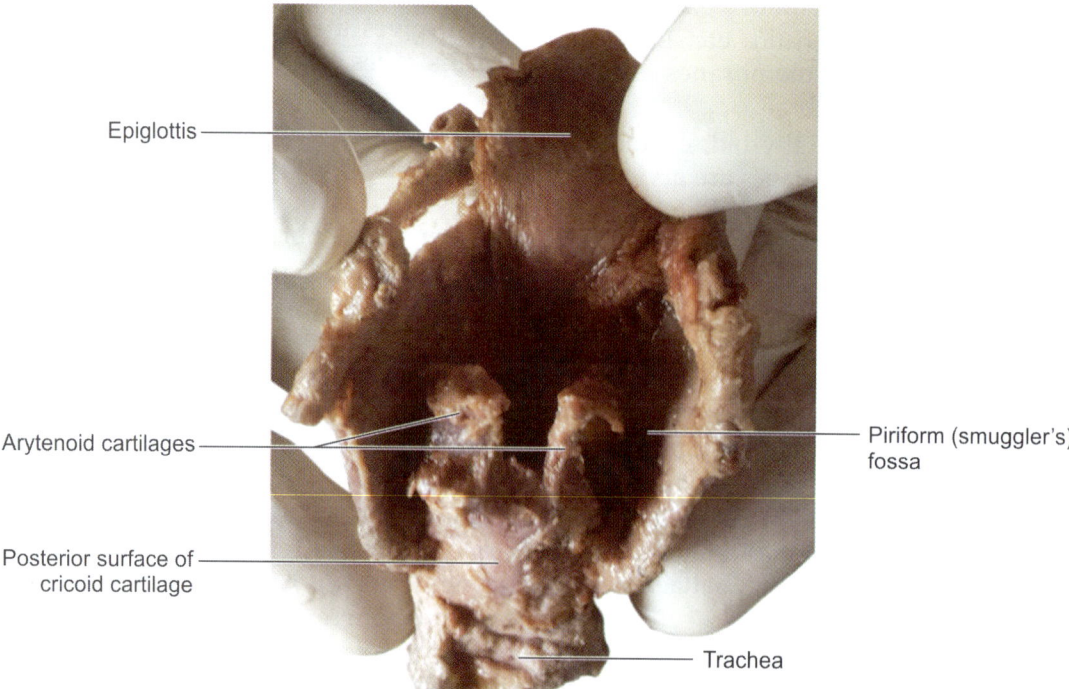

Epiglottis

Arytenoid cartilages

Piriform (smuggler's) fossa

Posterior surface of cricoid cartilage

Trachea

Fig. 60.2: Other cartilages of larynx (superior view)

adductors of vocal cords (recurrent laryngeal nerve). Aryepiglottic closes the inlet of larynx (recurrent laryngeal nerve). Thyroepiglottic opens the inlet of larynx (recurrent laryngeal nerve).

Sternohyoid and sternothyroid pull the larynx down (C2, C3).

Thyrohyoid and mylohyoid pull the larynx upward (C1 and V3 respectively).

The cartilages of larynx form joints. These are:

i. Cricothyroid joints—plane joint of synovial variety. Thyroid cartilage glides forward and backward on these two joints. Forward movement results in vocal cords becoming tense, while backward movement results in relaxation of vocal cords.

ii. Cricoarytenoid joints are also plane joints of synovial variety. These allow following movements:

   a. Sliding of arytenoids towards each other

   b. Sliding of arytenoids away from each other

   c. Tilting anteriorly

   d. Tilting posteriorly

   e. Rotation

> **Competency achievement:** The student should be able to:
>
> **AN 38.1** Describe the morphology, identify structure of the wall, nerve supply, blood supply and actions of intrinsic and extrinsic muscles of the larynx.

STEPS OF DISSECTION

- Identify the suprahyoid muscles seen earlier:
  1. Geniohyoid (C1)
  2. Mylohyoid (V3) (see Fig. 48.4)
  3. Stylohyoid (VII)
  4. Digastric (VII) (see Fig 48.2)
- Identify infrahyoid muscles seen earlier (see Fig. 48.2):
  1. Sternohyoid (Ansa cervicalis C1–C3)
  2. Superior belly of omohyoid (superior root of ansa cervicalis C1)
  3. Sternothyroid (Ansa cervicalis C1–C3)
  4. Thyrohyoid (C1)
- Identify internal laryngeal nerve (X) and superior laryngeal artery piercing thyrohyoid membrane as well as external laryngeal nerve innervating cricothyroid muscle.
- Locate the cricothyroid muscle, the only intrinsic muscle of larynx placed outside (Fig. 60.3a).

- Now move the head forwards so that the chin rests against the thoracic wall.
- Incise the posterior wall of pharynx (if not already done) and see the posterior surface of larynx (see Fig. 58.2).
- Identify piriform fossa between medial side of thyroid lamina and intrinsic muscles of larynx.
- Look for internal laryngeal nerve in this fossa.
- With blunt dissection, remove the mucosa from lamina of cricoid cartilage and see the most important posterior cricoarytenoid muscle (Fig. 60.3b). It is the *only abductor* of vocal folds.
- Superior to posterior cricoarytenoid identify transverse arytenoid and oblique arytenoid muscles. Trace the fibres of oblique arytenoid into aryepiglottic muscle (Fig. 60.3c).
- Identify cricothyroid joint (Fig. 15.4). See recurrent laryngeal nerve entering larynx by passing behind this joint.
- Now on the right side, disarticulate cricothyroid joint. Cut the right lamina of thyroid cartilage and free it from cricothyroid muscle.
- On the medial aspect of removed thyroid lamina identify lateral cricoarytenoid muscle an adductor of vocal cords.
- Also identify thyroarytenoid above lateral cricoarytenoid muscle. This muscle is a relaxor of vocal cords.
- Identify and look at vocal folds: The rima glottidis is the interval between right and left vocal cords.
- Identify and examine epiglottis (Figs 60.3c and 60.4). See its anterior attachment to back of thyroid cartilage. It moves posteriorly during swallowing to prevent food/fluid entering the larynx. Most of the time it points above towards the tongue so that the passage of air is patent for breathing.

Interior of Larynx

- See that cavity of larynx has following parts:
  i. Vestibule is the depression between vestibular folds and vocal cords
  ii. Infraglottic cavity lies below the vocal folds and continues with trachea.
- See the mucosa lining the internal aspect of larynx. Identify the vestibular fold above and vocal folds below.

Intrinsic Muscles of Larynx

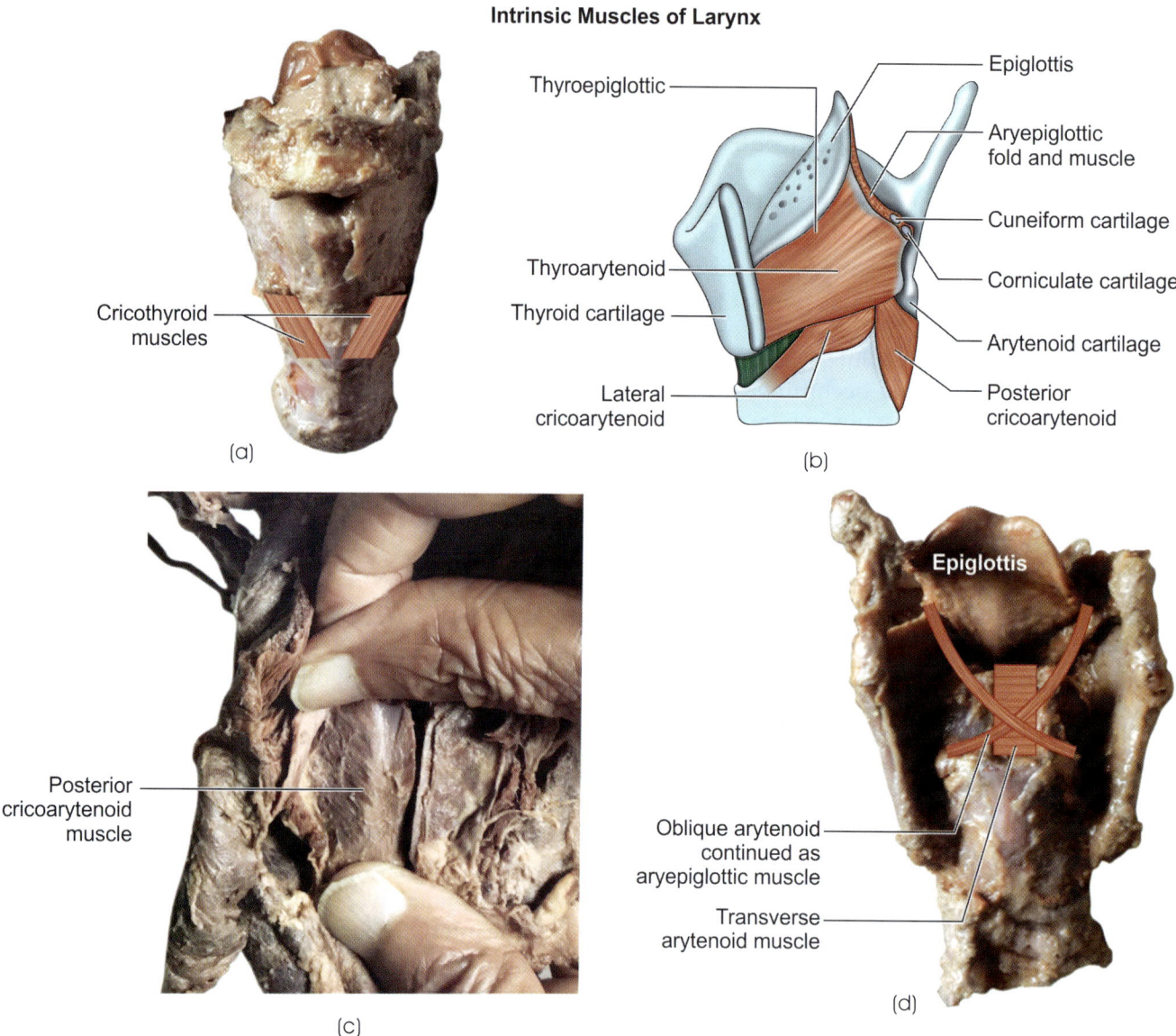

Fig. 60.3: Muscles of larynx: (a) Cricothyroid, (b) Thyroarytenoid, (c) Posterior cricoarytenoid, (d) Oblique arytenoid

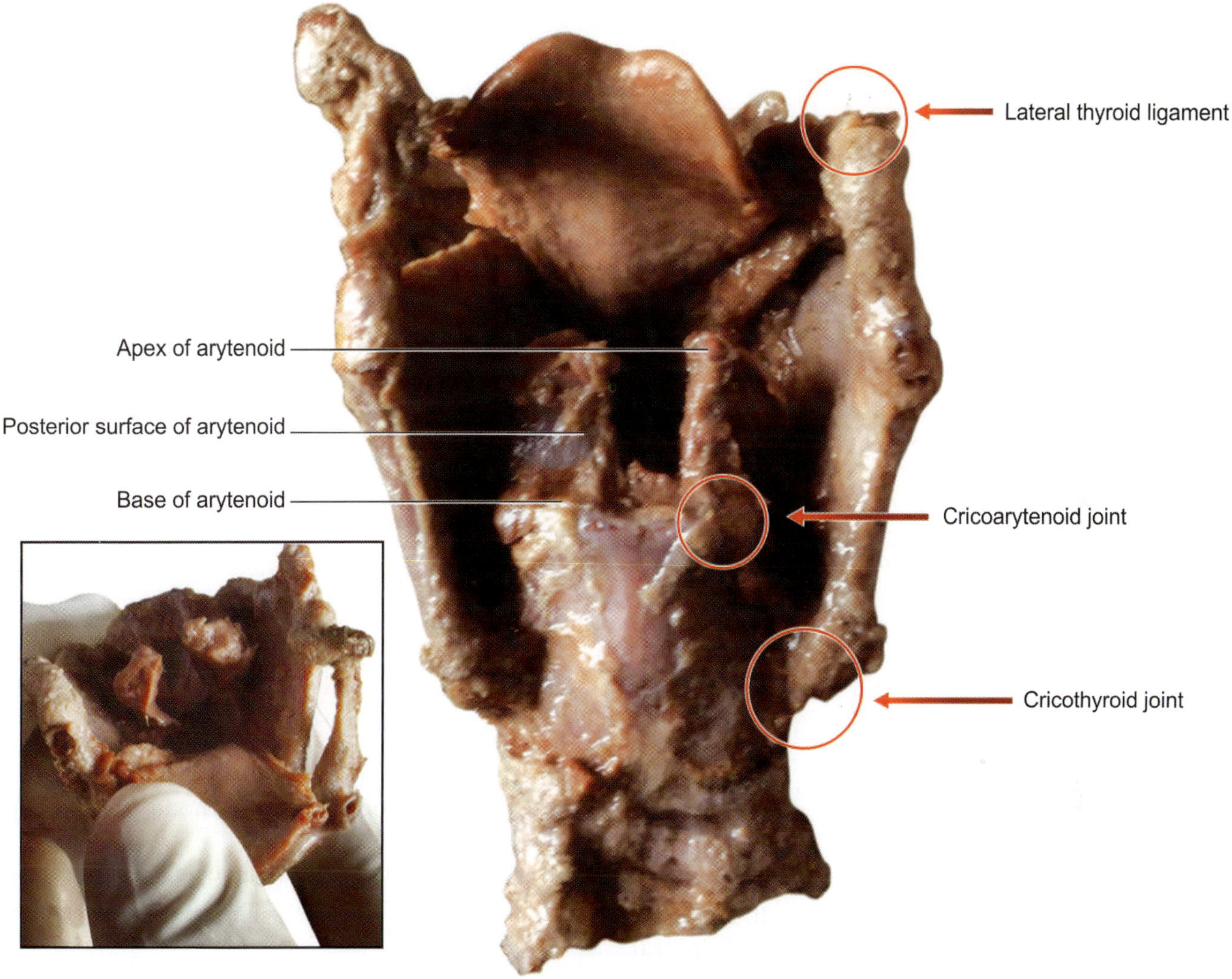

Lateral thyroid ligament

Apex of arytenoid

Posterior surface of arytenoid

Base of arytenoid

Cricoarytenoid joint

Cricothyroid joint

Fig. 60.4: Joints between laryngeal cartilages

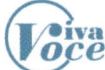

Viva Voce

- How much is the angle of thyroid laminae in male and female?
- Name the paired and unpaired cartilages of the larynx.
- Name the boundaries of piriform fossa. What is its importance?
- Where and why do the singer's nodules develop?
- Name the intrinsic muscles of larynx.
- Which is a life-saving muscle and why?
- Which is the only muscle supplied by external laryngeal nerve?
- What are the boundaries of inlet of larynx?

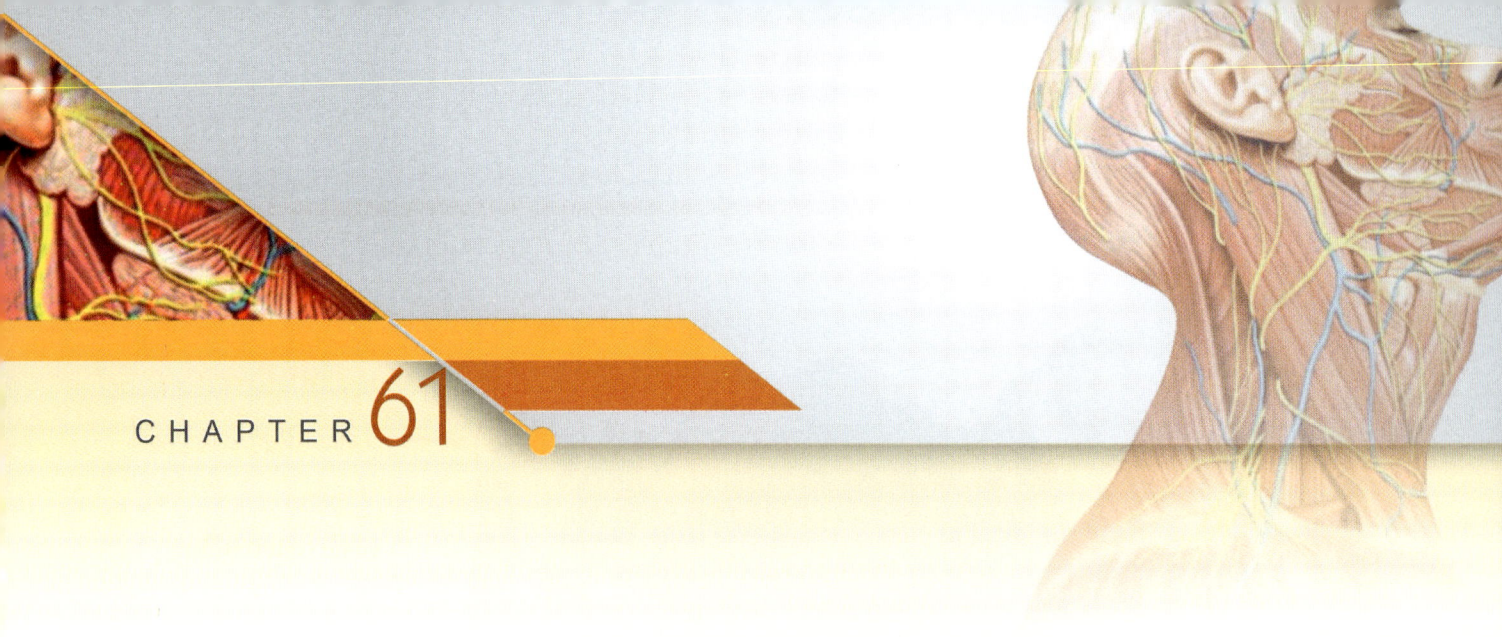

CHAPTER 61

Tongue

Learning Objectives

One should be able to

1. Name the extrinsic and intrinsic muscles of tongue with their nerve supply.
2. Name the types of papillae.
3. Which nerves innervate the taste buds of the tongue?

OVERVIEW

The muscular speaking pink tongue is 3" long with dorsal and ventral surfaces. Dorsal rough surface is divided into anterior 2/3 oral part and posterior 1/3 the pharyngeal part separated by sulcus terminalis (Figs 61.1 and 61.2). Ventral part is smooth. Tongue is connected to epiglottis by median and 2 lateral glossoepiglottic folds.

See your tongue in the mirror and identify the filiform, fungiform papillae, circumvallate papillae and lymphoid follicles on it (Fig. 61.2). Then view the tongue of your friends and identify the same.

Tongue is not swallowed into the oesophagus as it is supported and connected by muscles. These are styloglossus, palatoglossus, hyoglossus and genioglossus. Besides these four pairs of extrinsic muscle there are four pairs of intrinsic muscles. These are superior longitudinal, inferior longitudinal, transverse and vertical muscles. Out of these eight muscles on each side, seven are innervated by hypoglossal nerve. Only palatoglossus gets innervated by vago-accessory complex.

Tongue is richly supplied by lingual artery a branch of external carotid. In addition it also supplies blood to the neighbouring muscles. The lymph from tongue mostly drains into submandibular lymph nodes and then to jugulo-omohyoid lymph node of the deep cervical chain.

Nerve supply is sensory, special sensory and motor. It is subdivided according to the development of tongue. *Anterior 2/3rd:* General sensory nerve is lingual (V$_3$) and special sensory is chorda tympani (VII). *Posterior 1/3rd:* General sensory is IX and special sensory is also IX. This nerve also carries taste from the circumvallate papillae.

From posterior most part, the general and special sensory sensations are carried by internal laryngeal of X.

All the muscles are supplied by hypoglossal nerve except palatoglossus which is innervated by vago-accessory complex.

Competency achievement: The student should be able to:

AN 39.1 Describe and demonstrate the morphology, nerve supply, embryological basis of nerve supply, blood supply, lymphatic drainage and actions of extrinsic and intrinsic muscles of tongue.

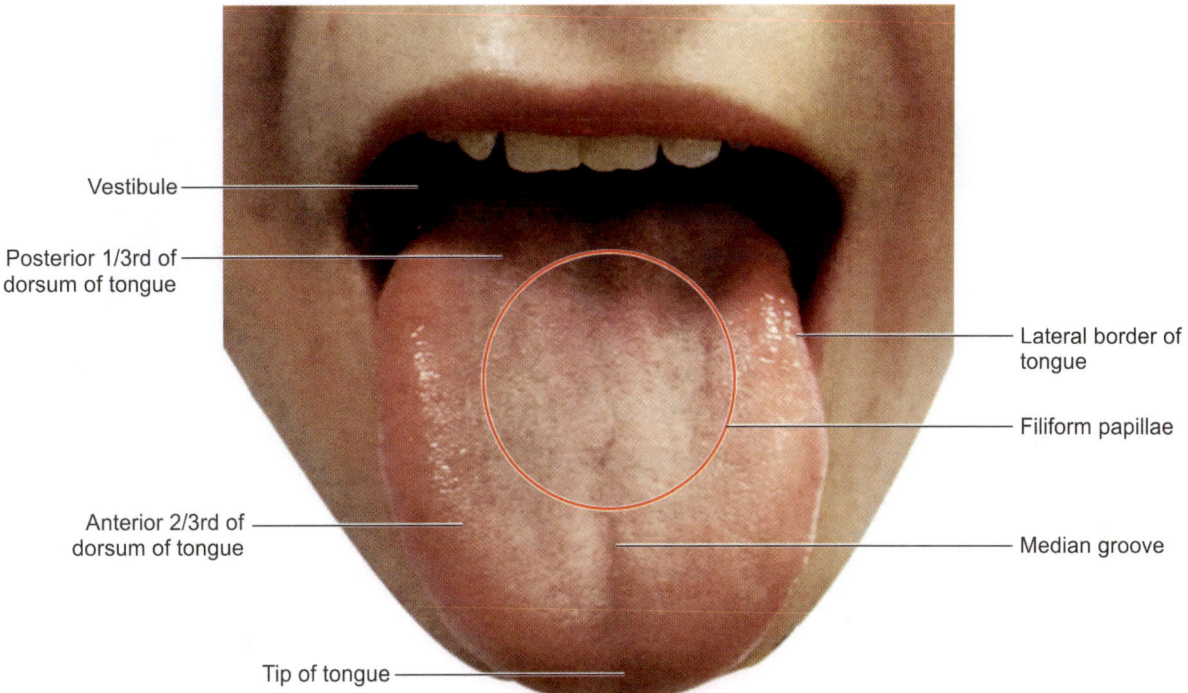

Fig. 61.1: Dorsum of tongue

Vestibule

Posterior 1/3rd of dorsum of tongue

Anterior 2/3rd of dorsum of tongue

Tip of tongue

Lateral border of tongue

Filiform papillae

Median groove

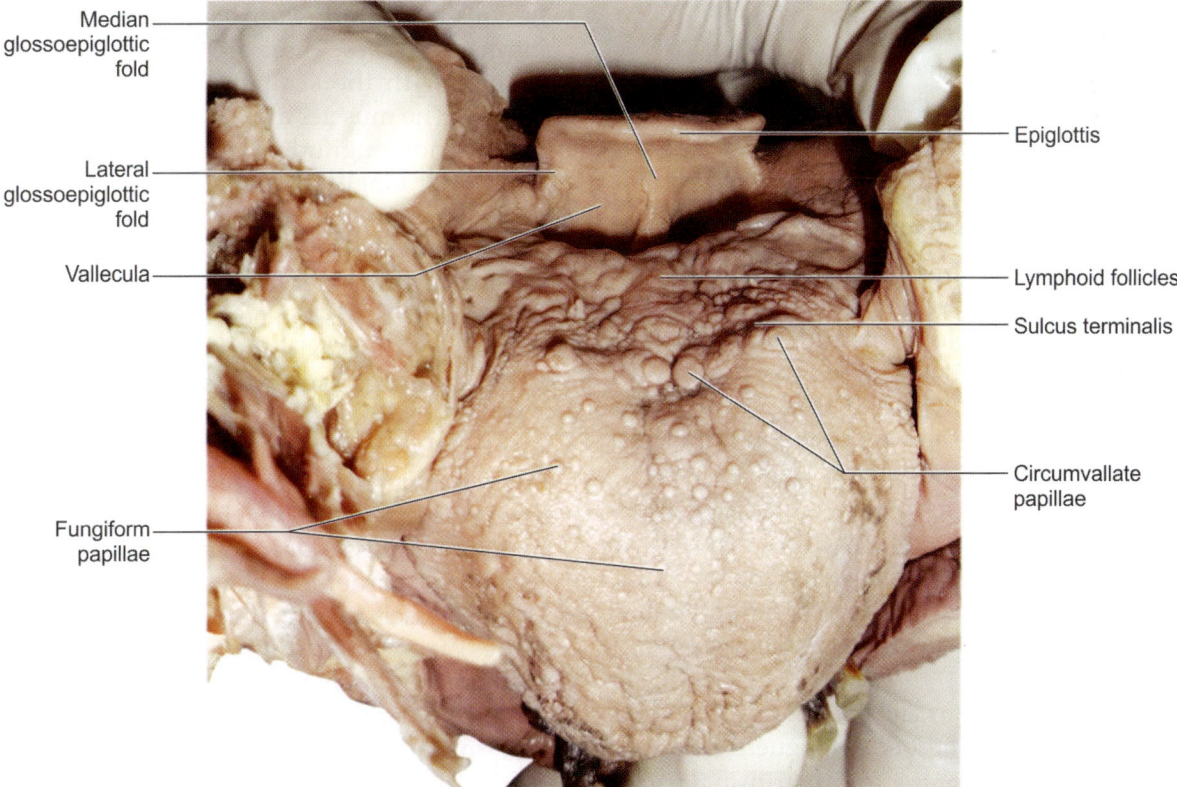

Fig. 61.2: Papillae on the dorsum of tongue

Median glossoepiglottic fold

Lateral glossoepiglottic fold

Vallecula

Fungiform papillae

Epiglottis

Lymphoid follicles

Sulcus terminalis

Circumvallate papillae

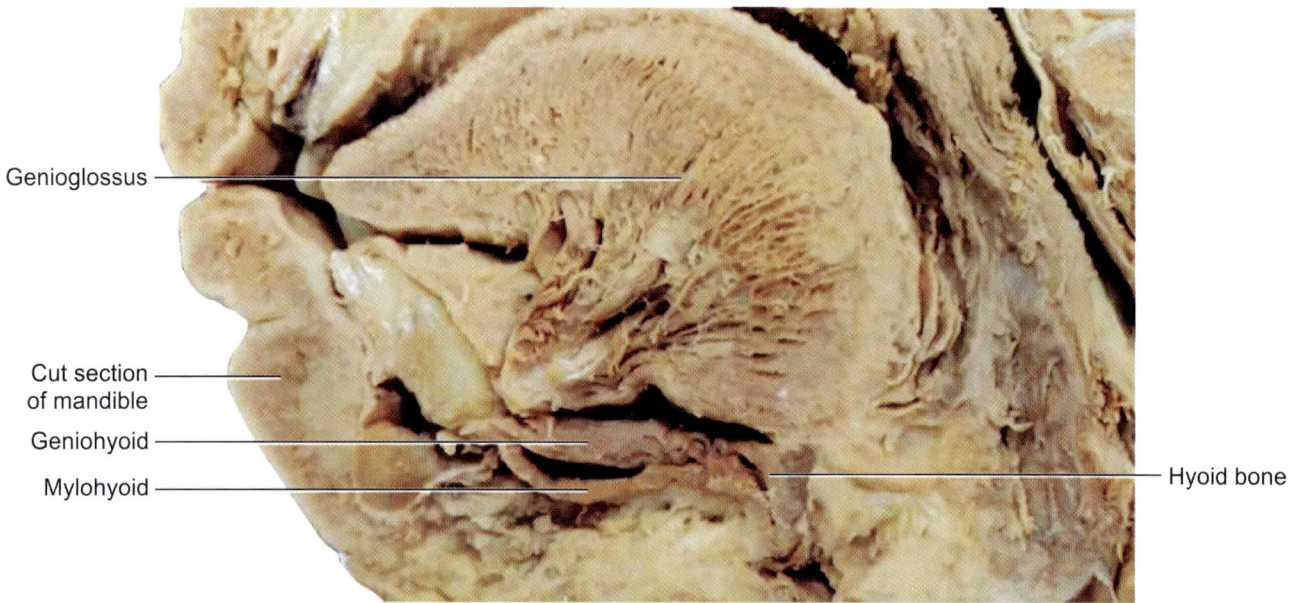

Genioglossus

Cut section of mandible

Geniohyoid

Mylohyoid

Hyoid bone

Fig. 61.3: Genioglossus muscle

STEPS OF DISSECTION

- In the sagittal section of head and neck, the cut part of tongue is seen (*see* Fig. 58.1).
- Expose the part of submental triangle.
- With the help of scalpel, cut only mylohyoid muscle along the median raphe. Separate mylohyoid muscle from deeper structures. Identify geniohyoid muscle between the lower genial tubercle and hyoid bone.
- Since mandible has already been bisected, look for big genioglossus muscle (Fig. 61.3), attached to upper genial tubercle of mandible and root of tongue including the hyoid bone, innervated by XII nerve. It is a *life saving muscle* as it protrudes the tongue and keeps the air way patent. It is the most important muscle of the tongue.
- Identify rectangular hyoglossus muscle between greater cornua of hyoid bone and the lateral side of tongue, innervated by XII nerve (*see* Fig. 51.3).
- Identify palatoglossus muscle between soft palate above and tongue below. It is supplied by vago-accessory complex.
- Trace the styloglossus muscle from the styloid process to the upper border of tongue.
  Note that three out of the four extrinsic muscles are innervated by XII nerve and only one, i.e.

palatoglossus is innervated by vagoaccessory complex.

- Besides these four extrinsic muscles identify four intrinsic muscles. These are seen by scrapping the tongue with the scalpel above and below the tongue. The muscles are:
  i. Superior longitudinal
  ii. Inferior longitudinal
  iii. Transverse
  iv. Vertical

  All muscles are innervated by XII nerve. Thus XII/hypoglossal nerve is the nerve of tongue supplying 7/8 muscles. All its extrinsic muscles have the suffix glossus, e.g. hyoglossus, palatoglossus, genioglossus and styloglossus.
- Identify the artery of tongue—the tortuous lingual artery (*see* Fig. 50.2). It is a branch of external carotid artery, runs up to reach posterior border of hyoglossus, passes deep to hyoglossus, then along its anterior border to reach substance of tongue.
- Lymph vessels from tip drain into submental lymph nodes, from lateral surface and dorsum into submandibular lymph nodes and from root of tongue bilaterally into deep cervical nodes.
- The main lymph node of tongue is jugulo-omohyoid, where omohyoid muscle crosses over the internal jugular vein.

- Identify all these lymph nodes.
- Try to see the sensory and special sensory nerves of tongue. Posterior most part is innervated by internal laryngeal branch of vagus, posterior

1/3rd by glossopharyngeal nerve and anterior 2/3rd general sensation by lingual and special sensation by chorda tympani branch of facial nerve.

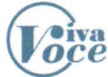

Viva Voce

- What are the parts of the tongue?
- How many types of papillae are there in the tongue? Which ones have the maximum number of taste buds?
- Name the extrinsic muscles of tongue with their nerve supply.
- Name the intrinsic muscles of tongue with their nerve supply.

- Which is the lymph node of the tongue?
- What is the importance of genioglossus muscle? What is its other name?
- If right XII nerve is injured, which side will the tip of tongue deviate on protrusion and why?
- Which drug is put sublingually during angina pectoris and why?

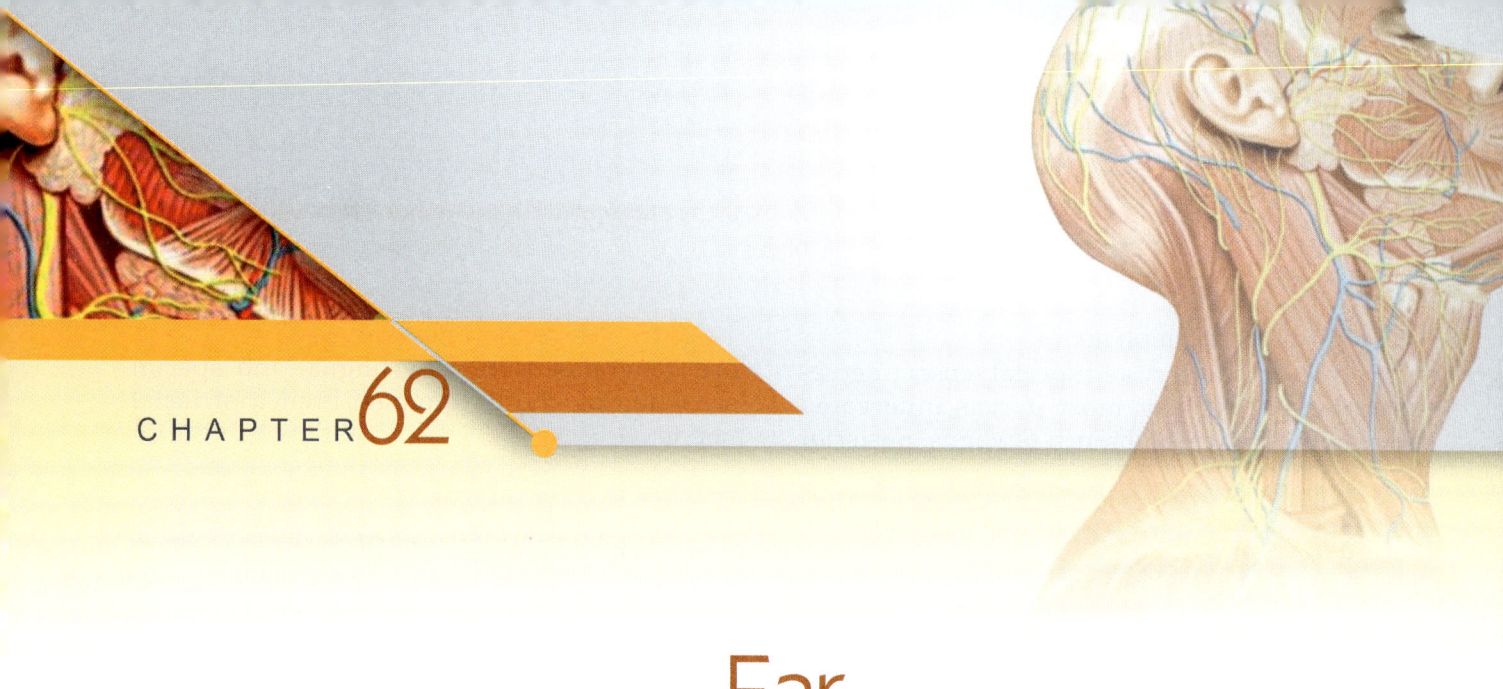

CHAPTER 62

Ear

Learning Objectives

One should be able to

1. Name the structures present in the medial wall of the middle ear
2. What are the features of posterior wall of middle ear?
3. Name the muscles of middle ear. What is their nerve supply?

OVERVIEW

The ear is an organ for hearing and is also responsible for maintaining the balance of the body. It comprises external ear, middle ear and internal ear.

External ear consists of an elastic pinna and an external auditory meatus. The meatus is 8 mm cartilaginous and 16 mm bony and impinges on the tympanic membrane.

Middle ear is a box like cavity with roof, floor, anterior, posterior, lateral and medial walls. Besides few nerves and vessels, it contains 3 bony ossicles: Malleus, incus and stapes. Malleus and incus are derived from 1st pharyngeal arch and incus is derived from 2nd pharyngeal arch. The pharyngotympanic tube connects the anterior wall of middle ear to the nasopharynx. Through nose, nasopharynx and tube air reaches the inner aspect of tympanic membrane. Air reaches the outer aspect of tympanic membrane via the auricle and external auditory meatus. This equalizes pressure on both sides of tympanic membrane. Thus infection from nasopharynx can spread to middle ear resulting in otitis media.

Internal ear is present inside the petrous temporal bone. It comprises bony and membranous labyrinth.

Bony labyrinth consists of cochlea anteriorly, vestibule in the middle and semicircular canals posteriorly.

Similarly membranous labyrinth consists of spiral duct of cochlea in cochlea; utricle and saccule within vestibule and semicircular ducts within semicircular canals.

Cochlear nerve is the nerve of hearing while vestibular nerve is for the balance.

Competency achievement: The student should be able to:

AN 40.1 Describe and identify the parts, blood supply and nerve supply of external ear.

EXTERNAL EAR

1. Pinna/auricle comprises chiefly of the elastic cartilage. Parts of the auricle are:

   a. Helix—outer rim (Fig. 62.1)

   b. Antihelix—rim inner to helix

   c. Concha—deepest part/well of auricle

   d. Tragus—lid of external auditory meatus

   e. Lobule—soft lowest part of auricle, deficient in cartilage.

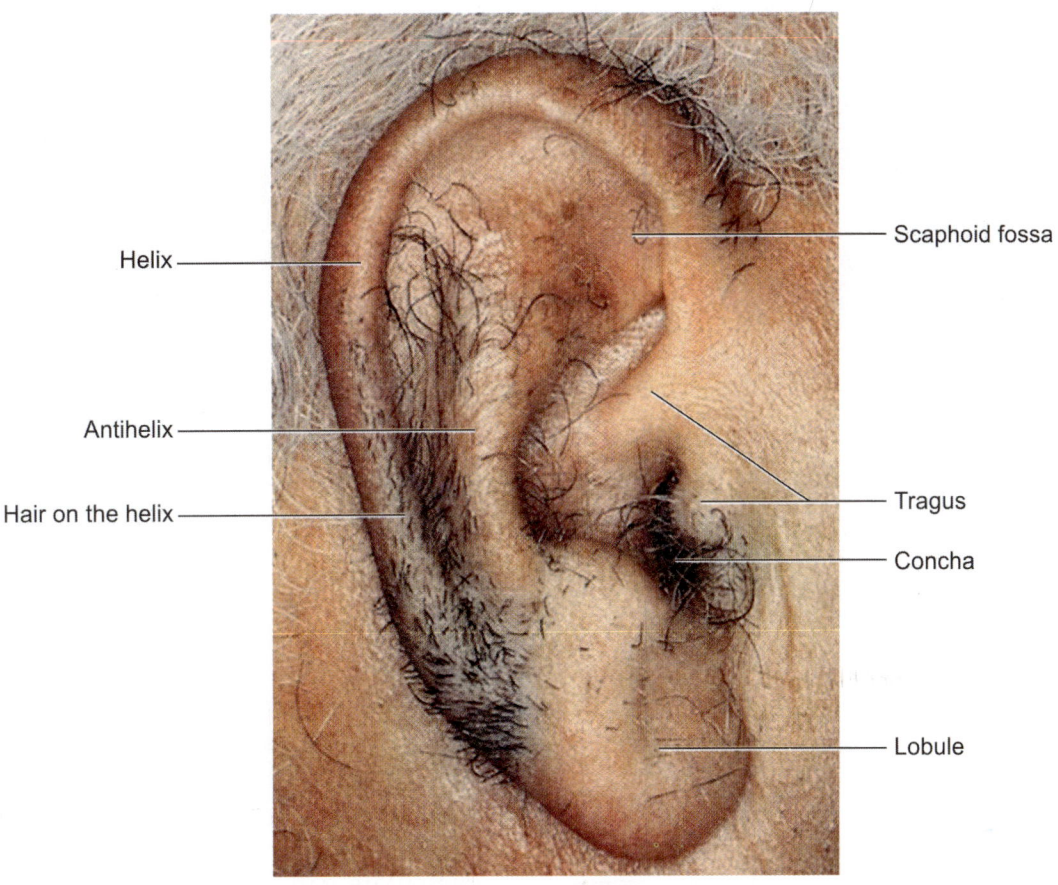

Helix

Antihelix

Hair on the helix

Scaphoid fossa

Tragus

Concha

Lobule

Fig. 62.1: Parts of auricle(pinna)

Nerve supply and lymphatic drainage is shown in Fig. 62.2a and b.

2. External auditory meatus—it begins at the deepest part of the concha and ends at the tympanic membrane. It is 'S' shaped with a length of 25 mm; lateral one-third is cartilaginous and medial two-thirds is bony. To make the meatus straight one has to pull the auricle upwards, backwards and laterally in an adult. Then only one can visualize the tympanic membrane.

> *Competency achievement:* The student should be able to:
>
> **AN 40.2** Describe and demonstrate the boundaries, contents, relations and functional anatomy of middle ear and auditory tube.

MIDDLE EAR/ TYMPANIC CAVITY

Middle ear is narrow air filled box like cavity within temporal bone. Its walls are:

i. *Roof:* Formed by tegmen tympani. It also forms roof of canal for tensor tympani muscle present on the anterior face of petrous temporal bone.

ii. *Floor* is a thin plate of bone anterior to jugular foramen.

iii. *Anterior wall:* Formed by canal for tensor tympani muscle and groove for pharyngotympanic tube.

iv. *Posterior wall:* Formed by aditus to mastoid antrum (Fig. 62.3), pyramid with stapedius muscle and posterior canaliculus of chorda tympani nerve.

v. *Lateral wall* by tympanic membrane and epitympanic recess above the membrane.

vi. *Medial wall:* Formed by promontory/an inward bulge/projection by basal turn of cochlea. Above promontory is oval window. Still above the oval window is a bulge formed by facial canal. Inferior to promontory is the round window.

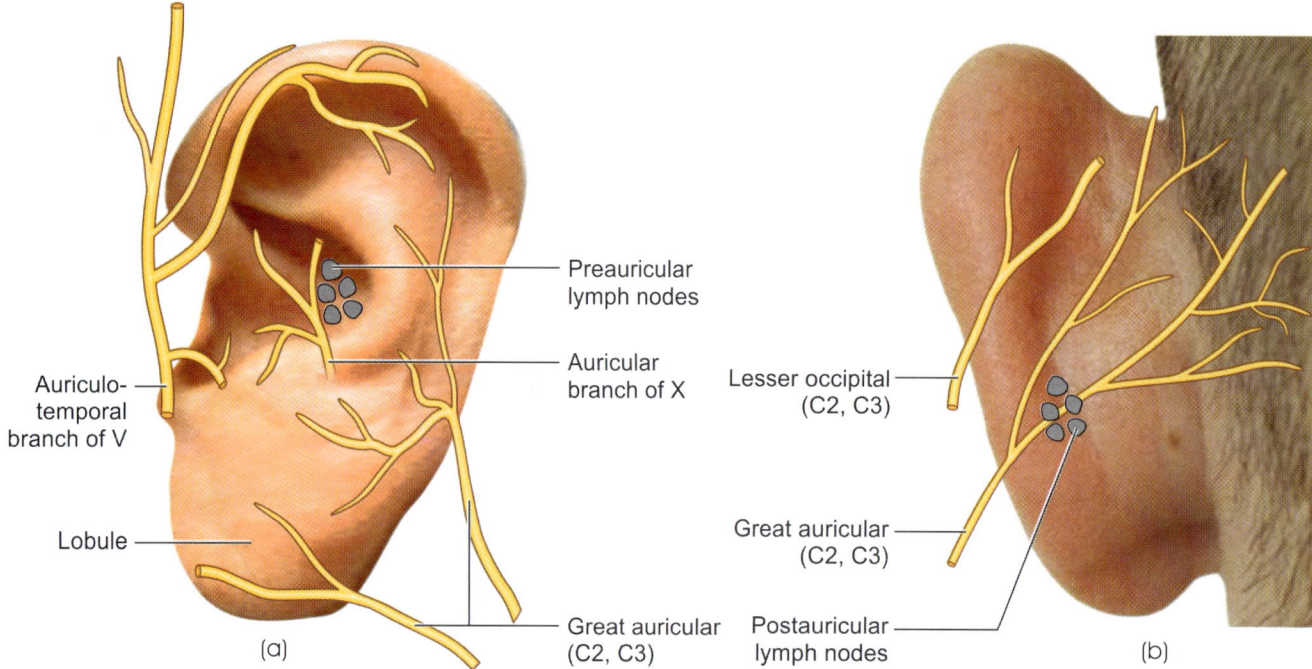

Fig. 62.2: Nerve supply and lymphatic drainage of auricle: (a) Lateral surface; (b) Medial surface

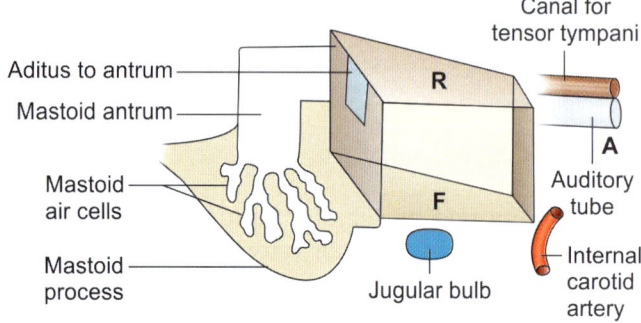

Fig. 62.3: Anterior and posterior walls of middle ear

Steps of Dissection

- Remove the tegmen tympani of the petrous part of temporal bone. It can be easily done in a decalcified bone if available. Identify greater petrosal nerve lying in sulcus of same name. The greater petrosal nerve lies between the bone and dura mater.
- Identify the internal acoustic meatus on the posterior surface of petrous temporal bone.
- Remove the roof of internal acoustic meatus. Look for VII and VIII nerves and labyrinthine vessels entering this meatus.

- Trace the facial nerve laterally till it makes a bend in posterior direction. Locate a tiny swelling, the geniculate ganglion, and beginning of greater petrosal nerve.
- Follow greater petrosal nerve through hiatus and groove of same name. This nerve joins deep petrosal nerve formed from sympathetic plexus around internal carotid artery. These two nerves join to form "nerve of pterygoid canal" which courses through the foramen lacerum to reach pterygo-palatine fossa.
- Trace the facial nerve in the facial canal at geniculate ganglion. It runs for a short distance in postero-lateral direction, and then the nerve turns inferiorly to exit the skull at the stylomastoid foramen.
- The position of cochlea can be understood as it lies in the angle formed by facial nerve, geniculate ganglion and greater petrosal nerve. In some cases the modiolus may also be visible.
- Identify the arcuate eminence on the anterior surface of petrous temporal bone. The superior semicircular canal lies under it.
- After removing the tegmen tympani, look for the 3 bony ossicles (Fig. 62.4). Malleus is attached to

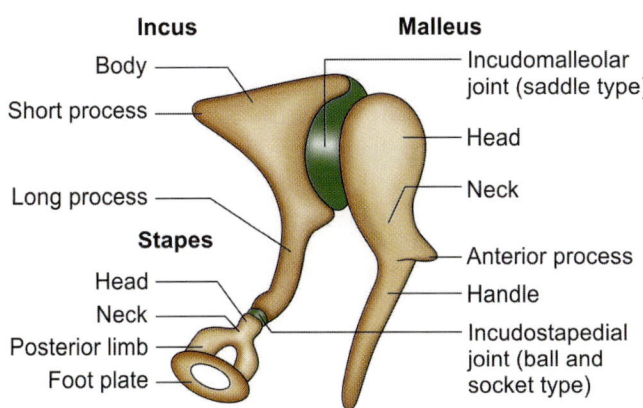

Fig. 62.4: Bony ossicles

tympanic membrane. Incus is in between malleus and stapes. The stapes is seen to fit into the oval window of medial wall.

- Identify the tympanic membrane on lateral wall of middle ear with convexity on medial side. One may be able to see tendon of tensor tympani (supplied by V_3) getting attached to handle of malleus. The other muscle is stapedius in relation to posterior wall. It is supplied by facial nerve.

- Trace the chorda tympani nerve (branch of VII) from posterior canaliculus in posterior wall of middle ear, across the medial aspect of tympanic membrane, between stapes and malleus, to reach petrotympanic fissure (Fig. 62.5). This nerve leaves the cranial cavity through petrotympanic fissure to join lingual nerve in submandibular region.

- See that the structures in the middle ear are covered with mucous membrane, which is innervated by IX nerve. This nerve forms a tympanic plexus which gives origin to lesser petrosal nerve conveying secretomotor fibres to the parotid gland.

INTERNAL EAR

See the structures of internal ear from models, as it is difficult to dissect.

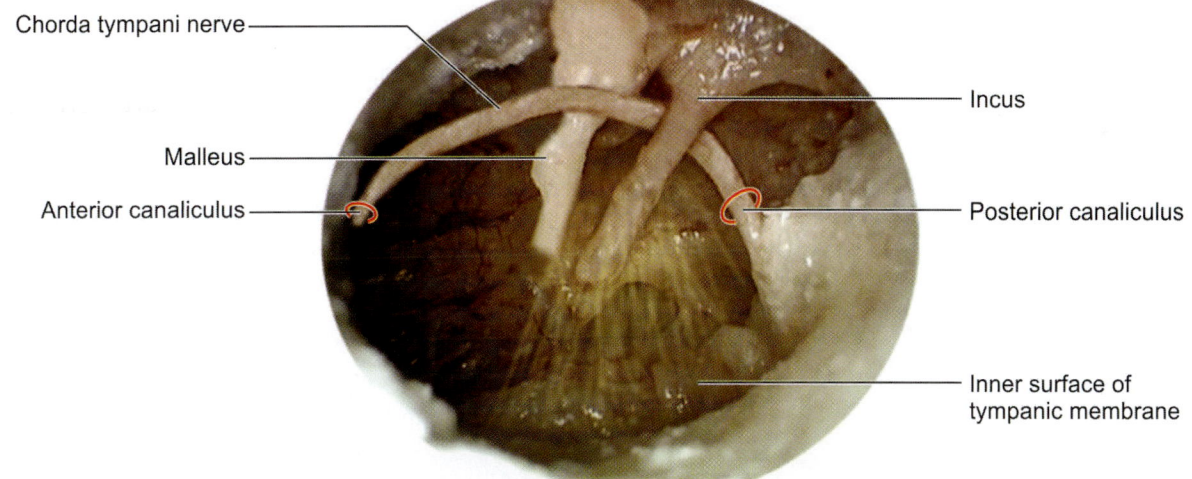

Fig. 62.5: Course of chorda tympani nerve through the middle ear

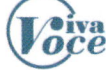 **Viva Voce**

- What is the nerve supply of tympanic membrane on both its surfaces?
- Name the bony ossicles and the types of joints formed between them.
- Name the muscles of the middle ear with their nerve supply.
- How can syringing of the ear cause nausea and bradycardia?

- Which structures form posterior wall of the middle ear?
- Which two tubes lie in the anterior wall of the middle ear?
- What is the receptor in saccule and utricle?
- Enumerate the reasons for 'earache'.
- Enumerate the complications of otitis media.

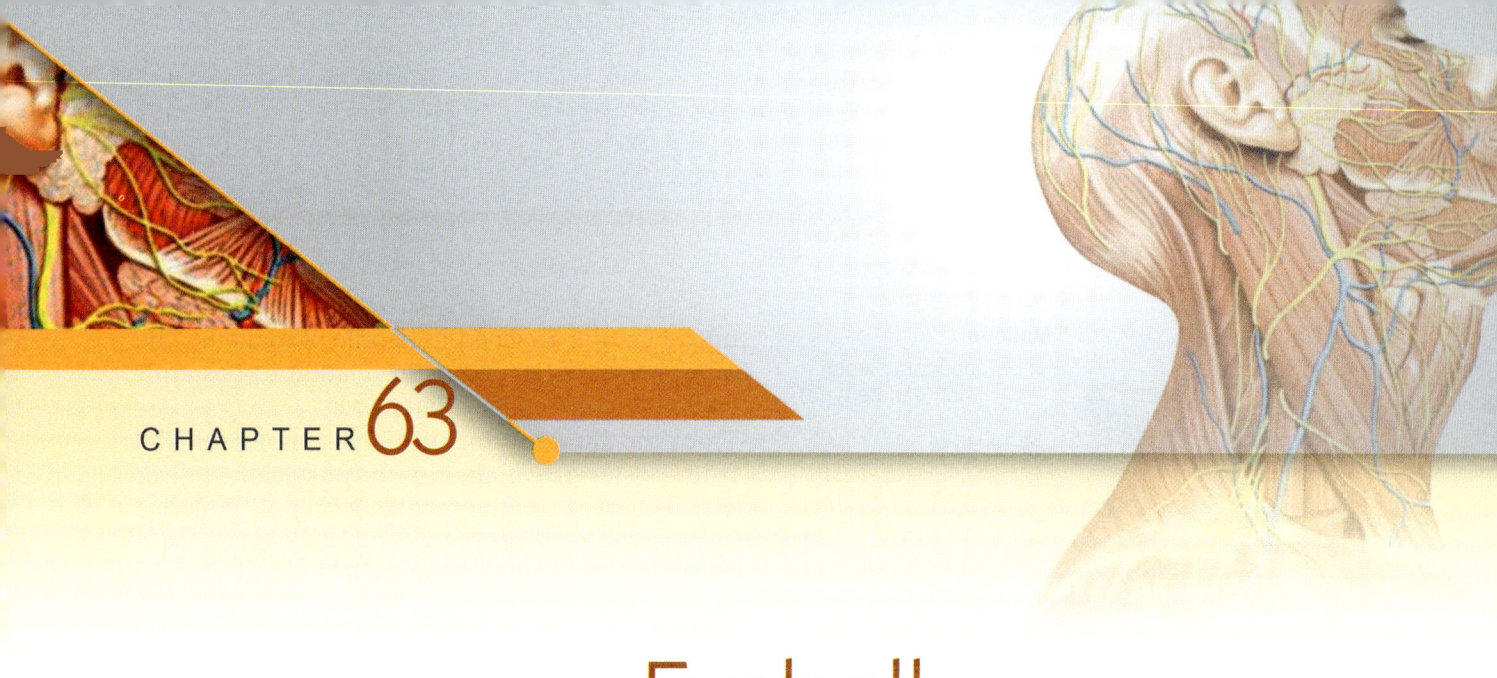

CHAPTER 63

Eyeball

Learning Objectives

One should be able to
1. Name the structures piercing sclera around exit of optic nerve.
2. Trace the light impulses from temporal field of right eye till the occipital cortex.
3. Name the parts of the middle coat of eyeball.

OVERVIEW

Eyeball is responsible for sense of sight. It comprises three layers: Outer coat is sclera (opaque) and cornea (transparent); middle coat is vascular choroid, ciliary body with smooth muscles and iris with a central hole, the pupil (Fig. 63.1a and b).

Eyeball is made of anterior segment and posterior segment. Anterior segment is subdivided into anterior chamber and posterior chamber both containing a circulating fluid the aqueous humor. The posterior segment contains a static vitreous humor.

Inner coat is the retina and is photosensitive layer. The images of the objects seen fall on the retina and

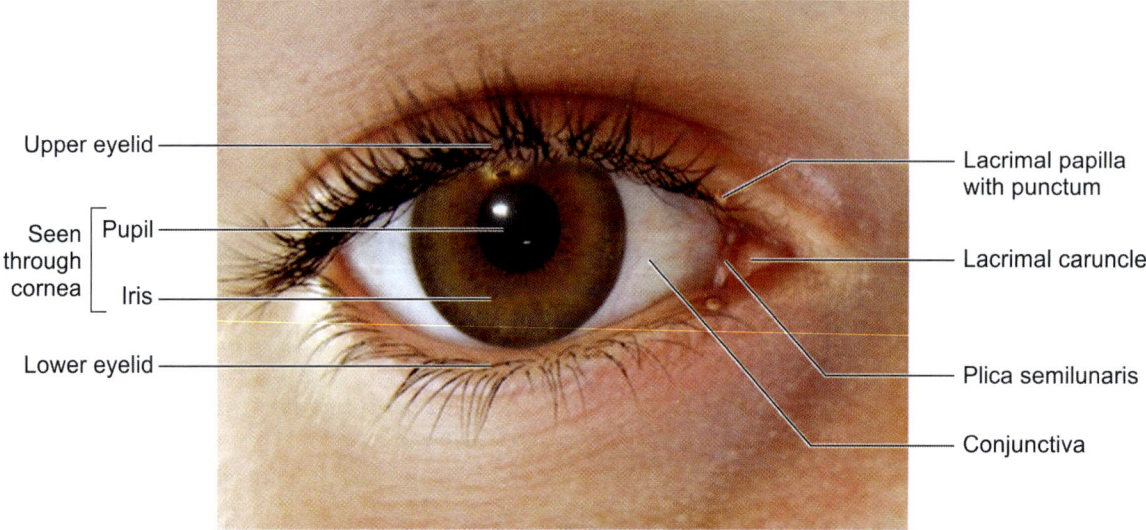

Seen through cornea — Pupil, Iris

Upper eyelid

Lower eyelid

Lacrimal papilla with punctum

Lacrimal caruncle

Plica semilunaris

Conjunctiva

Fig. 63.1a: External features of eye

are carried by optic nerve, optic chiasma, optic tract, lateral geniculate body, optic radiation to the occipital cortex.

Lens is biconvex transparent structure placed between the anterior and posterior segments of the eye. The central points of anterior and posterior surfaces are called anterior and posterior poles.

Lens is suspended by suspensory ligament of lens. Contraction of ciliary muscle relaxes the suspensory ligament the lens. It becomes more convex for near vision.

Competency achievement: The student should be able to:

AN 41.1 Describe and demonstrate parts and layers of eyeball.

STEPS OF DISSECTION

- Use the fresh eyeball of goat for dissection. Clean the eyeball by removing all the tissues from its surface.
- Cut through the fascial sheath around the margin of cornea.
- Clean and identify the optic nerve with posterior ciliary arteries and ciliary nerves close to the posterior pole of eyeball.
- Identify 4 venae vorticosae piercing the sclera just behind the equator.
- Incise only the equator and then cut through it all around and carefully strip it off from the choroid. Anteriorly the ciliary muscles are attached to the sclera offering some resistance.

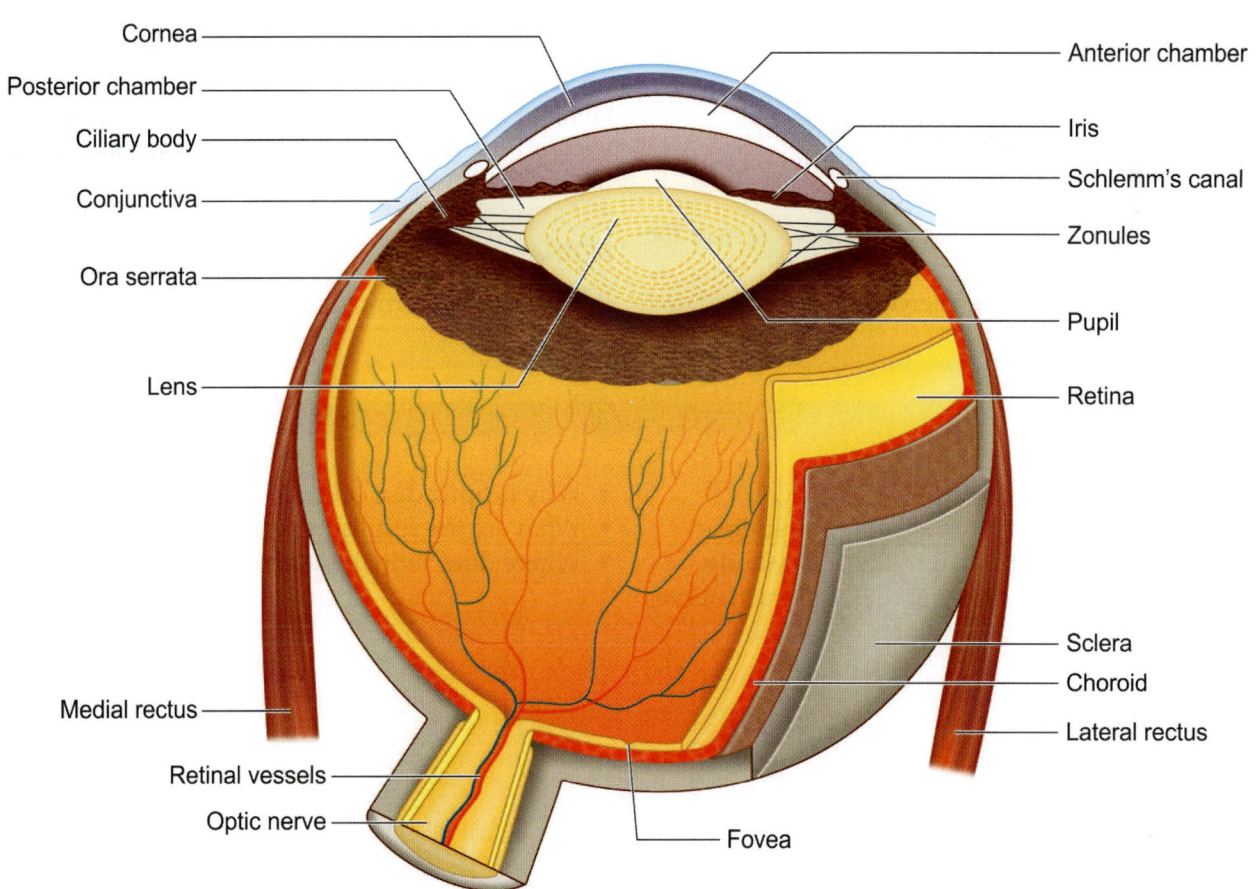

Fig. 63.1b: Layers of the eyeball

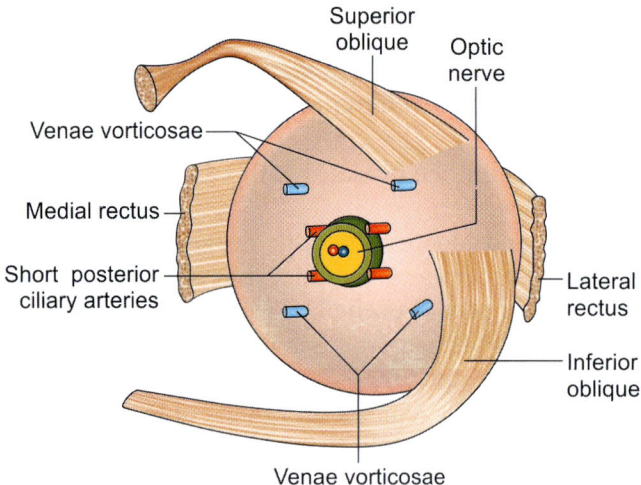

Fig. 63.2: Structures piercing the sclera

- As the sclera is separated the aqueous humour will escape from the anterior chamber of the eye. On dividing the optic nerve fibres, the posterior part of the sclera can be removed.
- See that the following structures pierce the sclera:
  1. Optic nerve pierces a little inferomedial to the posterior pole of the eyeball (Fig. 63.2).
  2. Posterior ciliary arteries and ciliary nerves pierce around the entrance of optic nerve.
  3. Anterior ciliary arteries pierce the sclera near the corneoscleral junction.
  4. Four venae verticosae pierce just behind equator.

CORNEA AND MIDDLE COAT

- Identify the cornea. Make an incision around the corneoscleral junction and remove the cornea so that the iris is exposed for examination.
- Identify the middle coat, i.e. choroid, ciliary body and iris deep to the sclera (Fig. 63.1b).
- Identify the ciliary body lateral to the iris. Ciliary body is composed of ciliary muscles and ciliary processes. The ciliary muscles along with constrictor pupillae are innervated by para-sympathetic fibres from Edinger Westphal nucleus via III nerve.
- Strip the iris, ciliary processes and anterior part of choroid. Dilator pupillae is supplied by sympathetic fibres.
- Remove the lens and put it in water. As the lens is removed, the vitreous body also escapes. Now only the posterior part of choroid and subjacent retina is left.

LENS

Give an incision in the anterior surface of lens and with a little pressure of fingers and thumb express the body of lens outside from the capsule.

RETINA

Retina is the innermost photosensitive layer.

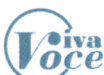

- Name the layers of the eyeball.
- Enumerate the structures piercing the sclera.
- Name the muscles present in the ciliary body.
- Name the muscles present in the iris. Which nerves supply these muscles?

- Why is optic disc called the 'blind spot'?
- What are the results of Horner's syndrome?
- Where does retinal detachment occur?

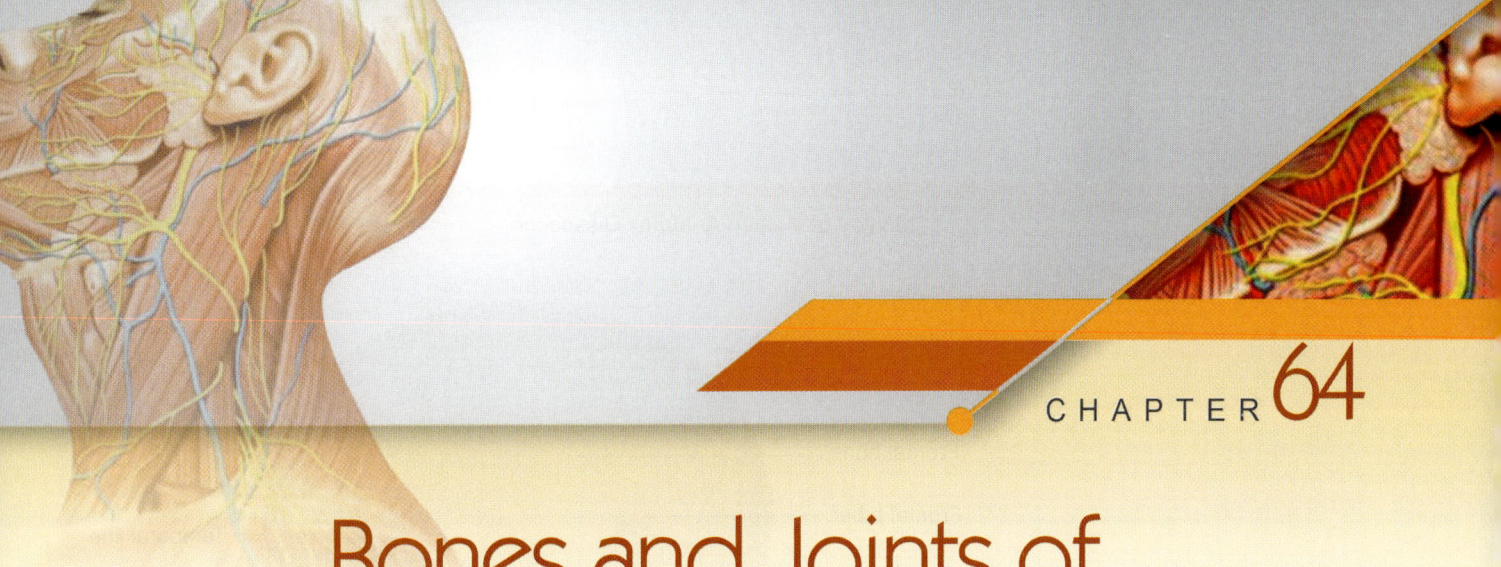

CHAPTER 64

Bones and Joints of Head and Neck

Learning Objectives

One should be able to

1. Show movements of the lower cervical vertebrae.
2. Name the structures passing through foramen magnum.

Head and neck contains numerous bones like skull, hyoid and 7 cervical vertebrae (Fig. 64.1).

Skull itself comprises 22 bones. Most of these bones are united to each other by fibrous joints known as sutures (Fig. 64.2). The teeth also articulate with maxilla and mandible to form fibrous joints known as gomphosis (Fig. 64.3). Both gomphosis and sutures are immobile joints.

Main mobile joint in the skull is the temporomandibular joint with typical and important movements, described earlier (*see* Figs 50.2 and 50.3). Even between the three bony ossicles of middle ear there are synovial joints (Fig. 64.4).

Hyoid bone is a visceral bone which does not articulate with any other bone or cartilage (Fig. 64.5).

The seven cervical vertebrae articulate with each other via intervertebral discs. Their bodies also articulate laterally with adjacent vertebrae through small joints—Luschka or uncovertebral joints (Fig. 64.6). The articular processes slope backwards to articulate with similar processes to form facet joints, permitting rotation of neck.

Movements between cervical vertebrae are flexion, extention and lateral flexion. Table 64.1 shows the movements and muscles responsible for them.

Table 64.1: Movements with muscles at lower cervical vertebrae

• Flexion	Longus capitis
• Extension	Splenius cervicis, semispinalis cervicis
• Lateral flexion	Splenius cervicis, semispinalis cervicis of one side.

Other important joints are atlantooccipital and atlantoaxial joints.

Atlantooccipital Joints

These two joints, one of each side, are synovial joints of ellipsoid variety. These move to say the movement of "YES" (Fig. 64.7). Table 64.2 shows the movements with their muscles.

Table 64.2: Movements with muscles at atlantooccipital joints

• Flexion	Longus capitis, rectus capitis anterior
• Extension	Rectus capitis posterior major and minor, semispinalis capitis, splenius capitis, upper part of trapezius.
• Lateral flexion	Rectus capitis lateralis, splenius capitis, semispinalis capitis, sternocleidomastoid, trapezius

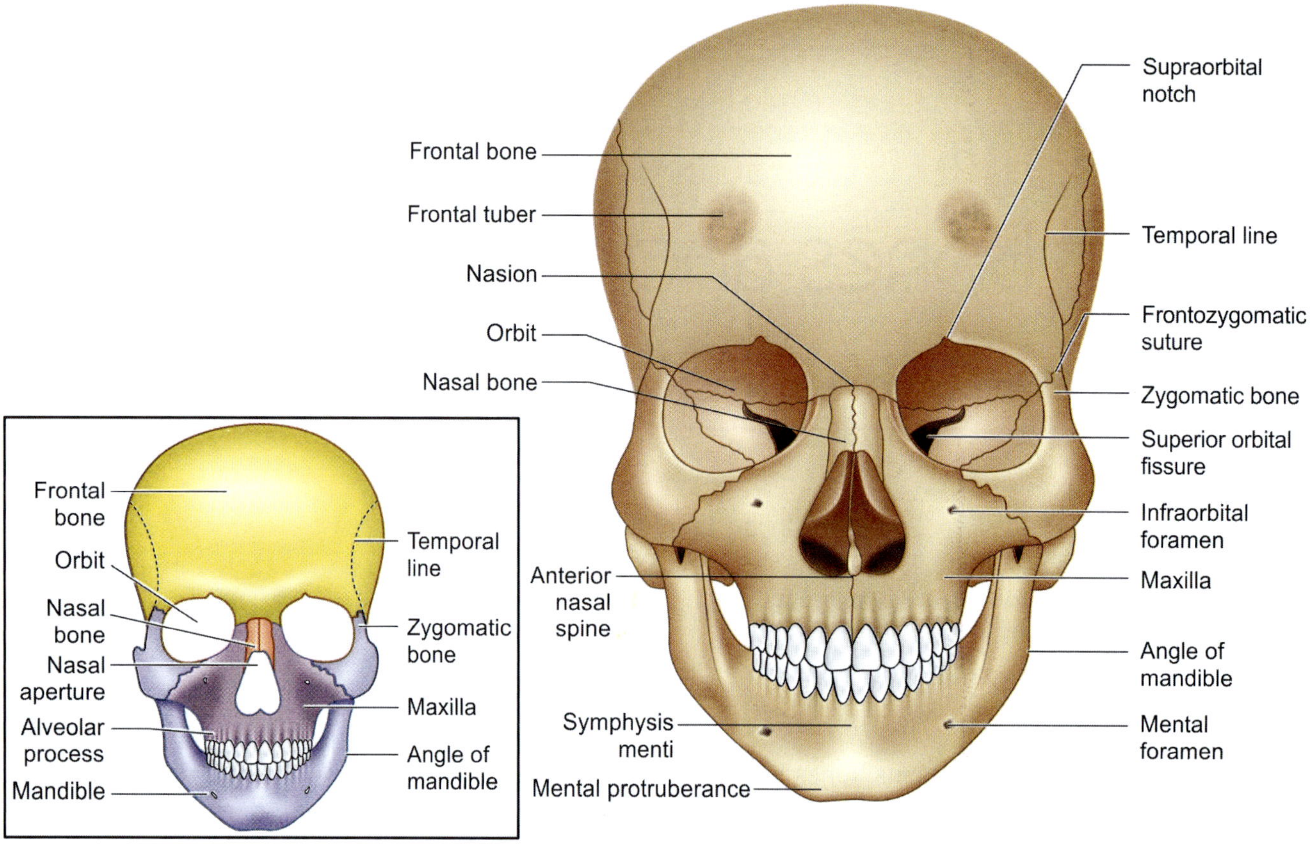

Frontal bone

Frontal tuber

Nasion

Orbit

Nasal bone

Supraorbital notch

Temporal line

Frontozygomatic suture

Zygomatic bone

Superior orbital fissure

Infraorbital foramen

Maxilla

Angle of mandible

Mental foramen

Anterior nasal spine

Symphysis menti

Mental protruberance

Frontal bone

Orbit

Nasal bone

Nasal aperture

Alveolar process

Mandible

Temporal line

Zygomatic bone

Maxilla

Angle of mandible

Fig. 64.1: Norma frontalis: Walls of orbit and nasal aperture. Inset showing apertures

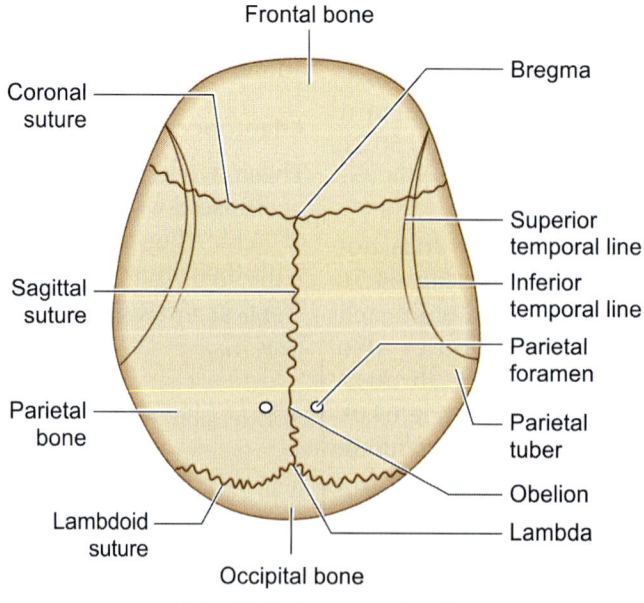

Frontal bone

Coronal suture

Sagittal suture

Parietal bone

Lambdoid suture

Bregma

Superior temporal line

Inferior temporal line

Parietal foramen

Parietal tuber

Obelion

Lambda

Occipital bone

Fig. 64.2: Norma verticalis

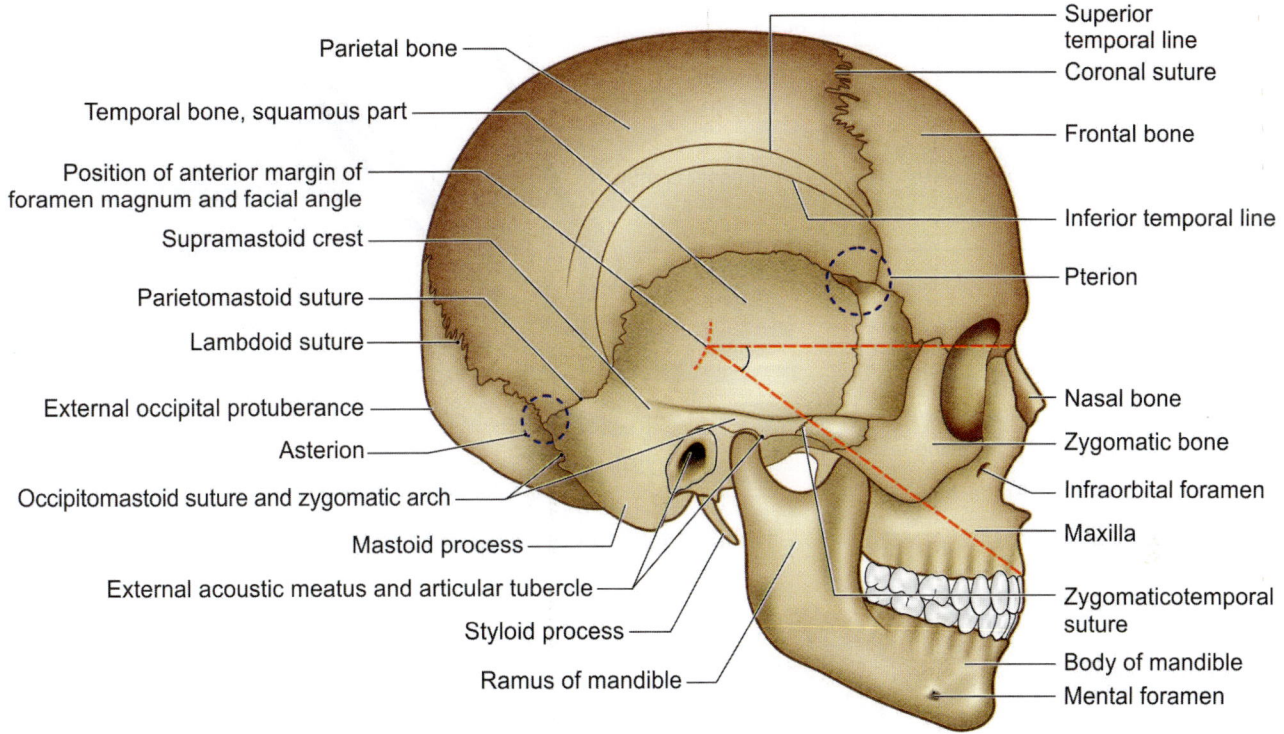

Fig. 64.3: Norma lateralis with facial angle

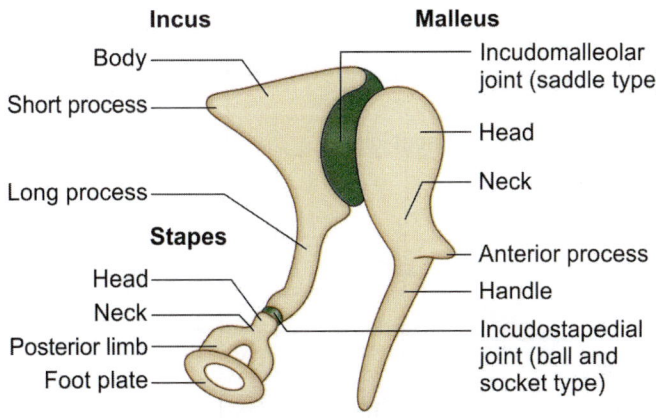

Fig. 64.4: Ossicles of the left ear, seen from the medial side

Atlantoaxial Joints

Atlantoaxial joints are three in number. Two are lateral atlantoaxial joints which move with the movements of neck. Extremely important is the median atlantoaxial joint (Fig. 64.8). This is a synovial joint of pivot variety.

Dens of the axis (C2) is held between the posterior surface of anterior arch of atlas (C1) and the transverse band of the cruciate ligament. This joint is mainly responsible for saying the movement of "NO". As atlas rotates on the dens, it rotates the skull as well.

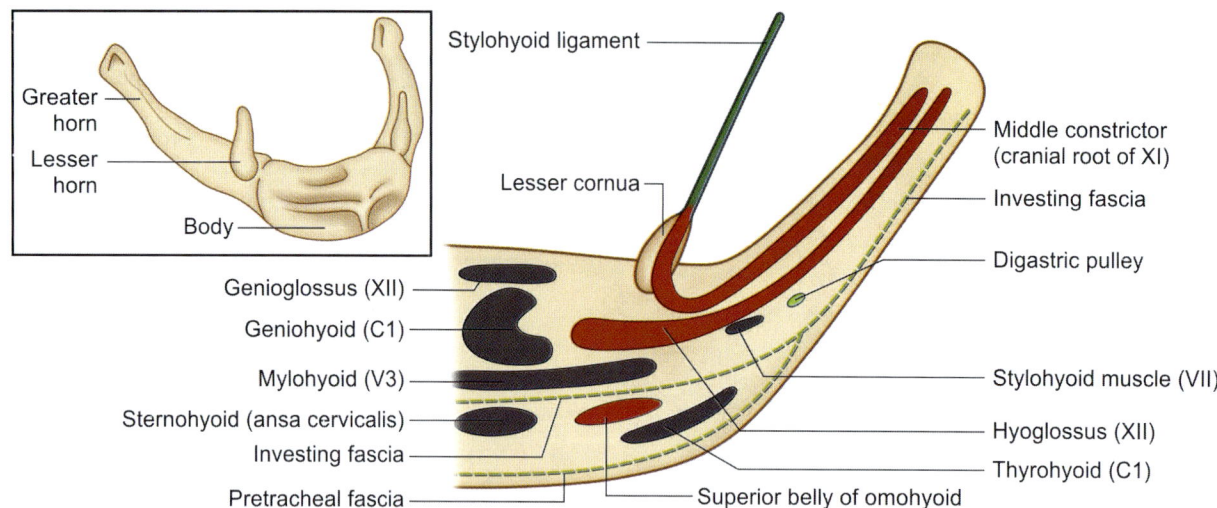

Fig. 64.5: Anterosuperior view of the left half of hyoid bone showing its attachments (Inset: Hyoid bone)

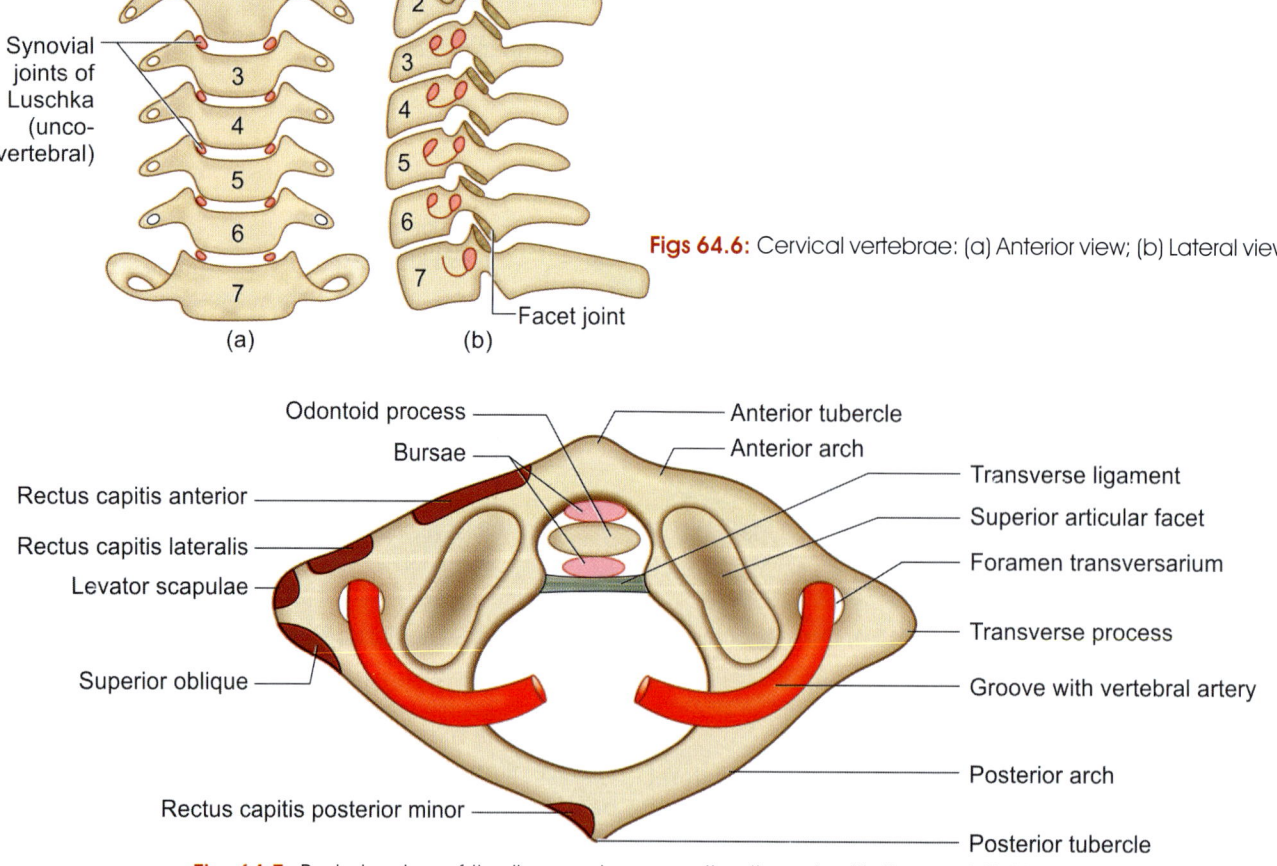

Figs 64.6: Cervical vertebrae: (a) Anterior view; (b) Lateral view

Fig. 64.7: Posterior view of the ligaments connecting the axis with the occipital bone

Muscles Responsible

Rotatory movements at median and two lateral atlantoaxial joints are brought about by obliquus capitis inferior, rectus capitis posterior major and splenius capitis of one side and sternocleidomastoid of the opposite side.

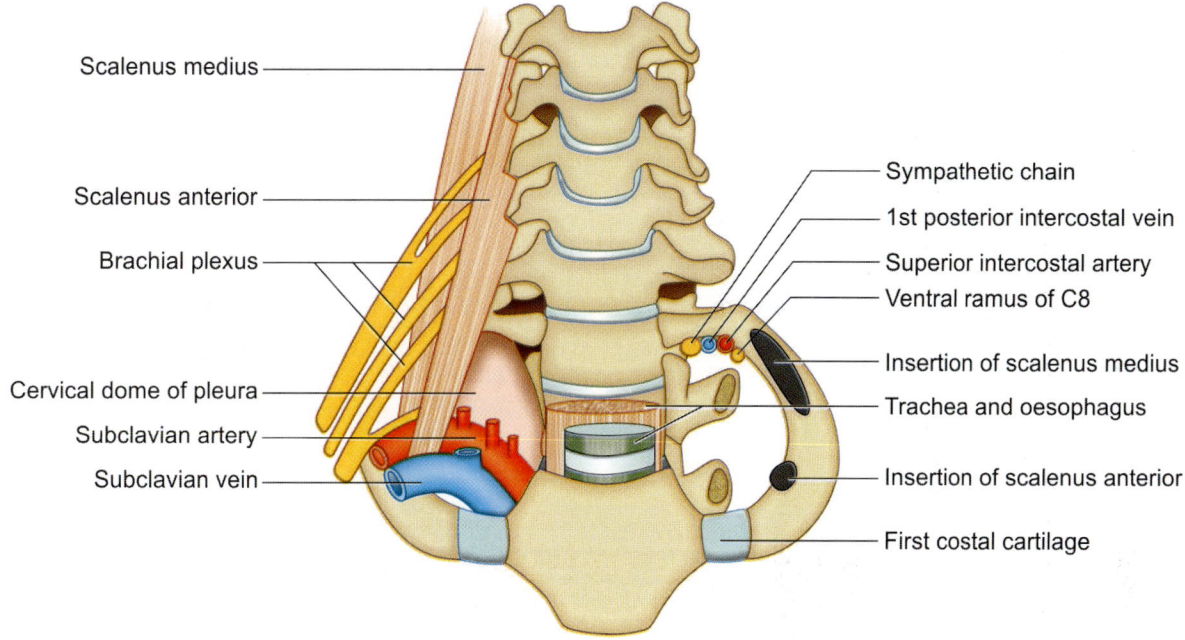

Scalenus medius

Scalenus anterior

Brachial plexus

Cervical dome of pleura

Subclavian artery

Subclavian vein

Sympathetic chain

1st posterior intercostal vein

Superior intercostal artery

Ventral ramus of C8

Insertion of scalenus medius

Trachea and oesophagus

Insertion of scalenus anterior

First costal cartilage

Fig. 64.8: Atlas vertebra seen from above

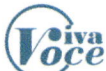

- Name the fibrous joints in skull.
- What type of joint is median atlantoaxial joint. What movement occurs here?
- Name the artery on the posterior arch of atlas vertebra.
- What are Luschka's joints

1. Identify the muscle
   a. What is its nerve supply?
   b. Enumerate its actions.

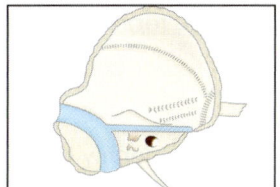

2. a. Identify the meatus.
   b. Name structures passing through it.

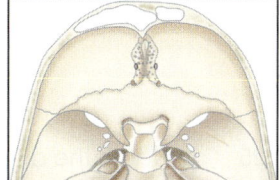

3. a. Name the structure lying in the anterior ethmoidal canal.
   b. What are the branches of that structure?

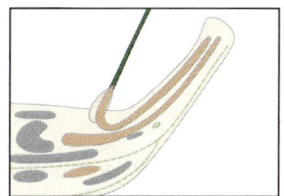

4. a. Identify the structure.
   b. From which pharyngeal arch does this develop?

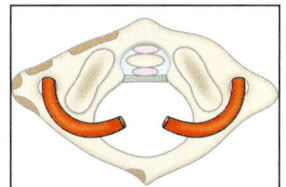

5. a. Identify the structure.
   b. Name its parts. What is the extent of its 2nd part?

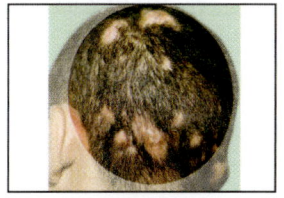

6. a. Identify the numerous swellings.
   b. Why do these appear in the scalp?

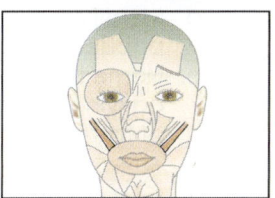

7. a. Identify the muscle.
   b. What is its nerve supply? What is its action?

8. a. Name the nerve and site of paralysis of the nerve.
   b. Which side of injury to corticonulcear fibres result in this paralysis?

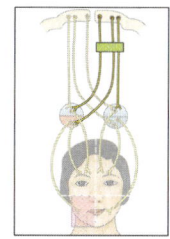

9. a. Identify the duct.
   b. Name the structures pierced by the duct before it opens?

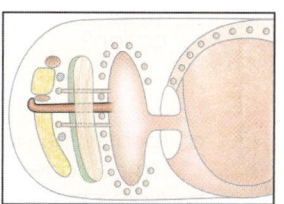

10. a. Identify the sheath.
    b. What structures lie anterior and posterior to this sheath?

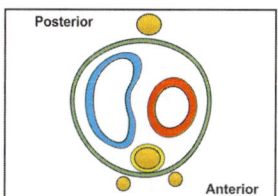

11. a. Identify the structure shown.
    b. Name the muscles innervated by it.

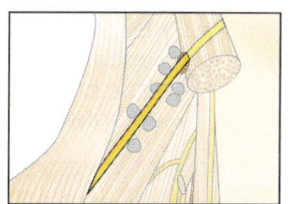

12. a. Identify the structure.
    b. What is its nerve supply?
    c. What is its relation to posterior triangle of neck?

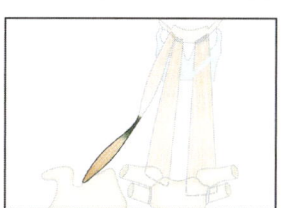

13. a. Identify the artery.
    b. How many parts does it have?
    c. What is its relation to XII nerve?

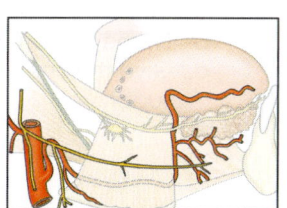

14. a. Identify the nerve.
    b. Enumerate its branches.

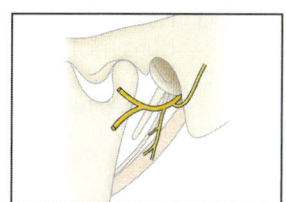

15. a. Identify these two arteries.
    b. What is their clinical importance?

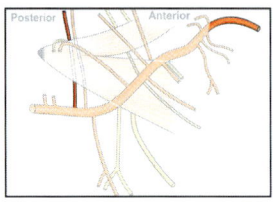

16. a. Identify the muscle. What is its nerve supply?
    b. What is its exclusive action?

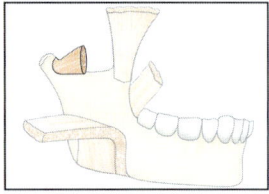

17. a. Identify the group of lymph nodes.
    b. Name the areas drained by it.
    c. Cancer of which organ can metastasize in these lymph nodes.

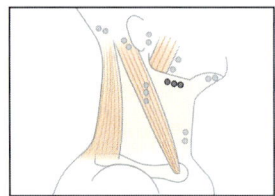

18. a. Identify highlighted artery
    b. Why are the glandular branches of the artery ligated separately?

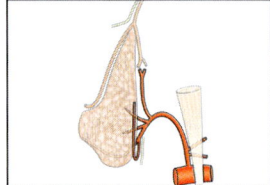

19. a. Identify the highlighted glands.
    b. Why do these glands descend downwards?

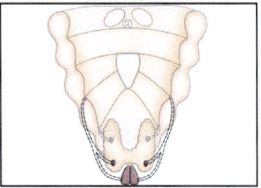

20. a. Identify the bone.
    b. Name the 3 muscles.
    c. Give their nerve supply.

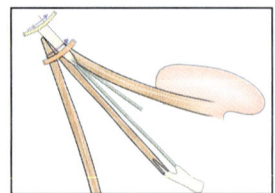

21. a. Name the fold of dura mater.
    b. Name the venous sinuses related to it.

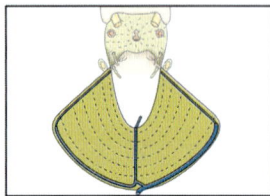

22. a. Identify the nerve.
    b. Name the muscles innervated by it. Which ganglion is associated with this nerve?

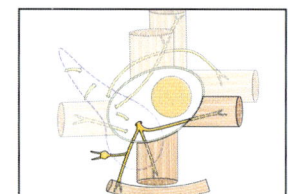

23. Name the ring.
    a. Identify the cleft. What does it represent?

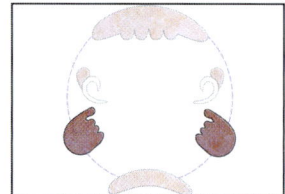

24. a. Identify the muscle.
    b. What is its nerve supply?

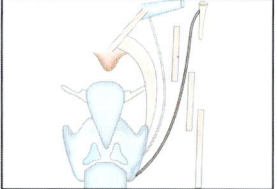

25. a. Name the arteries supplying nasal septum.
    b. Which artery is called the artery of epistaxis?

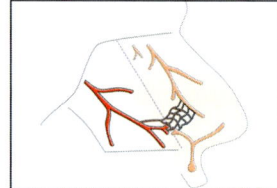

26. a. Name the ganglion.
    b. Identify the branch.

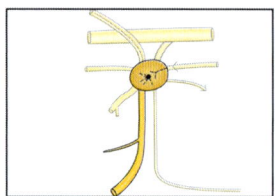

27. a. Identify the muscle.
    b. What is its nerve supply?

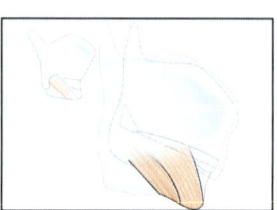

28. a. Identify the papillae.
    b. Name the nerve carrying sensation of taste.

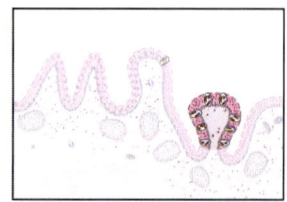

ANSWERS: HEAD AND NECK

1. a. Masseter muscle. Mandibular division of trigeminal nerve.
   b. Elevation at temporomandibular joint, protrusion of the mandibule and side to side movements of TMJ.

2. a. Internal acoustic meatus.
   b. Facial nerve, vestibulocochlear nerve and labyrinthine vessels.

3. a. Anterior ethmoidal nerve lies in the canal.
   b. Its branches are for anterior and middle ethmoidal sinuses, lateral wall of nose, septum of nose and its external nasal branch supplies tip of nose.

4. a. Stylohyoid ligament.
   b. It develops from second pharyngeal arch.

5. a. The highlighted artery is vertebral artery.
   b. It is subdivided into 1st, 2nd, 3rd and 4th parts.
   The second part starts from foramen transversarium of 6th cervical vertebra and ascends through same foramina of 5th → 4th → 3rd → 2nd → 1st cervical vertebrae.

6. a. Sebaceous cysts.
   b. Skin of scalp is very rich in sebaceous glands. Blockage of their ducts result in sebaceous cysts.

7. a. Zygomaticus major muscle supplied by zygomatic branch of facial nerve.
   b. It is known as smiling and laughing muscles.

8. a. Due to paralysis of the corticonuclear fibres of facial nerve on the left side.
   b. Paralysis of only lower quarter of facial muscles on the contralateral side (i.e. right side).

9. a. Theduct is parotid duct.
   b. It pierces buccal pad of fat, buccopharyngeal fascia, buccinator muscle and mucous membrane of mouth to open into the vestibule of mouth opposite the crown of second upper molar tooth.

10. a. This is carotid sheath.
    b. Anterior to it lies the ansa cervicalis. Posterior to the sheath lies the sympathetic trunk.

11. a. Spinal root of accessory nerve.
    b. It supplies sternocleidomastoid and trapezius muscles.

12. a. Inferior belly of omohyoid.
    b. It is supplied by a branch of descendens cervicalis (C2, C3)
    c. It divides the posterior triangle into an upper occipital part and lower supraclavicular/subclavian parts.

13. a. Lingual artery.
    b. It is subdivided into 4 parts
    c. Its first looped part is crossed by hypoglossal nerve.

14. a. The nerve shown is facial nerve coming out from stylomastoid foramen.
    b. It gives posterior auricular nerve for muscles of pinna,branches to stylohyoid and posterior belly of digastric and two main branches in parotid gland-temporofacial and cervicofacial.

15. a. The arteries are middle meningeal and sphenopalatine.
    b. Injury to middle meningeal artery causes extradural haemorrhage. Sphenopalatine is the artery of epistaxis.

16. a. The muscle highlighted is lateral pterygoid muscle.
    b. It is supplied by a branch of anterior division of mandibular nerve
    c. Its exclusive action is depression of temporomandibular joint.

17. a. The group of lymph nodes is submandibular.
    b. It drains central part of tongue, cheek, upper lip, part of lower lip.
    c. Cancer of upper surface of anterior 2/3rd of tongue excluding the tip can metastasize into these lymph nodes.

18. a. The artery is inferior thyroid artery.
    b. Its glandular branches are ligated individually, so that arterial supply to parathyroid glands does not suffer.

19. a. The glands are inferior parathyroid and thymus.
    b. As thymus descends downwards, it pulls the inferior parathyroid gland with it.

20. a. Bone is styloid process
    b. Muscles are styloglossus—XII nerve
       Stylohyoid—VII nerve
       Stylopharyngeus—IX nerve.

21. a. The dural fold is tentorium cerebelli.
    b. The venous sinuses related to it are straight sinus, right and left transverse sinuses, right and left supeior petrosal sinuses and confluence of sinuses.

22. a. The nerve is lower division of oculomotor nerve.
    b. It innervates medial rectus, inferior rectus and inferior oblique muscles. Ciliary ganglion is associated with the nerve to inferior oblique muscle.

23. a. The ring is Waldeyer's lymphatic ring.
    b. The cleft is intratonsillar cleft in the palatine tonsil. It represents remnant of 2nd pharyngeal pouch.

24. a. The muscle is stylopharyngeus.
    b. It is supplied by IX—the glossopharyngeal nerve.

25. a. The arteries are: Sphenopalatine, anterior ethmoidal, and branches of facial.
    b. The sphenopalatine artery is known as artery of epistaxis.

26. a. The ganglion is pterygopalatine ganglion.
    b. The branch shown is anterior palatine nerve.

27. a. The muscle is cricothyroid.
    b. Its nerve supply is from external laryngeal nerve, a branch of superior laryngeal nerve from vagus.

28. a. The papilla shown is circumvallate papilla.
    b. The taste from the taste buds of this papilla is conveyed by IX—the glossopharyngeal nerve.

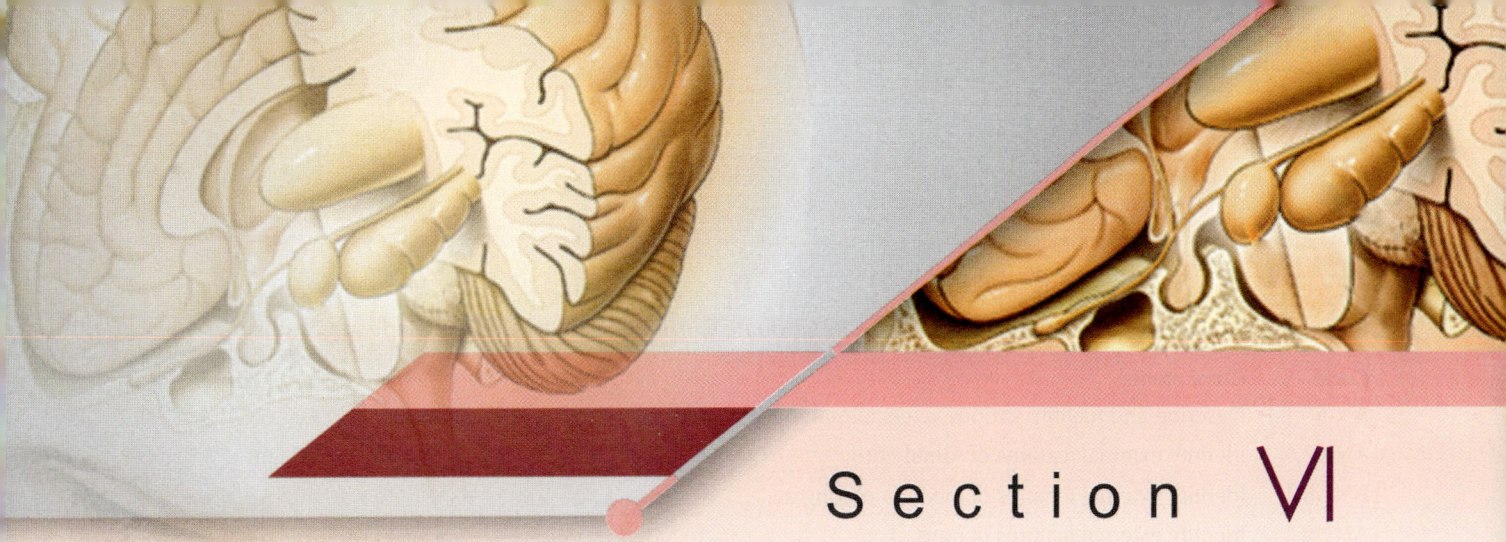

Section VI

Brain

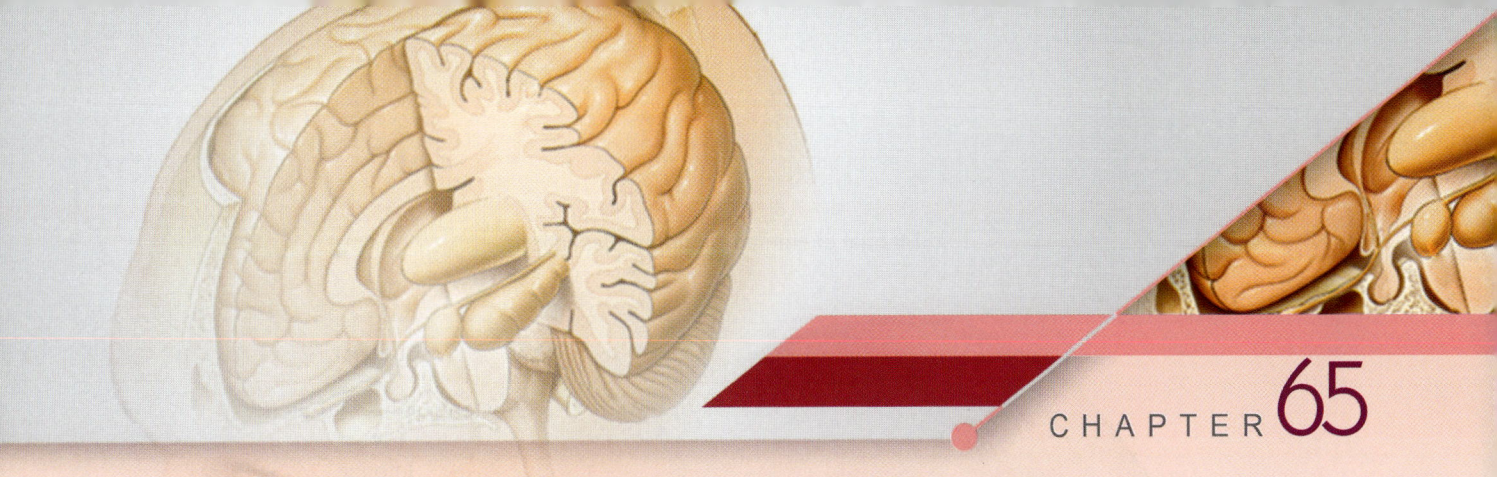

CHAPTER 65

Meninges

Learning Objectives

One should be able to
1. Name the four folds of dura mater.
2. Name various subarachnoid spaces.
3. Enumerate venous sinuses present in relation to the dural folds.

OVERVIEW

The central nervous system gets extra protection by the bony coverings, meninges, and cerebrospinal fluid (CSF). The meninges are dura mater, arachnoid mater and pia mater. Between arachnoid and pia maters lies the important CSF. The cranial cavity in addition contains an endosteum between the inner table of skull and the dura mater. The dura mater sends in four folds between parts of the brain, to prevent pressure of one lobe over the other one. In addition, in the regions of the folds the space between endosteum and dura mater encloses various venous sinuses. Arachnoid mater is cobweb like thin delicate layer. Subarachnoid space in important and is enlarged at places to form cisterns. These protect the structures present in these areas. Dura and arachnoid maters end at level of sacral 2 vertebra. Pia mater fuses with periosteum of the coccyx.

Competency achievement: The student should be able to:

AN 56.1 Describe and identify various layers of meninges with its extent and modifications.

STEPS OF DISSECTION

- Cut through the fused endosteum and dura mater on the ventral aspect of brain from the inferolateral

borders extending along the superolateral margin. See the branches of middle meningeal artery (Fig. 65.1).
- Pull upwards the endosteum along with the fold of dura mater presents between the adjacent medial surfaces of cerebral hemispheres, extending from the frontal lobe till the occipital lobe. This is falx cerebri (Figs 65.2 and 65.3).
- Pull backwards a similar but much smaller fold between two adjacent lobes of cerebellum—the falx cerebelli (Fig. 65.3).
- Separating the cerebrum and the cerebellum is another fold of dura mater called the tentorium cerebelli. Pull it on a horizontal plane (Figs 65.2 to 65.4). Another horizontal fold overlies the hypophysis cerebri. This fold is the diaphragma sellae.
- Thus, the fused endosteum and dura mater get separated from the underlying subarachnoid mater, pia mater and the brain.
- Identify various venous sinuses between the endosteum and folds of dura mater (Figs 65.2 and 65.3).
- Underneath the dura mater and separated by a flimsy subdural space is the cobweb like arachnoid

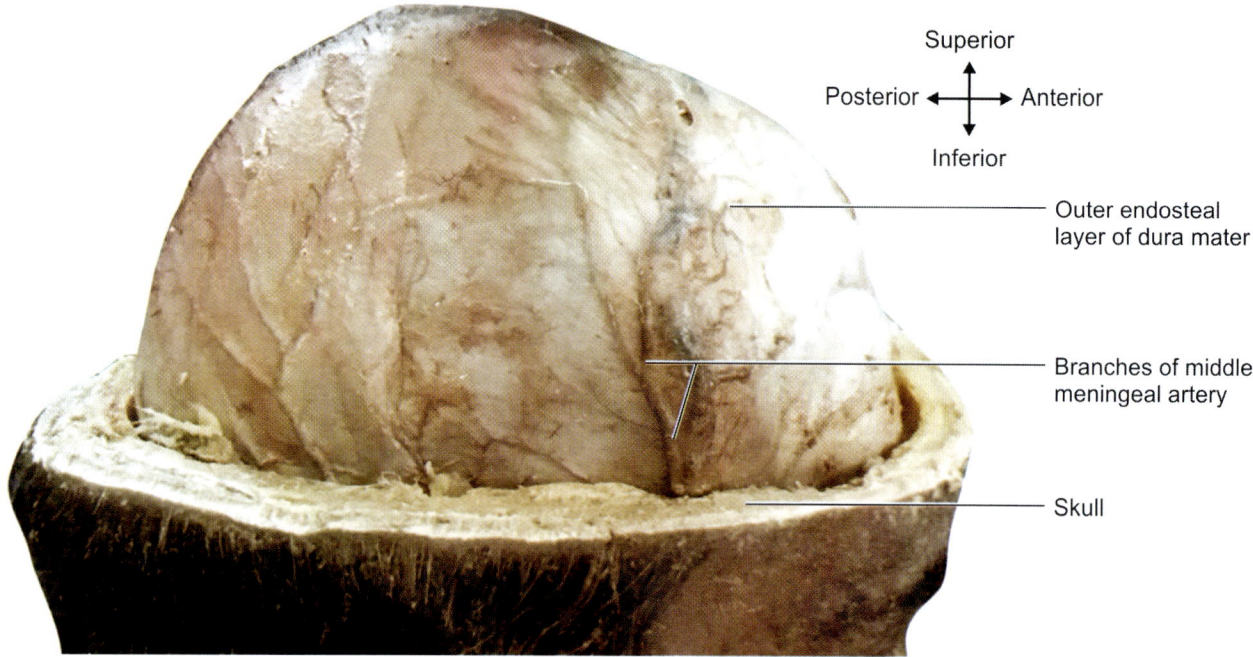

Superior

Posterior ←→ Anterior

Inferior

Outer endosteal layer of dura mater

Branches of middle meningeal artery

Skull

Fig. 65.1: Fused endosteal and meningeal layers of dura mater with blood vessels

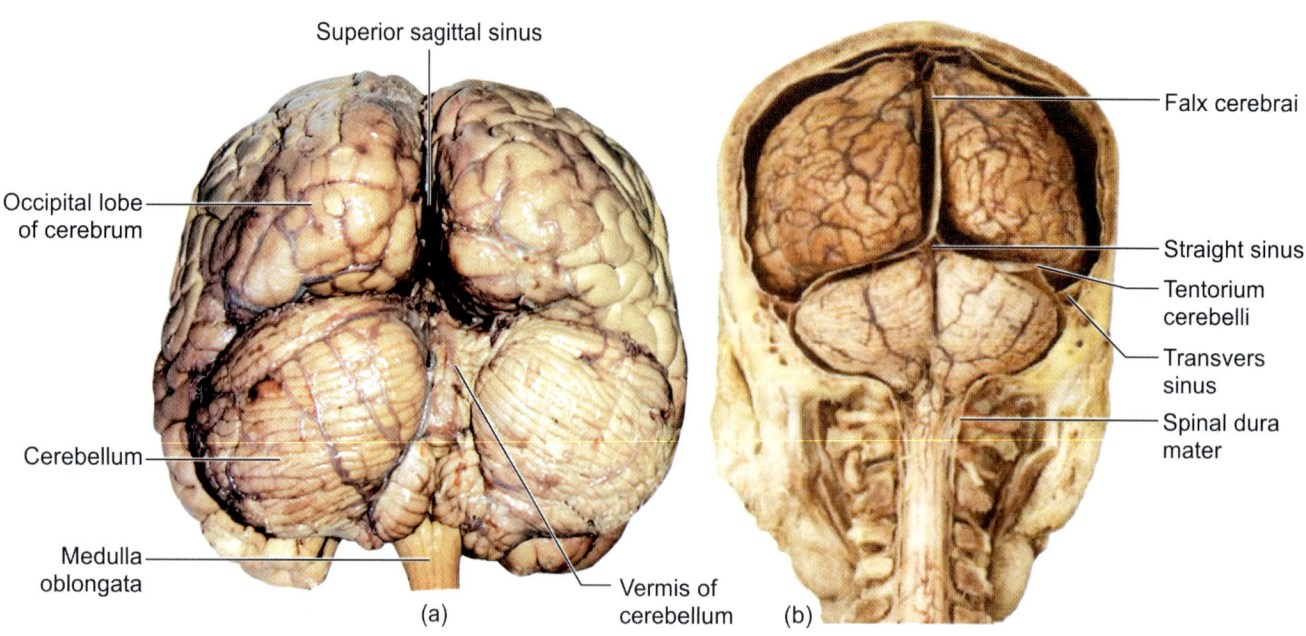

Superior sagittal sinus

Occipital lobe of cerebrum

Cerebellum

Medulla oblongata

Vermis of cerebellum

(a)

Falx cerebrai

Straight sinus

Tentorium cerebelli

Transvers sinus

Spinal dura mater

(b)

Fig. 65.2a and b: Folds of meningeal layer of dura mater

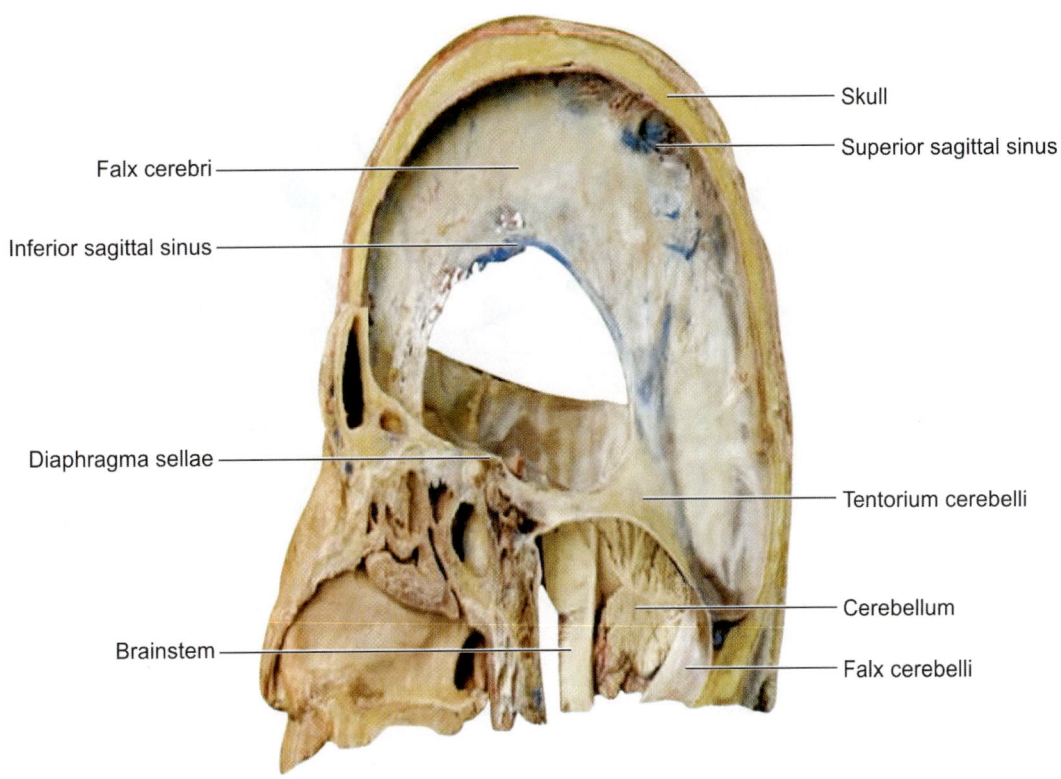

Fig. 65.3: Folds of meningeal layer of dura mater with venous sinuses

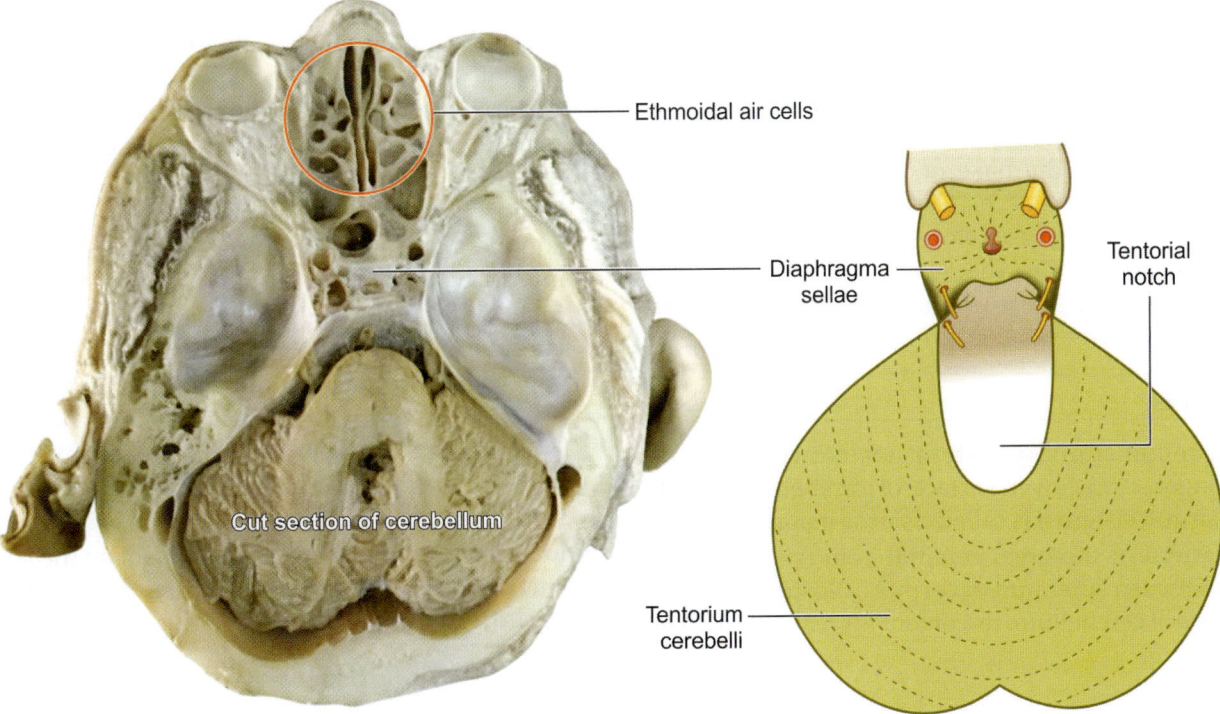

Fig. 65.4: Horizontal folds of dura mater

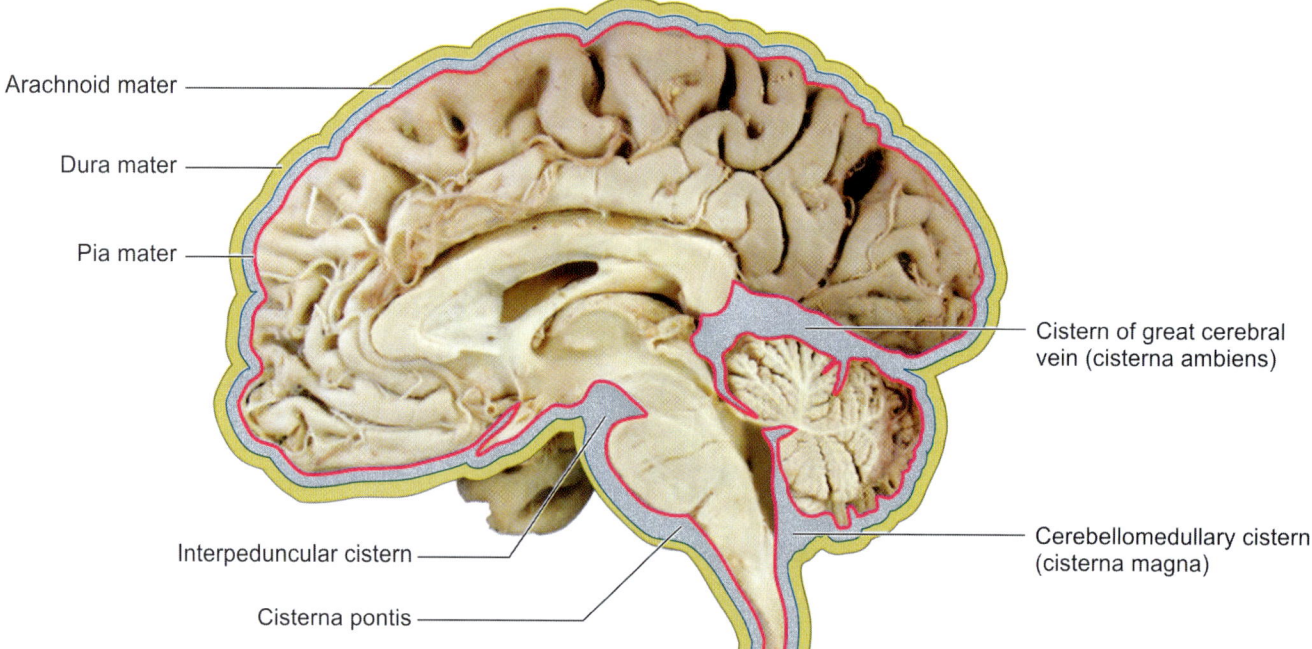

Arachnoid mater

Dura mater

Pia mater

Cistern of great cerebral vein (cisterna ambiens)

Cerebellomedullary cistern (cisterna magna)

Interpeduncular cistern

Cisterna pontis

Fig. 65.5: Position of three meninges including the cisterns

mater. It is separated from the underlying pia mater by the subarachnoid space, containing cerebrospinal fluid and blood vessels of the brain. Cranial nerves also pass through this space. Near the superior sagittal sinus, arachnoid mater forms arachnoid villi.

- The subarachnoid space is dilated around the brain stem and at the base of the brain forming the subarachnoid cisterns. Cerebrospinal fluid formed by choroid plexuses flows through the ventricles of the brain into the subarachnoid space to be absorbed via subarachnoid villi into the superior sagittal sinus.

CISTERNS

Cerebellomedullary cistern lies between medulla oblongata and lower surface of cerebellum. As it is the largest cistern it is called cisterna magna (Fig. 65.5).

Cistern of the great cerebral vein (vein of Galen) lies between splenium of corpus callosum and upper surface of cerebellum. Its content is great cerebral vein.

Cisterna pontis lies on the ventral surface of pons. It contains basilar artery and its branches.

Interpeduncular cistern lies on the base of brain between the temporal lobes. Its content is the circle of Willis.

Cistern of lateral sulcus (sylvian cistern) lies in the stem of lateral sulcus. It contains the middle cerebral artery.

- Divide the arachnoid mater over the stem of the lateral sulcus and strip it off both superiorly and inferiorly.
- Identify the veins on the superolateral surface of cerebrum. Lying in the lateral sulcus is the superficial middle cerebral vein (Fig. 65.6).
- See 8–10 superior cerebral veins present on the upper part of superolateral surface of cerebral hemisphere, draining into the superior sagittal sinus.
- Identify inferior cerebral veins present on the lateral surface of the hemisphere. These drain into the superficial middle cerebral vein.

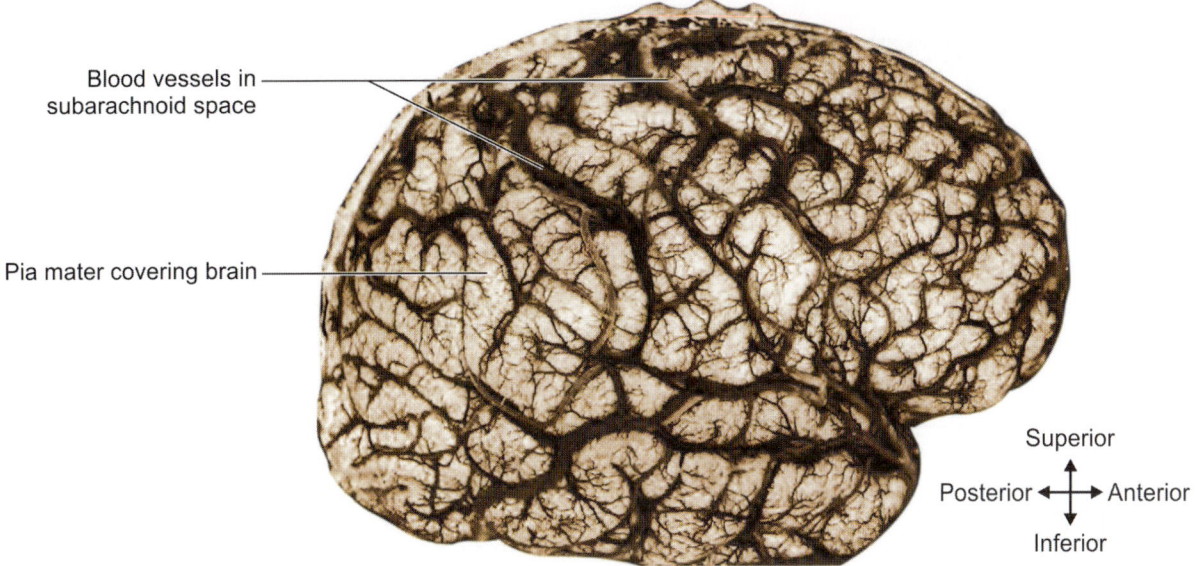

Blood vessels in subarachnoid space

Pia mater covering brain

Superior

Posterior ←→ Anterior

Inferior

Fig. 65.6: Blood vessels in subarachnoid space

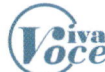

- Name the meninges of the cranial cavity.
- What venous sinuses lie at the attachments of the tentorium cerebelli?
- Name the cisterns of the brain. Enumerate their contents as well.

- What is the function of diaphragma sellae?
- What artery lies in extradural space?
- What is extradural haematoma?
- Enumerate the functions of CSF.

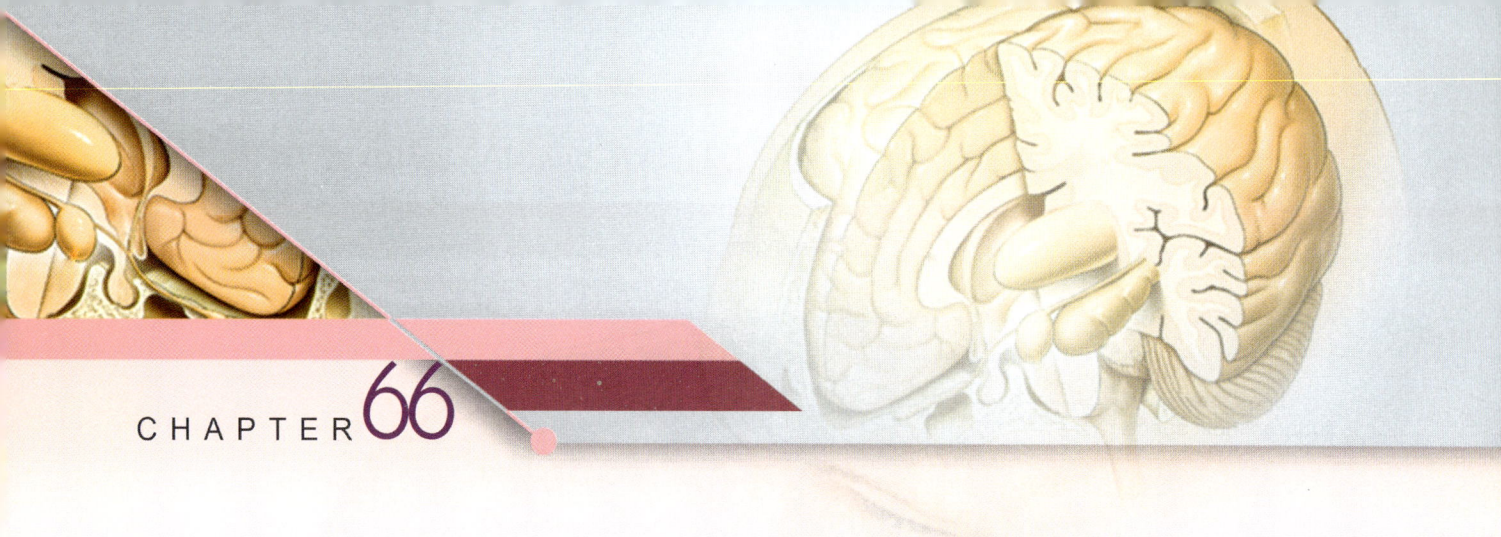

CHAPTER 66

Spinal Cord

Learning Objectives

One should be able to

1. Draw a diagram showing external features of the spinal cord.
2. Place the ascending and descending tracts in a diagram of spinal cord.
3. Enumerate symptoms produced in syringomyelia and tabes dorsalis

OVERVIEW

Spinal cord is the lower part of central nervous system (Fig. 66.1). It gives passage to the ascending/afferent/sensory and descending/efferent/motor tracts. It is also responsible for various reflex activities. Since it ends at lower border of L1 vertebra while the meninges extend till S2, the lower part of subarachnoid space is used for doing the lumbar puncture, if required. Spinal cord shows enlargements for nerves of upper and lower limbs.

Grey matter inside comprises dorsal and ventral horns throughout, and lateral horns only from T1 to L2 segments of spinal cord. Ascending and descending tracts are present in posterior, lateral and anterior funiculi of white matter of spinal cord.

Competency achievement: The student should be able to:

AN 57.1 Identify external features of spinal cord.

STEPS OF DISSECTION

• Study the spinal cord as it has been removed from vertebral canal and separated from the dura mater and arachnoid mater.

• See that spinal cord extends from upper border of C1 vertebra to lower border of L1 vertebra in an adult. In children, the spinal cord extends till L3 vertebra.

The lower end of spinal cord is known as *conus medullaris*, which continues as *filum terminale* till the first coccyx vertebra. The dura mater, arachnoid mater along with subarachnoid space containing CSF extends up to S2 vertebra.

• See that spinal cord is much shorter than the vertebral canal. So the spinal segments do not lie opposite the corresponding vertebrae.

The level of vertebral levels and spinal segments is as follows:

Vertebral levels	Spinal segments
C1–C7	C1–C8
T1–T4	T1–T6
T5–T9	T7–T12
T10, T11	L1–L5
T12, L1	S1–S5, Co1

• Observe that cervical nerves formed by dorsal and ventral nerve roots are horizontal in position. The thoracic nerves are oblique as these leave their

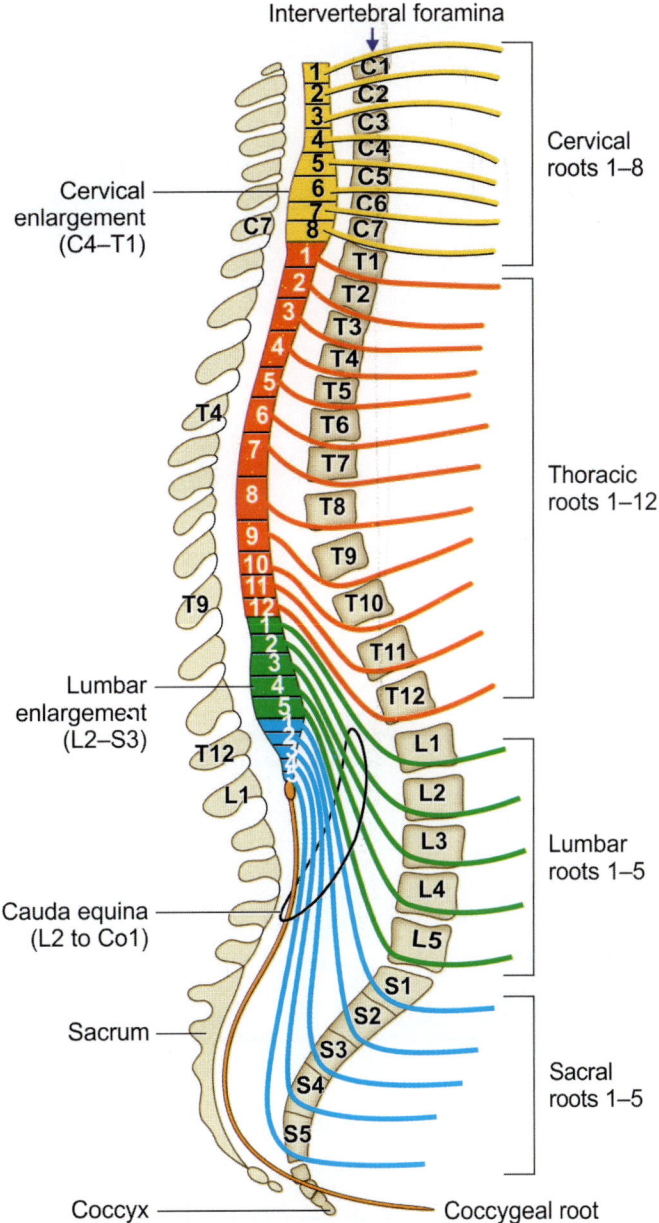

Fig. 66.1: Position of spinal cord with 31 pairs of spinal nerves

respective intervertebral foramina. The lumbar, sacral and coccygeal nerve roots are vertical as these descend to exit from their intervertebral foramina. These nerve roots together are called *cauda equina*.

Enlargements

- Observe that the spinal cord is not uniform in size. In lower cervical region it is thicker to form cervical enlargement. This enlargement extends from C4–T1 spinal segments with maximum diameter of 38 mm at C6 level. This enlargement has more neurons for the supply of upper limb muscles.

- Observe another enlargement, the lumbar enlargement extending from L2–S3 segments. The maximum diameter is 35 mm at the level of S1 segment. It is for the supply of muscles of the lower limb.

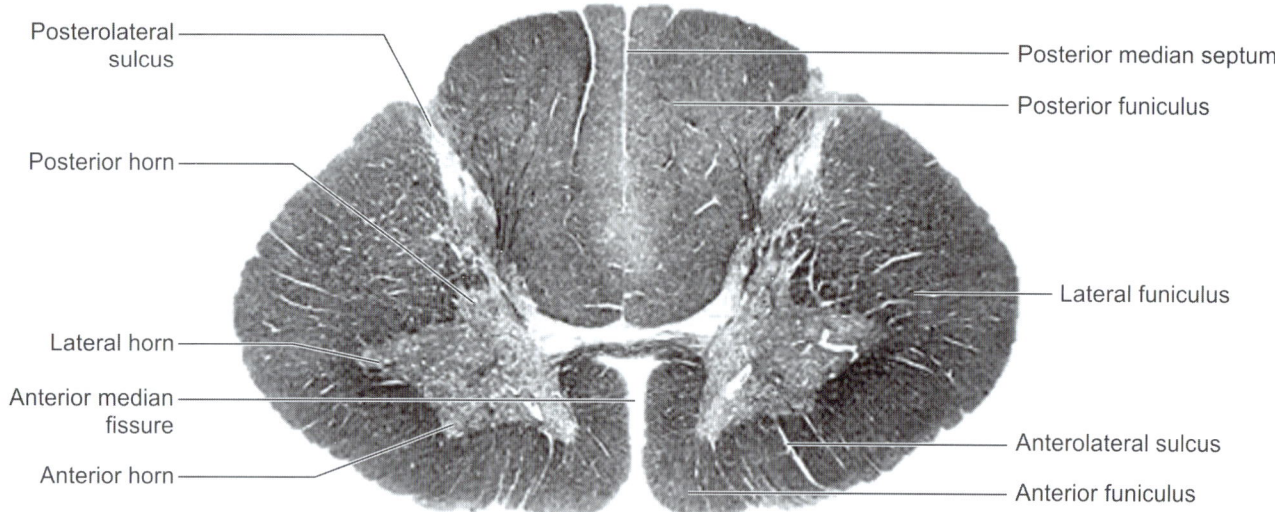

Posterolateral sulcus

Posterior horn

Lateral horn

Anterior median fissure

Anterior horn

Posterior median septum

Posterior funiculus

Lateral funiculus

Anterolateral sulcus

Anterior funiculus

Fig. 66.2: Gross features of spinal cord in a transverse section

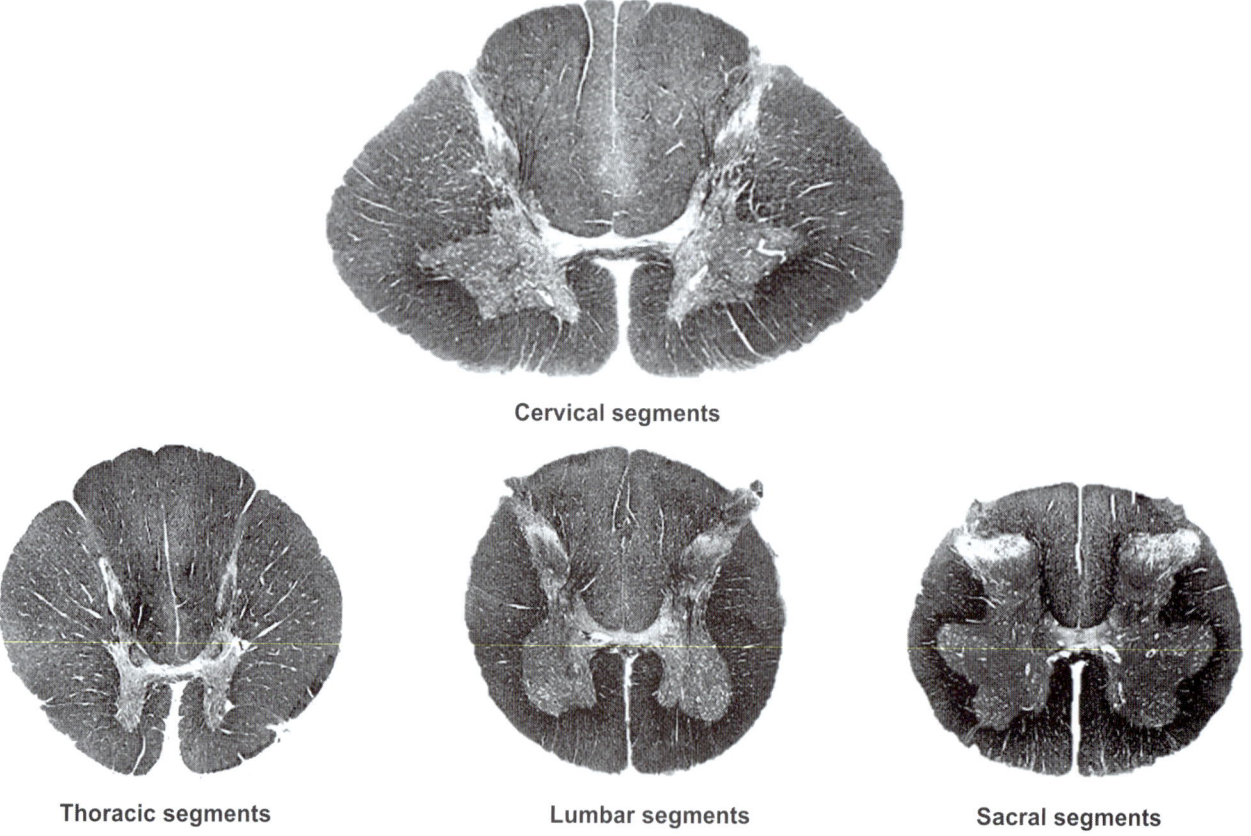

Cervical segments

Thoracic segments

Lumbar segments

Sacral segments

Fig. 66.3: Sections of spinal cord at various levels

External Features

- See that there is anterior median fissure in the anterior region of spinal cord (Fig. 66.2). It lodges the anterior spinal artery.
- See and identify the posterior median sulcus from which a septum runs to depth of spinal cord.
- See that each half of spinal cord is subdivided into anterior, lateral and posterior regions by anterolateral and posterolateral sulci.
- From anterolateral sulcus exits the motor nerve roots. The sensory roots enter the spinal cord from the posterolateral sulcus.
- Make transverse sections of spinal cord at cervical, thoracic, lumbar and sacral segments (Fig. 66.3).

Internal Features

- The grey mater lies in the centre and is 'H' shaped (cell bodies of neurons). The white mater is outside and contains the fibres (axons and dendrites).

- The grey mater comprises an anterior horn and a posterior horn in all the 31 segments. See that only in the segments T1–L2 and S2–S4 there is an additional lateral horn. The lateral horn of the T1–L2 segments is for preganglionic fibres of sympathetic nervous system. The lateral horn of S2–S4 segments is for preganglionic fibres of sacral component of parasympathetic nervous system.
- *Note that in:*
  - *Upper cervical segments:* Both anterior and posterior horns are narrow
  - *Lower cervical segments:* The anterior horn is broad
  - *Thoracic segments:* Both anterior and posterior horns are very narrow. Additional lateral horn is present in all 12 segments.
  - *Lumbar segments:* Both posterior horn and anterior horns are bulbous. Only L1 and L2 segments show lateral horn.
  - *Sacral segments:* Both the anterior and posterior horns are bulbous.

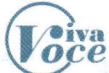

- Where does spinal cord end in an adult and in a child.
- What is vertebral level of C1–C8 spinal nerves.
- Where does spinal segments S1–S5 and Co 1 lie in relation to the vertebrae.
- How many processes are there in ligamentum denticulatum?
- Which segments of spinal cord have the lateral horns? Where do these lie in relation to vertebral levels?
- Name the ascending tracts of spinal cord.

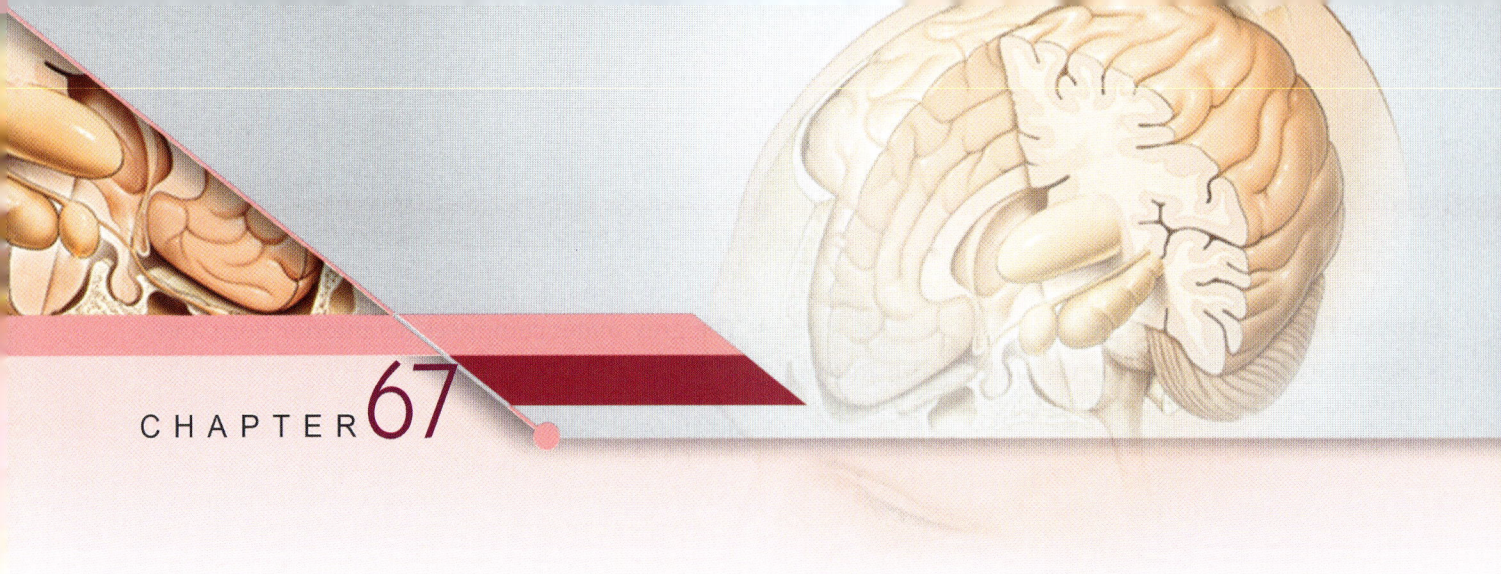

CHAPTER 67

Brainstem

Learning Objectives

One should be able to
1. Draw transverse sections of medulla oblongata at level of motor decussation, sensory decussation and floor of 4th ventricle.
2. Draw TS of pons at level of facial colliculus and at level of trigeminal nerve nuclei.
3. Draw TS of midbrain at level of inferior colliculus and superior colliculus.

OVERVIEW

Medulla oblongata, pons and midbrain constitute the brainstem (Fig. 67.1).

Medulla oblongata is the lowest part of brainstem. Last 4 cranial nerves, i.e. IX–XII are attached to its ventral surface. The tracts of spinal cord ascend/descend through the medulla, also called "bulb". It is connected to the cerebellum via the inferior cerebellar peduncles.

Lowest part of medulla shows motor/pyramidal decussation. Middle part shows great sensory decussation. Upper part forms part of floor of 4th ventricle.

Pons (bridge) forms a communication between cerebrum above and cerebellum below. V–VIII cranial nerves are attached to the pons. It is connected to cerebellum via middle cerebellar peduncle.

Midbrain is the cranial most part of the brainstem. III and IV cranial nerves are attached to it. Midbrain is connected to the cerebellum via superior cerebellar peduncles. Its cavity is the narrow aqueduct of Sylvius.

Competency achievement: The student should be able to:

AN 58.1 Identify external features of medulla oblongata.

STEPS OF DISSECTION

- Put the brain in a way that its ventral aspect is visible. Identify interpeduncular fossa between the two temporal lobes.
- Incise the crus cerebri on each side.
- Separate brainstem with cerebellum including the 4th ventricle as a separate piece for further dissection.
- Identify the cranial nerves emerging in relation to parts of brainstem (Fig. 67.2).
- 3rd cranial nerve, the oculomotor nerve, lies medial to crus cerebri in ventral surface of midbrain.
- 4th cranial nerve, the trochlear nerve, is seen emerging from dorsal surface of midbrain.
- 5th cranial nerve, the trigeminal nerve, is seen at junction of ventral surface of pons with middle cerebellar peduncle.
- 6th cranial nerve, the abducent nerve, is seen at lower border of pons at level of pyramid of medulla oblongata.

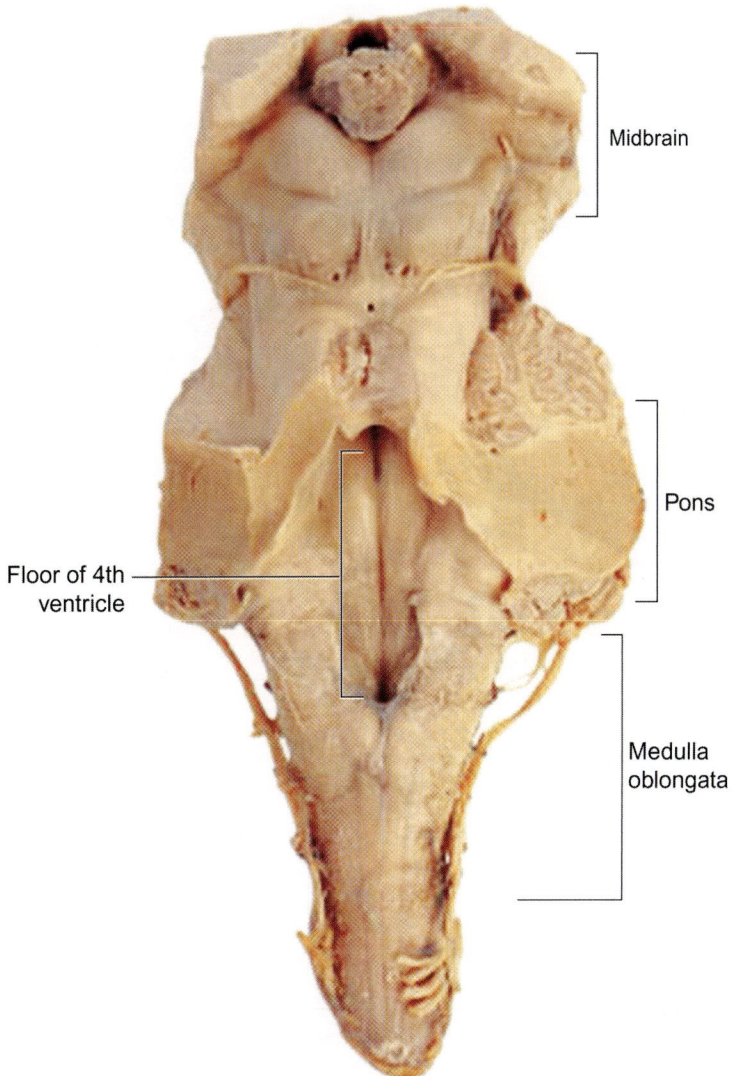

Fig. 67.1: Parts of brainstem

- 7th cranial nerve, the facial nerve, and 8th cranial nerve, the vestibulocochlear nerve, are seen at lower border of pons at level of olive of medulla oblongata.
- 9th, 10th and 11th (cranial root) cranial nerves are seen as rootlets in the posterolateral sulcus between olive and inferior cerebellar peduncle. These rootlets are in order: 9th—glossopharyngeal is highest, 10th—the vagus is in the middle and 11th—cranial root of accessory is lowest.
- 12th cranial nerve, the hypoglossal nerve, is seen as rootlets in anterolateral groove between pyramid and olive.

- Thus cranial nerves III–XII are attached to various parts of the brainstem (Fig. 67.2).
- Look for the median groove on the central aspect of pons containing single basilar artery formed by union of right and left vertebral arteries.

MEDULLA OBLONGATA

- The lower part of medulla oblongata is closed part while its upper part is open. Medulla oblongata contains important vasomotor, respiratory and cardiac centres.
- Identify ventral surface of medulla oblongata by following structures:

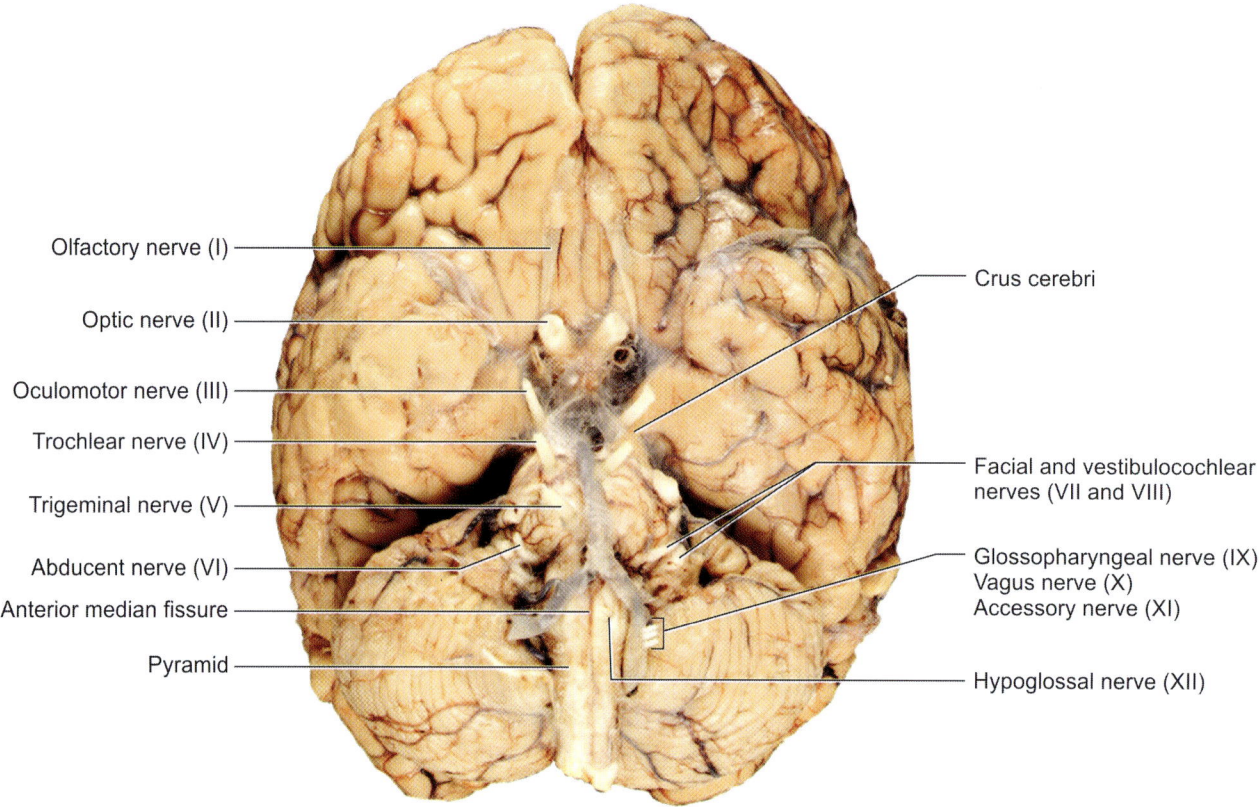

Olfactory nerve (I)

Optic nerve (II)

Oculomotor nerve (III)

Trochlear nerve (IV)

Trigeminal nerve (V)

Abducent nerve (VI)

Anterior median fissure

Pyramid

Crus cerebri

Facial and vestibulocochlear nerves (VII and VIII)

Glossopharyngeal nerve (IX)
Vagus nerve (X)
Accessory nerve (XI)

Hypoglossal nerve (XII)

Fig. 67.2: Attachment of cranial nerves to the brainstem

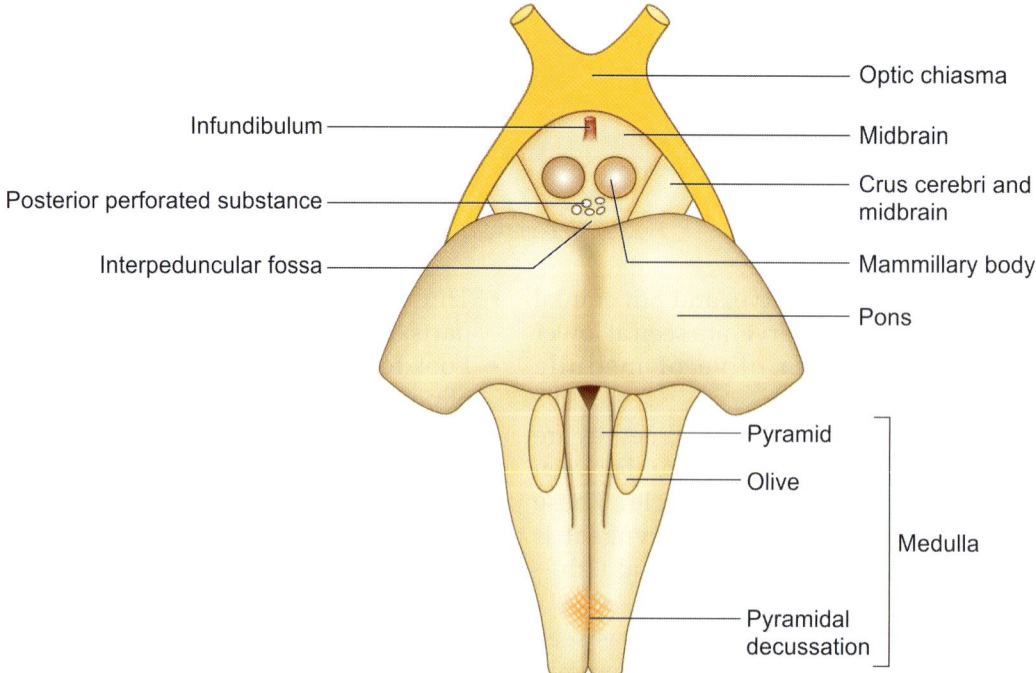

Infundibulum

Posterior perforated substance

Interpeduncular fossa

Optic chiasma

Midbrain

Crus cerebri and midbrain

Mammillary body

Pons

Pyramid

Olive

Medulla

Pyramidal decussation

Fig. 67.3: Section through midbrain including optic chiasma

- Pyramid-elongated swellings on each side of anteromedian fissure (Fig. 67.2).
- Olive-rounded swellings on each side of pyramids. Between pyramid and olive is anterolateral groove. It contains rootlets of XII cranial nerve. Posterior to olive is posterolateral sulcus.
- In the posterolateral sulcus are attached rootlets of IX—glossopharyngeal; rootlets of X—vagus in between; and rootlets of cranial root of XI—accessory nerve.

INFERIOR CEREBELLAR PEDUNCLE

- In caudal part posterolateral to olive is a bundle of fibres connecting medulla oblongata to the cerebellum, called inferior cerebellar peduncle.
- The dorsal surface is subdivided into 2 parts:
  A. Closed part
  B. Open part

A. Closed Part

In the closed part look for:
  i. Fasciculus gracilis ending in gracile tubercle medially
 ii. Fasciculus cuneatus ending in cuneate tubercle
iii. Tubercinerium lying lateral to cuneate tubercle. It is produced by spinal nucleus of V nerve
 iv. Inferior cerebellar peduncle.

B. Open Part

It shows nuclei of XII and X nerves. It will be seen in details in dissection of IV ventricle.

Competency achievement: The student should be able to:

AN 59.1 Identify external features of pons.

PONS

Pons acts as a bridge between midbrain and medulla oblongata. It mainly contains cortico-ponto-cerebellar fibres.

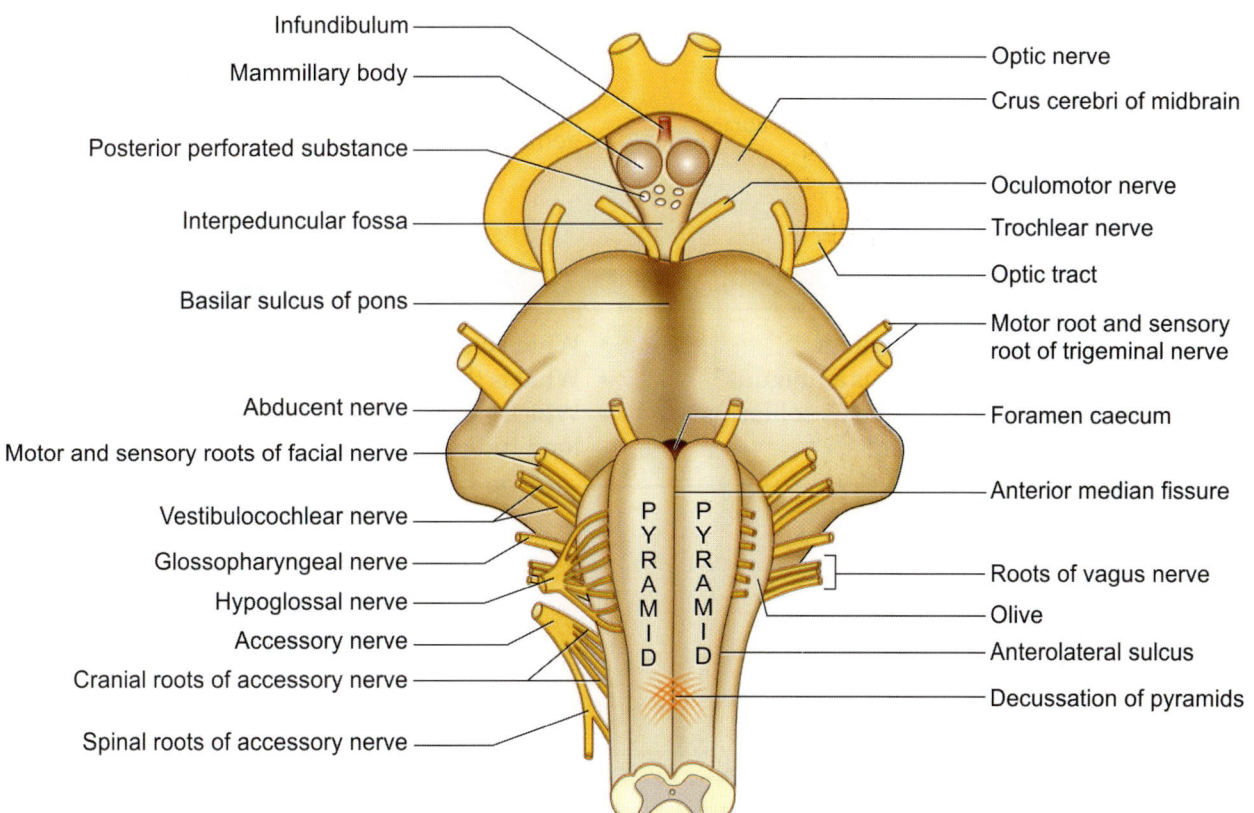

Fig. 67.4: Surface features of brainstem as seen from the front

A. Ventral Surface of Pons (Fig. 67.3)

- Identify a median ventral basilar groove lodging the basilar artery.
- See V nerve attached at junction of pons and middle cerebellar peduncle. Motor root is medial to larger sensory root placed laterally.
- Look for cerebral peduncles at junction of pons and midbrain.
- Identify VI, VII and VIII nerves attached to lower border of pons at its junction with medulla oblongata.

B. Dorsal Surface of Pons

- Look for facial colliculus in median plane.
- Identify vestibular area lateral to facial colliculus.
  Borders of pons
- Upper border lies at junction of pons and midbrain. Superior cerebellar arteries curve around this border.
- Inferior/lower border lies at junction of pons and medulla oblongata. Anterior inferior cerebellar arteries curve around this border.

Competency achievement: The student should be able to:

AN 61.1 Identify external and internal features of midbrain.

Midbrain

Midbrain is the most cranial and shortest part of brainstem. It contains a cavity—the aqueduct between its ventral and dorsal parts.

Ventral Surface

- Identify the crus cerebri forming ventral aspect of midbrain. It forms posterolateral boundary of interpeduncular fossa.
- Look for III cranial nerve at the medial side of crus cerebri (Fig. 67.2).
- Look for IV cranial nerve winding around the lateral aspect of cerebral peduncle and seen cranial to III nerve.

Dorsal Surface

- Identify 2 superior colliculi. These are reflex centres for visual pathways. These are connected by 2 superior brachia to the lateral geniculate bodies.
- Below superior colliculi identify 2 inferior colliculi. These are reflex centres for auditory pathways and are connected by 2 inferior brachia to the medial geniculate bodies.

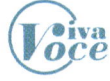

- Name the components of brainstem.
- Which nerves arise from nucleus ambiguus?
- Which cranial nerves end in tractus solitarius?
- What is law of neurobiotaxis?

- Which cranial nerve has a dorsal attachment?
- What is the function of Edinger-Westphal nucleus.
- Which cranial nerve nuclei are connected by medial longitudinal bundle?

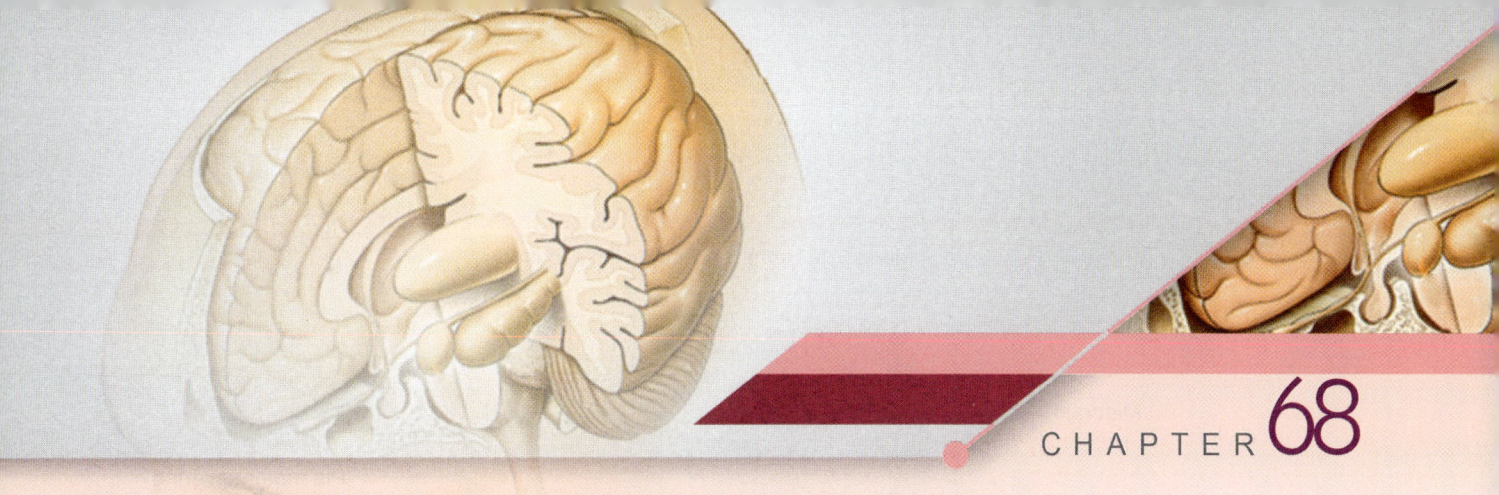

CHAPTER 68

Cerebellum

Learning Objectives

One should be able to
1. Draw the histological layers of cerebellum.
2. Name the symptoms of neocerebellar syndrome.
3. Name the deep nuclei of cerebellum.
4. Name the three cerebellar peduncles. Which parts are connected by these peduncles.

OVERVIEW

Cerebellum is the little brain located in posterior cranial fossa beneath the occipital lobe of cerebrum. These are separated by a double fold of meningeal layer of dura mater—the tentorium cerebelli. The tentorium lifts off the weight of big cerebrum from the little cerebellum. It is comprised of two small hemispheres united by a vermis. It is the older part of the brain. It is made of archicerebellum (vestibular part); paleocerebellum (spinal part) and neocerebellum (new part). Though cerebellum does not initiate movements, still it controls movements of the body by modifying input of various motor tracts on the spinal cord. The cerebellum has uniform structure and controls the same side of the body. Thus it has ipsilateral control. It is connected to all three components of the brainstem via 3 × 2 cerebellar peduncles

Midbrain → superior cerebellar peduncle → cerebellum

Pons → middle cerebellar peduncle → cerebellum

Medulla oblongata → inferior cerebellar peduncle → cerebellum

Competency achievement: The student should be able to:

AN 60.1 Describe and demonstrate external and internal features of cerebellum.

STEPS OF DISSECTION

- Remove the meninges from the lobe of cerebellum (Fig. 68.1).
- Identify the right and left lobes of the cerebellum.
- The midline structure between the two lobes is the vermis.
  - Vermis on the superior surface—superior vermis
  - Vermis on the inferior surface—inferior vermis.
- The superior vermis is identified as a slightly raised area in midline bounded by right and left cerebellar hemispheres.
- Identify the inferior surface of hemisphere by a deep notch—the vallecula (valley) (Fig. 68.2). The inferior vermis lies in the vallecula.
- Look for anterior cerebellar notch. This notch is broad and shallow. This notch accommodates the pons and cerebellum.
- On the posterior aspect of cerebellum identify deep and narrow posterior cerebellar notch.

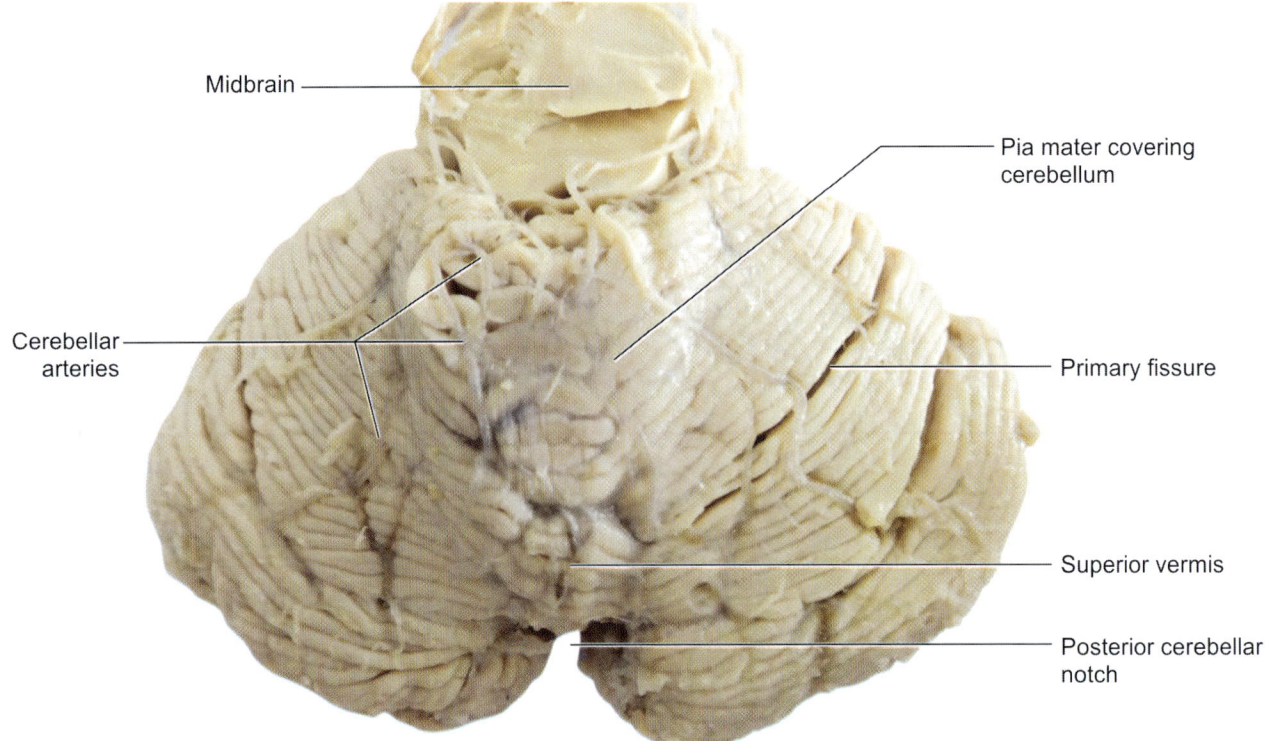

Midbrain

Pia mater covering
cerebellum

Cerebellar
arteries

Primary fissure

Superior vermis

Posterior cerebellar
notch

Fig. 68.1: Superior surface of cerebellum

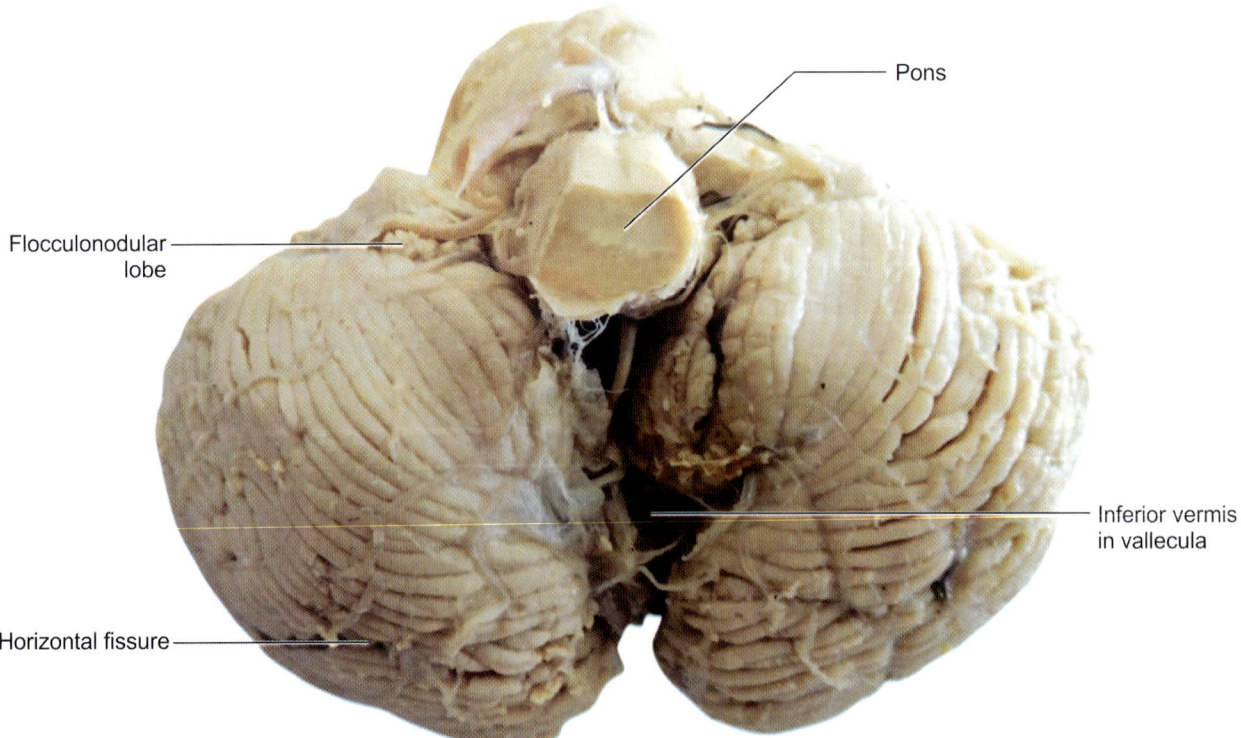

Pons

Flocculonodular
lobe

Inferior vermis
in vallecula

Horizontal fissure

Fig. 68.2: Inferior surface of cerebellum

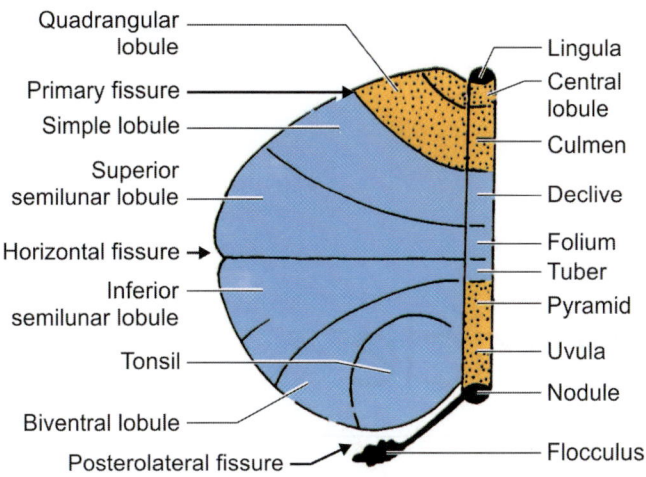

Quadrangular lobule — Lingula
Primary fissure — Central lobule
Simple lobule —
Superior semilunar lobule — Culmen
Horizontal fissure → — Declive
Inferior semilunar lobule — Folium
Tonsil — Tuber
Biventral lobule — Pyramid
Posterolateral fissure — Uvula
— Nodule
— Flocculus

Fig. 68.3: Scheme to show subdivision of cerebellum. Parts above horizontal fissure form superior surface and those below this fissure are seen on inferior surface

- Identify the falx cerebelli present in this posterior notch.
- Identify the horizontal fissure between superior and inferior surfaces of cerebellum (Fig. 68.3).
- Look for a "V" shaped fissura prima on the superior surface of cerebellum. Anterior lobe lies anterior to

fissura prima. Middle/posterior lobe is partly situated behind fissura prima.

- On the inferior surface of cerebellum, identify the posterolateral fissure which separates flocculo-nodular lobe from part of middle/posterior lobe.
- Identify the small anterior lobe of cerebellum lying anterior to fissura prima.
- Identify the smallest lobe—the flocculonodular lobe lying anterior to posterolateral fissure.
- See the largest lobe—middle/posterior lobe presents both on superior and inferior surfaces of the cerebellum.
- Depress the superior surface of cerebellum and identify the superior cerebellar peduncles between tectum and the cerebellum.
- Identify middle cerebellar peduncles between the lateral parts of pons to cerebellum on each side.
- Lastly identify inferior cerebellar peduncles on posterolateral aspects of medulla oblongata connecting it with cerebellum.
- Scrape the cerebellum on one hemisphere gently till one is able to locate the deep nucleus—the dentate nucleus. It looks like a crumpled bag (Fig. 68.4).

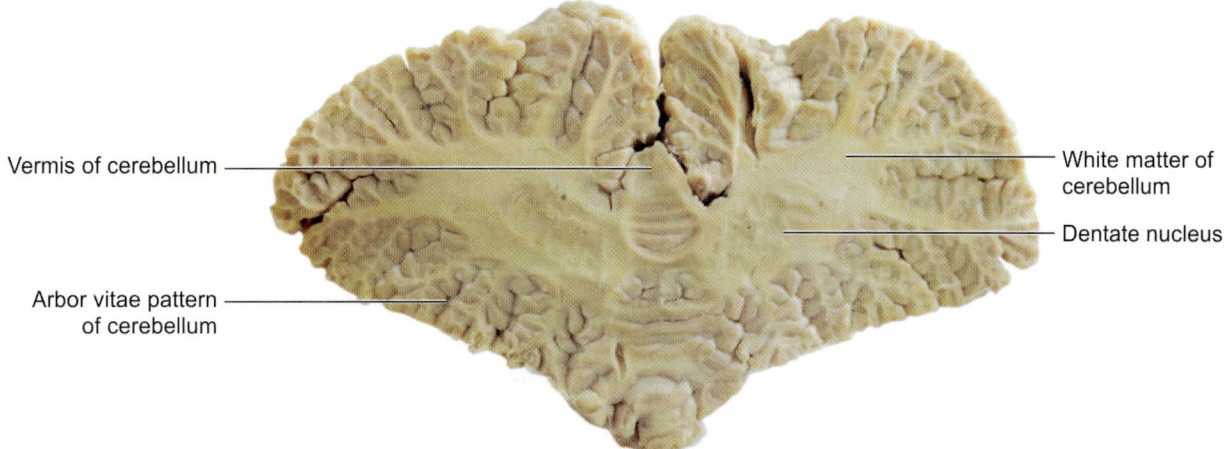

Vermis of cerebellum — White matter of cerebellum
— Dentate nucleus
Arbor vitae pattern of cerebellum

Fig. 68.4: Dentate nucleus of cerebellum, arbor vitae pattern of cerebellum seen

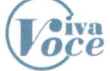

- Name the nuclei present in white matter of the cerebellum.
- Name the peduncles which connect cerebellum to 3 parts of the brainstem.
- What are the symptoms of anterior lobe lesion of the cerebellum.
- Name the three functional zones with their respective functions.
- Name the characteristic cell seen in a histological slide of cerebellum.
- What are the symptoms of neocerebellar lesion.
- Name the morphological divisions of cerebellum.

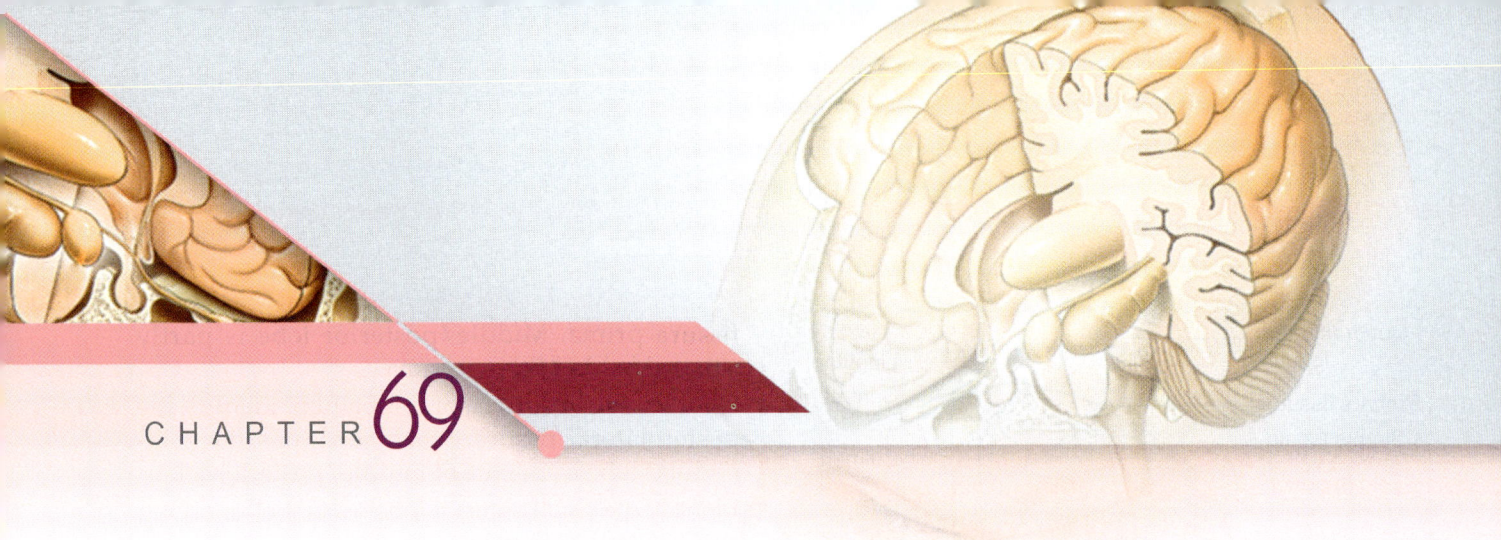

Fourth Ventricle

OVERVIEW

Fourth ventricle is a diamond shaped cavity in the hindbrain. It is thus the cavity of rhombencephalon. It is located dorsal to pons and medulla oblongata, but ventral to cerebellum. It communicates above with aqueduct of midbrain and below with central canal of spinal cord.

The roof of IV ventricle is very thin. The floor comprises an upper pontine part and a lower medullary part. It has three openings: One median opening, opening into cerebellomedullary cistern; two lateral openings, one on each side opening into subarachnoid space.

Competency achievement: The student should be able to:

AN 63.1 Describe and demonstrate parts, boundaries and features of IIIrd, IVth and lateral ventricle.

STEPS OF DISSECTION

- Cut the cerebellum through the vermis and see its right and left hemispheres.
- Appreciate the leaf-like pattern of cerebellum—the arbor vitae pattern (*see* Fig 68.4). It provides more space for the grey matter (neurons) in a limited space.
- As the cerebellum is being cut, identify roof of IV ventricle. See the position of median aperture of IV ventricle.
- Incise all three peduncles on both sides so that cerebellum gets separated from brainstem.
- Identify the boundaries as:
  - Upper lateral wall
  - Lower lateral wall
  - Roof and recesses
  - Floor and angles
- Identify the cut ends of superior cerebellar peduncles forming upper and lateral walls
- Look for the cut ends inferior cerebellar peduncles forming lower and lateral walls.
- Observe that roof is formed by:
  i. Superior medullary velum joining right and left superior cerebellar peduncles
  ii. Inferior medullary velum forms small part of roof lateral to nodule. In the lower part roof is formed by pia mater and ependyma.

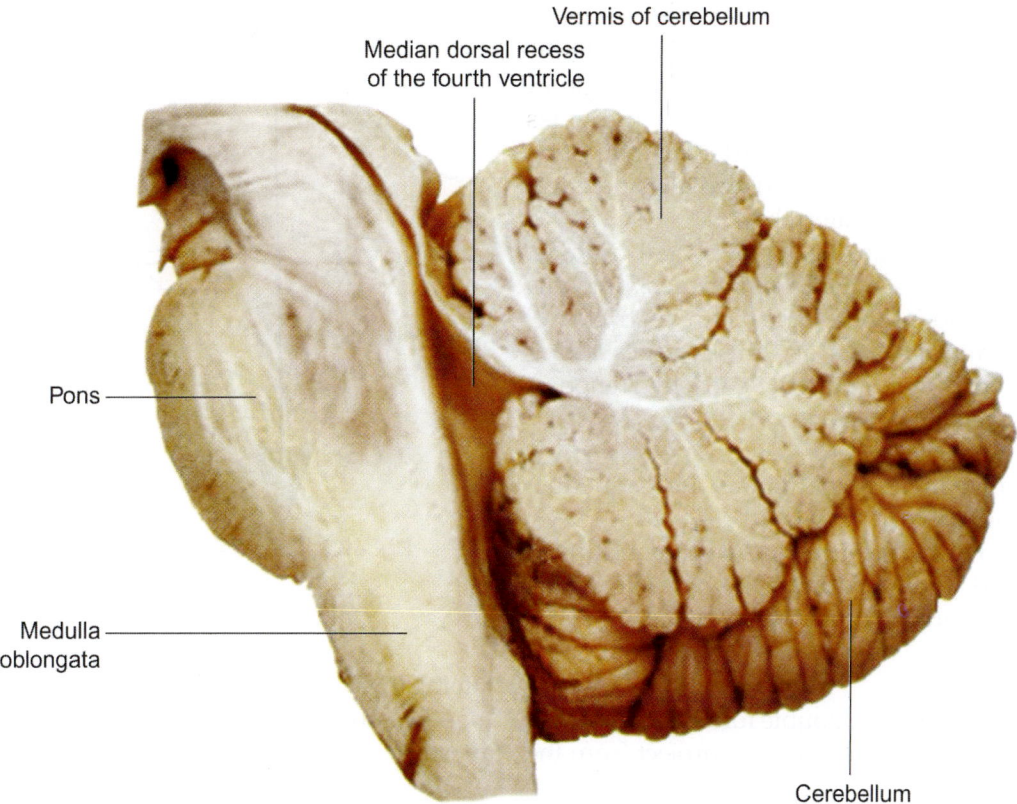

Fig. 69.1: Median dorsal recess of cerebellum

iii. An opening is seen in the lower part. This opening is called foramen of Magendie and it opens into the subarachnoid space of the cerebellomedullary cistern.

- Look for the recesses of the roof of IV ventricle:
  i. One median dorsal recess extends towards nodule of vermis of cerebellum (Fig. 69.1).
  ii. Two lateral dorsal recesses extend dorsally lateral to nodule (Fig. 69.2).
  iii. Two lateral recesses extend laterally between inferior cerebellar peduncle and peduncle of flocculus. These recesses exhibit apertures at their ends and are known as foramen of Luschka.
- Floor is seen as a diamond shaped area. Posterior surfaces of lower part of pons and upper part of medulla oblongata form the floor (Fig. 69.3).
- Identify the following structures:
  i. Pontine part of floor:
    - Identify median sulcus in median plane

- Medial eminence formed by facial colliculus (*see* Fig. 67.1)
- Sulcus limitans lies lateral to median eminence. At upper end of sulcus limitans identify superior fovea.

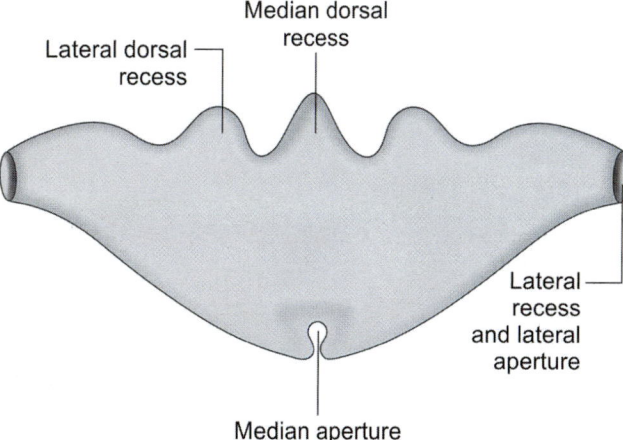

Fig. 69.2: Roof of 4th ventricle with recesses and apertures

ii. Vestibular part is seen lateral to sulcus limitans. Nuclei of vestibular part of VIII nerve lie here.

iii. Medullary part-inferior fovea is the angle of inverted "V" shaped sulcus limitans. It divides medial eminence into two parts. The two parts are hypoglossal triangle (XII) medially and vagal triangle below and laterally.

iv. Funiculus separans lies below vagal triangle. Area postrema is a small area between funiculus separans and inferior angle of 4th ventricle.

v. Taenia may be seen as white ridges along inferolateral margin of 4th ventricle. The point where taenia meet is obex.

vi. Angles:
   a. Superior angle is continuous with aqueduct (*see* Fig. 67.1)
   b. Inferior angle is continuous with central canal
   c. Lateral angle extends laterally towards inferior cerebellar peduncle.

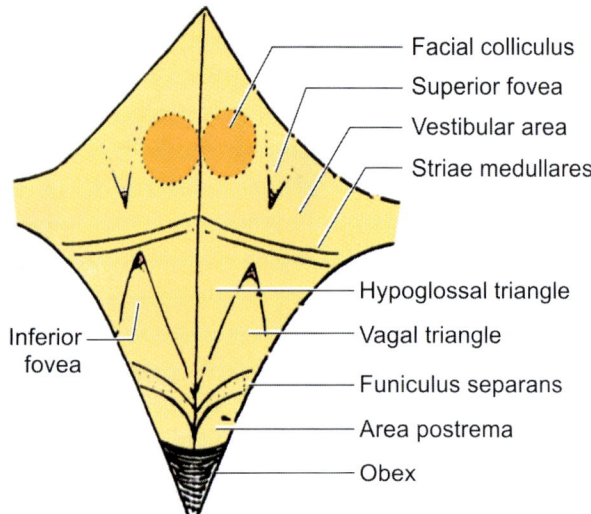

Fig. 69.3: Structures in the floor of IV ventricle

Tela Choroidea

See the tela choroidea as a double fold of pia mater. It is "π shaped", the two lateral angles project from the lateral apertures. The vertical bands are also two, run together and may be seen projecting from median aperture of the ventricle.

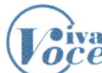

- How are the lateral boundaries of IVth ventricle formed?
- Name the apertures in roof of IVth ventricle.
- Name the recesses in roof of IVth ventricle.

Cerebrum

OVERVIEW

Cerebrum contains the highest centres of the body. Cerebrum comprises two cerebral hemispheres. Between the two hemispheres is a longitudinal fissure extending anteriorly from frontal pole to the occipital pole posteriorly. On the dorsal surface the longitudinal fissure separates the hemispheres partially. These are joined in the lower part by corpus callosum. On the ventral surface of the brain the two hemispheres are joined at the interpeduncular fossa.

Cerebrum forms major part of the central nervous system. It is protected by endosteum, three meninges and CSF. It is divided into 2 cerebral hemispheres by a longitudinal fissure. Each hemisphere comprises 4 lobes—frontal, parietal, occipital and temporal; 3 surfaces—superolateral convex surface, medial flat surface and inferior surface divided into orbital and tentorial; 3 borders—superomedial, inferolateral and medial. The surface area is increased greatly due to the presence of sulci and gyri. Structure of the areas is different in different areas, i.e. it is heterotypical. Cerebrum controls the opposite side of the body, i.e.

its control is contralateral in contrast to that of the cerebellum.

> *Competency achievement:* The student should be able to:
> **AN 62.2** Describe and demonstrate surfaces, sulci, gyri, poles and functional areas of cerebral hemisphere.

STEPS OF DISSECTION

- With a sharp knife, cut through the parts of corpus callosum starting from its posterior part, the splenium, towards the trunk and genu.
- Extend the incision into tela choroidea of the lateral and third ventricles and the interthalamic adhesion connecting the medial surfaces of the two thalami.
- Identify the thin septum pellicidum connecting the inferior surface of corpus callosum to a curved band of white mater—anterior column of fornix. Look for anterior commissure just at the anterior end of the anterior column of fornix.
- Turn the brain upside down and identify optic chiasma.
- Divide the optic chiasma, infundibulum, a thin groove between the adjacent mammillary bodies

and posterior cerebral artery close to its origin. Carry the line of division around the midbrain to join the two ends of the median cut. Separate the right and left cerebral hemispheres.

- In each hemisphere, sulci (grooves) and gyri (raised areas between sulci) are almost identical.
- Identify:
  - 3 surfaces—superolateral, medial and inferior
  - 3 poles—frontal, temporal and occipital
  - 4 borders—superomedial, inferolateral, medial orbital and medial occipital borders
- Identify each of the following.

Surfaces

- Identify the superolateral surface. It is convex and is related to cranial vault (Fig. 70.1).
- Medial surface is flat and vertical. Falx cerebri and longitudinal fissure separate the opposite medial surfaces. Corpus callosum unites these surfaces partially (Fig. 70.2). The inferior surface is irregular (Fig. 70.3). Look for a deep cleft—stem of lateral sulcus which divides the surface into an anterior flat orbital part and a posterior concave tentorial part.

Borders

These are easily identifiable.

- Superomedial border is the longest border, separating superolateral and medial surfaces (Fig. 70.4)
- Inferolateral border separates the large superolateral surface from the inferior surface
- Medial occipital border separates the medial surface from the orbital surface
- Medial occipital border separates the medial surface from the tentorial surface.

Poles

- There are three poles in each hemisphere (more than the poles of the Earth) (Fig. 70.5).
- Anterior pole is rounded
- Posterior pole is pointed
- Temporal pole is on the lateral side

Lobes

There are four lobes.
1. Anteriorly—frontal lobe (Fig. 70.4)
2. Superiorly—parietal lobe

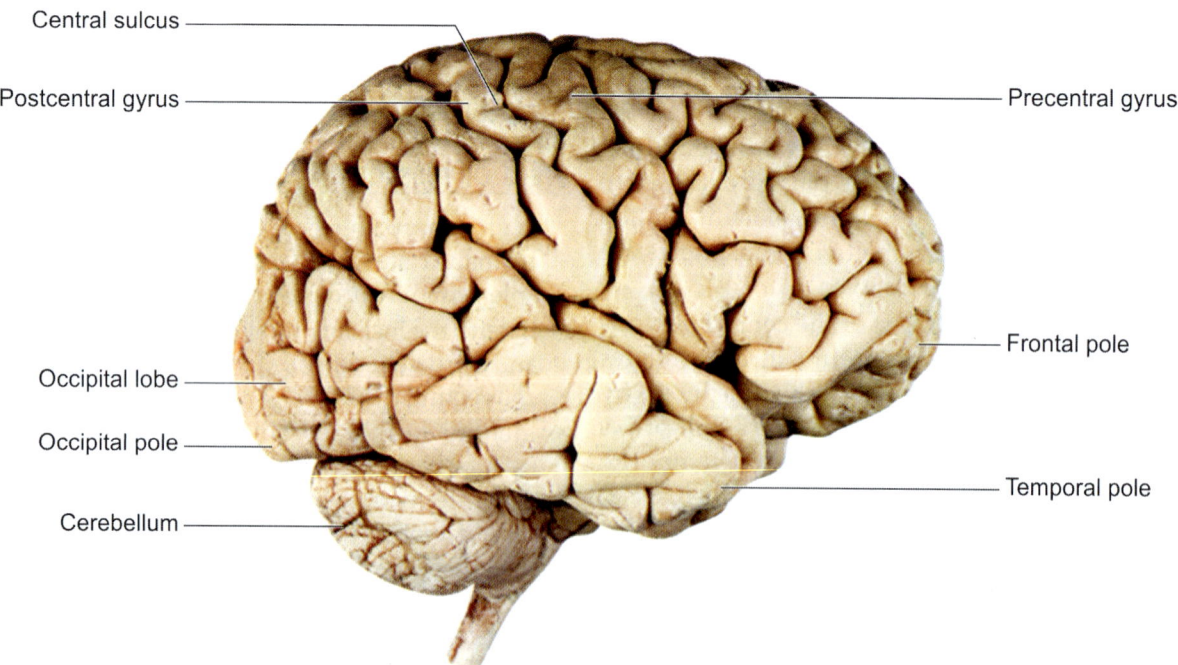

Fig. 70.1: Superior view of brain showing its superolateral surface

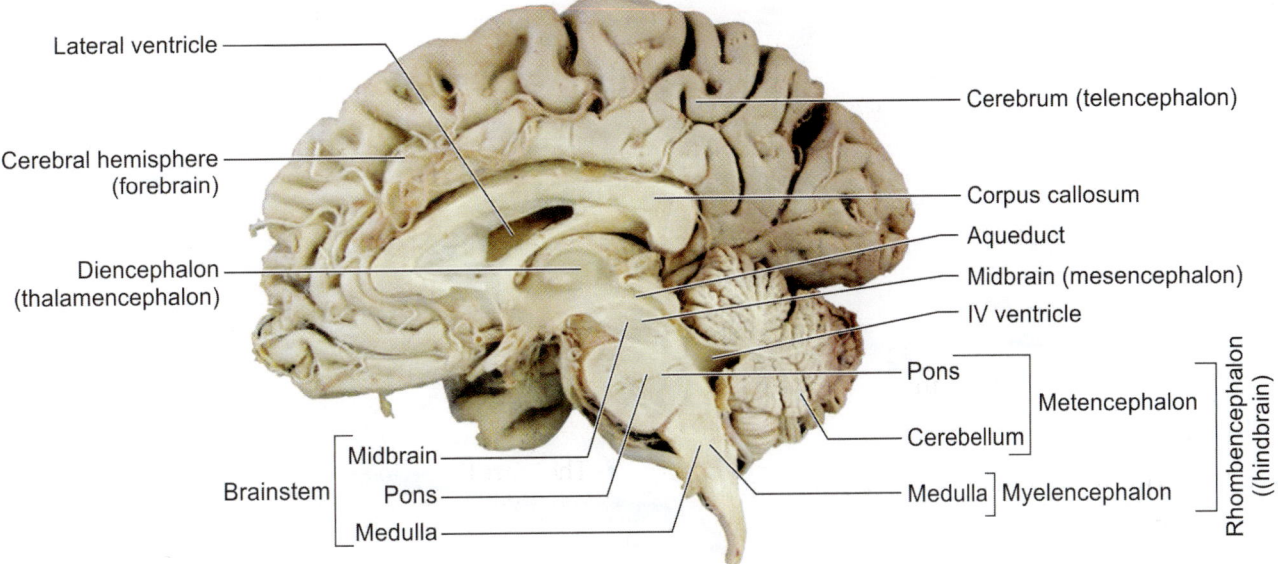

Lateral ventricle

Cerebral hemisphere
(forebrain)

Diencephalon
(thalamencephalon)

Cerebrum (telencephalon)

Corpus callosum

Aqueduct

Midbrain (mesencephalon)

IV ventricle

Pons

Metencephalon

Cerebellum

Rhombencephalon
((hindbrain)

Brainstem
Midbrain
Pons
Medulla

Medulla Myelencephalon

Fig. 70.2: Medial surface of cerebral hemisphere including midbrain and hindbrain

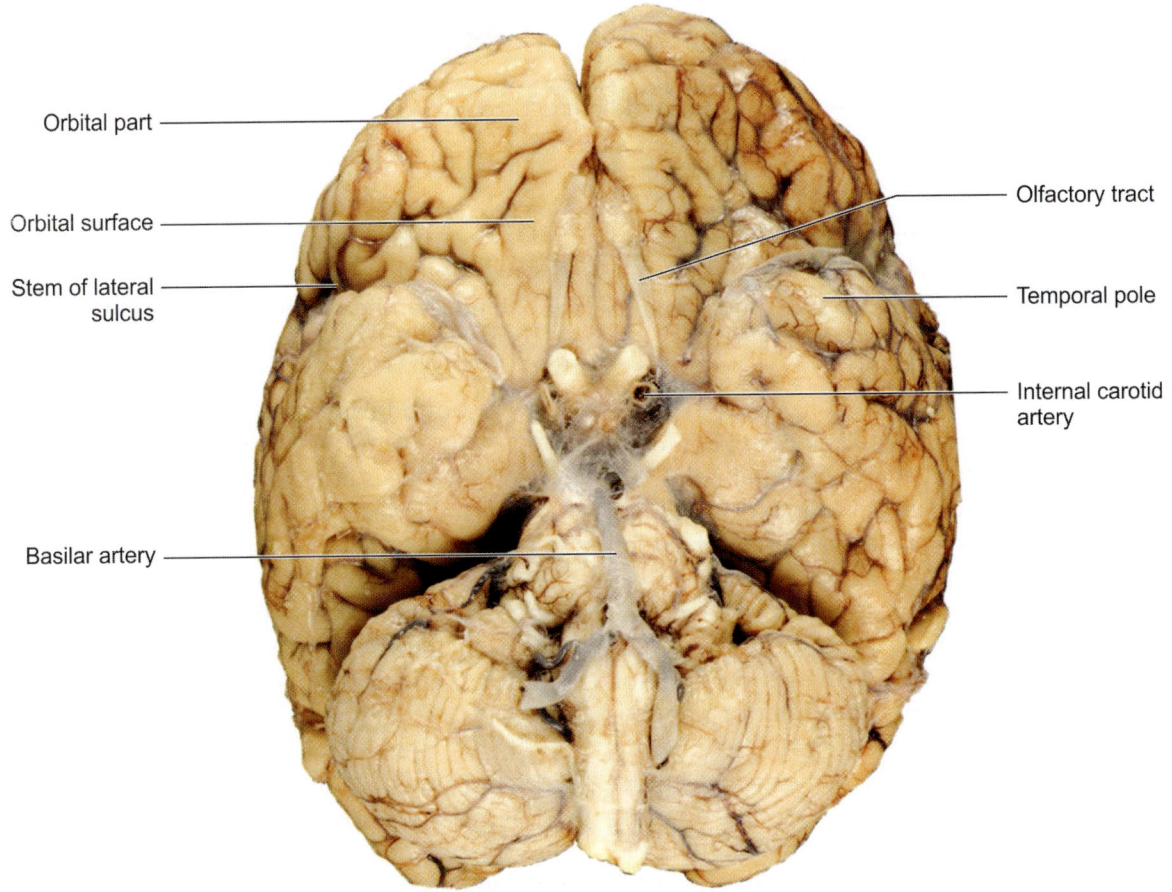

Orbital part

Orbital surface

Stem of lateral
sulcus

Olfactory tract

Temporal pole

Internal carotid
artery

Basilar artery

Fig. 70.3: Inferior surface of brain

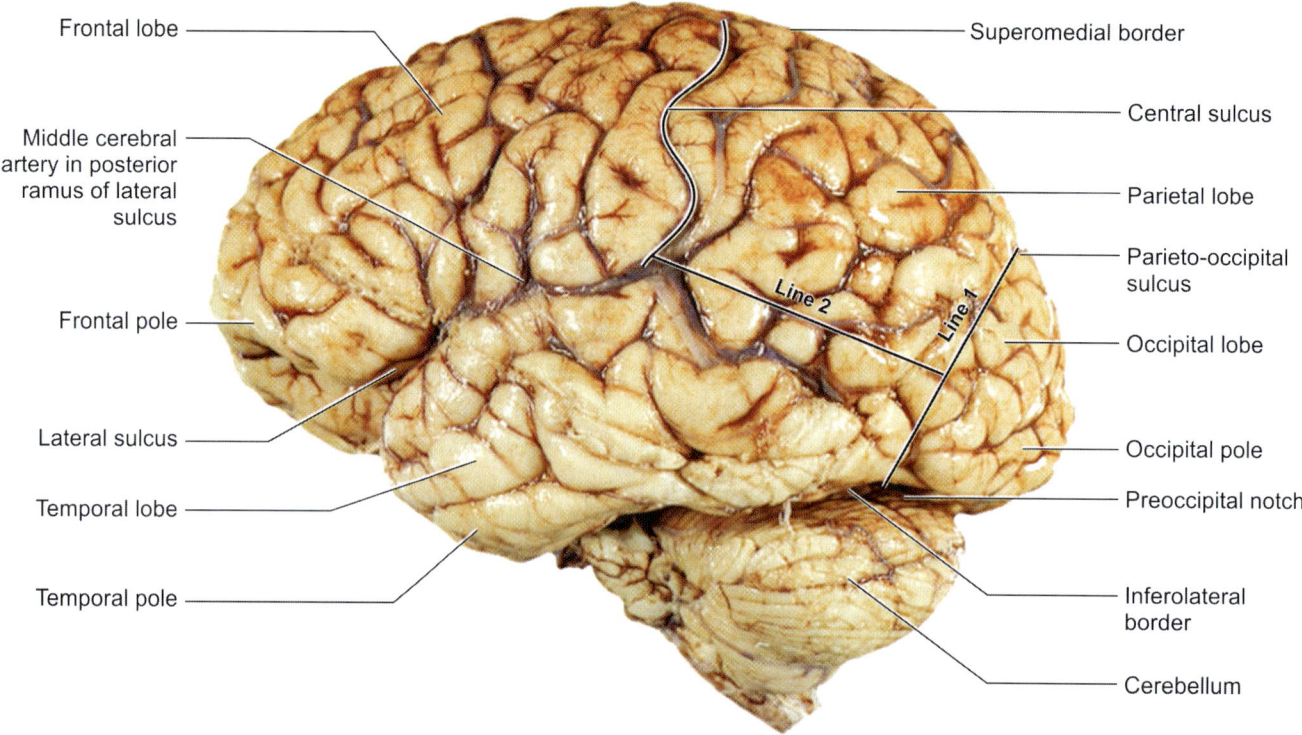

Fig. 70.4: Superolateral surface of cerebral hemisphere showing borders and lobes (with lines drawn for demarcating its lobes)

3. Laterally—temporal lobe
4. Posteriorly—occipital lobe

These are separated, some by sulci and some by drawing a few lines.

Sulci

1. Central sulcus—identify a sulcus 1 cm behind the midpoint between frontal and occipital poles. See it running obliquely downwards and forwards and ending a little above posterior ramus of lateral sulcus (Fig. 70.6a).
2. Lateral sulcus—it separates orbital and tentorial parts of inferior surface. It ascends to reach superolateral surface where it divides into anterior, ascending and posterior rami. Posterior ramus is the longest.
3. Parieto-occipital sulcus starts on the medial surface from middle of calcarine sulcus. It ascends up to the superomedial border 5 cm anterior to occipital pole.
4. Preoccipital notch is a slight depression on the inferolateral border, 5 cm in front of occipital pole.

5. Draw a line joining parieto-occipital sulcus to preoccipital notch.
6. Extend the line of posterior rami of lateral sulcus backwards till it meets the line drawn just before it (Fig. 70.4).

Now boundaries of all four lobes are clear on superolateral surface as follows:

1. Frontal lobe is anterior to central sulcus
2. Occipital lobe lies behind line number 1
3. Temporal lobe between posterior rami of lateral sulcus and its extension till line 1 and inferolateral border from temporal pole to preoccipital notch.
4. Parietal lobe is the area between central sulcus, line 1, line 2 and superomedial border.

Insula

- Identify insula lying deep in the floor of lateral fissure surrounded by a circular sulcus and overlapped by adjacent cortical areas (Fig. 70.7).
- It comprises anterior and posterior parts. Anterior insular cortex has a role in olfaction and taste.

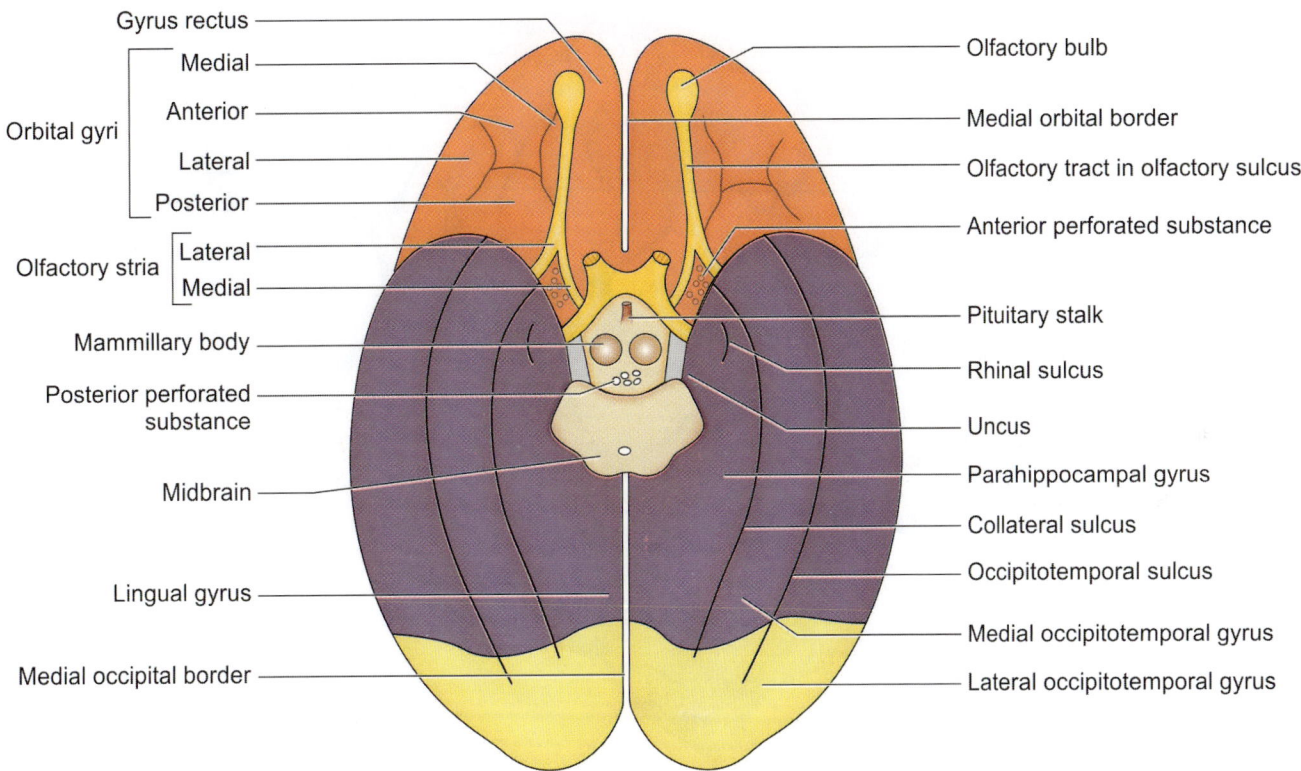

Gyrus rectus

Orbital gyri
— Medial
— Anterior
— Lateral
— Posterior

Olfactory stria
— Lateral
— Medial

Mammillary body

Posterior perforated substance

Midbrain

Lingual gyrus

Medial occipital border

Olfactory bulb

Medial orbital border

Olfactory tract in olfactory sulcus

Anterior perforated substance

Pituitary stalk

Rhinal sulcus

Uncus

Parahippocampal gyrus

Collateral sulcus

Occipitotemporal sulcus

Medial occipitotemporal gyrus

Lateral occipitotemporal gyrus

Fig. 70.5: Gyri and sulci on the inferior aspect of cerebral hemisphere

Posterior insular cortex has a role in language function.

Important Sulci and Gyri

- Identify central sulcus. Anterior to it is precentral gyrus and precentral sulcus. This is the motor area (area 4) (Fig. 70.6a). Anterior to precentral sulcus are three horizontal gyri. These are superior frontal gyrus, middle frontal gyrus and inferior frontal gyrus separated by superior and inferior frontal gyri. See all these parts. Motor speech area is located in the inferior frontal gyrus (areas 44, 45).

- Identify the temporal lobe. See superior temporal gyrus, middle temporal gyrus and inferior temporal gyrus separated by superior and inferior temporal sulci.

- Open up the posterior ramus of lateral sulcus and look for two transverse temporal gyri. The anterior gyrus is the auditory or hearing area (areas 41, 42).

- Identify parietal lobe and look for postcentral gyrus and postcentral sulcus. The postcentral gyrus is the main sensory area (areas 3, 1, 2).

- Identify interparietal sulcus which divides rest of parietal lobe into superior parietal lobule (areas 5, 7) and inferior parietal lobule.

- Identify the superomarginal and angular gyri around the upturned margin of posterior ramus of lateral sulcus and superior temporal sulcus. These gyri contain the Wernicke's sensory speech area.

- Identify the posteriorly placed occipital lobe. See the calcarine sulcus starting just behind splenium of corpus callosum to the centre of occipital lobe. The area on each side of calcarine sulcus is area 17. This is the visual area. On each side of area 17 is areas 18 and 19. These are visuopsychic areas.

- Look for sulci and gyri on inferior surface. Identify olfactory sulcus which lodges the olfactory bulb and olfactory tract.

- Look for anterior perforated substance situated between the two split roots of olfactory tract. Rest of the flat orbital surface is divided into anterior, posterior, lateral and medial gyri.

- Identify the gently concave tentorial surface. Look for inturned projection—the uncus which is part of parahippocampal gyrus (Fig. 70.5).

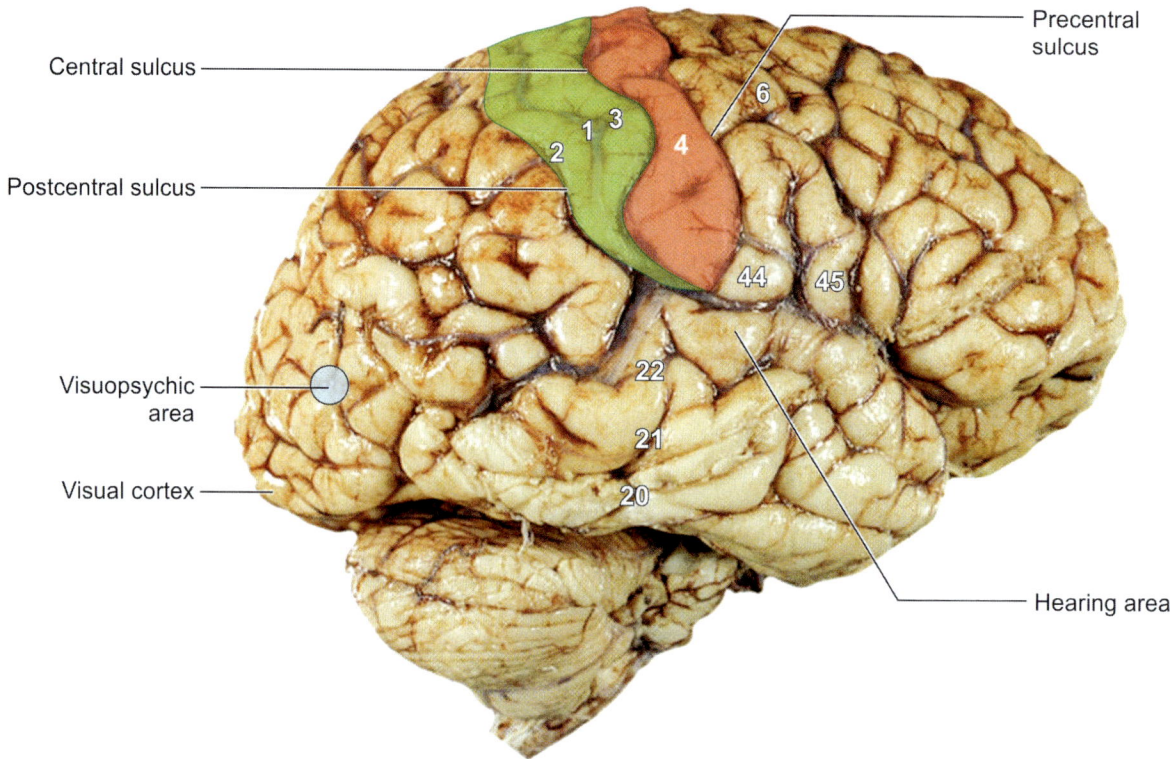

Central sulcus

Postcentral sulcus

Visuopsychic area

Visual cortex

Precentral sulcus

Hearing area

Fig. 70.6a: Functional areas on superolateral surface of brain

- Lateral to it is collateral sulcus, followed by medial occipitotemporal gyrus, occipitotemporal sulcus and lateral occipitotemporal gyrus.
- Uncus is the higher centre for smell. Hippocampus present within parahippocampal gyrus is for recent memory.
- Now turn the hemisphere so that its medial surface is visible.
- Identify the bundle of white mater—the corpus callosum joining the identical areas of two hemispheres (Fig. 70.6b). It is closer to frontal pole of hemisphere.
- Look for parts of corpus callosum: Anterior part is rostrum, the bend is genu, the body or trunk is main part and posterior end is splenium.

- Above the corpus callosum is callosal sulcus. Above this sulcus is cingulate gyrus. Still above is cingulate sulcus.
- Identify paracentral lobule between cingulate sulcus and superomedial border. Central sulcus lies in the centre of paracentral lobule.
- Motor area (area 4) extends into anterior part of the lobule while sensory area (areas 3,1,2) extends into the posterior part of the lobule.
- Locate medial frontal gyrus above and anterior to cingulate gyrus. Behind paracentral lobule locate precuneus which forms medial aspect of parietal lobe.
- Trace one deep sulcus—calcarine sulcus from just below splenium to the occipital lobe.

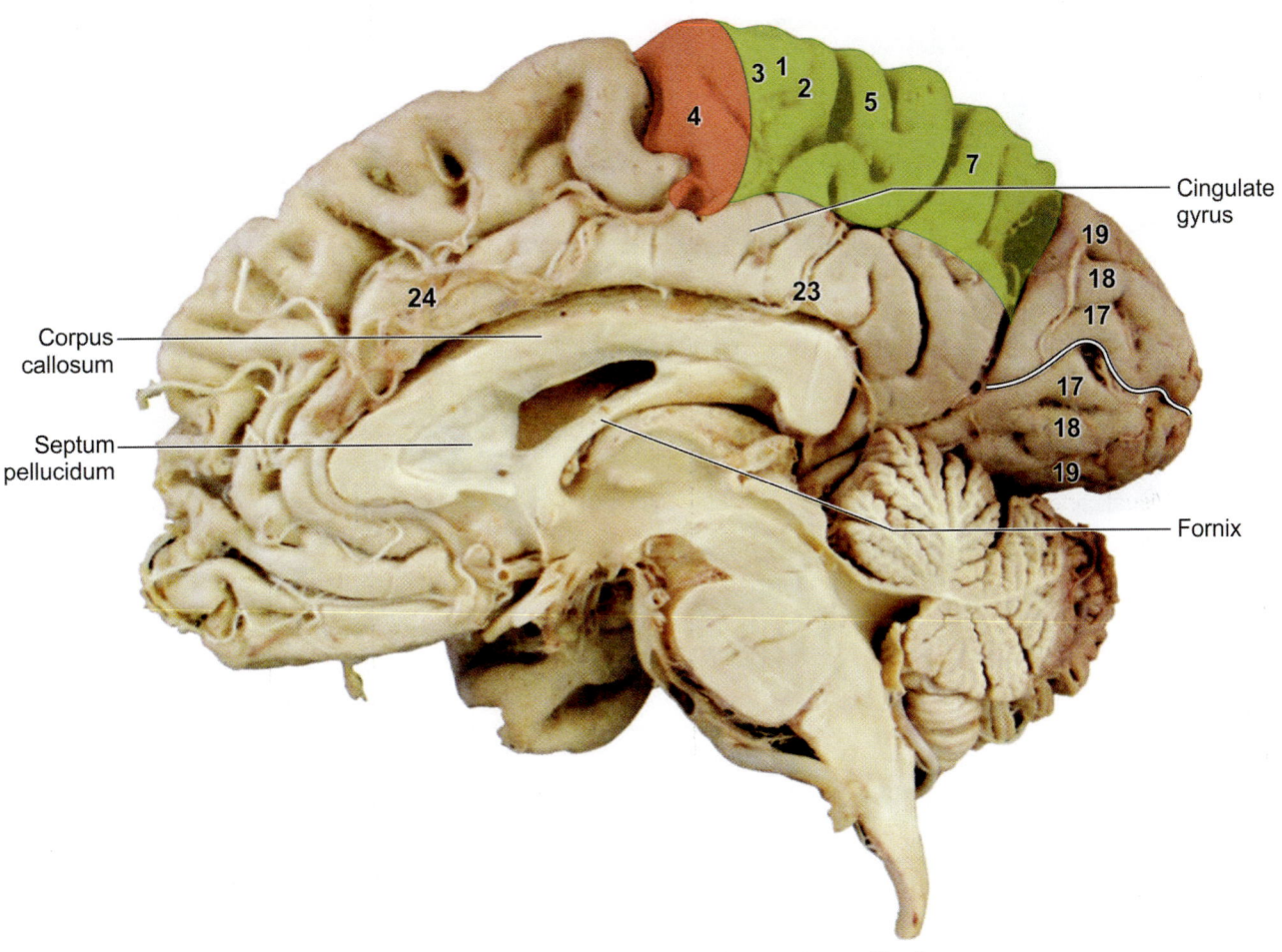

Fig. 70.6b: Functional areas on medial surface of brain

- Identify and trace a parieto-occipital sulcus starting from middle of calcarine sulcus, ascending up to reach superomedial border.
- Make thin slices through the part of calcarine sulcus posterior to its junction with the parieto-occipital sulcus. Identify the striae running through it. On cutting series of thin slices try to trace the extent of visual stria.

- Identify a thin membrane—the septum pellucidum present inferior to corpus callosum.
- Fornix is a bundle of fibres attached to the inferior margin of septum pellucidum.
- Try to locate the interventricular foramen between anterior part of fornix and anterior end of thalamus. This is a communication between lateral ventricle and third ventricle of brain.

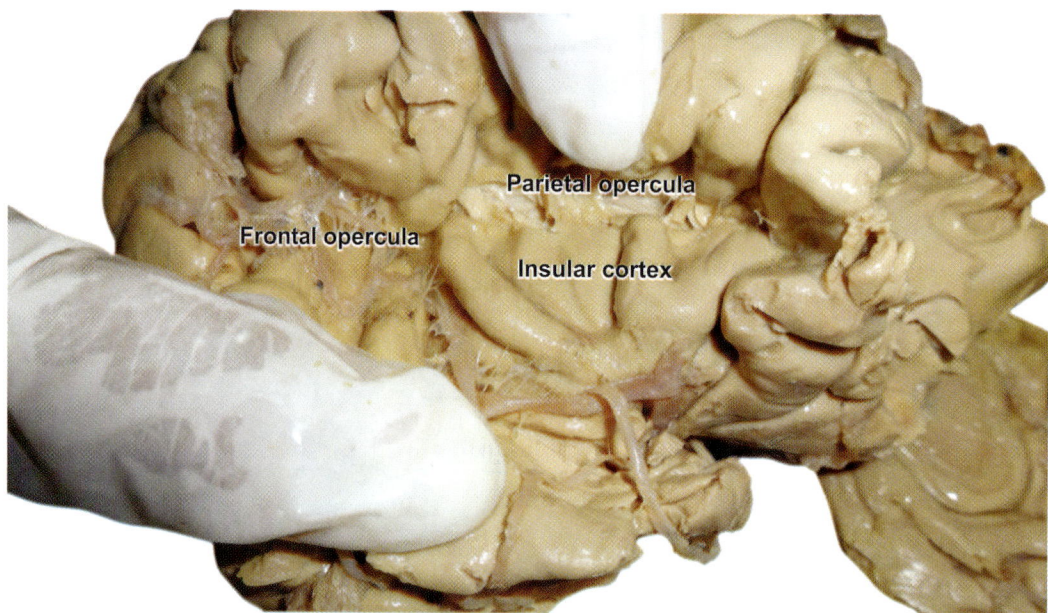

Fig. 70.7: Insular cortex

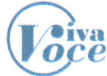

- Name the poles and lobes of cerebral hemisphere.
- Name the borders and surfaces of cerebral hemisphere.
- Where is motor speech area present?
- What is the function of primary motor area?
- What is the number of visual area?

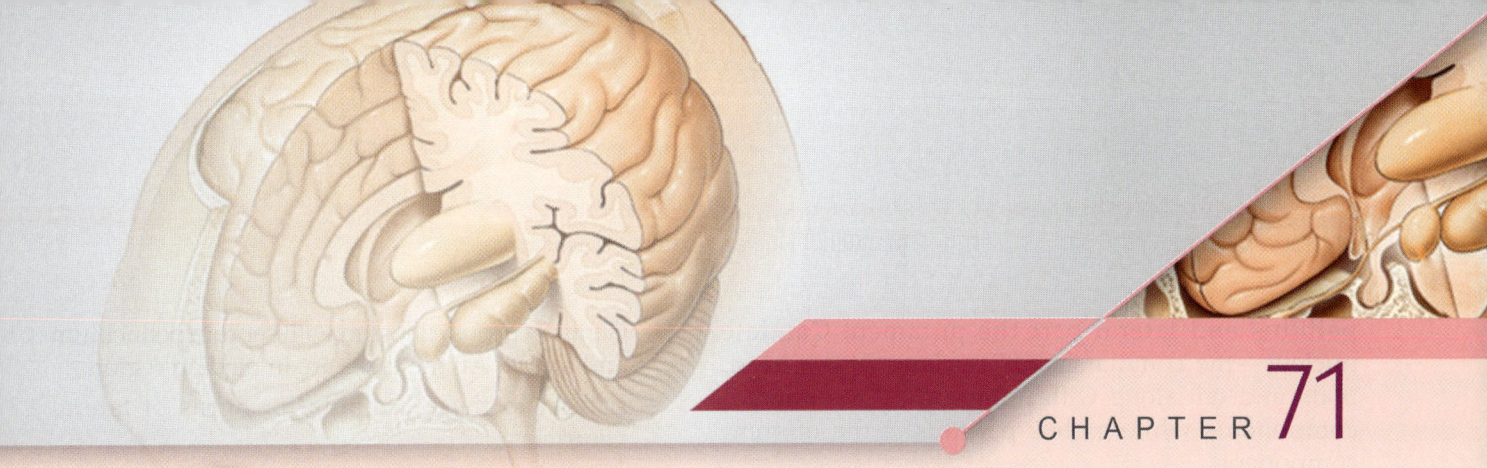

Diencephalon, Basal Ganglia and White Matter

DIENCEPHALON

Overview

It is placed deep in the cerebrum. Its cavity is the third ventricle. Its parts are—thalamus, epithalamus, hypothalamus and subthalamus. Thalamus (inner chamber) is a mass of grey matter 4 cm in all its dimensions. It lies in the lateral wall of 3rd ventricle and floor of central part of lateral ventricle. Thalamus comprises 2 ends—anterior and posterior; 4 surfaces—superior, inferior, medial and lateral. Anterior end forms the posterior boundary of interventricular foramen of Monro. Posterior end is wide and overlies medial and lateral geniculate bodies.

Its superior surface is related to floor of central part of lateral ventricle on its lateral aspect and third ventricle on the medial aspect. Its inferior surface rests on subthalamus and hypothalamus. Medial surface forms lateral wall of third ventricle. The medial surfaces of two thalami are interconnected by the interthalamic adhesion. Its lateral surface forms

medial boundary of posterior limb of the internal capsule. Nuclei of thalamus are—anterior, medial, lateral, ventral, intralaminar, midline, reticular, centromedian, medial and lateral geniculate bodies. For connections and functions *see* BD Chaurasia's *Human Anatomy*. Epithalamus comprises pineal body and posterior commissure.

Hypothalamus comprises many nuclei which function for temperature regulation, biological clock, reproductive cycle, endocrine control and autonomic nervous system control.

BASAL GANGLIA

Overview

Basal ganglia are collection of neurons in the depth of the white matter. These are corpus striatum composed of caudate nucleus and lentiform nucleus, amygdaloid body, etc.

The corpus striatum is the main part. Lentiform nucleus is divided into medial 2 parts, the globus pallidus and lateral part the putamen. Caudate nucleus—the comma shaped nucleus with a head, body and tail along with putamen are the afferent components while globus pallidus is the efferent component.

Main neurotransmitter in this region is the dopamine. Lack of dopamine leads to a typical disease called the parkinsonism.

Other basal ganglia are claustrum, amygdaloid body, red nucleus, substantia nigra and subthalamus.

Competency achievement: The student should be able to:

AN 62.4 Enumerate parts and major connections of basal ganglia and limbic lobe.

Steps of Dissection

- Take one of the two hemispheres. Make one horizontal incision with a brain knife at the level of interventricular foramen.
- Identify the following structures in median and medial regions, anterior to posterior sides in anterior half of the section:
  – Grey matter of frontal lobe on the surface
  – White matter of frontal lobe

  – Genu of corpus callosum with septum pellucidum and fornix. All the three are in median region.
  – Lateral to these are anterior horns of lateral ventricle.
  – Caudate nucleus is a mass of grey matter. The head of caudate is seen in this section forming lateral boundary of anterior horn. Other parts of caudate nucleus are body and tail.

- Just posterior to the fornix in median plane lies the narrow cavity of 3rd ventricle. On both sides of this narrow cavity are big masses of grey matter known as thalamus; forming the lateral boundaries of 3rd ventricle (Fig. 71.1a and b).
- Lateral to caudate nucleus and thalamus, separated by a band of white matter is a lens like mass of grey matter—the lentiform nucleus (Fig. 71.2). See that this nucleus is divided into an outer dark part, the putamen and an inner lighter part, the globus pallidus by white matter plate—the external medullary lamina.
- Lateral to lentiform nucleus is external capsule. Still lateral to the external capsule is the grey matter of claustrum.

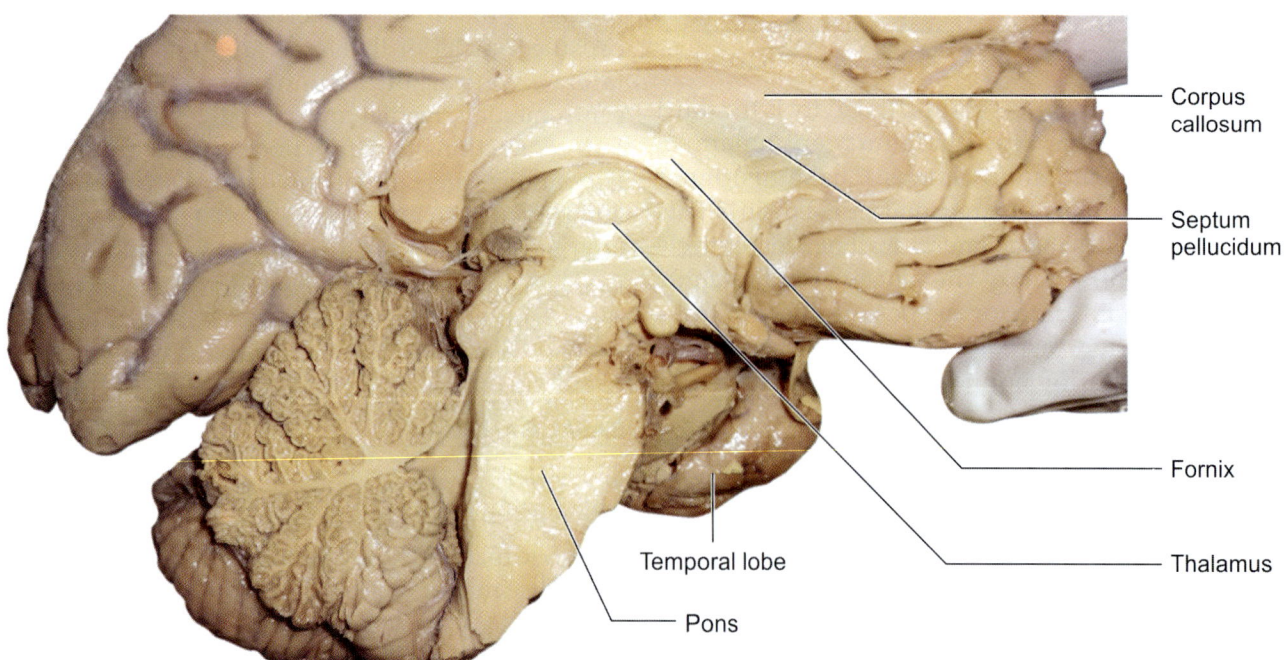

Corpus callosum

Septum pellucidum

Fornix

Temporal lobe

Thalamus

Pons

Fig. 71.1a: Medial surface of brain showing thalamus

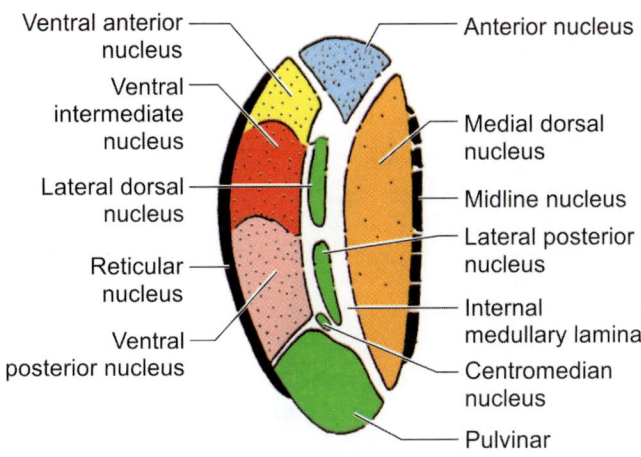

Fig. 71.1b: Various nuclei of thalamus

Competency achievement: The student should be able to:

AN 62.3 Describe the white matter of cerebrum.

WHITE MATTER OF CEREBRUM

Overview

White matter is divided into:

i. Association fibres—connecting different parts of some hemisphere;

ii. Commissural fibres—connecting identical parts of the same hemisphere;

iii. Projection fibres—connecting upper areas of brain with lower areas. These fibres constitute the "internal capsule". Since the motor, sensory, autonomic fibres are placed close together, being supplied by central branches, it is subjected to various maladies, leading to contralateral hemiplegia.

Steps of Dissection

Association fibres

• Scrape the grey matter between adjacent gyri till the white matter connecting the adjacent gyri is visible. This will expose the short association fibres (Fig. 71.3). Identify the cingulate gyrus on the medial surface of the left hemisphere. Scrape the grey matter of this gyrus till a band of white matter—the cingulum is exposed. Define the extent of cingulum from the anterior end of corpus callosum, around its convex trunk and splenium into the parahippocampal gyrus.

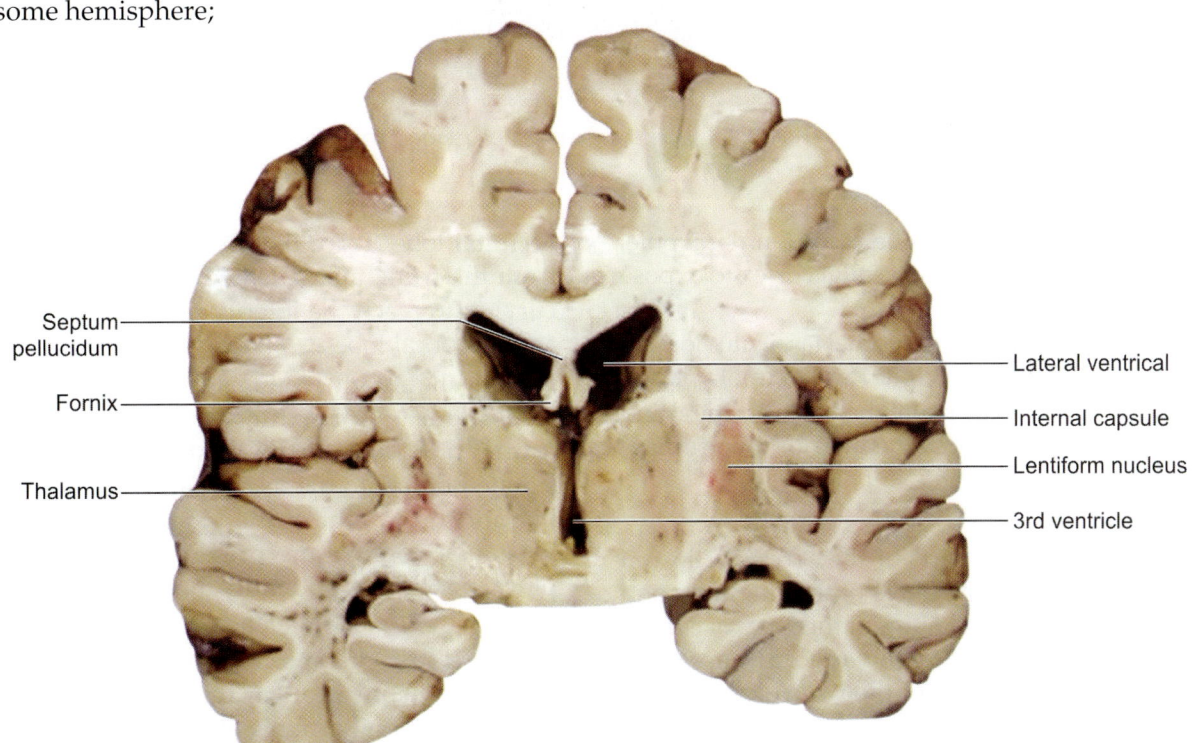

Fig. 71.2: Coronal section of brain showing basal ganglia, parts of ventricles and internal capsule

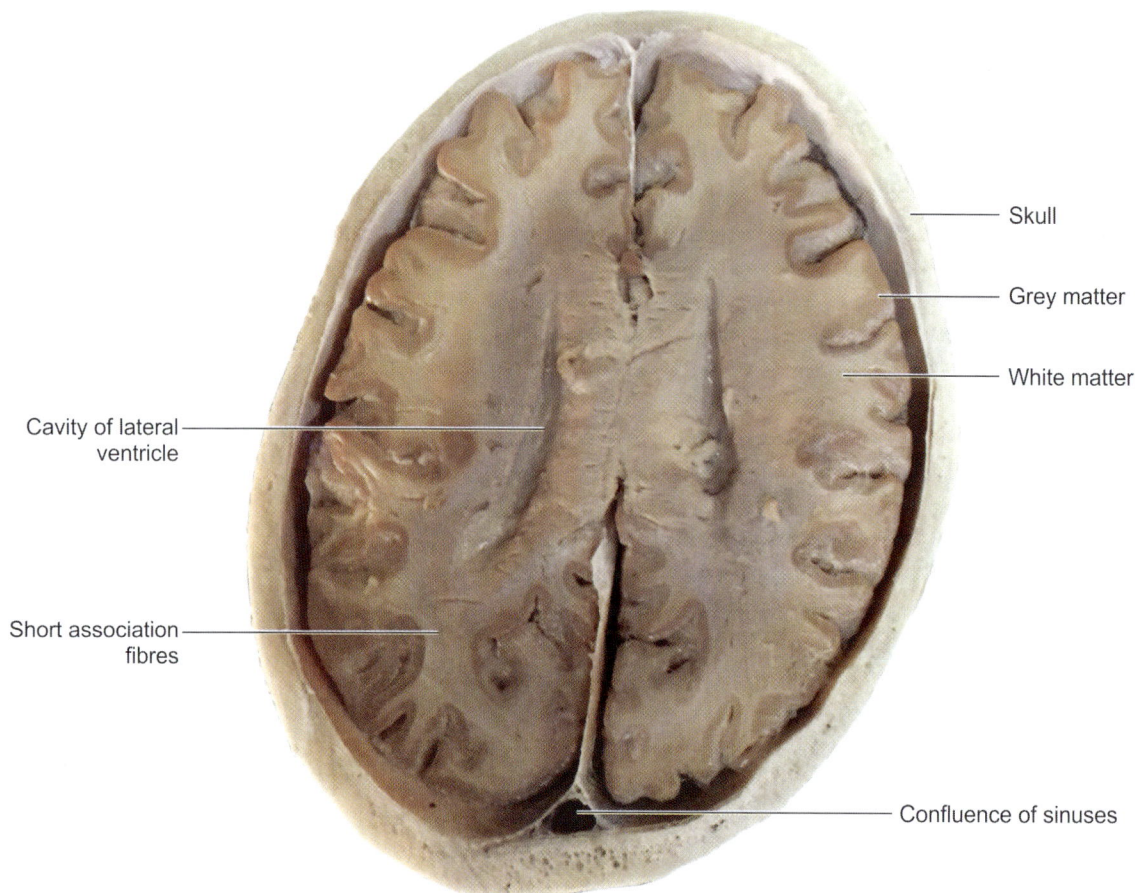

Skull

Grey matter

White matter

Cavity of lateral ventricle

Short association fibres

Confluence of sinuses

Fig. 71.3: Horizontal section showing short association fibres

- Similarly scrape the cortex between temporal pole, motor speech area and the orbital cortex to expose uncinate fasciculus.
- Also expose superior longitudinal fasciculus joining the frontal lobe to the occipital and temporal lobes.
- Lastly, scrape the grey matter between occipital and temporal lobes to expose the inferior longitudinal fasciculus.

Commissural fibres
- Identify the various parts of the corpus callosum (Fig. 71.4). Remove the fibres of the cingulum and identify the superficial fibres of the genu of corpus callosum passing into the medial aspect of hemisphere. Such fibres of the two sides form the forceps minor.
- Expose the band of fibres passing from splenium of corpus callosum towards the superior part of occipital lobe. Trace the fibres of tapetum arising from the trunk and splenium of corpus callosum curving to reach the inferior parts of the occipital and temporal lobes.
- Identify the anterior commissure lying just anterior to column of fornix and the interventricular foramen. Examine the posterior commissure situated dorsal to the upper part of aqueduct and inferior to the root of the pineal body. Look for habenular commissure present at the root of the pineal body. Lastly, identify the commissure of the fornix and the hypothalamic commissures.
- Lift up a strip of superficial fibres of the genu of corpus callosum and tear these laterally. Identify the intersectioning fibres of corpus callosum and those of the vertically disposed fibres of the corona radiata.

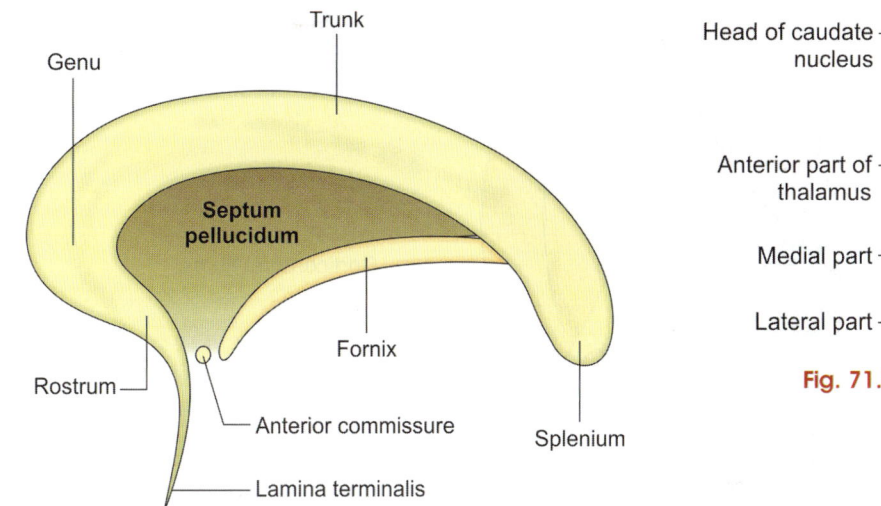

Genu

Trunk

Septum pellucidum

Rostrum

Anterior commissure

Fornix

Splenium

Lamina terminalis

Fig. 71.4: Parts of corpus callosum as seen in a sagittal section

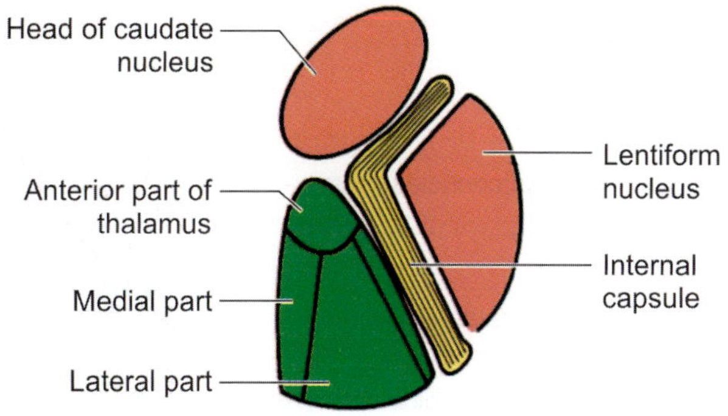

Head of caudate nucleus

Anterior part of thalamus

Medial part

Lateral part

Lentiform nucleus

Internal capsule

Fig. 71.5: Position of internal capsule

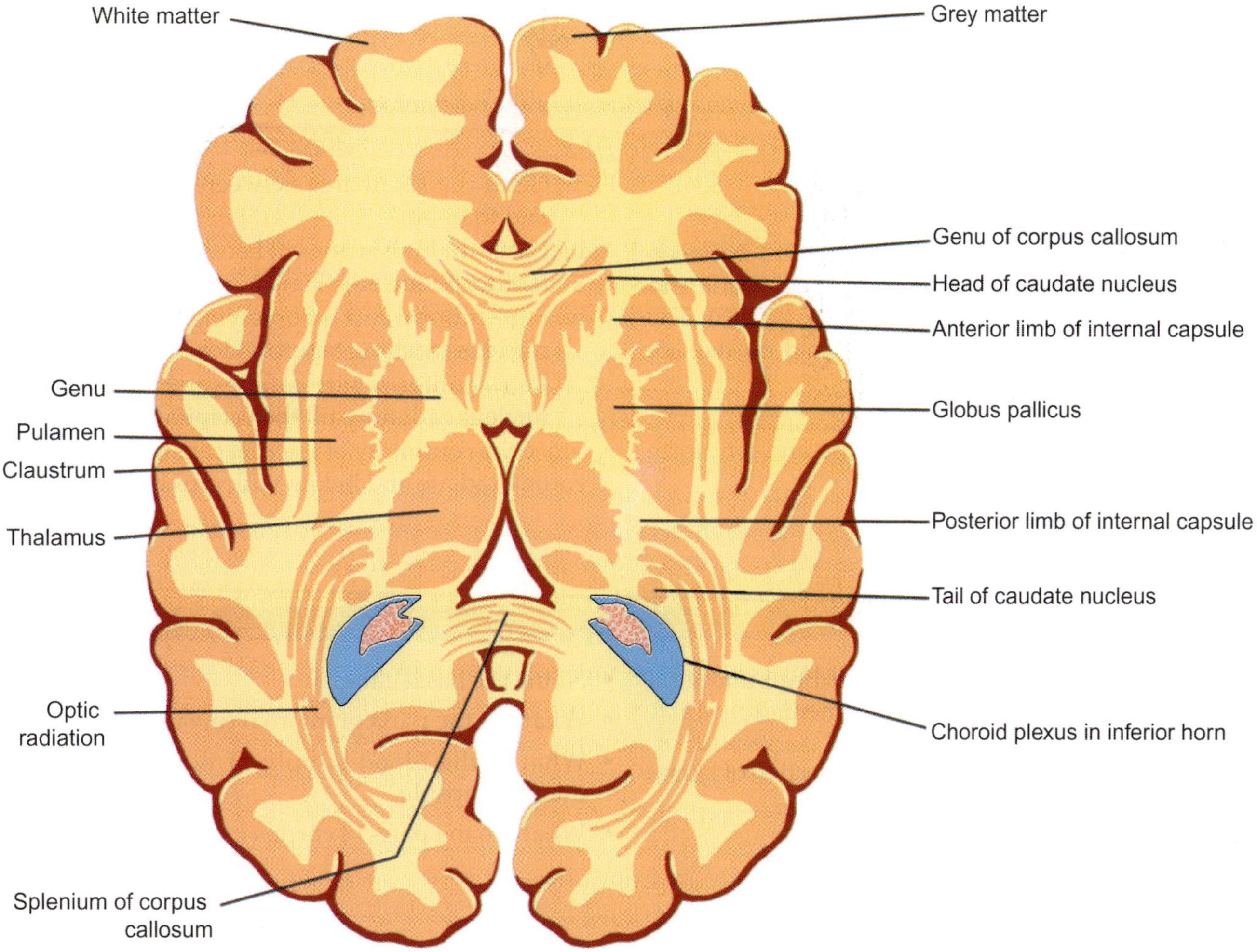

White matter

Grey matter

Genu of corpus callosum

Head of caudate nucleus

Anterior limb of internal capsule

Genu

Pulamen

Claustrum

Thalamus

Globus pallicus

Posterior limb of internal capsule

Tail of caudate nucleus

Optic radiation

Choroid plexus in inferior horn

Splenium of corpus callosum

Fig. 71.6: Internal capsule as seen in horizontal section

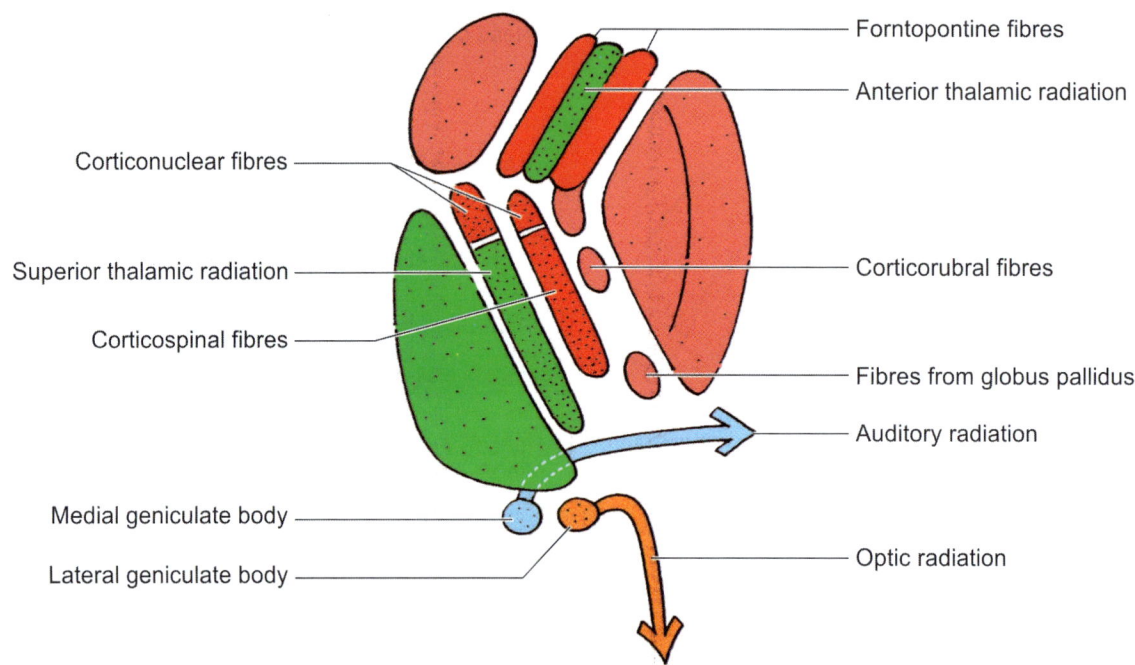

Fig. 71.7: Scheme to show fibres of internal capsule

Projection fibres

Internal capsule

- Identify compact layer of white fibres between caudate nucleus and thalamus on medial side and lentiform nucleus on lateral side (Fig. 71.5). The shape of internal capsule is "V" laid on its side (Fig. 71.2).
- *See its various parts:*
    i. Anterior limb between caudate and lentiform nuclei (Fig. 71.6)

ii. Genu is a small area between caudate nucleus and thalamus
iii. Posterior limb is present between thalamus and lentiform nucleus (Fig. 71.7)
iv. Sublentiform part is fibres lying below lentiform nucleus reaching temporal lobe
v. Retrolentiform part is fibres behind lentiform nucleus radiating till the occipital lobe.
- Trace the continuity of internal capsule above with corona radiate and below with crus cerebri.

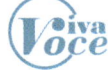 **Viva Voce**

- Name the biggest commissural fibre bundle on medial surface of cerebral hemisphere.
- Name the nuclei of the thalamus.
- Name the afferent and efferent connection of lateral geniculate body.
- Name the features of parkinsonism
- Name the basal ganglia
- What are the parts of internal capsule?
- What is the blood supply of posterior limb of internal capsule?
- What are the parts of corpus callosum?

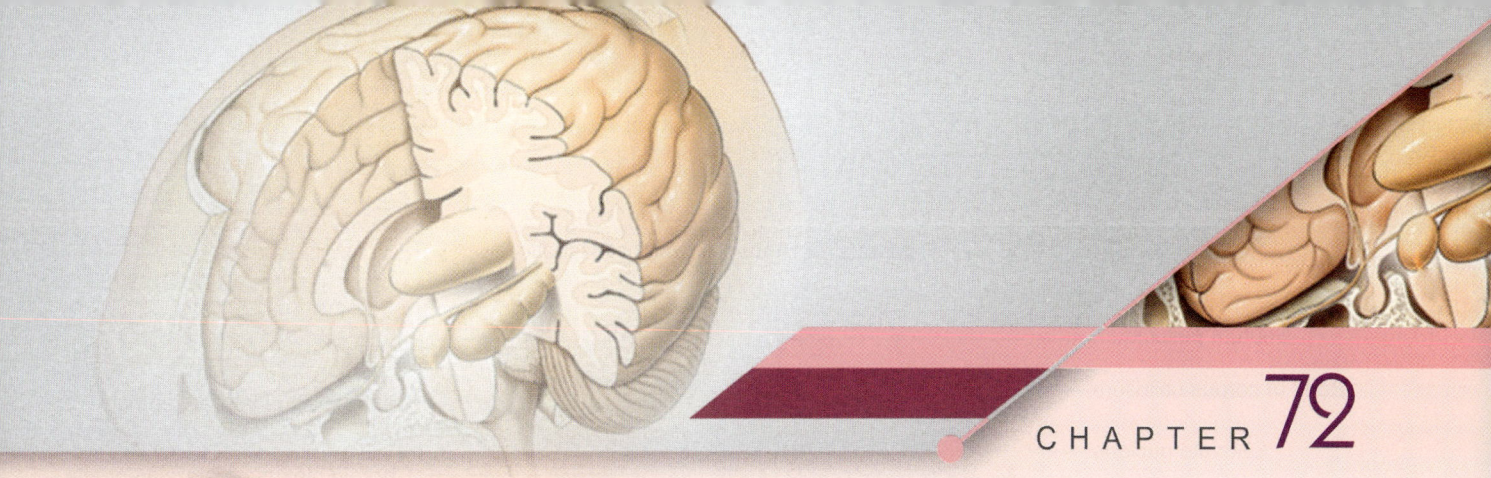

Third Ventricle and Lateral Ventricle

THIRD VENTRICLE

Overview

Third ventricle is a narrow cavity of diencephalon. It lies between the right and left thalami. The interventricular foramina from right and left ventricles open into the third ventricle. It continues caudally into the aqueduct of midbrain (Fig. 72.1a and b)

Anterior wall: Lamina terminalis, anterior commissure, and anterior column of fornix

Posterior wall: Pineal body, posterior commissure and cerebral aqueduct

Roof: Body of fornix and choroid plexus

Floor: Optic chiasma, tubercinerium, infundibulum, mammillary bodies, posterior perforated substance and tegmentum of midbrain

Lateral wall: Medial surface of thalamus, hypothalamic sulcus and hypothalamus.

Competency achievement: The student should be able to:
AN 63.1 Describe and demonstrate parts, boundaries and features of IIIrd, IVth and lateral ventricle.

Steps of Dissection

- Identify the extent of the third ventricle from the lamina terminalis anteriorly to the upper end of the aqueduct and root of pineal body posteriorly.
- Examine its anterior wall, posterior wall, roof, floor and lateral walls.

LATERAL VENTRICLE

Overview

The lateral ventricle (LV) is the cavity of telencephalic vesicle of forebrain. This ventricle also has 4 parts corresponding to the lobes of the cerebral hemisphere. All the four parts are continuous with each other (Fig. 72.2).

The parts are:
- The body of lateral ventricle in relation to parietal lobe
- Anterior horn of left ventricle in relation to frontal lobe
- Posterior horn of left ventricle in relation to occipital lobe

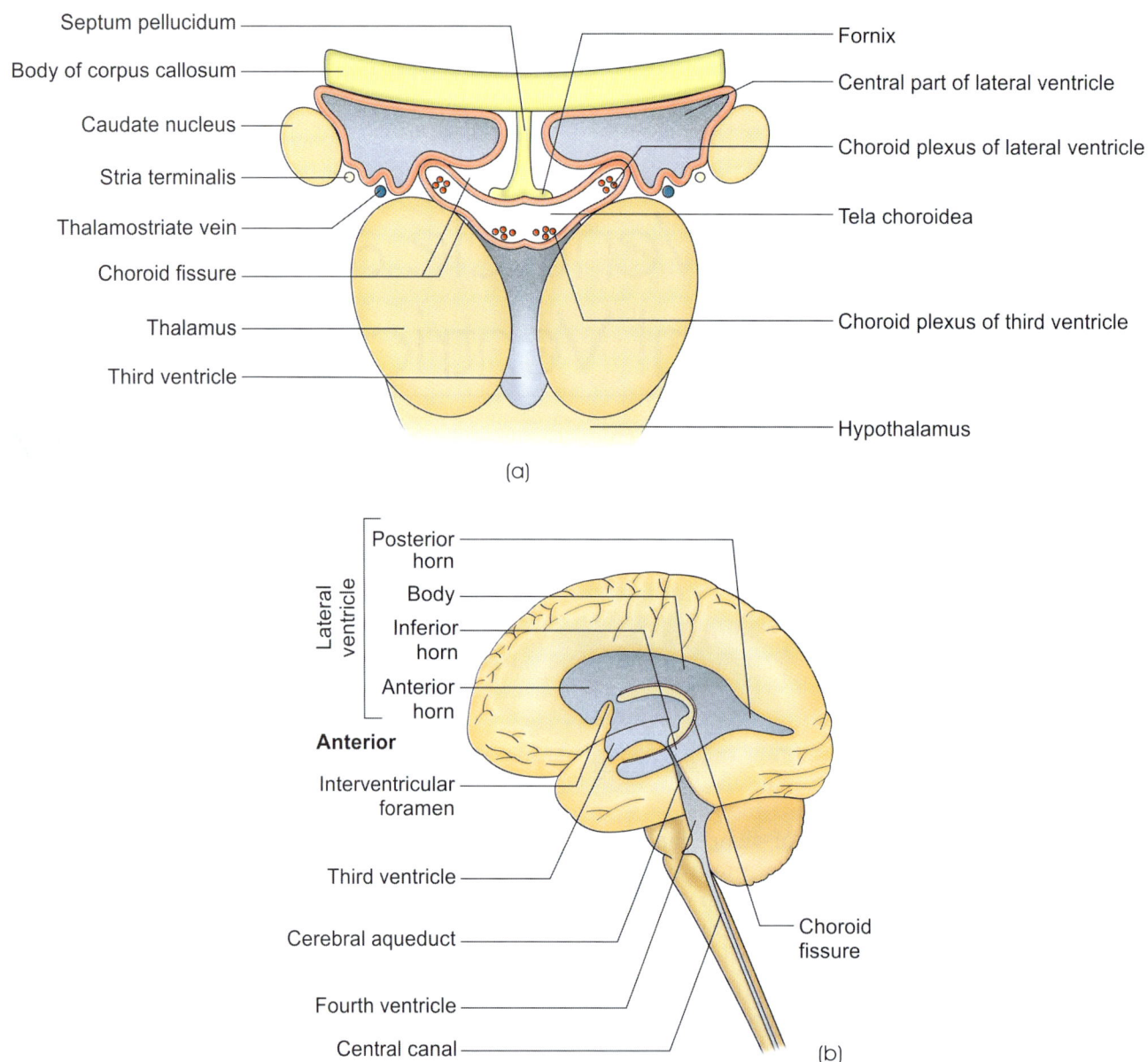

Fig. 72.1a and b: (a) Parts of lateral ventricle; (b) Lateral view of ventricular system

- Inferior horn of left ventricle in relation to temporal lobe

Their boundaries are:

Central part
- Roof: Under surface of corpus callosum
- Floor: Body of caudate nucleus, stria terminalis, thalamostriate vein, lateral portion of upper

surface of thalamus, choroid plexus, part of body of fornix
- Medial wall: Septum pellucidum and body of fornix.
- Anterior horn
  - Roof: Genu and rostrum of corpus callosum
  - Floor: Head of caudate nucleus
  - Medial wall: Septum pellucidum and column of fornix

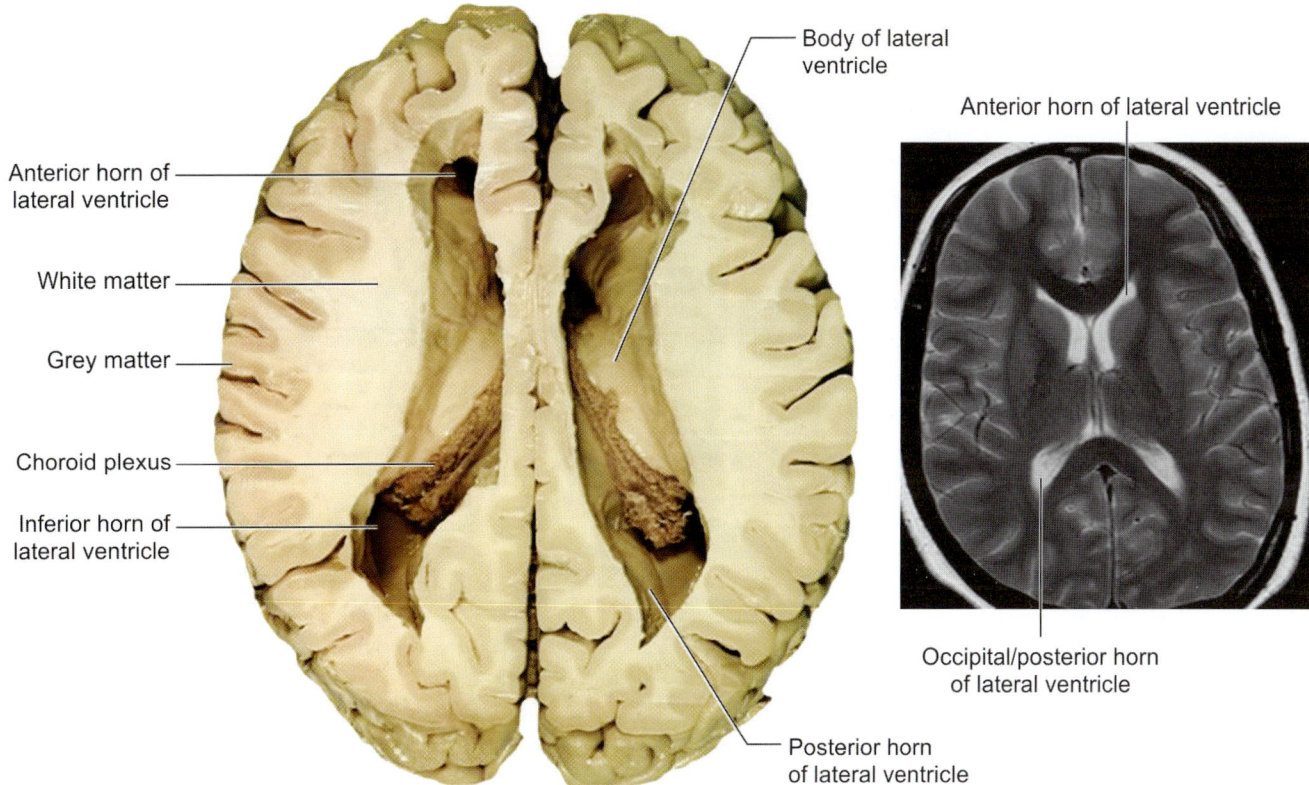

Fig. 72.2: Parts of lateral ventricle in horizontal section. MRI also seen

Posterior horn

Floor and medial wall—bulb of posterior horn raised by forceps major and calcar avis produced by calcarine sulcus.

Roof and lateral wall—tapetum and fibres of optic radiation.

Inferior horn

Roof and lateral wall—tapetum, tail of caudate nucleus, stria terminalis and amygdaloid body.

Floor: Collateral eminence raised by collateral sulcus and hippocampus

The ventricle opens by an interventricular foramen (IVF) into the narrow third ventricle. Look for the boundaries of IVF. These are column of fornix anteriorly and anterior end of thalamus posteriorly.

Steps of Dissection

- Take the right hemisphere and put the tip of the knife at the interventricular foramen. Give a vertical incision through the fornix, septum pellucidum,

body of corpus callosum, the medial surface of the hemisphere till the superomedial border (Fig. 72.3a).
- Turn the brain so that superolateral surface points towards you. Continue the previous incision on this surface for 2 cm. Carry the incision posteriorly and then curve it downwards till the end of the posterior ramus of the lateral sulcus (Fig. 72.3b).
- Expose the insula by depressing the temporal lobe. Cut through the medial part of the gyri situated on the superior surface of the temporal lobe till the stem of the lateral sulcus (Fig. 72.3c).
- Now try to separate the frontal lobe from the temporal lobe, and open up the stem of the lateral sulcus. Put the knife in the anterior part of stem of the lateral sulcus and extend the incision medially to the inferior part of stem of the lateral sulcus. Keep on opening the cut while making it and identify the choroid plexus entering the inferior horn of the lateral ventricle from its medial side.
- Now brain is easily separable into an upper frontal part and a lower occipitotemporal part. Lift the

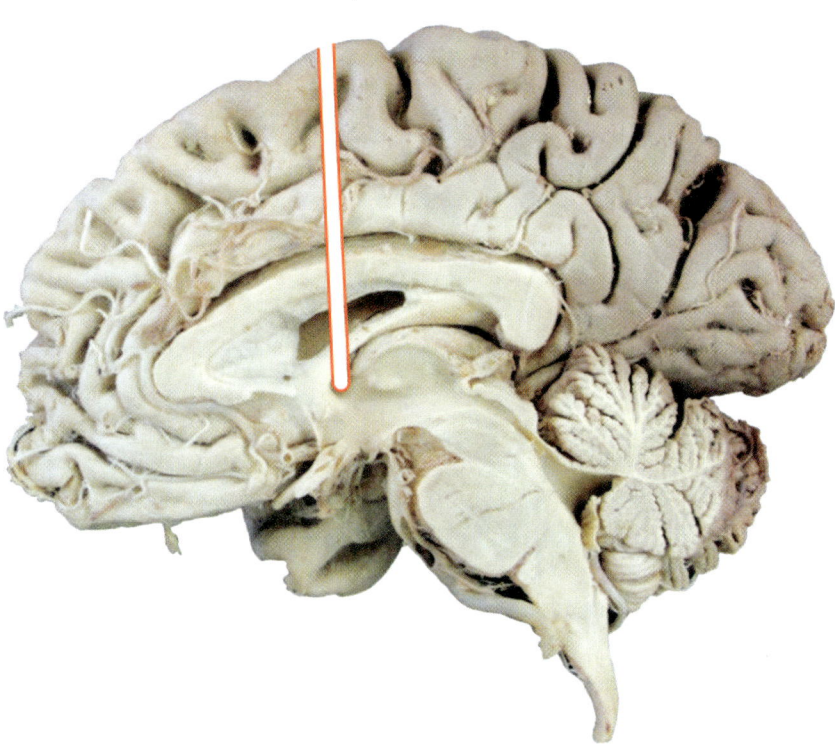

Fig. 72.3a: 1st part of incision

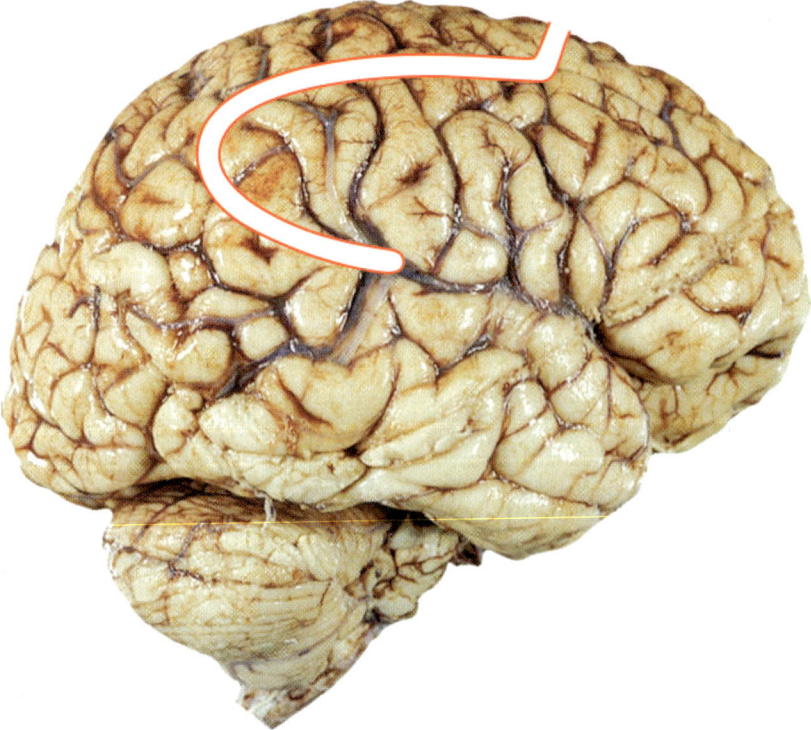

Fig. 72.3b: 2nd part of incision

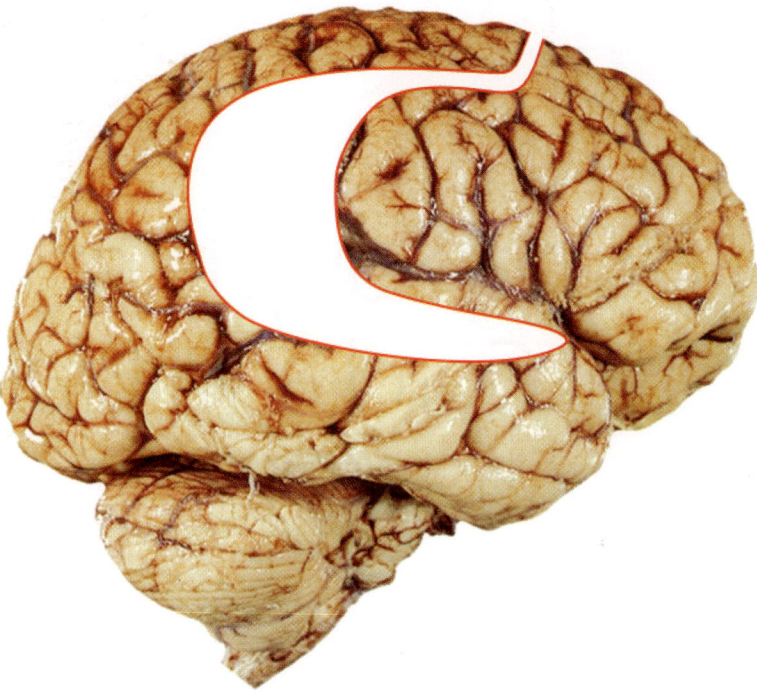

Fig. 72.3c: 3rd part of incision to complete the exposure of lateral ventricle

fornix from the thalamus, separating the fornix from the choroid plexus. Identify the choroidal branches of the posterior cerebral artery.

- Identify structures in all horns of lateral ventricle with the help of the two parts, i.e. frontal and occipitotemporal parts of the cerebral hemisphere.

- Expose the anterior column of fornix by scrapping the ependymal of anterior part of third ventricle. Trace the anterior column of fornix till the mammillary body. Trace another bundle, the mammillothalamic tract till the anterior nucleus of the thalamus.

- Name the anterior and posterior boundaries of third ventricle.

- Name the structures present in the floor of central part of lateral ventricle of brain.

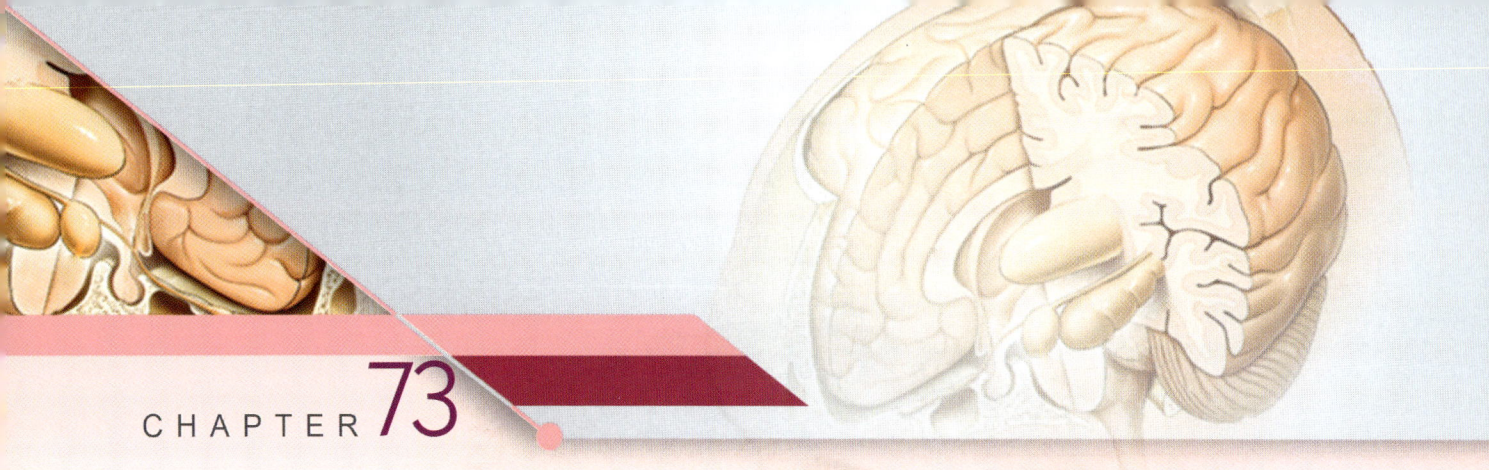

CHAPTER 73

Blood Supply of Spinal Cord and Brain

Learning Objectives

One should be able to

1. Trace the course of anterior, middle and posterior cerebral arteries.

2. Enumerate the branches and areas of distribution of these arteries.

BLOOD SUPPLY OF SPINAL CORD

Overview

Arteries to spinal cord are one anterior spinal artery and two posterior spinal arteries. These are supplemented by regional arteries (Fig. 73.1).

Veins are in six longitudinal channels. These drain into various segmental veins via internal vertebral venous plexus.

ARTERIES OF BRAIN

Overview

Brain gets maximum blood supply per unit tissue in the body. It is functioning all the time. Its functions are motor, sensory control, control of all special sense, emotional control, control of attention concentration, innovative thoughts, etc. Two arteries on each side supply cerebral hemisphere. These are a pair of vertebral and internal carotid arteries. These four arteries and their branches form an important circle of Willis. Branches from the circle are cortical for the cerebral cortex, central for deeper nuclei and choroidal

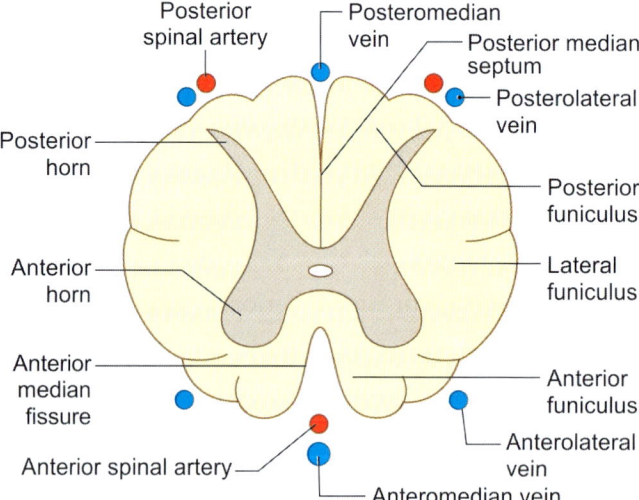

Fig. 73.1: Blood supply of spinal cord

branches for the choroid plexuses which in turn secrete CSF.

Posterior cerebral artery is the artery of vision located in the occipital lobe. Middle cerebral artery supplies most of the motor, sensory, auditory, taste areas. Anterior cerebral artery supplies orbital surface, prefrontal surface and a small strip on the superolateral surface.

Competency achievement: The student should be able to:

AN 62.6 Describe and identify formation, branches and major areas of distribution of circle of Willis.

Steps of Dissection

- Vertebral arteries enter through foramen magnum. Each vertebral artery runs forwards and medially to join with each other to form single basilar artery (Fig. 73.2).
- Identify branches of vertebral artery. These are:
  - Meningeal
  - Medullary
  - Posterior spinal
  - Anterior spinal
  - Posterior inferior cerebellar

- See single basilar artery running in the basilar groove of pons (Fig. 73.2). Its branches are:
  - Two anterior inferior cerebellar
  - 5–6 pairs of pontine branches
  - Two labyrinthine arteries
  - Two superior cerebellar arteries
  - Two posterior cerebral arteries

Internal Carotid Arteries (ICA)

Each ICA enters cranial cavity through carotid canal to reach superior aspect of foramen lacerum. Then it passes through cavernous venous sinus, pierces its roof and ends just lateral to optic chiasma. There it gives ophthalmic artery which accompanies optic nerve in the optic canal.

Then the artery bends backwards close to anterior perforated substance.

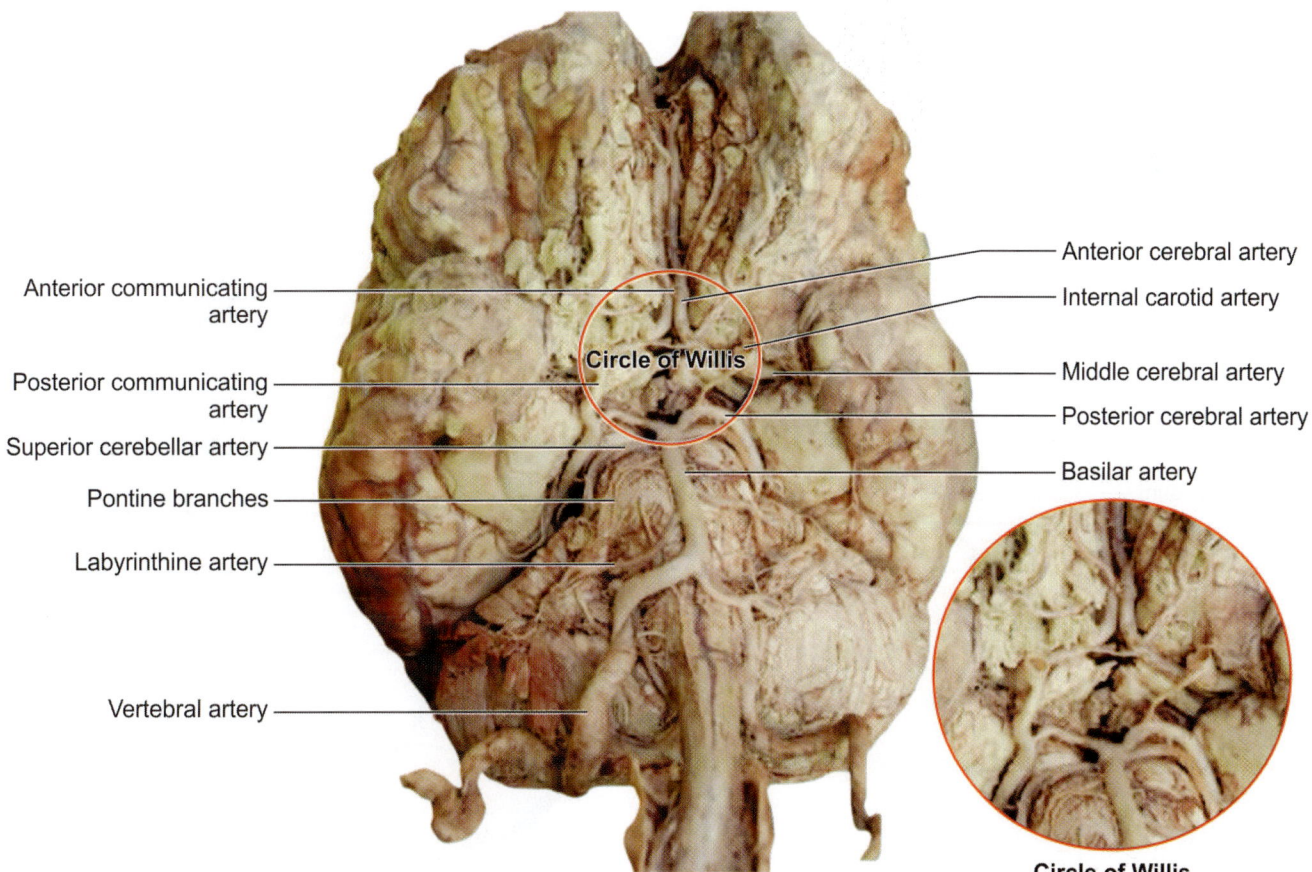

Fig. 73.2: Basilar artery and circle of Willis

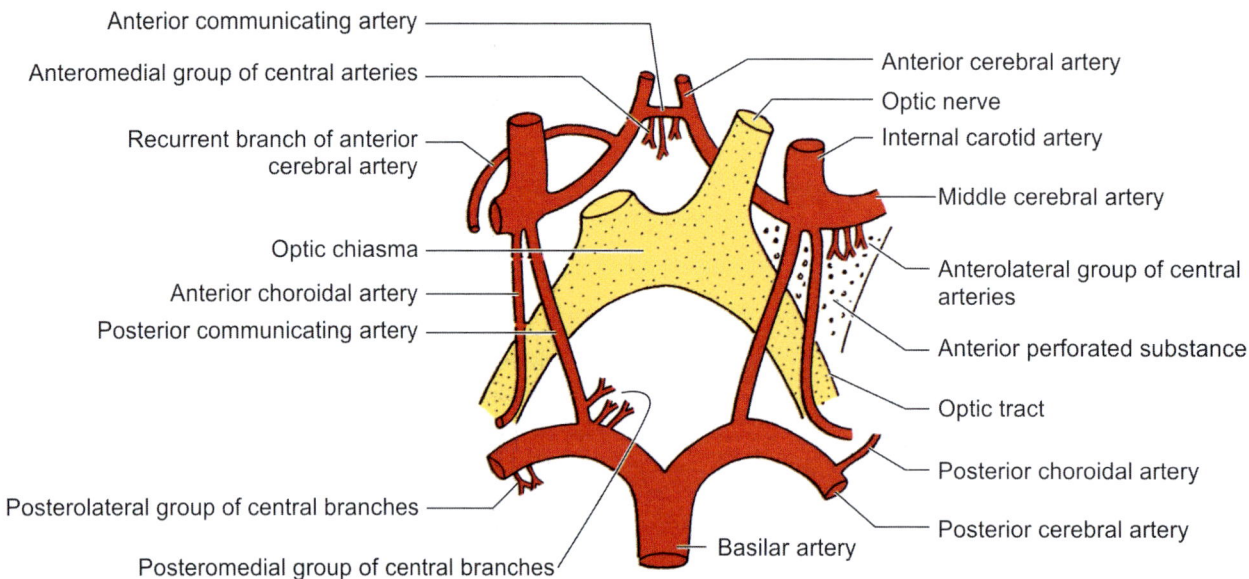

Fig. 73.3: Circle of Willis

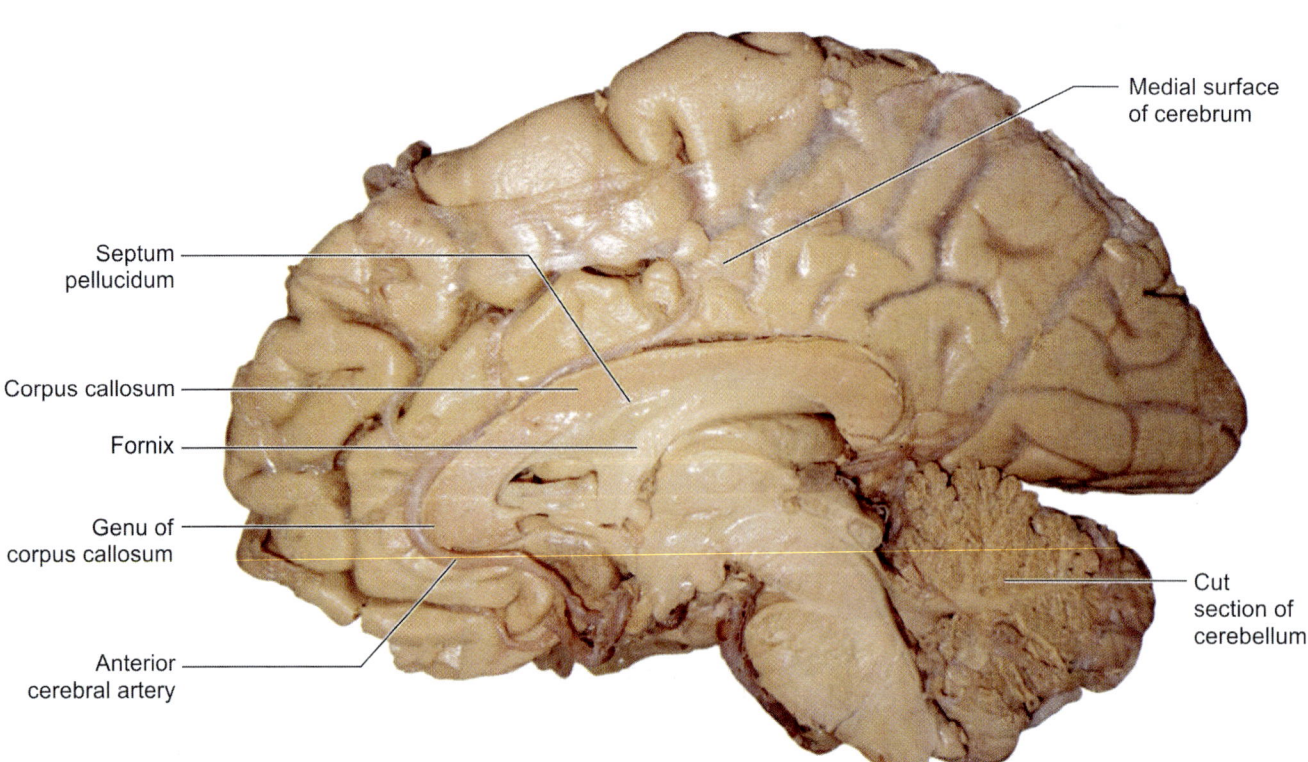

Fig. 73.4: Anterior cerebral artery seen on medial surface of brain

Here it gives:

- Anterior cerebral (Figs 73.3 and 73.4)
- Posterior communicating, which joins the posterior cerebral artery
- Anterior choroidal

  It continues as middle cerebral artery.

Circle of Willis

The circle is hexagonal in shape. It is formed by:

  i. Anteriorly by anterior communicating artery

 ii. Anterolaterally by anterior cerebral arteries

iii. Laterally by internal carotid arteries

 iv. Posterolaterally by posterior cerebral arteries

  v. Posteriorly by medial parts of posterior cerebral arteries.

The branches given off by the cerebral arteries are of following types:

- Cortical for surface of cerebral hemisphere
- Central for deeper nuclei like caudate nucleus, thalamus, lentiform nucleus
- Choroidal for the supply of blood to choroid plexus of the various ventricles. These plexuses secrete the cerebrospinal fluid.

For details of the course of arteries *see* BD Chaurasia's *Human Anatomy*.

Veins of Brain

Veins are in:

  i. External cerebral veins which are in two sets—the superior cerebral veins and inferior cerebral veins

 ii. Internal cerebral veins, formed by union of thalamostriate and choroidal veins (Fig. 73.5a and b).

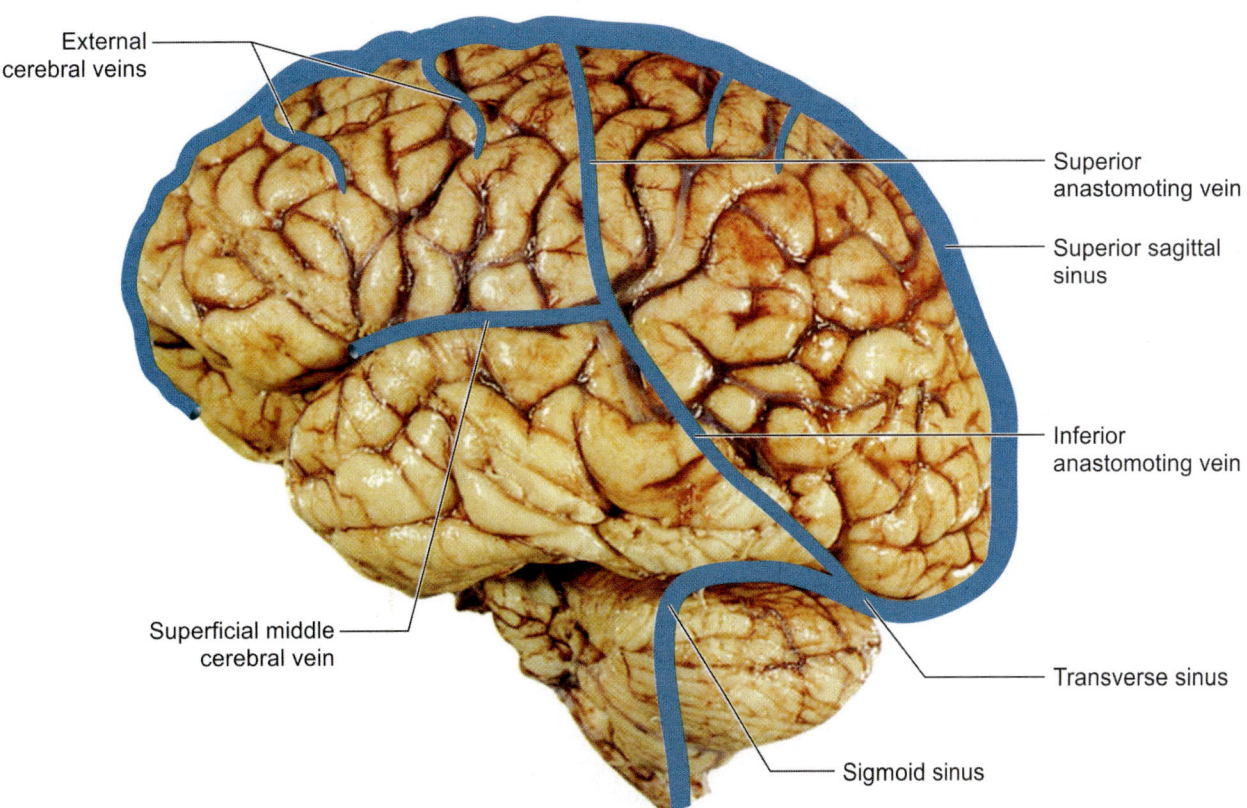

Fig. 73.5a: Veins on the superolateral surface of cerebral hemisphere

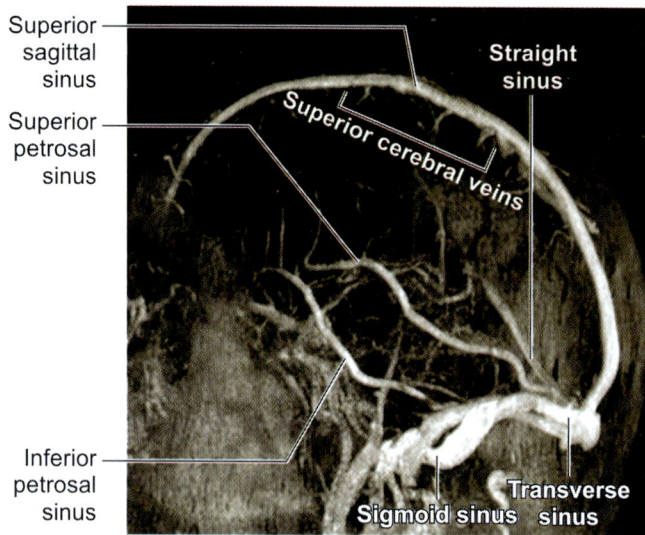

Superior sagittal sinus
Superior petrosal sinus
Inferior petrosal sinus
Straight sinus
Superior cerebral veins
Sigmoid sinus
Transverse sinus

Fig. 73.5b: MRI of veins

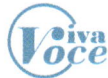

- Name the arteries and veins present in relation to the spinal cord.
- Name the branches of vertebral and basilar arteries.
- How is the circle of Willis formed?
- Does middle cerebral artery take part in formation of circle of Willis?
- Which artery is predominant on medial surface?
- Which artery is predominant on superolateral surface?
- Which artery is predominant on the inferior surface?
- Name the artery involved in hemiplegia.
- Name the functional areas of brain supplied by middle cerebral artery.
- Name the paired and unpaired venous sinuses.

CHAPTER 74

Cranial Nerves

Learning Objectives

One should be able to
1. Trace the course of III nerve. Enumerate its branches.
2. Name all the branches of VII nerve.
3. Enumerate the branches of XII nerve.

OVERVIEW

There are 12 pairs of cranial nerves numbered I to XII. I,II,VIII are mostly sensory in function. III, IV, VI, XI and XII are mostly motor in function. Remaining V, VII, IX and X are mixed nerves. Flowcharts for these cranial nerves are given in this chapter. Diagrams have to be seen from BD Chaurasia's *Human Anatomy*.

Course of olfactory nerve

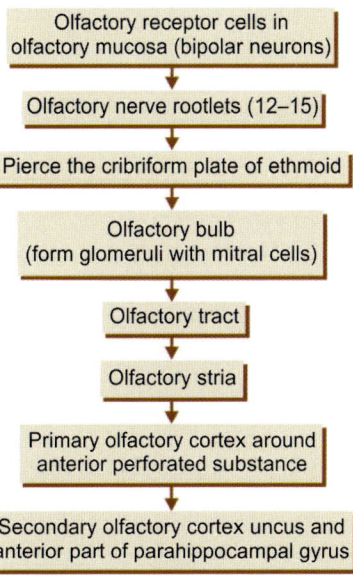

Olfactory receptor cells in olfactory mucosa (bipolar neurons)
↓
Olfactory nerve rootlets (12–15)
↓
Pierce the cribriform plate of ethmoid
↓
Olfactory bulb (form glomeruli with mitral cells)
↓
Olfactory tract
↓
Olfactory stria
↓
Primary olfactory cortex around anterior perforated substance
↓
Secondary olfactory cortex uncus and anterior part of parahippocampal gyrus

Course of optic nerve

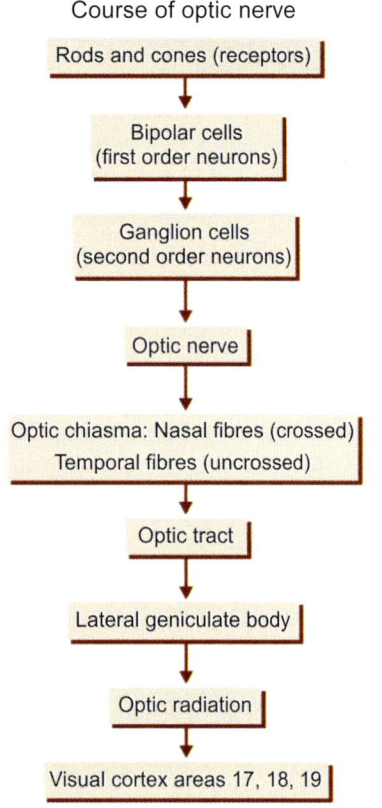

Rods and cones (receptors)

↓

Bipolar cells
(first order neurons)

↓

Ganglion cells
(second order neurons)

↓

Optic nerve

↓

Optic chiasma: Nasal fibres (crossed)
Temporal fibres (uncrossed)

↓

Optic tract

↓

Lateral geniculate body

↓

Optic radiation

↓

Visual cortex areas 17, 18, 19

Course of oculomotor nerve

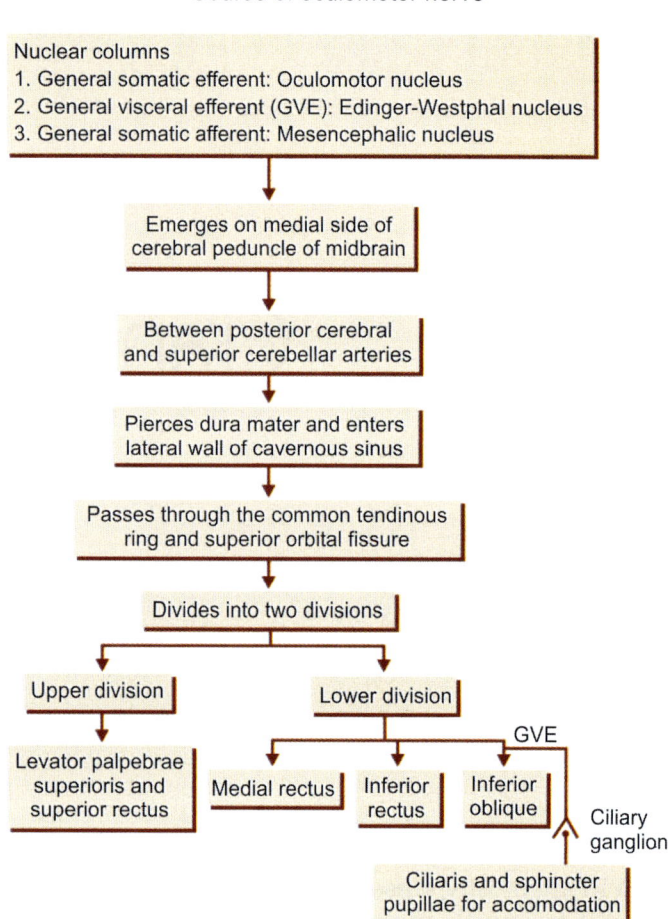

Nuclear columns
1. General somatic efferent: Oculomotor nucleus
2. General visceral efferent (GVE): Edinger-Westphal nucleus
3. General somatic afferent: Mesencephalic nucleus

↓

Emerges on medial side of
cerebral peduncle of midbrain

↓

Between posterior cerebral
and superior cerebellar arteries

↓

Pierces dura mater and enters
lateral wall of cavernous sinus

↓

Passes through the common tendinous
ring and superior orbital fissure

↓

Divides into two divisions

Upper division   Lower division

Levator palpebrae   Medial rectus   Inferior   Inferior   GVE
superioris and   rectus   oblique
superior rectus

Ciliary
ganglion

Ciliaris and sphincter
pupillae for accomodation

Course of trochlear nerve

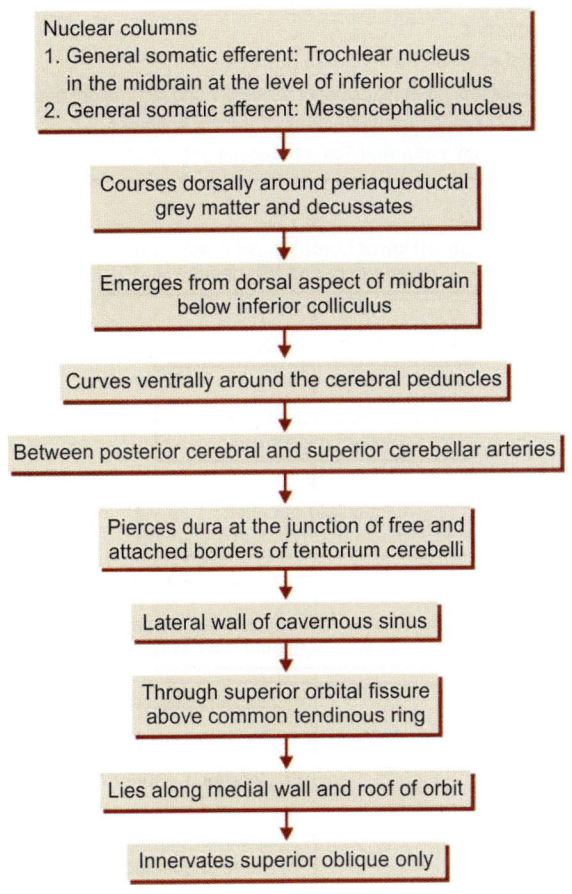

Nuclear columns
1. General somatic efferent: Trochlear nucleus in the midbrain at the level of inferior colliculus
2. General somatic afferent: Mesencephalic nucleus

↓

Courses dorsally around periaqueductal grey matter and decussates

↓

Emerges from dorsal aspect of midbrain below inferior colliculus

↓

Curves ventrally around the cerebral peduncles

↓

Between posterior cerebral and superior cerebellar arteries

↓

Pierces dura at the junction of free and attached borders of tentorium cerebelli

↓

Lateral wall of cavernous sinus

↓

Through superior orbital fissure above common tendinous ring

↓

Lies along medial wall and roof of orbit

↓

Innervates superior oblique only

Course of trigeminal nerve

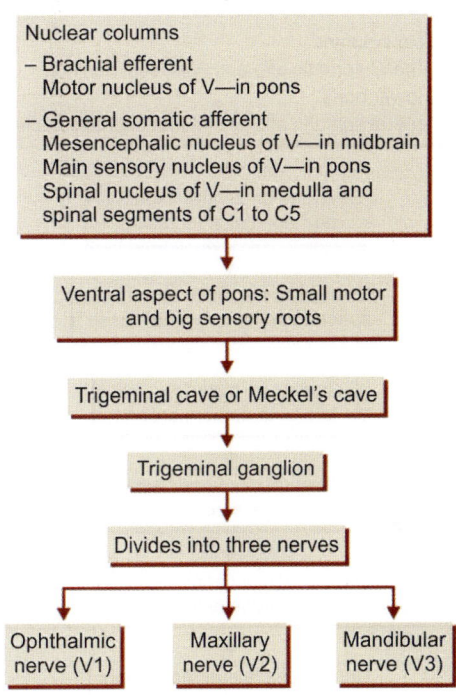

Nuclear columns
– Brachial efferent
  Motor nucleus of V—in pons
– General somatic afferent
  Mesencephalic nucleus of V—in midbrain
  Main sensory nucleus of V—in pons
  Spinal nucleus of V—in medulla and spinal segments of C1 to C5

↓

Ventral aspect of pons: Small motor and big sensory roots

↓

Trigeminal cave or Meckel's cave

↓

Trigeminal ganglion

↓

Divides into three nerves

↓

| Ophthalmic nerve (V1) | Maxillary nerve (V2) | Mandibular nerve (V3) |

Course of abducent nerve

Nuclear columns
1. General somatic efferent: Abducent nucleus
   in lower pons
2. General somatic afferent: Mesencephalic nucleus

↓

Emerges on ventral aspect of
pontomedullary junction

↓

Passes laterally in subarachnoid
space of posterior cranial fossa

↓

Pierces dura mater at a point
lateral to dorsum sellae

↓

Passes through cavernous sinus lateral
to internal carotid artery

↓

Passes through superior orbital fissure
(within common tendinous ring)

↓

Innervates lateral rectus only

Course of facial nerve

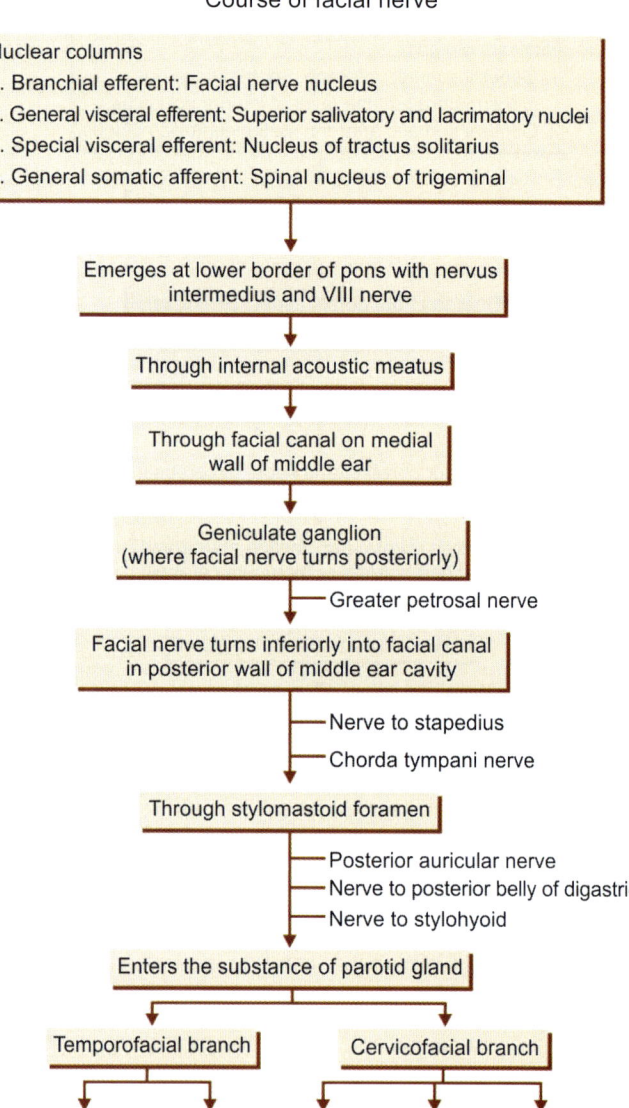

Nuclear columns
1. Branchial efferent: Facial nerve nucleus
2. General visceral efferent: Superior salivatory and lacrimatory nuclei
3. Special visceral efferent: Nucleus of tractus solitarius
4. General somatic afferent: Spinal nucleus of trigeminal

↓

Emerges at lower border of pons with nervus
intermedius and VIII nerve

↓

Through internal acoustic meatus

↓

Through facial canal on medial
wall of middle ear

↓

Geniculate ganglion
(where facial nerve turns posteriorly)
— Greater petrosal nerve

↓

Facial nerve turns inferiorly into facial canal
in posterior wall of middle ear cavity
— Nerve to stapedius
— Chorda tympani nerve

↓

Through stylomastoid foramen
— Posterior auricular nerve
— Nerve to posterior belly of digastric
— Nerve to stylohyoid

↓

Enters the substance of parotid gland

Temporofacial branch   Cervicofacial branch

Temporal   Zygomatic   Buccal   Marginal   Cervical
branch   branch   branch   mandibular branch
                                branch

Comparison of V and VII cranial nerves

Trigeminal nerve (V)	Facial nerve (VII)
Nerve of 1st pharyngeal arch	Nerve of 2nd pharyngeal arch
Derived from 2 nuclear/functional columns	Derived from 4 nuclear/functional columns
SVE: Nucleus in upper part of pons	SVE: Nucleus is in lower part of pons
GSA: Nuclei are (a) nucleus of spinal tract of V; (b) superior sensory nucleus; (c) mesencephalic nucleus	GVE: Nerves are greater petrosal nerve and part of chorda tympani nerve, which are secretomotor
	GVA: Afferents from 2 salivary glands and nasal, palatal and pharyngeal glands
	SVA: Nucleus is upper part of tractus solitarius in medulla oblongata
V nerve gives 3 main branches which give lots (30) of branches, both motor and sensory.	VII nerve gives 10 branches which are motor
Four parasympathetic ganglia are provided by sensory roots by branches of V nerve	Two parasympathetic ganglia are provided secretomotor roots by branches of VII nerve
Mandibular branch innervates 4 muscles of mastication and 4 other muscles	Facial nerve innervates 6 groups of muscles of facial expression. In addition it also supplies muscles which elevate hyoid bone
Innervates tensor tympani of anterior wall of middle ear	Innervates stapedius of posterior wall of middle ear
Innervates anterior belly of digastric muscle	Innervates posterior belly of digastric muscle
Nucleus receives fibres from contralateral motor cortex only	Lower part of nucleus of VII nerve which innervates muscles of upper ½ of face receive fibres from ipsilateral and contralateral motor cortices

Course of vestibulocochlear nerve

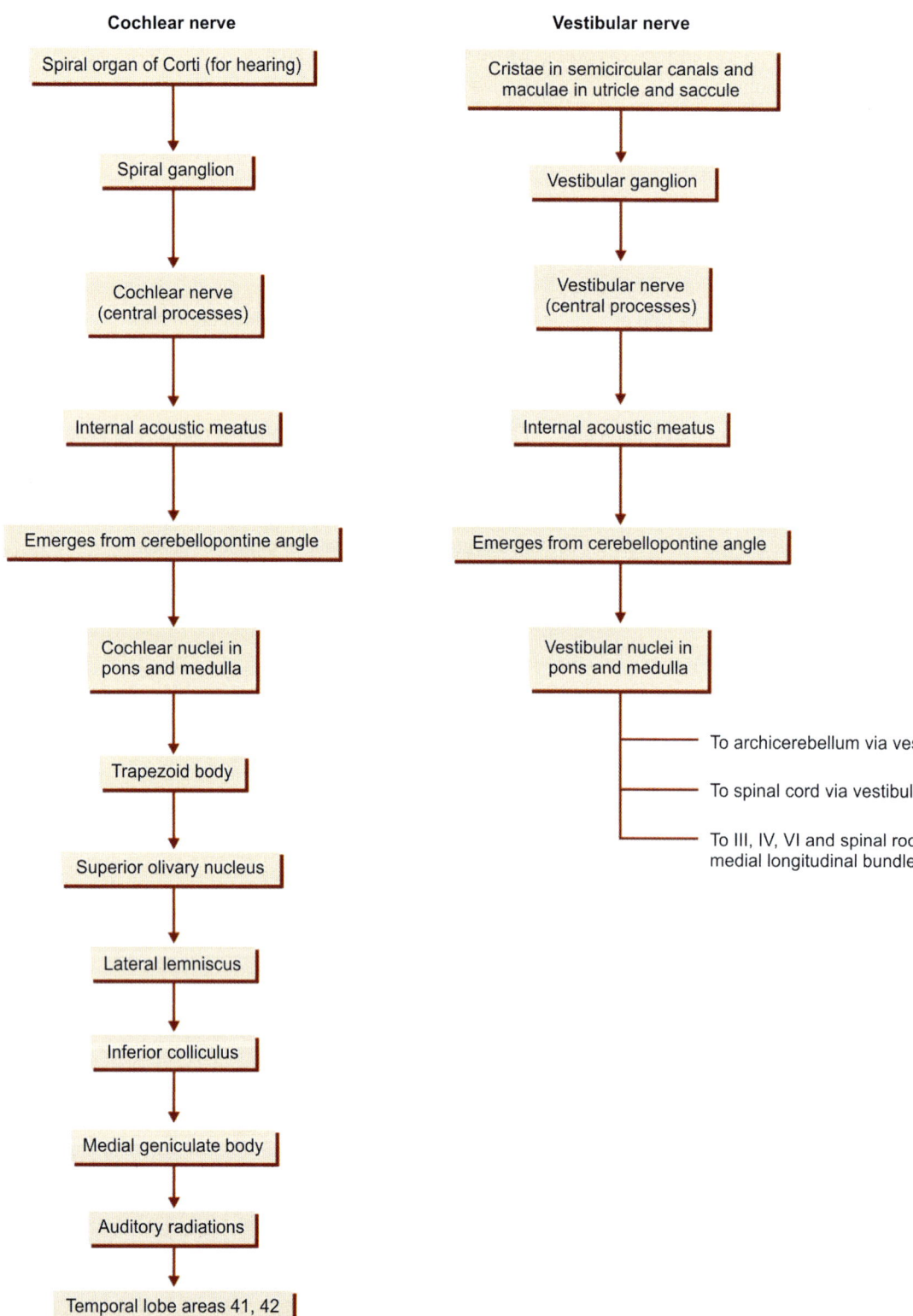

Course of glossopharyngeal nerve

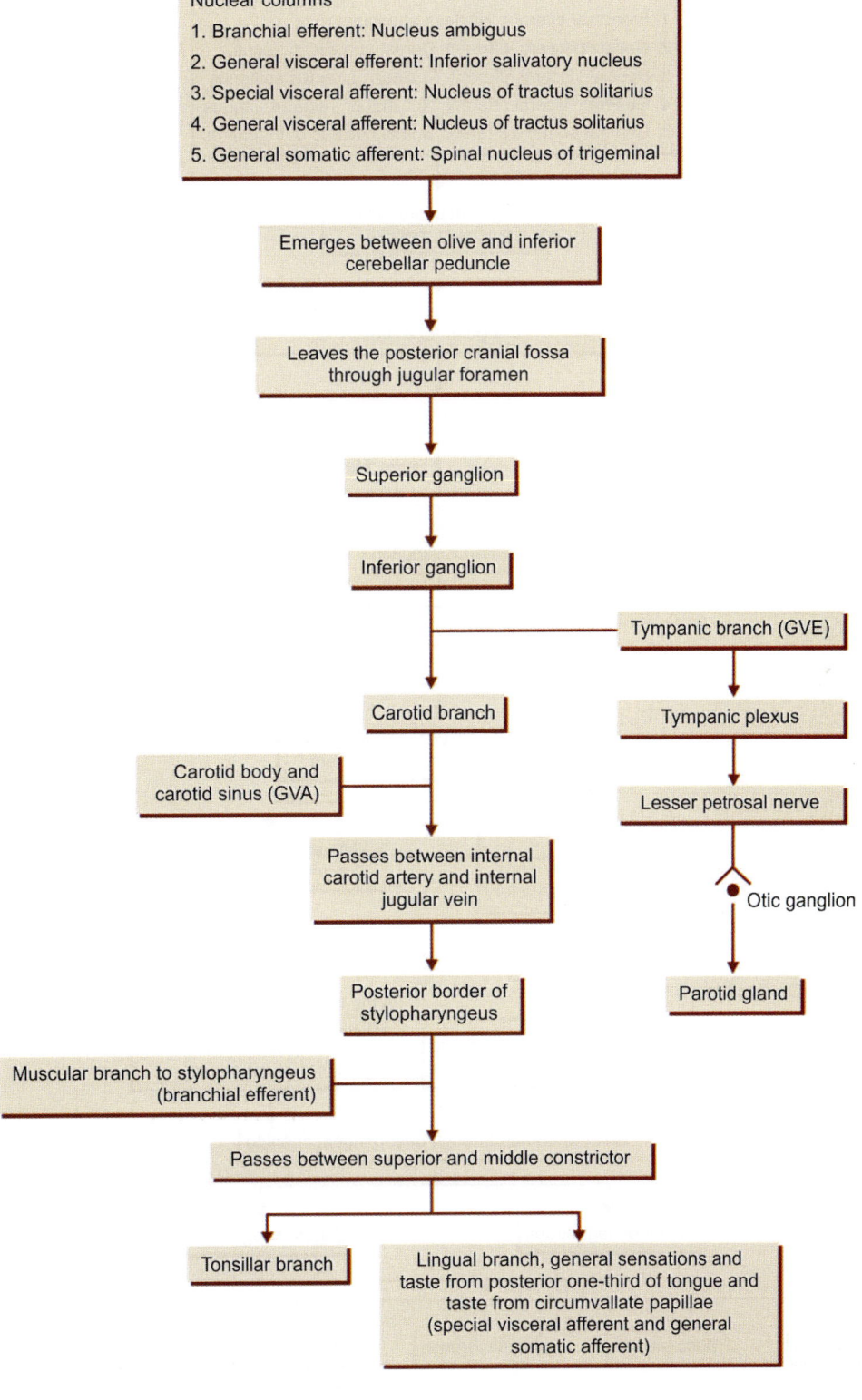

Course of vagus nerve

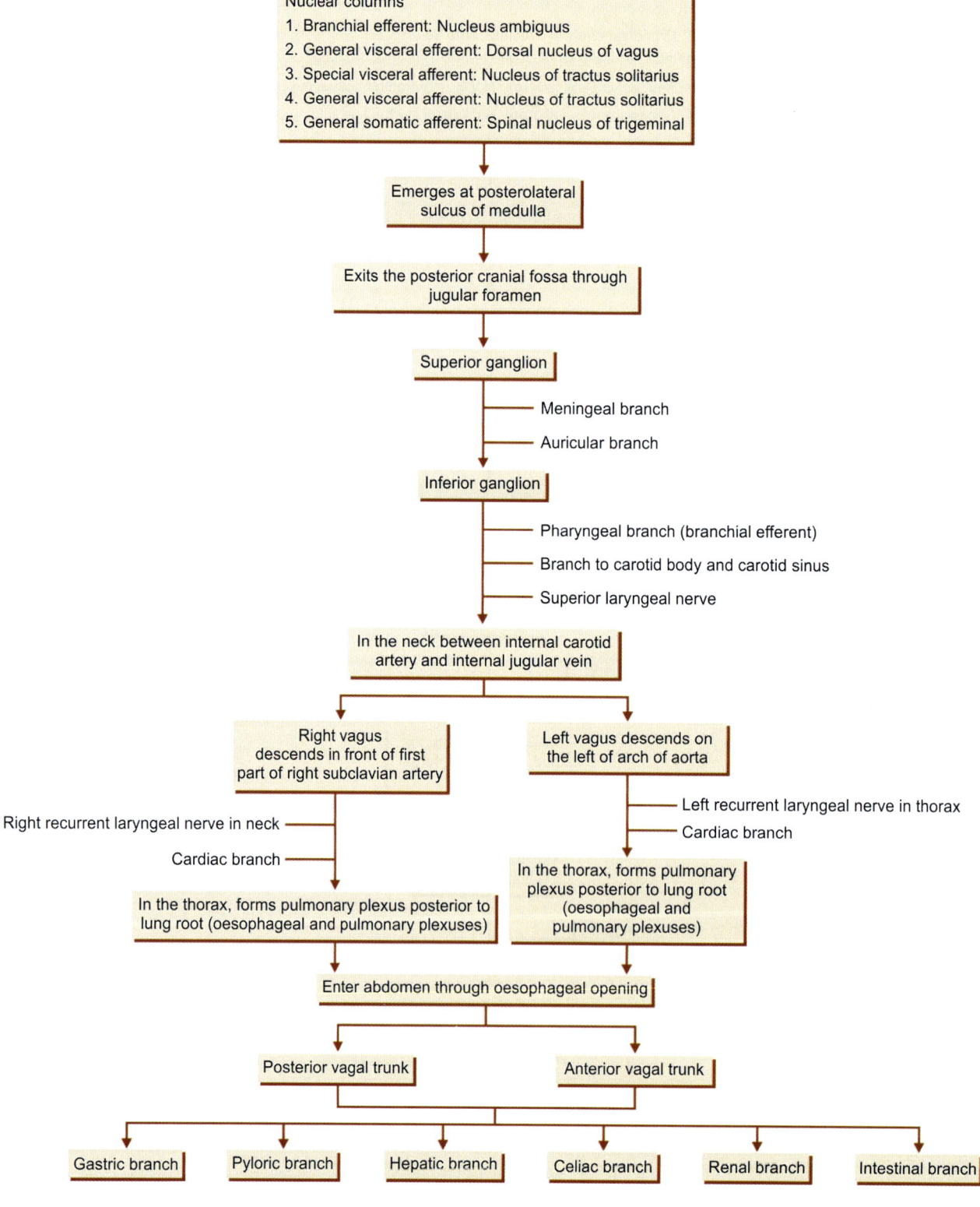

Course of accessory nerve

Cranial root
Branchial efferent: Nucleus ambiguus in the medulla

Spinal root
Branchial efferent: Ventral horns of cervical segments of spinal cord C1 to C5

Emerges on anterior surface of medulla

Emerges from spinal cord between ligamentum denticulatum and dorsal nerve roots

Between olive and interior cerebellar peduncle

Ascends into the posterior cranial fossa through foramen magnum

Cranial root and spinal root join and exit the posterior cranial fossa through jugular foramen

Two roots separate (divorce)

Cranial root
Joins with the vagus at inferior ganglion

Spinal root

Sternocleidomastoid and trapezius

Pharyngeal, palatal and laryngeal muscles
1. Pharyngeal: Superior constrictor, middle constrictor, inferior constrictor, salpingopharyngeus, palatopharyngeus
2. Palatal muscles: Levator veli palatini, palatoglossal, musculus uvulae
3. Laryngeal muscles: Cricothyroid, thyroarytenoid, vocalis, posterior cricoarytenoid, lateral cricoarytenoid, transverse arytenoid, oblique arytenoid, aryepiglottic and thyroepiglottic

Course of hypoglossal nerve

General somatic efferent: Hypoglossal nucleus in medulla

Emerges from the anterolateral sulcus between pyramid and olive

Exits the posterior cranial fossa through the hypoglossal canal

— Meningeal branch

Between internal carotid artery and internal jugular vein

Deep to posterior belly of digastric

— Descendens hypoglossi
— Joins descendens cervicalis
— Forms ansa cervicalis

Passes forwards lateral to internal carotid, external carotid and loop of lingual artery

— Nerve to thyrohyoid and geniohyoid from cervical 1

On lateral surface of hyoglossus

On lateral surface of genioglossus muscle

All muscles of tongue except palatoglossus

Muscles of tongues
Extrinsic muscles: Styloglossus, genioglossus, hyoglossus
Intrinsic muscles: Superior longitudinal, inferior longitudinal, transverse and vertical

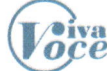

Viva Voce

- Name the ganglia associated with trigeminal nerve.
- Which cranial nerves are sensory?
- Which cranial nerves are motor?
- Which cranial nerves are mixed?
- Right XII nerve is injured, which side will the tongue deviate on protrusion?

- Name the cranial nerve which supplies all muscles of tongue except palatoglossus.
- Name the cranial nerve which is paralysed most frequently.

1. a. Identify the corpuscle.
   b. Which sensation is carried by this corpuscle?

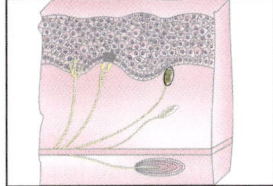

2. a. Identify the flexure.
   b. Structures developing from the part above and part below this flexure.

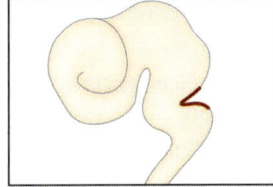

3. a. Name the cistern
   b. Which artery lies in this cistern?

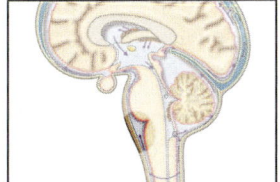

4. a. Identify the tract
   b. Where does it start and what sensations are carried by it?

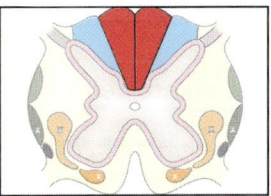

5. a. Identify the nerves in the lateral wall
   b. Name the ganglion associated with the lowest nerve.

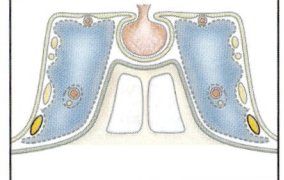

6. a. Name the artery in the internal acoustic meatus.
   b. What is it a branch of?

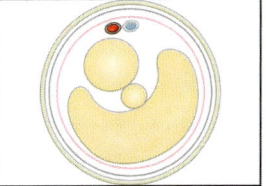

7. a. Which syndrome results due to lesion of the highlighted are?
   b. Which muscles get paresis in this syndrome?

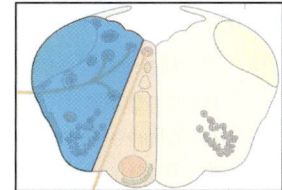

8. a. Identify the highlighted area.
   b. How is this produced?

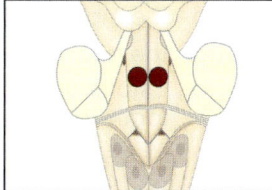

9. a. Name the highlighted area.
   b. Enumerate the functions of this area?

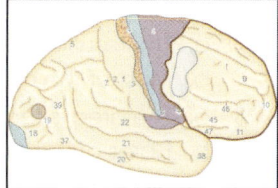

10. a. Identify the part of internal capsule.
    b. Name the ascending and descending tracts present here.

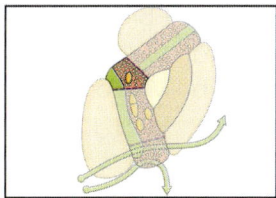

11. a. Name the highlighted artery.
    b. Enumerate the areas supplied by this artery.

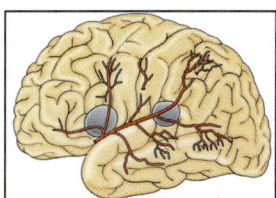

ANSWERS: BRAIN

1. a. Meissner's corpuscle
    b. It carries the sensation of touch.
2. a. Marked flexure is pontine flexure.
    b. The part above pontine flexure is metencephalon which gives rise to pons and cerebellum. Part below the flexure is myelencephalon which gives rise to the medulla oblongata.
3. a. Cisterna pontis.
    b. The main structure in this cistern is the basilar artery.
4. a. The tract is fasciculus gracilis.
    b. It starts from sacral, lumbar and lower thoracic regions. Carries deep touch, pressure, tactile localisation, tactile discrimination, stereognosis and sense of vibration.
5. a. Nerves are oculomotor, trochlear, ophthalmic and maxillary.
    b. The ganglion associated with lowest, i.e. maxillary nerve is pterygopalatine ganglion.
6. a. Artery is labyrinthine artery.
    b. This artery is a branch of basilar artery.
7   a. The resulting syndrome is lateral medullary syndrome.
    b. Most of the muscles of soft palate, pharynx and larynx get paresis.
8   a. The area is facial colliculus.
    b. Fibres of facial nerve going around the nucleus of VI nerve cause facial colliculus.
9   a. The area is prefrontal lobe.
    b. It is responsible for attention, concentration, judgement, intelligence, for initiative and for emotions.
10. a. Genu of internal capsule.
    b. Fibres are corticonuclear and anterior part of superior thalamic radiations.
11. a. Middle cerebral artery.
    b. Most of motor and sensory areas, Broca's motor speech area, Wernicke's sensory speech area and hearing area.

Index